Pathological and Clinical Aspects of Liver Cancer

Pathological and Clinical Aspects of Liver Cancer

Editor: Eddie Goblin

AMERICAN
MEDICAL PUBLISHERS
www.americanmedicalpublishers.com

AMERICAN
MEDICAL PUBLISHERS
www.americanmedicalpublishers.com

Cataloging-in-Publication Data

Pathological and clinical aspects of liver cancer / edited by Eddie Goblin.
p. cm.
Includes bibliographical references and index.
ISBN 979-8-88740-230-7
1. Liver--Cancer. 2. Liver--Cancer--Pathogenesis. 3. Liver--Cancer--Treatment. I. Goblin, Eddie.
RC280.L5 P38 2023
616.994 36--dc23

American Medical Publishers,
41 Flatbush Avenue,
1st Floor, New York,
NY 11217, USA

ISBN 979-8-88740-230-7 (Hardback)

Contents

Preface

This book has been a concerted effort by a group of academicians, researchers and scientists, who have contributed their research works for the realization of the book. This book has materialized in the wake of emerging advancements and innovations in this field. Therefore, the need of the hour was to compile all the required researches and disseminate the knowledge to a broad spectrum of people comprising of students, researchers and specialists of the field.

Liver cancer refers to a cancer that affects the liver. It is grouped in two categories, namely, primary liver cancer and secondary liver cancer. Primary cancer develops in the liver and is classified into three types, namely, hepatocellular carcinoma (HCC), intrahepatic cancer (IHC), and angiosarcoma. Secondary liver cancer or liver metastasis begins in other parts of the body and reaches the liver. Cirrhosis is the primary cause of liver cancer, which is caused due to hepatitis B or hepatitis C. Some common symptoms of liver cancer are jaundice, nausea, fatigue, unexplained weight loss, etc. A few of the treatment methods for this medical condition are liver transplantation, hepatic arterial embolization and ablation. Treatment may also include therapies like targeted therapy, chemotherapy, immunotherapy and radioembolization. This book outlines the pathological and clinical aspects of liver cancer in detail. It is a valuable compilation of topics, ranging from the basic to the most complex advancements in the management of this disease. The book will serve as a valuable source of reference for graduate and post graduate students.

At the end of the preface, I would like to thank the authors for their brilliant chapters and the publisher for guiding us all-through the making of the book till its final stage. Also, I would like to thank my family for providing the support and encouragement throughout my academic career and research projects.

Editor

1

Pre- and Postoperative Models for Prediction of Recurrence in Non-B, Non-C Hepatocellular Carcinoma

Kongying Lin[1†], Qizhen Huang[2†], Lei Wang[3†], Jianxing Zeng[1], Zongren Ding[1], Hongzhi Liu[1], Jun Fu[1], Pengfei Guo[4], Zhenwei Chen[4], Yongyi Zeng[1], Weiping Zhou[5] and Jingfeng Liu[1,3*]*

[1] Department of Hepatopancreatobiliary Surgery, Mengchao Hepatobiliary Hospital of Fujian Medical University, Fuzhou, China, [2] Department of Radiation Oncology, Mengchao Hepatobiliary Hospital of Fujian Medical University, Fuzhou, China, [3] Department of Radiation Oncology, Fujian Medical University Cancer Hospital, Fujian Cancer Hospital, Fuzhou, China, [4] The Big Data Institute of Southeast Hepatobiliary Health Information, Mengchao Hepatobiliary Hospital of Fujian Medical University, Fuzhou, China, [5] The Third Department of Hepatic Surgery, Eastern Hepatobiliary Surgery Hospital, Second Military Medical University, Shanghai, China

Correspondence:
Jingfeng Liu
drjingfeng@126.com
Weiping Zhou
ehphwp@126.com

[†]These authors have contributed equally to this work

Background and Aims: The incidence of non-B, non-C hepatocellular carcinoma (NBNC-HCC) is increasing. Like in hepatitis B virus (HBC)/HCV-associated HCC, treatment of NBNC-HCC after resection is challenging due to its high recurrence rate. However, few studies on the recurrence of NBNC-HCC have been published in the past decades. Hence, we aimed to investigate the risk factors for recurrence of NBNC-HCC and construct pre- and postoperative prognostic models for predicting recurrence in these patients who underwent curative resection.

Methods: We retrospectively analyzed 608 patients who underwent liver resection for NBNC-HCC. A multivariate Cox proportional hazard regression analysis was conducted to identify the independent risk factors of recurrence, based on which the prediction nomogram models were constructed and validated. The predictive performance of the models was assessed using the concordance index, time-dependent receiver operating characteristic curve, prediction error cure, and calibration curve. To facilitate clinical use, we stratified the patients into three distinct risk groups based on the score of the models. The cutoff scores of the models were determined by a survival tree analysis.

Results: Multivariable analysis identified neutrophil-to-lymphocyte ratio, alpha fetoprotein, tumor number, and tumor diameter as independent preoperative risk factors for recurrence. In addition to these variables, microvascular invasion was an independent postoperative risk factor for recurrence. The pre- and postoperative nomograms were constructed based on these variables. The C-index of the pre- and postoperative nomograms was 0.689 and 0.702 in the training cohort, 0.682 and 0.688 in the validation cohort, respectively, which were both higher than those of the conventional Barcelona Clinic Liver Cancer (BCLC) and 8th edition of the American Joint Committee on Cancer (AJCC^{8th}) staging systems. In addition, the pre- and postoperative nomograms could also re-stratify patients with BCLC stage 0/A or AJCC[8th] stage IA/IB/II into distinct risk groups.

Conclusions: We constructed pre- and postoperative prognostic models for predicting recurrence in patients with NBNC-HCC who underwent curative resection. They can play a supplementary role to the traditional staging system.

Keywords: non-B non-C hepatocellular carcinoma, resection, recurrence, inflammation, nomogram

INTRODUCTION

Hepatocellular carcinoma (HCC) is the fifth most common cancer and third leading cause of cancer-related deaths worldwide (1). Chronic infections with hepatitis B (HBV) and C viruses (HCV) are the prominent etiological factors for HCC. However, with the adoption of HBV immunization programs and control of HCV transmission, the incidence of HBV\HCV-associated HCC has decreased in recent years (2, 3). The number of patients with HCC who are seronegative for both HBV and HCV, so called "NBNC-HCC," is gradually increasing (4, 5).

Due to the shortage of donor organs, surgical resection remains the main treatment strategy for patients with HCC who have a good liver function and resectable tumors (6). However, long-term survival after surgery remains unsatisfactory due to the high incidence of tumor recurrence (7). Owing to the heterogeneity of HCC, some highly selected patients may benefit from a prognostic prediction model, well-selected therapeutic assignment, and strict postoperative monitoring (8, 9). There are several studies on constructed prognostic models for HCC; however, very few studies have specifically focused on the recurrence of patients with NBNC-HCC. Considering the different clinical manifestations and prognostic outcomes of NBNC-HCC and viral-associated HCC, the study of its risk factors and establishment of prognostic models may provide important insight into novel strategies for the treatment and postoperative monitoring of NBNC-HCC.

Host inflammatory response to cancer and tumor-mediated systemic inflammation promote migration, invasion, and metastasis of malignant cells (10, 11); they are prognostic factors for HCC (12). Recent studies have demonstrated that preoperative inflammatory indices, such as the neutrophil-to-lymphocyte ratio (NLR) (13), neutrophil times γ-glutamyl transpeptidase-to-lymphocyte ratio (NγLR) (14), platelet-to-lymphocyte ratio (PLR) (15), prognostic nutritional index (PNI) (16), aspartate aminotransferase-to-neutrophil ratio (ANRI) (17), γ-glutamyl transpeptidase-to-platelet ratio (GPR) (18), aspartate aminotransferase-to-lymphocyte ratio index (ALRI) (19) and platelet times neutrophil-to-lymphocyte ratio (PNLR) (20) are independent prognostic factors for patients with HCC who have undergone liver resection and have been used in the construction of several prognosis prediction models; however, the relationship between these inflammatory indexes and prognosis of NBNC-HCC, and the inflammatory index with the highest prognostic significance remain unclear.

In our study, we aimed to: (1) investigate the relationship between inflammatory indexes and recurrence of NBNC-HCC, (2) investigate the pre- and postoperative risk factors for recurrence of NBNC-HCC, and (3) construct a pre- and postoperative nomogram model for the prediction of recurrence of NBNC-HCC.

Abbreviations: NBNC-HCC, Non-B non-C hepatocellular carcinoma; NAFLD, non-alcoholic fatty liver disease; ALD, alcoholic liver disease; BCLC, Barcelona Clinic Liver Cancer staging system; HBcAb, hepatitis B virus core antibody; RBCs, red blood cells; WBCs, white blood cells; Hb, hemoglobin; ALT, alanine aminotransferase; AST, aspartate aminotransferase; GGT, γ-glutamyl transpeptidase; NLR, neutrophil to lymphocyte ratio; PLR, platelet to lymphocyte ratio; PNI, prognostic nutritional index; ANRI, aspartate aminotransferase to neutrophil ratio index; ALRI, aspartate aminotransferase to Lymphocyte ratio index; PNLR, platelet times neutrophil to lymphocyte ratio; GPR, γ-glutamyl transpeptidase to platelet ratio; NγLR, neutrophil times γ-glutamyl transpeptidase to lymphocyte ratio; DNLR, derived neutrophil to lymphocyte ratio; AFP, alpha fetoprotein; MVI, microvascular invasion.

MATERIALS AND METHODS

Patients

Data from patients diagnosed with NBNC-HCC who underwent hepatectomy as a primary anti-cancer therapy between April 28, 2008 and December 30, 2015 were extracted from the primary liver cancer big data (PLCBD) (21, 22). In this study, patients with HCC who were seronegative for hepatitis B surface antigen, HBV- deoxyribonucleic acid (DNA), hepatitis C antibody, and HCV-RNA test were considered patients with NBNC-HCC (23). All data in this study were verified by three independent researchers, and the study was approved by the institutional ethics committee of Mengchao Hepatobiliary Hospital of Fujian Medial University.

Patients with Child Pugh A or B7 liver function, no extrahepatic metastasis, no macroscopic vascular invasion, and who underwent R0 resection (complete removal of all detectable tumor nodes with tumor-free margins confirmed by histological examination) were included. Patients who underwent palliative tumor resection or any preoperative anti-HCC therapy, with a history of other cancers, or incomplete clinical data were excluded.

Preoperative Assessment, Hepatectomy, and Follow-Up

All patients underwent routine preoperative examinations, which included hepatitis B and C immunology, HBV-DNA load, alpha-fetoprotein (AFP) levels, liver and kidney function examinations, chest radiography, abdominal ultrasonography, contrast-enhanced computed tomography, and magnetic resonance imaging. HCC was diagnosed according to the practice guidelines recommended by the American Association for the Study of Liver Diseases (24). The choice of performing anatomical or partial hepatectomy is commonly based on the patient's liver function status, tumor number, and location. In simple terms, anatomical hepatectomy was preferentially performed for patients with a good liver function and tumors located within a segment, sector, and hemiliver. Partial hepatectomy was performed for tumors that were peripherally located or patients with unsatisfactory liver function. Intraoperative liver ultrasonography was routinely used to ensure that all detectable tumors were completely removed. The follow-up of patients after discharge was performed in the outpatient clinic. The follow-up program and diagnostic criteria for tumor recurrence are reported in a previous study (9).

Clinicopathologic Variables

For hematological investigations, we used the results of the most recent test that was performed within 15 days prior to surgery. The formulae of the indices (NLR, PLR, GPR, PNLR, PNI, ANRI, ALRI, DNLR, and NγLR) are reported in a previous study (14, 18, 25–27). The preoperative imaging data, including tumor number and diameter was obtained from contrast-enhanced Computed Tomography or contrast-enhanced magnetic resonance imaging. Tumor diameter was the diameter of the largest tumor. Histologic grading of the tumor was done according to the Edmondson-Steiner classification. The definition of microvascular invasion (MVI) from a previous study was used (28). The pathological review of all resected specimens was carried out independently by two pathologists.

Statistical Analysis

Categorical variables were expressed as number (percentage) and compared using the $\chi 2$ test or Fisher's exact test. Continuous variables were expressed as mean (standard deviation SD) and compared using the Student t test or the Mann–Whitney U test. Univariate and multivariate Cox proportional hazard regression analyses were performed to determine the independent prognostic factors for recurrence. Clinical variables considered to be potentially relevant ($p<0.05$ in univariate analyses) were entered in the multivariate Cox proportional hazard regression analyses, and the final independent risk factors for recurrence were identified by the multivariable analyses with stepwise backward selection method.

The nomograms were constructed based on the results of multivariable analyses of recurrence in the training cohort. The R code used for construction of nomogram was shown in the supporting information. The preoperative nomogram was developed on the available preoperative clinicopathologic data. The postoperative nomogram was based on all available clinicopathologic variables. The predictive performance of the nomograms was measured using Harrell's concordance index (C-index), time-dependent areas under the receiver operating characteristic curve (tdAUC), prediction error curve, and calibration plot (29, 30). The cutoff of models was determined by a survival tree analysis (29). The cumulative recurrence between each risk group was assessed and tested using Kaplan-Meier curves and the log-rank test, respectively. All statistical tests were two-tailed, and $P < 0.05$ was considered statistically significant. Statistical analyses were performed using SPSS version 20.0 and R version 3.0 (http://www.r-project.org/); the R packages of "table1," "rms," "CsChange," "survminer," "survival," "pec," "riskRegression," "timeROC," and "party" were used.

RESULTS

Patients' Characteristics

A total of 608 eligible patients were included in the study. They were randomly divided into a training cohort (n=456) and validation cohort (n=152) in a 3:1 ratio. A comparison of the clinicopathologic characteristics between the two cohorts is shown in **Table 1**. There were no significant differences in the clinicopathologic features between the two cohorts. The mean age was 59.2 ± 11.2 years and 58.3 ± 11.7 years in the training and validation cohorts, respectively. Most of the patients were male (85.5–87.5%), and few patients had cirrhotic livers (32.9–35.5%). The mean tumor diameter was 7.06 ± 3.99 cm and 6.80 ± 4.12 cm in the training and validation cohorts, respectively. Most of the patients harbored solitary tumors (86.2–83.6%).

POSTOPERATIVE PROGNOSIS

The median follow-up period was 44.3 (range, 2.1–114.7) months and 45.3 months (range, 1.9–114.7) months in the training cohort and validation cohort, respectively. In the training cohort, the postoperative 1-, 3-, and 5-year overall survival (OS) rates were 91.7, 72.8, and 57.4%, respectively, and the corresponding cumulative recurrence rates were 24.2, 37.5, and 48.6%, respectively. In the validation cohort, the postoperative 1-, 3-, and 5-year OS rates were 87.2, 67.7, and 54.5%, respectively, and the corresponding cumulative recurrence rates were 28.8, 43.3, and 48.0%, respectively.

Construction of Pre- and Postoperative Nomograms for Prediction of Recurrence

All the variables shown in **Table 1** were included in the univariate and multivariate Cox proportional hazard regression analyses to identify independent risk factors for recurrence. Results of the univariate analysis are shown in **Table 2**. On univariate analysis, there was a significant relationship between six inflammatory indexes (NLR, PLR, ALRI, PNLR, NγLR, and DNLR) and recurrence. Other significant variables were neutrophil count, lymphocyte count, aspartate aminotransferase, AFP, tumor diameter, tumor number, MVI, and satellite nodules.

To construct the preoperative model, presence of MVI and satellite nodules, which were recorded only postoperatively, were

TABLE 1 | Baseline clinical characteristics of patients.

	Training cohort (n=456)	Validation cohort (n=152)	P-value
Age, Mean (SD), years	59.2 (11.2)	58.3 (11.7)	0.402
Gender			
Female	66 (14.5%)	19 (12.5%)	0.636
Male	390 (85.5%)	133 (87.5%)	
Alcohol consumption			0.407
No	321 (70.4%)	113 (74.3%)	
Yes	135 (29.6%)	39 (25.7%)	
Cigarette smoking			0.065
No	278 (61.0%)	106 (69.7%)	
Yes	178 (39.0%)	46 (30.3%)	
Hypertension			0.959
Absent	321 (70.4%)	108 (71.1%)	
Present	135 (29.6%)	44 (28.9%)	
Diabetes			0.126
Absent	389 (85.3%)	121 (79.6%)	
Present	67 (14.7%)	31 (20.4%)	
Fatty liver			0.501
Absent	403 (88.4%)	138 (90.8%)	
Present	53 (11.6%)	14 (9.2%)	
Cirrhosis			0.620
Absent	306 (67.1%)	98 (64.5%)	
Present	150 (32.9%)	54 (35.5%)	
BCLC staging system			0.684
0	9 (2.0%)	3 (2.0%)	
A	396 (86.8%)	128 (84.2%)	
B	51 (11.2%)	21 (13.8%)	
AJCC staging system^{8th}			0.961
IA	9 (2.0%)	3 (2.0%)	
IB	295 (64.7%)	96 (63.2%)	
II	105 (23.0%)	35 (23.0%)	
IIIA	47 (10.3%)	18 (11.8%)	
HbcAb			0.370
Negative	57 (12.5%)	24 (15.8%)	
Positive	399 (87.5%)	128 (84.2%)	
WBCs, Mean (SD), 10^9/L	5.85 (1.92)	5.67 (1.85)	0.320
RBCs, Mean (SD), 10^9/L	4.55 (0.57)	4.52 (0.53)	0.559
Hb, Mean (SD), g/L	138.27 (17.47)	136.80 (16.15)	0.343
Neutrophil Count, Mean (SD), 10^9/L	3.68 (1.62)	3.53 (1.48)	0.305
Lymphocyte Count, Mean (SD), 10^9/L	1.66 (0.61)	1.64 (0.61)	0.640
Platelets, Mean (SD), 10^9/L	194.37 (75.32)	194.85 (85.53)	0.951
Total bilirubin, Mean (SD), umol/L	13.4 (5.29)	13.2 (5.10)	0.604
Albumin, Mean (SD), g/L	42.7 (3.71)	42.1 (3.60)	0.069
ALT, Mean (SD), U/L	31.1 (24.9)	29.7 (24.6)	0.538
AST, Mean (SD), U/L	34.0 (27.0)	30.7 (26.1)	0.186
GGT, Mean (SD), U/L	76.3 (111)	89.7 (169)	0.360
NLR	2.47 (1.43)	2.36 (1.18)	0.371
PLR	127.27 (59.35)	127.87 (59.36)	0.914
PNI	51.00 (5.31)	50.24 (5.24)	0.127
ANRI	10.63 (9.47)	9.99 (8.50)	0.436
ALRI	23.89 (22.33)	21.53 (17.55)	0.182
PNLR	491.55 (419.79)	471.33 (360.71)	0.567
GPR	0.887 (1.40)	1.170 (2.79)	0.232
NγLR	195.32 (341.11)	185.94 (261.38)	0.724
DNLR	1.76 (1.44)	1.75 (0.75)	
AFP, ng/ml			0.482
≤20	236 (51.8%)	73 (48.0%)	
>20	220 (48.2%)	79 (52.0%)	
Intraoperative blood transfusion			0.882
No	406 (89.0%)	134 (88.2%)	
Yes	50 (11.0%)	18 (11.8%)	
Tumor size*, Mean (SD), cm	6.92 (3.91)	6.68 (4.07)	0.522
Tumor number*			0.380
Solitary	396 (86.8%)	127 (83.6%)	
Multiple	60 (13.2%)	25 (16.4%)	
Tumor size, Mean (SD), cm	7.06 (3.99)	6.80 (4.12)	0.501
Tumor number			0.506
Solitary	393 (86.2%)	127 (83.6%)	
Multiple	63 (13.8%)	25 (16.4%)	
MVI			0.709
Absent	339 (74.3%)	110 (72.4%)	
Present	117 (25.7%)	42 (27.6%)	
Satellite nodules			0.587
Absent	304 (66.7%)	97 (63.8%)	
Present	152 (33.3%)	55 (36.2%)	
Tumor capsule			0.272
Complete	92 (20.2%)	39 (25.7%)	
Incomplete	268 (58.8%)	79 (52.0%)	
None	96 (21.1%)	34 (22.4%)	
Edmondson-Steiner classification			0.727
I/II	91 (20.0%)	33 (21.7%)	
III/IV	365 (80.0%)	119 (78.3%)	

BCLC, Barcelona Clinic Liver Cancer staging system; AJCC, American Joint Committee on Cancer; HBcAb, hepatitis B virus core antibody; RBCs, red blood cells; WBCs, white blood cells; Hb, hemoglobin; ALT, alanine aminotransferase; AST, aspartate aminotransferase; GGT, gamma-glutamyl transpeptidase; NLR, neutrophil to lymphocyte ratio; PLR, platelet-to-lymphocyte ratio; PNI, prognostic nutritional index; ANRI, AST to neutrophil ratio index; ALRI, AST to Lymphocyte ratio index; PNLR, platelet–neutrophil–lymphocyte ratio; GPR, gamma-glutamyl transpeptidase (GGT) to platelet ratio; NγLR, neutrophil times γ-glutamyl transpeptidase to lymphocyte ratio; DNLR, derived neutrophil to lymphocyte ratio; AFP, alpha fetoprotein; MVI, microvascular invasion.

**Preoperative images were obtained from contrast-enhanced Computed Tomography or contrast-enhanced magnetic resonance imaging.*

excluded, and the remaining 12 factors were entered into the multivariate Cox regression analysis using a stepwise method. All 14 risk factors that could be acquired preoperatively were entered in the multivariate analysis.

Multivariate analyses revealed that multiple tumor number [hazard ratio with 95% confidence interval (CI)=3.381 (2.401–4.761), P<0.001], large tumor diameter [1.072 (1.035–1.111), P<0.001], elevated AFP levels [1.624 (1.218–2.166), P=0.001], and elevated NLR [1.142 (1.046–1.246), P=0.003] were independent preoperative risk factors for recurrence of NBNC-HCC (**Table 3**); Multivariate analysis of the postoperative variables revealed that multiple tumor number [3.187 (2.273–4.470), P<0.001], large tumor diameter [1.069 (1.033–1.106), P<0.001], presence of MVI [1.587 (1.153–2.186), P=0.005], elevated AFP levels [1.428 (1.057–1.930), P=0.02], and elevated NLR [1.144 (1.048–1.250), P=0.003] were independent postoperative risk factors for recurrence of NBNC-HCC (**Table 4**). These independent risk factors were then used to build the pre- and postoperative nomogram models (**Figures 1A, B**).

TABLE 2 | Univariate Cox regression analysis of risk factors of Recurrence in the training cohort.

Variable	B	SE	HR(95%CI)	P-value
Age, years	−0.003	0.006	0.997(0.985–1.009)	0.609
Gender, Male versus Female	−0.040	0.205	0.961(0.643–1.436)	0.846
Alcohol consumption, Yes versus No	0.084	0.159	1.088(0.797–1.485)	0.596
Cigarette smoking, Yes versus No	0.054	0.148	1.055(0.789–1.412)	0.716
Hypertension, present versus absent	0.070	0.157	1.072(0.789–1.458)	0.657
Diabetes, present versus absent	0.004	0.205	1.004(0.672–1.500)	0.984
Fatty liver, present versus absent	−0.234	0.242	0.791(0.492–1.272)	0.333
Cirrhosis, present versus absent	0.172	0.151	1.188(0.883–1.598)	0.255
HbcAb, Positive versus Negative	0.127	0.227	1.136(0.727–1.774)	0.576
WBCs, 10^9/L	0.059	0.033	1.060(0.994–1.131)	0.074
RBCs, 10^9/L	0.074	0.128	1.076(0.837–1.384)	0.566
Hb, g/L	−0.003	0.004	0.997(0.989–1.005)	0.450
Neutrophil count, 10^9/L	0.104	0.031	1.110(1.044–1.180)	0.001
Lymphocyte count, 10^9/L	−0.322	0.127	0.725(0.565–0.930)	0.011
Platelets, 10^9/L	0.001	0.001	1.001(0.999–1.003)	0.387
Total bilirubin, umol/L	0.003	0.014	1.003(0.976–1.031)	0.835
Albumin, g/L	0.004	0.020	1.004(0.966–1.043)	0.850
ALT, U/L	0.002	0.003	1.002(0.997–1.007)	0.426
AST, U/L	0.004	0.002	1.004(1.001–1.008)	0.025
GGT, U/L	0.001	0.001	1.001(0.999–1.002)	0.329
NLR	0.187	0.038	1.206(1.120–1.299)	<0.001
PLR	0.003	0.001	1.003(1.001–1.005)	0.002
PNI	−0.018	0.014	0.982(0.956–1.009)	0.187
ANRI	0.007	0.006	1.007(0.994–1.019)	0.288
ALRI	0.007	0.002	1.007(1.002–1.012)	0.006
PNLR	0.0004	0.0001	1.0004(1.000–1.001)	<0.001
GPR	0.043	0.048	1.044(0.950–1.147)	0.372
NγLR	0.001	0.0001	1.001(1.000–1.001)	<0.001
DNLR	0.176	0.071	1.193(1.037–1.372)	0.014
AFP, ng/ml, >20 versus ≤20	0.444	0.146	1.558(1.171–2.074)	0.002
Intraoperative blood transfusion, Yes versus No	0.374	0.219	1.454(0.947–2.234)	0.087
Tumor size*, cm	0.089	0.017	1.093(1.057–1.130)	<0.001
Tumor number*, Multiple versus Solitary	1.301	0.172	3.673(2.623–5.145)	<0.001
Tumor size, cm	0.088	0.016	1.091(1.057–1.127)	<0.001
Tumor number, Multiple versus Solitary	1.274	0.169	3.576(2.566–4.983)	<0.001
MVI, Present versus Absent	0.726	0.153	2.067(1.531–2.792)	<0.001
Satellite nodules, Present versus Absent	0.746	0.147	2.109(1.582–2.811)	<0.001
Tumor capsule				0.345
Complete	Ref	Ref	Ref	Ref
Incomplete	0.200	0.194	1.221(0.835–1.785)	0.303
None	0.332	0.228	1.394(0.891–2.179)	0.146
Edmondson-Steiner grading, I/II versus III/IV	0.310	0.190	1.363 (0.940–1.977)	0.102

HBcAb, hepatitis B virus core antibody; RBCs, red blood cells; WBCs, white blood cells; Hb, hemoglobin; ALT, alanine aminotransferase; AST, aspartate aminotransferase; GGT, gamma-glutamyl transpeptidase; NLR, neutrophil to lymphocyte ratio; PLR, platelet-to-lymphocyte ratio; PNI, prognostic nutritional index; ANRI, AST to neutrophil ratio index; ALRI, AST to Lymphocyte ratio index; PNLR, platelet–neutrophil–lymphocyte ratio; GPR, gamma-glutamyl transpeptidase (GGT) to platelet ratio; NγLR, neutrophil times γ-glutamyl transpeptidase to lymphocyte ratio; DNLR, derived neutrophil to lymphocyte ratio; AFP, alpha fetoprotein; MVI, microvascular invasion; B, coefficient; SE, stand error; CI, confidence interval; HR, hazard ratio.

**Preoperative images were obtained from contrast-enhanced Computed Tomography or contrast-enhanced magnetic resonance imaging.*

Performance of the Pre- and Postoperative Nomograms in Recurrence Prediction

In the training and validation cohorts, both nomograms had a satisfactory performance in recurrence prediction. The C-index of the preoperative nomogram in the training and validation cohorts was 0.689 (95% CI, 0.651–0.728) and 0.682 (0.618–0.746), respectively, which were significantly higher than the currently used Barcelona Clinic Liver Cancer (BCLC) staging system (31) [0.593 (0.564–0.622), p<0.001; 0.593 (0.544–0.641), p=0.001] and 8th edition of the American Joint Committee on Cancer (AJCC) staging system [0.645 (0.608–0.682), p=0.018; 0.624 (0.562–0.687), p=0.024]. For the postoperative nomogram model, the C-index values were 0.702 (0.664–0.739) in the training cohort and 0.688 (0.622–0.753) in the validation cohort, which were greater than those of the BCLC (p<0.001, p=0.001, respectively) and 8th edition of the AJCC (p<0.001, p=0.002, respectively) staging systems.

Time-dependent receiver operating characteristic curve analysis was also performed to assess the discriminative performance of the nomograms. For the preoperative nomogram model, the median tdAUCs for prediction of 1-, 2-, and 3 year recurrences were 0.725 (range, 0.706–0.749) in the

TABLE 3 | Multivariate Cox regression analysis of risk factors of Recurrence based on Preoperative data of the training cohort.

Variable	B	SE	HR(95%CI)	P-value
Tumor number*, Multiple versus Solitary	1.218	0.175	3.381(2.401–4.761)	<0.001
Tumor size*, cm	0.069	0.018	1.072(1.035–1.111)	<0.001
AFP, ng/ml, >20 versus ≤20	0.485	0.147	1.624(1.218–2.166)	0.001
NLR	0.132	0.045	1.142(1.046–1.246)	0.003

NLR, neutrophil to lymphocyte ratio; AFP, alpha fetoprotein; B, coefficient; SE, stand error; CI, confidence interval; HR, hazard ratio.
**Preoperative images were obtained from contrast-enhanced Computed Tomography or contrast-enhanced magnetic resonance imaging.*

TABLE 4 | Multivariate Cox regression analysis of risk factors of Recurrence based on Postoperative data of the training cohort.

Variable	B	SE	HR(95%CI)	P-value
Tumor number, Multiple versus Solitary	1.159	0.173	3.187(2.273–4.470)	<0.001
Tumor size, cm	0.066	0.017	1.069(1.033–1.106)	<0.001
MVI, Present versus Absent	0.462	0.163	1.587(1.153–2.186)	0.005
AFP, ng/ml, >20 versus ≤20	0.357	0.154	1.428(1.057–1.930)	0.02
NLR	0.135	0.045	1.144(1.048–1.250)	0.003

NLR, neutrophil to lymphocyte ratio; AFP, alpha fetoprotein; MVI, microvascular invasion; B, coefficient; SE, stand error; CI, confidence interval; HR, hazard ratio.

training cohort and 0.741 (0.677–0.743) in the validation cohort. For the postoperative nomogram model, the corresponding tdAUC was 0.751 (range, 0.722–0.753) in the training cohort and 0.755 (range, 0.687–0.768) in the validation cohort. Both models had higher tdAUCs than those of the BCLC and AJCC staging systems (**Figures 2A, B**). In addition, the prediction error curve analysis was used to assess the overall performance of the models. The nomogram models had a lower prediction error rate than the conventional staging systems (**Figures 2C, D**).

The calibration plots also displayed a good agreement between predictions of the pre- and postoperative nomogram models and the probability of 1-, 2-, and 3-year recurrence in the training and validation cohorts (**Figure 3**).

Risk Stratification Based on the Nomograms' Score

Each patient received an individualized risk score according to the individual scores calculated with the nomograms. We performed a survival tree analysis to determine the cutoff points of the risk score (**Figure 4**). Based on the cutoff points, the patients were stratified into three different risk subgroups (low-risk, intermediate-risk, and high-risk). The Kaplan-Meier analysis showed that the recurrence curves were widely separated among the three different risk groups in the training and validation cohorts, which further indicated that the nomograms had good discrimination ability for recurrence (**Figure 5**).

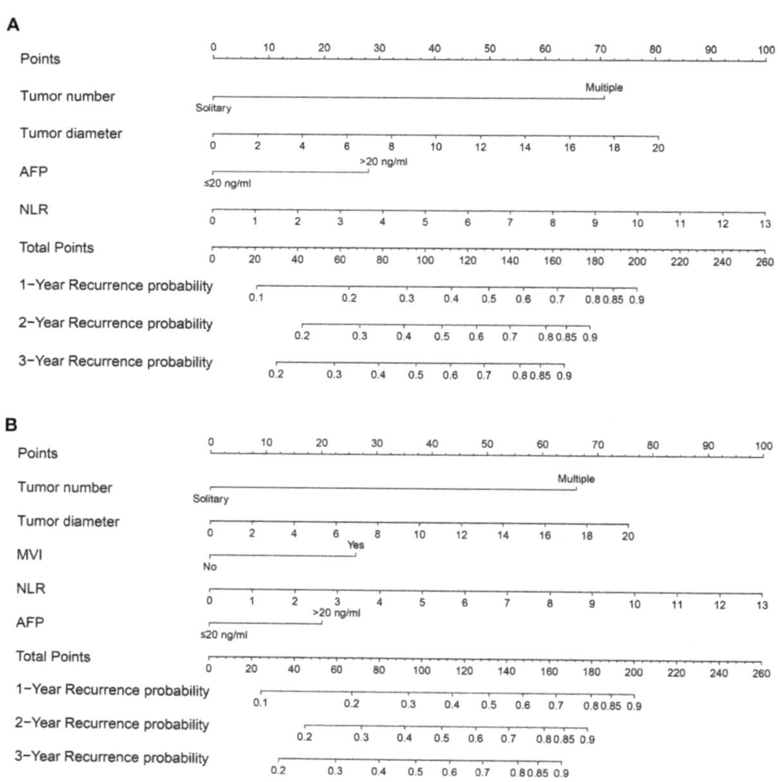

FIGURE 1 | Nomogram for preoperative prediction **(A)** and postoperative prediction **(B)** of Recurrence for NBNCHCC patients who underwent hepatectomy.

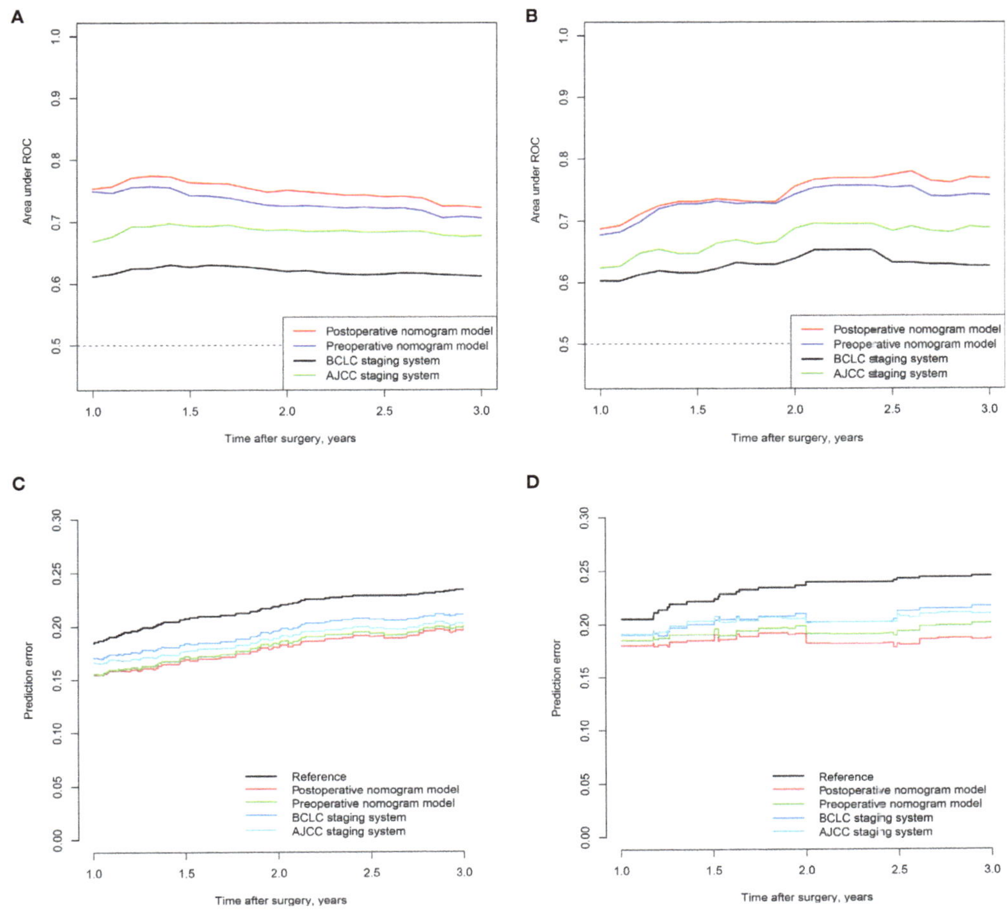

FIGURE 2 | Time-dependent AUC of pre- and postoperative of nomograms in the training **(A)** and validation **(B)** cohorts; prediction error curve of pre- and postoperative nomogram models in the training **(C)** and validation cohorts **(D)**.

In addition, we combined the models with the BCLC/AJCC^{8th} staging system and found that the models had a good re-stratification effect on the traditional staging systems. Because there were only 12 patients with BCLC stage 0 and AJCC stage IA tumors, these patients were incorporated into the group of patients with BCLC stage A or AJCC 8th stage IB. As shown in **Figure 6**, both models could re-stratify the patients with different recurrence risks in BCLC stages 0/A (p<0.001, preoperative nomogram model; p<0.001, postoperative nomogram model) well. The re-stratification ability of the models persisted in patients with BCLC B stage (p=0.044, preoperative nomogram model; p=0.037, postoperative nomogram model), but given that only a small number of patients were in the high-risk group, the re-stratification ability of models in patients with BCLC B stage needed be validated in a further large sample cohort. For the AJCC^{8th} staging system, we found that the models distinguished patients with stages IA/IB (p<0.001, preoperative nomogram model; p<0.001, postoperative nomogram model), and II (p<0.001, preoperative nomogram model; p=0.002, postoperative nomogram model) well (**Figure 7**).

DISCUSSION

In this study, we reported significant independent risk factors for recurrence of NBNC-HCC, which included large tumor diameter, multiple tumor number, elevated AFP levels, elevated NLR, and presence of MVI. We also constructed pre- and postoperative nomograms for individualized prediction of recurrence in patients with NBNC-HCC who underwent curative resection. Both nomograms had a better predictive performance than the currently used BCLC and AJCC^{8th} staging systems. Additionally, according to the individualized scores assessed using the nomograms, patients in cohorts can be stratified into three risk groups. These two easy-to-apply graphical models will be valuable in preoperative treatment planning, adjuvant therapy implementation, postoperative monitoring, and designing of clinical trials based on prognostic stratification.

Tumor diameter and number are important prognostic factors in the BCLC staging system; however, these tumor factors are insufficient to reflect the malignant characteristics

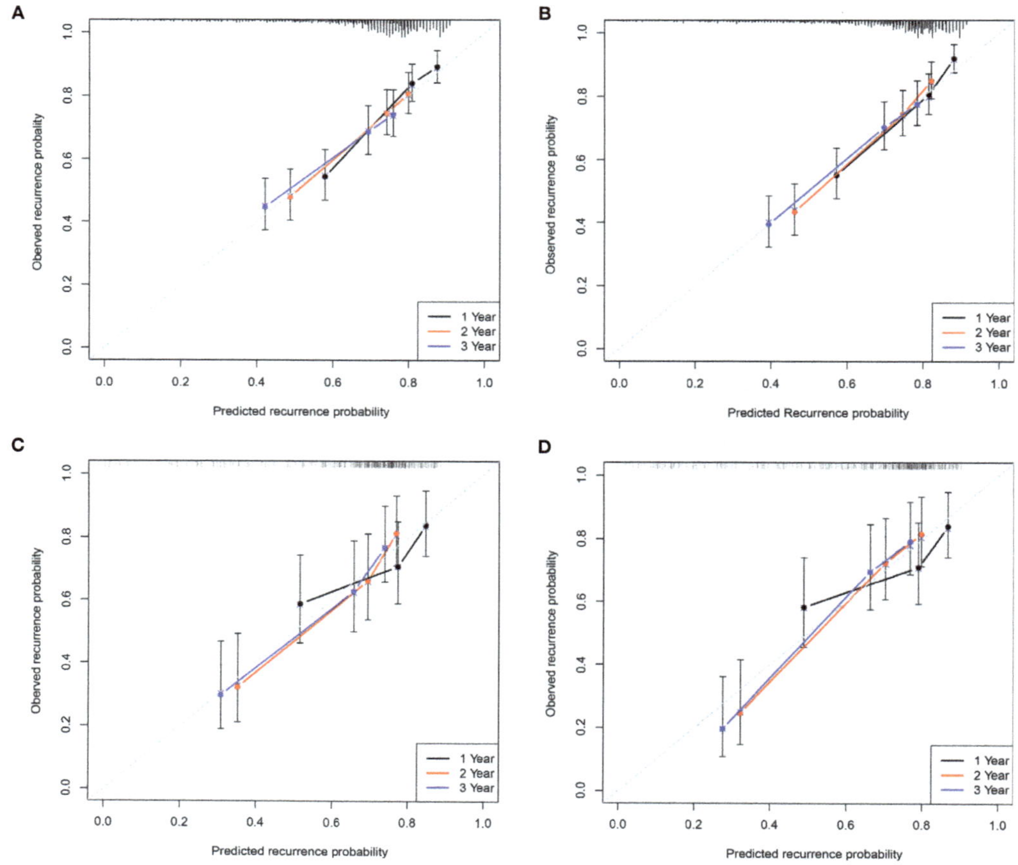

FIGURE 3 | The calibration curves for predicting the 1, 2, and 3-year Recurrence by the Pre- and postoperative nomogram in the training **(A, B)** and validation cohorts **(C, D)**.

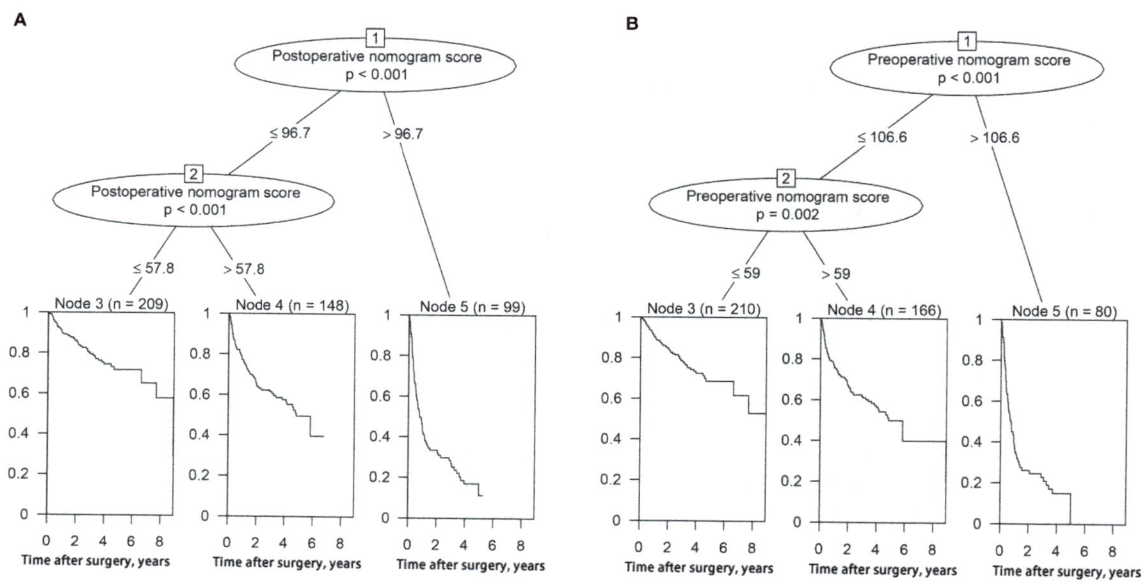

FIGURE 4 | Survival tree analysis of best cut-off scores in the training cohort. **(A)** postoperative nomogram model; **(B)** preoperative nomogram model.

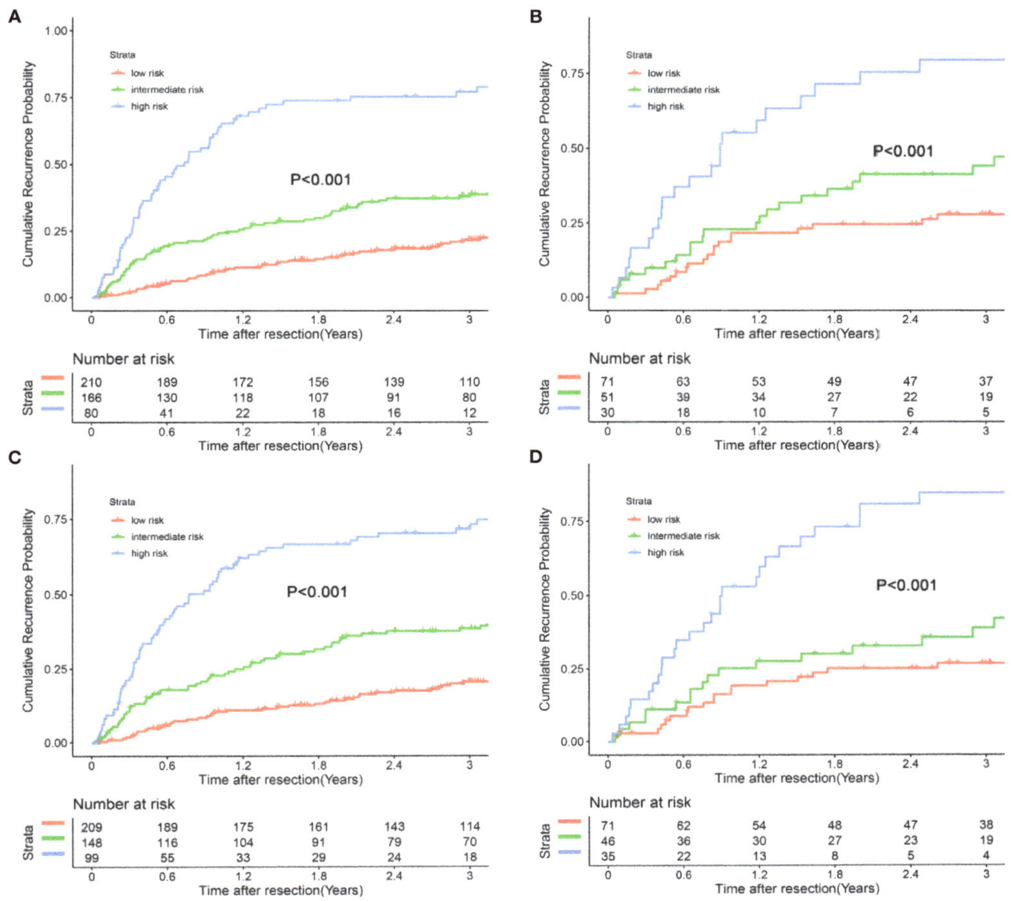

FIGURE 5 | Kaplan-Meier plots for cumulative recurrence rate of risk subgroups defined by the nomograms model scores. **(A)** preoperative nomogram model, training cohort; **(B)** preoperative nomogram model, validation cohort; **(C)** postoperative nomogram model, training Cohort; **(D)** postoperative nomogram model, validation Cohort.

of HCC (32). Compared to the BCLC staging system, the AJCC^{8th} staging system included the presence of MVI as a stratification criterion; however, given that MVI is a pathological feature that can only be diagnosed after surgery, it limits the applicability of this system in preoperative clinical decision making. Moreover, both the BCLC and AJCC^{8th} staging systems were not developed specifically for the prediction of HCC recurrence. The nomograms in this study integrated the independent risk factors for recurrence of NBNC-HCC, including the above three tumor-associated factors; serum tumor biomarker, AFP; and inflammatory index, NLR; thus, making them more accurate recurrence predictors.

Our recurrence nomograms were able to re-stratify patients in the same traditional staging system stages, and thus can play a supplementary role to the traditional staging system. The preoperative nomogram in this study, which had a significantly better predictive performance than the BCLC staging system, may be an additional tool for surgeons to identify high-risk patients before operation; thus, it may be valuable in preoperative treatment planning [e.g., preoperative transarterial chemoembolization (TACE), widened surgical margin]. Owing to the lack of consensus on follow-up procedures for the postoperative diagnosis of recurrence of HCC (33), using the postoperative nomogram can help surgeons to design stricter follow-up procedures (e.g., reduced interval of follow-up and more high-end imaging tests) and postoperative adjuvant therapy for the high-recurrence risk patients. For the current results, it is difficult to specify which model is better for the recurrence prediction. In terms of the predictive performance of the models, the C-index and tdAUC of the postoperative model were higher than those of the preoperative model, and the prediction error curve also shows that the postoperative model is better than the preoperative model, although the difference was not obvious, the postoperative model may be superior to the preoperative model considering that the postoperative model includes the indicator of MVI, MVI is currently widely recognized as an independent risk factor for recurrence in HCC. However, when the preoperative model shows poor prognosis of patients and the postoperative model

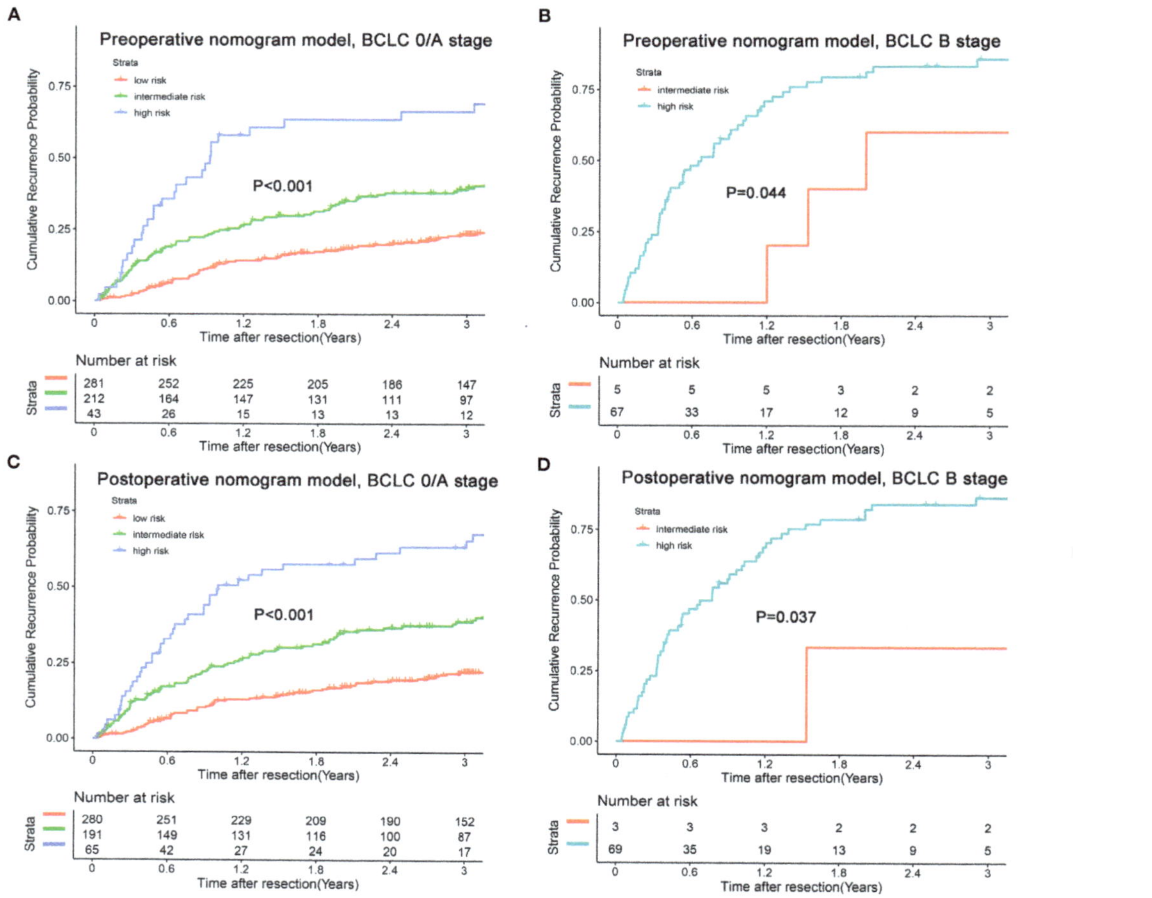

FIGURE 6 | Kaplan-Meier plots for cumulative recurrence rate of risk subgroups defined by the nomograms model scores in different BCLC stage. **(A)** preoperative nomogram model, BCLC 0/A stage; **(B)** preoperative nomogram model, BCLC B stage; **(C)** postoperative nomogram model, BCLC 0/A stage; **(D)** postoperative nomogram model, BCLC B stage.

shows good prognosis, it may more proper to choose the preoperative model. After all, the cost of shortening the follow-up interval is much less than the cost of finding recurrence of HCC too late. Further prospective studies may be needed to distinguish which model has better predictive power.

In addition, we included an inflammatory index in this study. To the best of our knowledge, this is the first study to investigate the association between a system inflammatory index and recurrence in NBNC-HCC. In this study, we analyzed nine inflammatory indices and found that the NLR was an independent risk factor for recurrence in NBNC-HCC. High NLR has been reported to be a poor prognostic factor for recurrence and OS in several malignancies, including HCC (13, 34). Given that NLR consists of serum neutrophil count and lymphocyte count, elevation of NLR can be reviewed as elevated neutrophil and lymphocyte counts. Neutrophilia can promote cancer cell growth and progression by releasing angiogenic factors and inflammatory mediators (28, 35, 36). On the other hand, lymphocytes play an anti-cancer role in host immunity by inducing cytotoxicity and inhibiting proliferation, invasion, and migration of cancer cells; lymphopenia may weaken this anti-cancer effect (37–39). All these factors included in the NLR were adverse factors for HCC, which could possibly explain why NLR could be used to evaluate the recurrence probability of patients with HCC. However, the mechanism underlying the association between NLR and recurrence of NBNC-HCC remains unclear and needs further elucidation.

This study had some limitations. First, it was limited by its retrospective nature and limited sample size; thus, selection bias was unavoidable. A large sample, outer validation cohort, and prospective study are needed to validate the nomograms in future. Second, postoperative adjuvant therapy information, such as postoperative adjuvant TACE (PA-TACE), has not been included in our study. Given that PA-TACE may improve the prognostic outcome of high-risk patients (40, 41), whether high-risk patients assessed by these nomograms can benefit from PA-TACE is to be determined. Third, the prognostic value of postoperative inflammatory indexes or the changed indexes after post-operation compared to pre-operation in HCC have been recognized in some studies, but this study did not include because the data of some postoperative inflammatory

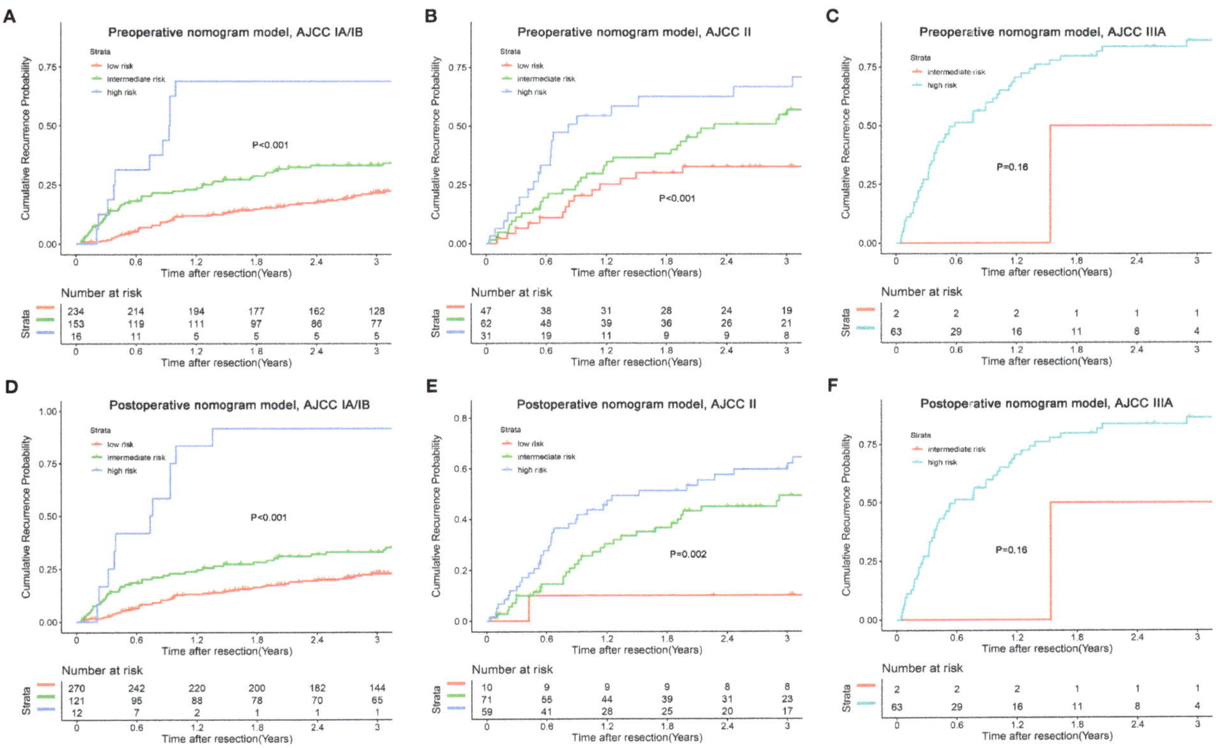

FIGURE 7 | Kaplan-Meier plots for cumulative recurrence rate of risk subgroups defined by the nomograms model scores in different AJCC[8th] stage. **(A)** preoperative nomogram model, AJCC IA/IB stage; **(B)** preoperative nomogram model, AJCC II stage; **(C)** preoperative nomogram model, AJCC IIIA stage; **(D)** postoperative nomogram model, AJCC IA/IB stage; **(E)** postoperative nomogram model, AJCC II stage; **(F)** postoperative nomogram model, AJCC IIIA stage.

indexes were missing. Last, the nomograms were generated using data of patients who underwent radical resection, which may not be applicable for patients receiving other therapies.

CONCLUSION

In summary, we developed pre- and postoperative nomograms for predicting the recurrence of patients with NBNC-HCC after resection. These two easy-to-apply graphical models will be valuable in guiding preoperative treatment planning, adjuvant treatment implementation, and postoperative monitoring for patients with NBNC-HCC.

AUTHOR CONTRIBUTIONS

KL, QH, LW, WZ, and JL: study conception, design, quality control of this study, drafting of the manuscript, and statistical analysis. JZ, ZD, HL, JF, PG, and ZC: data acquisition and data interpretation. YZ, WZ, and JL: resource and study supervision. All authors contributed to the article and approved the submitted version.

ACKNOWLEDGMENTS

We thank our colleagues and all the patients who participated in this study.

REFERENCES

1. Torre LA, Bray F, Siegel RL, Ferlay J, Lortet-Tieulent J, Jemal A. Global cancer statistics, 2012. *CA: Cancer J Clin* (2015) 65(2):87–108. doi: 10.3322/caac.21262
2. Bosetti C, Levi F, Boffetta P, Lucchini F, Negri E, La Vecchia C. Trends in mortality from hepatocellular carcinoma in Europe, 1980-2004. *Hepatol (Baltimore Md)* (2008) 48(1):137–45. doi: 10.1002/hep.22312
3. Goh GB, Chang PE, Tan CK. Changing epidemiology of hepatocellular carcinoma in Asia. *Best Pract Res Clin Gastroenterol* (2015) 29(6):919–28. doi: 10.1016/j.bpg.2015.09.007
4. Utsunomiya T, Shimada M, Kudo M, Ichida T, Matsui O, Izumi N, et al. A comparison of the surgical outcomes among patients with HBV-positive, HCV-positive, and non-B non-C hepatocellular carcinoma: a nationwide study of 11,950 patients. *Ann Surg* (2015) 261(3):513–20. doi: 10.1097/SLA.0000000000000821
5. Nishikawa H, Osaki Y. Non-B, non-C hepatocellular carcinoma (Review). *Int J Oncol* (2013) 43(5):1333–42. doi: 10.3892/ijo.2013.2061
6. Zhang X, Li C, Wen T, Yan L, Li B, Yang J, et al. Appropriate treatment strategies for intrahepatic recurrence after curative resection of hepatocellular carcinoma initially within the Milan criteria: according to the recurrence pattern. *Eur J Gastroenterol Hepatol* (2015) 27(8):933–40. doi: 10.1097/MEG.0000000000000383
7. Dhir M, Melin AA, Douaiher J, Lin C, Zhen WK, Hussain SM, et al. A Review and Update of Treatment Options and Controversies in the Management of Hepatocellular Carcinoma. *Ann Surg* (2016) 263(6):1112–25. doi: 10.1097/SLA.0000000000001556

8. Zhu SL, Chen J, Li H, Li LQ, Zhong JH. Efficacy of hepatic resection for huge (>/= 10 cm) hepatocellular carcinoma: good prognosis associated with the uninodular subtype. *Int J Clin Exp Med* (2015) 8(11):20581–8.
9. Yang P, Qiu J, Li J, Wu D, Wan X, Lau WY, et al. Nomograms for Pre- and Postoperative Prediction of Long-term Survival for Patients Who Underwent Hepatectomy for Multiple Hepatocellular Carcinomas. *Ann Surg* (2016) 263 (4):778–86. doi: 10.1097/SLA.0000000000001339
10. Mantovani A, Allavena P, Sica A, Balkwill F. Cancer-related inflammation. *Nature* (2008) 454(7203):436–44. doi: 10.1038/nature07205
11. Balkwill F, Mantovani A. Inflammation and cancer: back to Virchow? *Lancet (London England)* (2001) 357(9255):539–45. doi: 10.1016/S0140-6736(00) 04046-0
12. Hu B, Yang XR, Xu Y, Sun YF, Sun C, Guo W, et al. Systemic immune-inflammation index predicts prognosis of patients after curative resection for hepatocellular carcinoma. *Clin Cancer Res an Off J Am Assoc Cancer Res* (2014) 20(23):6212–22. doi: 10.1158/1078-0432.CCR-14-0442
13. Mano Y, Shirabe K, Yamashita Y, Harimoto N, Tsujita E, Takeishi K, et al. Preoperative neutrophil-to-lymphocyte ratio is a predictor of survival after hepatectomy for hepatocellular carcinoma: a retrospective analysis. *Ann Surg* (2013) 258(2):301–5. doi: 10.1097/SLA.0b013e318297ad6b
14. Li J, Liao Y, Suo L, Zhu P, Chen X, Dang W, et al. A novel prognostic index-neutrophil times gamma-glutamyl transpeptidase to lymphocyte ratio (NgammaLR) predicts outcome for patients with hepatocellular carcinoma. *Sci Rep* (2017) 7(1):9229. doi: 10.1038/s41598-017-09696-y
15. Ma W, Zhang P, Qi J, Gu L, Zang M, Yao H, et al. Prognostic value of platelet to lymphocyte ratio in hepatocellular carcinoma: a meta-analysis. *Sci Rep* (2016) 6:35378. doi: 10.1038/srep35378
16. Chan AW, Chan SL, Wong GL, Wong VW, Chong CC, Lai PB, et al. Prognostic Nutritional Index (PNI) Predicts Tumor Recurrence of Very Early/Early Stage Hepatocellular Carcinoma After Surgical Resection. *Ann Surg Oncol* (2015) 22(13):4138–48. doi: 10.1245/s10434-015-4516-1
17. Ji F, Fu S, Guo Z, Pang H, Chen D, Wang X, et al. Prognostic significance of preoperative aspartate aminotransferase to neutrophil ratio index in patients with hepatocellular carcinoma after hepatic resection. *Oncotarget* (2016) 7 (44):72276–89. doi: 10.18632/oncotarget.10848
18. Wang Y, Sun K, Shen J, Li B, Kuang M, Cao Q, et al. Novel Prognostic Nomograms Based on Inflammation-Related Markers for Patients with Hepatocellular Carcinoma Underwent Hepatectomy. *Cancer Res Treat Off J Korean Cancer Assoc* (2019) 51(4):1464–78. doi: 10.1136/gutjnl-2019-IDDFAbstracts.252
19. Yang Z, Zhang J, Lu Y, Xu Q, Tang B, Wang Q, et al. Aspartate aminotransferase-lymphocyte ratio index and systemic immune-inflammation index predict overall survival in HBV-related hepatocellular carcinoma patients after transcatheter arterial chemoembolization. *Oncotarget* (2015) 6(40):43090–8. doi: 10.18632/oncotarget.5719
20. Wang L, Lin N, Lin K, Xiao C, Wang R, Chen J, et al. The Clinical Value of Postoperative Transarterial Chemoembolization for Resectable Patients with Intermediate Hepatocellular Carcinoma After Radical Hepatectomy: a Propensity Score-Matching Study. *J Gastrointest Surg* (2020). doi: 10.1007/ s11605-020-04588-5
21. Wang L, Lin N, Lin K, Xiao C, Wang R, Chen J, et al. The Clinical Value of Postoperative Transarterial Chemoembolization for Resectable Patients with Intermediate Hepatocellular Carcinoma After Radical Hepatectomy: a Propensity Score-Matching Study. *J Gastrointest Surg Off J Soc Surg Aliment Tract* (2020). doi: 10.1007/s11605-020-04588-5
22. Huang Q, Lin K, Wang L, Zeng J, Liu H, Ding Z, et al. Postoperative Adjuvant Transarterial Chemoembolization Improves Short-Term Prognosis of Hepatocellular Carcinoma with Bile Duct Tumor Thrombus: A Propensity-Score Matching Study. *Cancer Manage Res* (2020) 12:9183–95. doi: 10.2147/ CMAR.S270467
23. Utsunomiya T, Shimada M, Kudo M, Ichida T, Matsui O, Izumi N, et al. Nationwide study of 4741 patients with non-B non-C hepatocellular carcinoma with special reference to the therapeutic impact. *Ann Surg* (2014) 259(2):336–45. doi: 10.1097/SLA.0b013e31829291e9
24. Bruix J, Sherman M. Practice Guidelines Committee AAftSoLD: Management of hepatocellular carcinoma. *Hepatol (Baltimore Md)* (2005) 42(5):1208–36. doi: 10.1002/hep.20933
25. Zheng J, Seier K, Gonen M, Balachandran VP, Kingham TP, D'Angelica MI, et al. Utility of Serum Inflammatory Markers for Predicting Microvascular Invasion and Survival for Patients with Hepatocellular Carcinoma. *Ann Surg Oncol* (2017) 24(12):3706–14. doi: 10.1245/s10434-017-6060-7
26. Zhang W, Tan Y, Jiang L, Yan L, Yang J, Li B, et al. Prognostic nomogram for patients with non-B non-C hepatocellular carcinoma after curative liver resection. *Int J Surg (London England)* (2017) 44:160–5. doi: 10.1016/ j.ijsu.2017.06.041
27. Johnson PJ, Berhane S, Kagebayashi C, Satomura S, Teng M, Reeves HL, et al. Assessment of liver function in patients with hepatocellular carcinoma: a new evidence-based approach-the ALBI grade. *J Clin Oncol Off J Am Soc Clin Oncol* (2015) 33(6):550–8. doi: 10.1200/JCO.2014.57.9151
28. Wislez M, Rabbe N, Marchal J, Milleron B, Crestani B, Mayaud C, et al. Hepatocyte growth factor production by neutrophils infiltrating bronchioloalveolar subtype pulmonary adenocarcinoma: role in tumor progression and death. *Cancer Res* (2003) 63(6):1405–12.
29. Zhang XP, Wang K, Gao YZ, Wei XB, Lu CD, Chai ZT, et al. Prognostic model for identifying candidates for hepatectomy among patients with hepatocellular carcinoma and hepatic vein invasion. *Br J Surg* (2020) 107 (7):865–77. doi: 10.1002/bjs.11524
30. Mogensen UB, Ishwaran H, Gerds TA. Evaluating Random Forests for Survival Analysis using Prediction Error Curves. *J Stat Softw* (2012) 50 (11):1–23. doi: 10.18637/jss.v050.i11
31. European Association for the Study of the Liver and Electronic address eee, European Association for the Study of the L. EASL Clinical Practice Guidelines: Management of hepatocellular carcinoma. *J Hepatol* (2018) 69 (1):182–236. doi: 10.1016/j.jhep.2018.03.019
32. Forner A, Reig ME, de Lope CR, Bruix J. Current strategy for staging and treatment: the BCLC update and future prospects. *Semin Liver Dis* (2010) 30 (1):61–74. doi: 10.1055/s-0030-1247133
33. European Association For The Study Of The L, European Organisation For R, Treatment Of C. EASL-EORTC clinical practice guidelines: management of hepatocellular carcinoma. *J Hepatol* (2012) 56(4):908–43. doi: 10.1016/ j.jhep.2011.12.001
34. Halazun KJ, Aldoori A, Malik HZ, Al-Mukhtar A, Prasad KR, Toogood GJ, et al. Elevated preoperative neutrophil to lymphocyte ratio predicts survival following hepatic resection for colorectal liver metastases. *Eur J Surg Oncol J Eur Soc Surg Oncol Br Assoc Surg Oncol* (2008) 34(1):55–60. doi: 10.1016/ j.ejso.2007.02.014
35. Queen MM, Ryan RE, Holzer RG, Keller-Peck CR, Jorcyk CL. Breast cancer cells stimulate neutrophils to produce oncostatin M: potential implications for tumor progression. *Cancer Res* (2005) 65(19):8896–904. doi: 10.1158/0008-5472.CAN-05-1734
36. Liang J, Piao Y, Holmes L, Fuller GN, Henry V, Tiao N, et al. Neutrophils promote the malignant glioma phenotype through S100A4. *Clin Cancer Res an Off J Am Assoc Cancer Res* (2014) 20(1):187–98. doi: 10.1158/1078-0432.CCR-13-1279
37. Dunn GP, Old LJ, Schreiber RD. The immunobiology of cancer immunosurveillance and immunoediting. *Immunity* (2004) 21(2):137–48. doi: 10.1016/j.immuni.2004.07.017
38. Kitayama J, Yasuda K, Kawai K, Sunami E, Nagawa H. Circulating lymphocyte number has a positive association with tumor response in neoadjuvant chemoradiotherapy for advanced rectal cancer. *Radiat Oncol (London England)* (2010) 5:47. doi: 10.1186/1748-717X-5-47
39. Diakos CI, Charles KA, McMillan DC, Clarke SJ. Cancer-related inflammation and treatment effectiveness. *Lancet Oncol* (2014) 15(11): e493–503. doi: 10.1016/S1470-2045(14)70263-3
40. Zhang X-P, Liu Y-C, Chen Z-H, Sun J-X, Wang K, Chai Z-T, et al. Postoperative Adjuvant Transarterial Chemoembolization Improves Outcomes of Hepatocellular Carcinoma Associated with Hepatic Vein Invasion: A Propensity Score Matching Analysis. *Ann Surg Oncol* (2019) 26 (5):1465–73. doi: 10.1245/s10434-019-07223-z
41. Wang YY, Wang LJ, Xu D, Liu M, Wang HW, Wang K, et al. Postoperative adjuvant transcatheter arterial chemoembolization should be considered selectively in patients who have hepatocellular carcinoma with microvascular invasion. *HPB* (2019) 21(4):425–33. doi: 10.1016/j.hpb.2018.08.001

2

A Somatic Mutation-Derived LncRNA Signature of Genomic Instability Predicts Prognosis for Patients with Liver Cancer

Cheng Guo[†], *Jie Zhou*[†], *Boyu Ma, Rui Wang, Yanli Ge, Zhe Wang, Bing Ji, Wei Wang, Junjie Zhang** *and Zhirong Wang**

Department of Gastroenterology, Tongji Hospital, Tongji University School of Medicine, Shanghai, China

***Correspondence:**
Junjie Zhang
junjie81@126.com
Zhirong Wang
wangzr929@126.com

[†] *These authors have contributed equally to this work*

Background: Genomic instability is considered as one of the hallmarks of hepatocellular carcinoma (HCC) and poses a significant challenge to the clinical treatment. The emerging evidence has revealed the roles of long non-coding RNAs (lncRNAs) in the maintenance of genomic instability. This study is aimed to develop a genomic instability-related lncRNA signature for determining HCC prognosis and the suitability of patients for immunotherapy.

Methods: In this study, data related to transcriptome profiling, clinical features, and the somatic mutations of patients with HCC were downloaded from The Cancer Genomic Atlas (TCGA). Bioinformatics analysis was performed to identify and construct a somatic mutation-derived genomic instability-associated lncRNA signature (GILncSig). Single-sample gene set enrichment analysis (ssGSEA) was applied to estimate the levels of immune cell infiltration. A nomogram was constructed, and calibration was performed to assess the effectiveness of the model.

Results: In the study, seven genomic instability-related lncRNAs were identified and used to define a prognostic signature. Patients with HCC were stratified into high- and low-risk groups with significant differences in the survival (median survival time = 1.489, 1.748 year; $p = 0.006$) based on the optimal cutoff value (risk score = 1.010) of the risk score in the training group. In addition, GILncSig was demonstrated to be an independent risk factor for the patients with HCC when compared to the clinical parameters ($p < 0.001$). According to the receiver operating characteristic (ROC) curve, nomogram, and calibration plot, the signature could predict the survival rate for the patients with HCC in the 1st, 3rd, and 5th years. Furthermore, ssGSEA revealed the potential of the signature in guiding decisions for administering clinical treatment.

Conclusions: In this study, we developed a novel prognostic model based on the somatic mutation-derived lncRNAs and validated it using an internal dataset. The independence of the GILncSig was estimated using univariate and follow-up multivariate analyses. Immunologic analysis was used to evaluate the complex factors involved in the HCC progression.

Keywords: hepatocellular carcinoma, long non-coding RNA, immune infiltration, prognosis, genomic instability

BACKGROUND

Hepatocellular carcinoma (HCC) is a malignant tumor with a high rate of recurrence and poor prognosis, constituting the fourth major cause of cancer-associated deaths worldwide (1). Surgical resection, transplantation, and radiofrequency ablation are the most effective treatment methods for patients with early-stage liver cancer (1). For a decade, sorafenib, an antiangiogenic tyrosine kinase inhibitor, is the only treatment strategy recognized by the Food and Drug Administration (FDA) for advanced liver cancer (2). However, the therapeutic efficacy of sorafenib is gradually weakening or restricting owing to the chemical resistance and recurrence (3, 4). Early diagnosis is essential for improving patient outcomes (4). The Liver Cancer Staging System, described in the eighth edition of the American Joint Committee on Cancer (AJCC 2017), is one of the most recognized staging systems globally (5). However, the accuracy of AJCC staging in predicting prognosis in patients with liver cancer requires improvement.

Genomic instability attributed to the somatic mutations is a hallmark of cancer cells (6). Genomic instability is observed frequently in HCC (6, 7). It is also a significant prognostic parameter, and an increase in the genomic instability ratio indicates a worse outcome (8–10). Although the mechanisms underlying genomic instability are not entirely clear, aberrant transcription and post-transcriptional modifications play important roles (11).

Non-coding RNAs with a length of more than 200 nucleotides, termed long non-coding RNAs (lncRNAs), are characterized as non-coding transcripts and do not encode proteins (12). The abnormal regulation, involving processes such as deletion or mutation, of lncRNA has been associated with many human diseases, including cancer (13). More importantly, lncRNAs are involved in chromatin interactions, transcriptional regulation, mRNA post-transcriptional regulation, and epigenetic regulation. New evidence has illustrated the vital roles of lncRNAs in regulating genomic stability (14–17). For example, Lee et al. (17) identified a specific non-coding RNA, NORAD, which alters genomic stability through the sequestration of PUMILIO proteins. Although several lncRNAs are associated with genomic instability, the regulatory role of lncRNAs associated with genomic instability in cancers remains elusive.

In this study, we developed a novel promising prognostic signature that is more effective than the AJCC staging system. In addition, our research showed the immune microenvironment and immune functions of patients with HCC.

Abbreviations: HCC, hepatocellular carcinoma; LncRNA, long non-coding RNA; TCGA, The Cancer Genomic Atlas; K-M, Kaplan-Meier; ROC, receiver operating characteristic; FDA, Food and Drug Administration; GU, genomic unstable; GS, genomic stable; GILncSig, genomic instability-related lncRNA signature; FDR, false discovery rate; OS, overall survival; C-index, the concordance index; SNP, single nucleotide polymorphism; AUC, the area under the curve; AFP, alpha-fetoprotein; PD-1, programmed cell death protein-1; PD-L1, programmed cell death protein ligand 1; MHC, major histocompatibility complex; ICI, immune checkpoint inhibitors.

METHODS

Data Source

RNA-seq expression data (FPKM), somatic mutation information, and the related clinical variables of 343 patients with liver cancer were obtained from The Cancer Genomic Atlas (TCGA, http://cancergenome.nih.gov/, accessed July 20, 2020). The lncRNA expression profile was extracted from the mRNA expression profile data based on the GTF file information downloaded from the GENECODE website.

Identification and Construction of the Genomic Instability-Associated lncRNA Signatures

Information on somatic variants observed in patients with HCC stored in the format of mutation annotation downloaded from TCGA was analyzed using the "maftools" R package (17). In order to identify the genomic instability-associated lncRNAs, first, after calculating the total number of mutations per patient, they were ranked in descending order (**Figure 1**). Second, according to a previous study (18), the top 25% and the last 25% were characterized as the genomic unstable (GU) group and genomic stable (GS) group, respectively. Third, the Wilcoxon test was employed for the comparison of the lncRNA expression matrix between the GU and GS groups. Finally, according to the definition, differentially expressed lncRNAs [$\log_2$ fold change $>|1|$ and false discovery rate (FDR) adjusted $p < 0.05$] were considered as the genomic instability-related lncRNAs.

Among the genomic instability-related lncRNAs, lncRNAs associated with the overall survival (OS) of patients with HCC were screened by employing univariate Cox regression analyses ($p < 0.05$). Next, the genomic instability-associated lncRNA signature (GILncSig) was constructed by performing multivariate Cox regression analysis. The risk score was determined for every patient by applying the following formula: GILncSig score $= \text{coef}_{\text{lncRNA1}} * \text{expr}_{\text{lncRNA1}} + \text{coef}_{\text{lncRNA2}} * \text{expr}_{\text{lncRNA2}} + \ldots + \text{coef}_{\text{lncRNA}n} * \text{expr}_{\text{lncRNA}n}$, based on a previous study (18). Linear integration of the expression levels of lncRNAs weighted by regression coefficients (coef) was used to assign the risk score. Log transformation of the hazard ratio (HR) from the multivariate Cox regression analysis was employed to calculate the coef value. Patients enrolled in the training group were divided into high and low-risk groups using the median score as a cutoff value. The Kaplan-Meier method was used to compare the survival rates between the high-risk and low-risk groups. The independence of the risk signature was estimated from other clinical features using the multivariate Cox regression.

ssGSEA Analysis

The immune-related term enrichment score was established by exploring the associations between the risk score of GILncSig and components of the immune system, such as innate or adaptive immune cell types, immune functions, or pathways using the ssGSEA program. The levels of immune infiltration were estimated using the "gsva" R package (19). Quantitative indicators of immune infiltration were determined for each patient with HCC. In addition, different distributions of immune

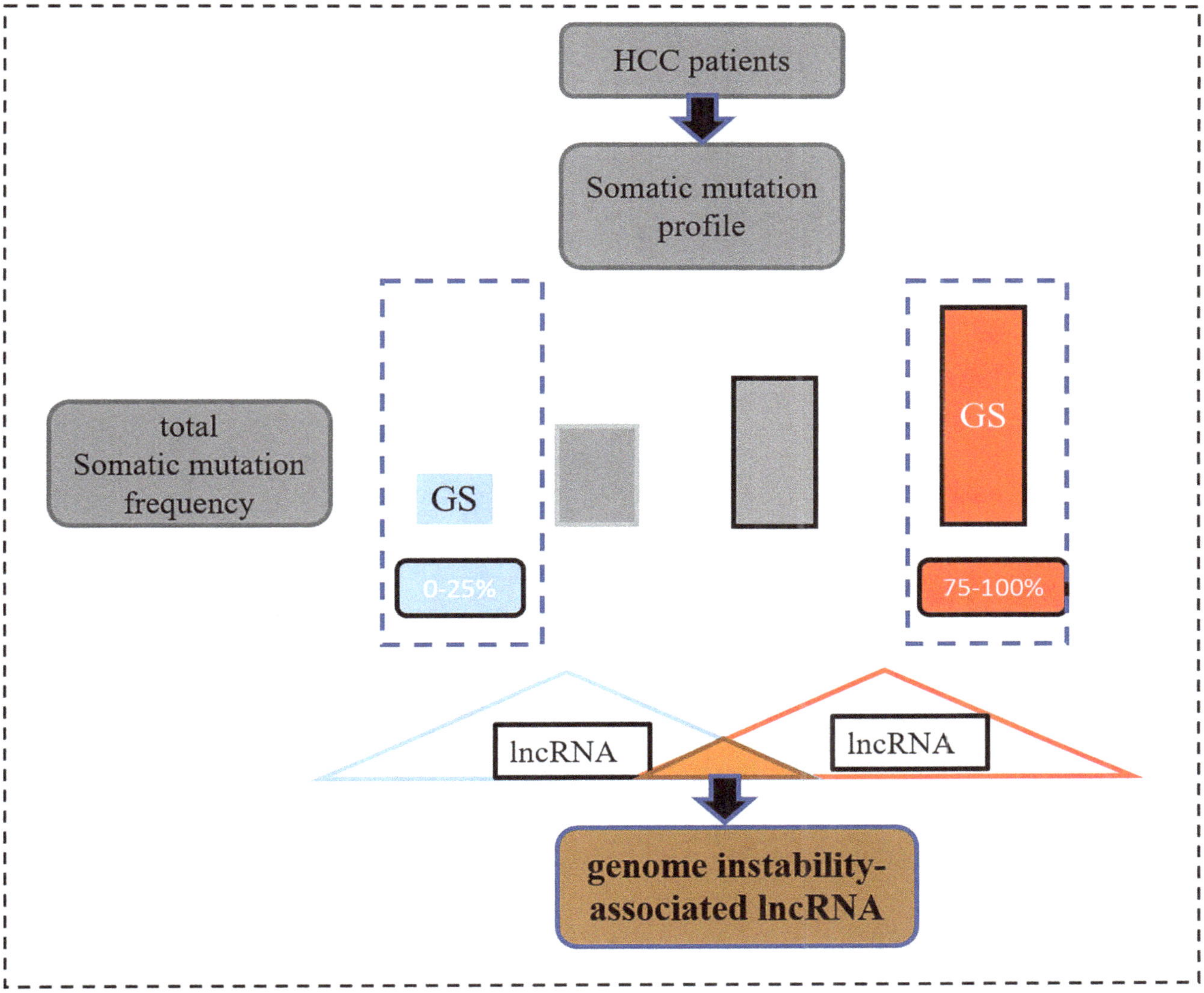

FIGURE 1 | The process of screening genomic instability-associated lncRNAs.

cell types or functions between the high and low-risk groups in the TCGA cohort were visualized using the "vioplot" R package (20).

Construction and Assessment of a Predictive Nomogram

A nomogram was constructed based on the clinical factors using multivariate regression analysis in the training group. The discrimination and calibration of the predictive nomogram were assessed by applying the concordance index (C-index) and the calibration curve. The construction of nomogram and calibration was performed using the "rms" package (21). The effectiveness of the signature was assessed by constructing a time-dependent receiver operating feature (ROC) curve using the "survivalROC" packages (22).

Statistical Analysis

All statistical analyses were performed using the RStudio (v.1.4.1106). Continuous data are presented as medians or mean ± SD. Statistical significance was set at $P < 0.05$.

RESULTS

Identifying the Genomic Instability-Related lncRNAs in Patients With HCC

Liver cancer is highly heterogeneous with respect to the mutated genes (23, 24). In **Figures 2A,B**, we illustrate the landscape of the HCC mutation profile including variant classification, type of variants, single nucleotide polymorphism (SNP) class, variants per sample, and the top 10 mutated genes. As shown in **Figure 2B**, SNP was the most common variant type. TP53 was the

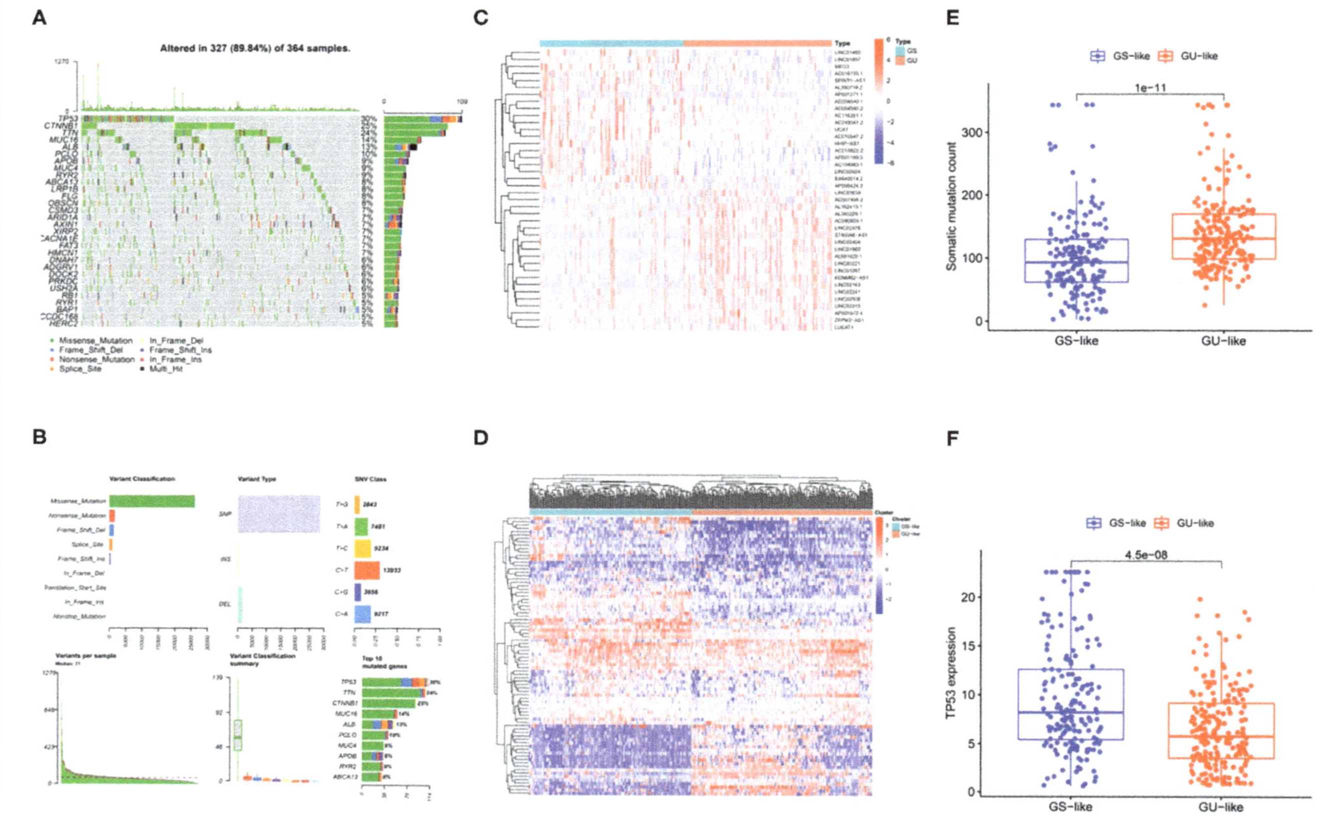

FIGURE 2 | Identification of genomic instability-related lncRNAs in patients with HCC. **(A)** Waterfall summarized mutational data from patients with HCC. **(B)** Mutational frequencies in the top 10 genes in the training and testing cohorts. **(C)** Differentially expressed lncRNAs between GS group and GU group. **(D)** Hierarchical cluster analyses of TCGA patients with liver cancer based on the expression pattern of 82 genomic instability-related lncRNAs. **(E)** Boxplots of somatic mutations in the GU-like and GS-like groups. **(F)** Boxplots of TP53 expression level in the GU-like and GS-like groups.

most mutated gene in the HCC, with an average of 30% mutation frequency. To identify lncRNAs related to the genomic instability, differential lncRNA expression profiles of patients with HCC between the GU and GS groups determined by different mutation patterns were compared. Wilcoxon's test was used to screen 82 lncRNAs with significant differences ($\log_2$ fold change $> |1|$ and FDR regulated $P < 0.05$; **Supplementary Table 1**). The expression of 53 of 82 lncRNAs was upregulated and that of the remaining lncRNAs was downregulated. The profiles of the top 20 lncRNAs with upregulated and downregulated expressions are shown in **Figure 2C**. In addition, all the patients were divided into two clusters based on the differential expression profiles of the 82 lncRNAs (**Figure 2D**). The group with higher somatic mutation frequency was regarded as the GS-like group, while the other group was regarded as the GU-like group. The somatic mutation patterns of the two groups were significantly different. Cumulative somatic mutations in the GS-like group were significantly lower than those in the GU-like group (**Figure 2E**, $p < 0.001$). In addition, the TP53 expression was significantly higher in the GS-like group than that in the GU-like group (**Figure 2F**, $p < 0.001$).

Construction of the Genomic Instability-Related lncRNA Signature

To investigate the prognostic effectiveness of these genomic instability-related lncRNAs, 343 patients with liver cancer from the TCGA database were randomly assigned to the training group ($n = 172$) and the testing group ($n = 171$). The inclusion standard included patients with complete prognostic information and pathologically confirmed HCC. The exclusion criterion was patients with equal to or <30 days of survival because they were more likely to die from non-tumor factors, such as post-operative bleeding or infection. No statistically significant differences were observed with respect to age ($p = 0.855$), gender ($p = 0.538$), AJCC stage ($p = 0.170$), histologic grade ($p = 1$), T ($p = 0.239$), M ($p = 1$), and N ($p = 1$) using the chi-square test (**Table 1**).

The association between the expression profiles of 82 genomic instability-related lncRNAs and the OS of patients with liver cancer in the training group was analyzed using the univariate Cox proportional hazard regression. The results revealed that 11 lncRNAs influenced the prognosis of patients with HCC ($p < 0.05$; **Supplementary Table 2**). These lncRNAs

TABLE 1 | Clinical information of the 343 patients with liver cancer.

Variables	Type	Entire group (n = 343)	Testing group (n = 172)	Training group (n = 171)	p-value
Age	<=65	216 (62.97%)	109 (63.74%)	107 (62.21%)	0.8554
	>65	127 (37.03%)	62 (36.26%)	65 (37.79%)	
Gender	Female	110 (32.07%)	58 (33.92%)	52 (30.23%)	0.5382
	Male	233 (67.93%)	113 (66.08%)	120 (69.77%)	
Histologic grade	G1-2	214 (62.39%)	106 (61.99%)	108 (62.79%)	1
	G3-4	124 (36.15%)	62 (36.26%)	62 (36.05%)	
	Unknown	5 (1.46%)	3 (1.75%)	2 (1.16%)	
AJCC stage	Stage I–II	238 (69.39%)	112 (65.5%)	126 (73.26%)	0.1695
	Stage III–IV	83 (24.2%)	47 (27.49%)	36 (20.93%)	
	Unknown	22 (6.41%)	12 (7.02%)	10 (5.81%)	
T	T1-2	252 (73.47%)	120 (70.18%)	132 (76.74%)	0.2386
	T3-4	88 (25.66%)	49 (28.65%)	39 (22.67%)	
	Unknown	3 (0.87%)	2 (1.17%)	1 (0.58%)	
M	M0	245 (71.43%)	121 (70.76%)	124 (72.09%)	1
	M1	3 (0.87%)	1 (0.58%)	2 (1.16%)	
	Unknown	95 (27.7%)	49 (28.65%)	46 (26.74%)	
N	N0	239 (69.68%)	118 (69.01%)	121 (70.35%)	1
	N1	2 (0.58%)	1 (0.58%)	1 (0.58%)	
	Unknown	102 (29.74%)	52 (30.41%)	50 (29.07%)	

were then incorporated into a multivariate Cox proportional hazards regression model to identify an optimal risk signature model without the risk of overfitting using the "glmnet" R package. Finally, 7 of 11 lncRNAs were used to construct the GILncSig based on the maximum value of the Akaike information criterion (AIC, AIC = 446.94) (**Table 2**). The GILncSig score was calculated using the following formula: value of LINC01287*0.035+ value of AC004540.1*0.259+ value of AC096996.2*0.338+ value of PRRT3-AS1*0.202+ value of AC004862.1*(−0.188) + value of AC245041.2*0.063+ value of AC010205.1*(−0.782). The coefficients of these lncRNAs represent the contribution of lncRNAs to the prognostic risk score obtained from the regression index of multivariate Cox analysis. The aforementioned formula was adopted to obtain the risk score of patients with liver cancer in the training group, and the median risk score (value = 1.010) was used as the cutoff value to cluster these patients into different groups. The group with a higher score was called the high-risk group, and the other group was called the low-risk group. The Kaplan-Meier analysis indicated that patients in the low-risk group showed better outcomes than those in the high-risk group (p = 0.006; p = 0.008; p < 0.001) (**Figure 3**).

The expression profiles of lncRNAs, the distribution of somatic mutation frequency, and TP53 expression in different cohorts are illustrated in **Figures 4A–C**. TP53 expression was significantly higher in the high-risk group than that in the low-risk group in the testing cohort as well as the entire cohort (p < 0.001; **Figures 4E,F**). Although the level of TP53 was not significantly different between the high-and low-risk groups in the training cohort, the p-value was close to 0.05 (**Figure 4D**).

TABLE 2 | Seven lncRNAs identified using the Cox regression model.

LncRNA	Coefficient	Hazard ratio (95% CI)	p-value
LINC01287	0.035	1.036 (1.002–1.071)	0.039
AC004540.1	0.259	1.296 (1.029–1.632)	0.028
AC096996.2	0.338	1.403 (1.065–1.847)	0.016
PRRT3-AS1	0.202	1.224 (1.091–1.374)	0.001
AC004862.1	−0.188	0.828 (0.663–1.035)	0.098
AC245041.2	0.063	1.066 (0.993–1.414)	0.076
AC010205.1	−0.782	0.457 (0.206–1.018)	0.055

Independence of the GILncSig From Other Clinical Parameters

The independence of the GILncSig in patients with HCC was assessed by performing Cox regression analyses. The univariate and follow-up multivariate analyses showed that AJCC stage (p = 0.002; p = 0.002; p < 0.001) and GILncSig risk scores (p < 0.001; p < 0.001; p = 0.002) were significantly related to OS and were independent factors for patients with liver cancer in the three groups (**Table 3**). In addition, according to the time-dependent ROC curve analysis, the area under the curve (AUC) for the risk score was 0.730, which was higher than the AUC values for age (AUC = 0.494), gender (AUC = 0.505), grade (AUC = 0.516), and stage (AUC = 0.704) in the training group (**Figure 5A**). The testing set and the entire set showed similar outcomes (**Figures 5B,C**).

Moreover, we investigated the association between the independent signature and clinical parameters by using the chi-square test. Tumor grade (p < 0.05), AJCC stage (p < 0.01), and

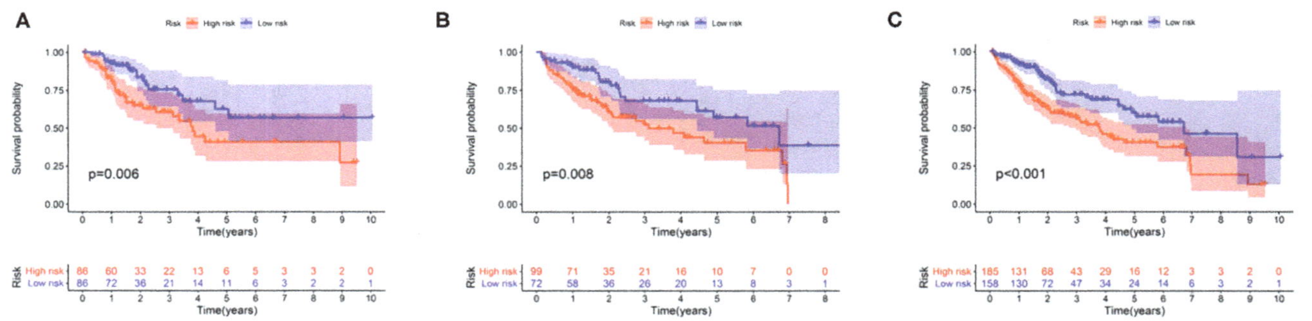

FIGURE 3 | Survival curve analysis between the high-risk and low-risk groups in the training group **(A)**, the testing group **(B)**, and the entire group **(C)**.

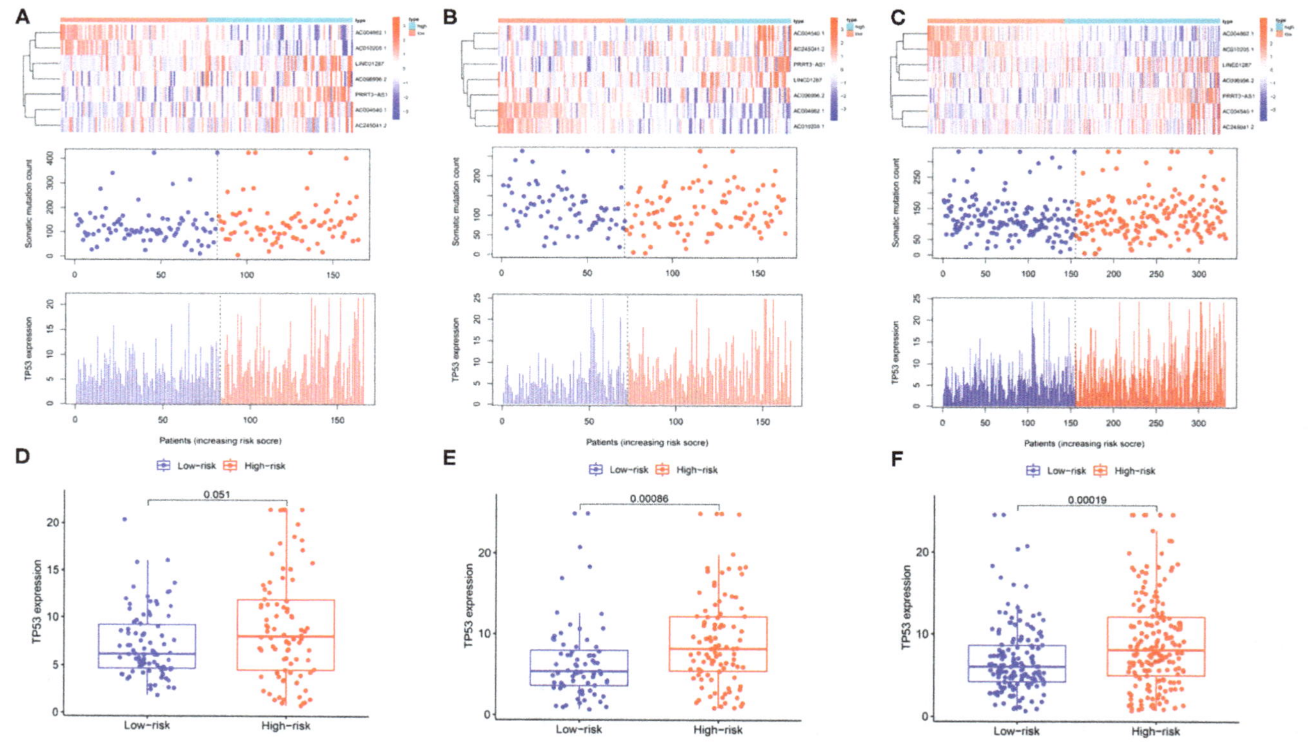

FIGURE 4 | Identification of the genomic instability-related lncRNA signature for outcome prediction. Heatmap of LncRNAs and the distribution of somatic mutation and TP53 expression with increasing risk score in the training group **(A,D)**, in the testing group **(B,E)**, and the entire group **(C,F)**.

T stage ($p < 0.05$) were significantly related to GILncSig in the training group (**Figure 5D**). Notably, the AJCC stage and the T stage were significantly associated with the GILncSig in the training, testing, and overall groups (**Figures 5D–F**).

Association Between the GILncSig and Immune Cell Infiltration

In the study, immune cell types, immune functions, or pathways were evaluated to assess immune cell infiltration among patients with HCC in an integrated fashion *via* ssGSEA analysis of the transcriptome profiles of patients with liver cancer. As shown in **Figures 6A,B**, GILncSig scores showed a significantly positive association with immune cell types, including various types of dendritic cells, T-helper cells, Treg cells, follicular helper T cells, macrophages, and tumor-infiltrating lymphocytes. In addition, patients in the high-risk group showed a higher proportion of APC co-stimulation, APC co-inhibition, CCR, check-point, HLA, MHC class I, para inflammation, T-cell co-stimulation, and T-cell co-inhibition. In addition, seven of the 13 types of immune functions were significantly higher in high-risk patients than in low-risk patients, while the expression of type II IFN response

TABLE 3 | The univariate and multivariate Cox regression analyses in the training, testing, and entire groups.

Variable	Univariate analysis			Multivariate analysis		
	HR	HR.95L-HR.95H	*p*	HR	HR.95L-HR.95H	*p*
Training set (*n* = 172)						
Age (<=65/>65)	1.005	0.983–1.027				
Gender (Female/male)	0.870	0.480–1.578				
Grade (G1–G4)	0.802	0.535–1.204				
Stage (I–IV)	1.776	1.293–2.440	**<0.001**	1.665	1.205–2.300	**0.002**
Risk score	1.131	1.087–1.177	**<0.001**	1.123	1.077–1.170	**<0.001**
Testing set (*n* = 171)						
Age (<=65/>65)	1.006	0.986–1.026				
Gender (Female/male)	0.696	0.413–1.174				
Grade (G1–G4)	1.460	1.037–2.056				
Stage (I–IV)	1.783	1.339–2.375	**0.030**	1.609	1.160–2.205	**0.002**
Risk score	1.009	0.980–1.038	**<0.001**	1.229	1.172–1.280	**<0.001**
Entire set (*n* = 343)						
Age (<=65/>65)	1.005	0.991–1.020				
Gender (Female/male)	0.758	0.513–1.118				
Grade (G1–G4)	1.121	0.865–1.454				
Stage (I–IV)	1.808	1.463–2.234	**<0.001**	1.775	1.436–2.194	**<0.001**
Risk score	1.028	1.010–1.047	**0.003**	1.025	1.005–1.046	**0.002**

HR, hazard ratio. Bold value means $p < 0.05$.

was the opposite. More importantly, the expression of HLA family genes and programmed cell death protein-1 (PD-1) in the high-risk group was significantly higher than that in low-risk patients with HCC (**Figures 6C,D**). The aforementioned results showed that abnormal immune infiltration and differences in the expression of immune checkpoints can be adopted as prognostic indices for patients with liver cancer with respect to immunotherapy with significant clinical implications.

Nomogram Construction and Validation

A nomogram was constructed by combining the age, gender, tumor grade, AJCC stage, and risk score (**Figure 7**). Each parameter in the nomogram was assigned a score. Based on the parameters of each patient, the score related to each prognostic element was added to obtain the total score, which corresponds to the corresponding scale. The survival rates of the patients were obtained at the 1st, 3rd, and 5th years.

The predictive ability of the nomogram model could be evaluated and quantified by measuring the extent of fit between the C-index forecast by the nomogram in the standard curve and the baseline time. The C-index in the training group was 0.770 (95% *CI*: 0.708–0.832), while that for the testing group and the whole group was 0.680 (95% *CI*: 0.610–0.750) and 0.686 (95% *CI*: 0.635–0.737), respectively. The calibration curves of the nomogram were remarkably consistent between the predicted OS rates and actual observations made at the 5th year in different groups (**Figures 8A–C**). Simultaneously, the ROC curve analysis showed that AUC was 0.735 after 1 year, 0.672 after 2 years, and 0.695 after 5 years in the training group (**Figure 8D**). The testing group and the whole group showed similar outcomes (**Figures 8E,F**).

DISCUSSION

Hepatocellular carcinoma is a malignant tumor with a highly heterogeneous immune microenvironment, gene expression profile and associated genetic variations, signal transduction pathways, and cancer stem cells (1, 25). The high heterogeneity of liver cancer poses a significant challenge for clinical treatment (6, 7). Tumor heterogeneity may result from genomic instability (26). Genomic instability is a common feature of most cancers and can act as a mutator, enhancing the frequency of mutations that extend the ability of the primary tumor to adapt, escape, and metastasize, ultimately contributing to tumor-specific immune response and resistant phenotypes (27, 28). Thus, genomic instability leads to tumor heterogeneity, which may act as a target for prognosis, prevention, and treatment (29). However, the quantitative analysis of genomic instability is a major problem. An emerging study illustrated that abnormal transcriptional or epigenetic changes may lead to genomic alterations (29, 30). LncRNAs exert a significant effect on the progression of liver cancer, such as regulating proliferation, migration, apoptosis, cell cycle, tumorigenesis, and metastasis (30, 31). An examination of the functional mechanism of lncRNA has shown that lncRNAs are also essential for genomic stability (30, 31).

In this study, the clinical outcomes of the patients with HCC were predicted by exploring the GILncSig. Patients with HCC, whose data are included in the TCGA database, can be distinguished effectively into high-risk and low-risk cohorts by applying the prognostic model risk scores. The Cox analysis showed that the prognostic GILncSig was an independent factor that could effectively predict HCC prognosis better than other clinical factors. A nomogram model was built for

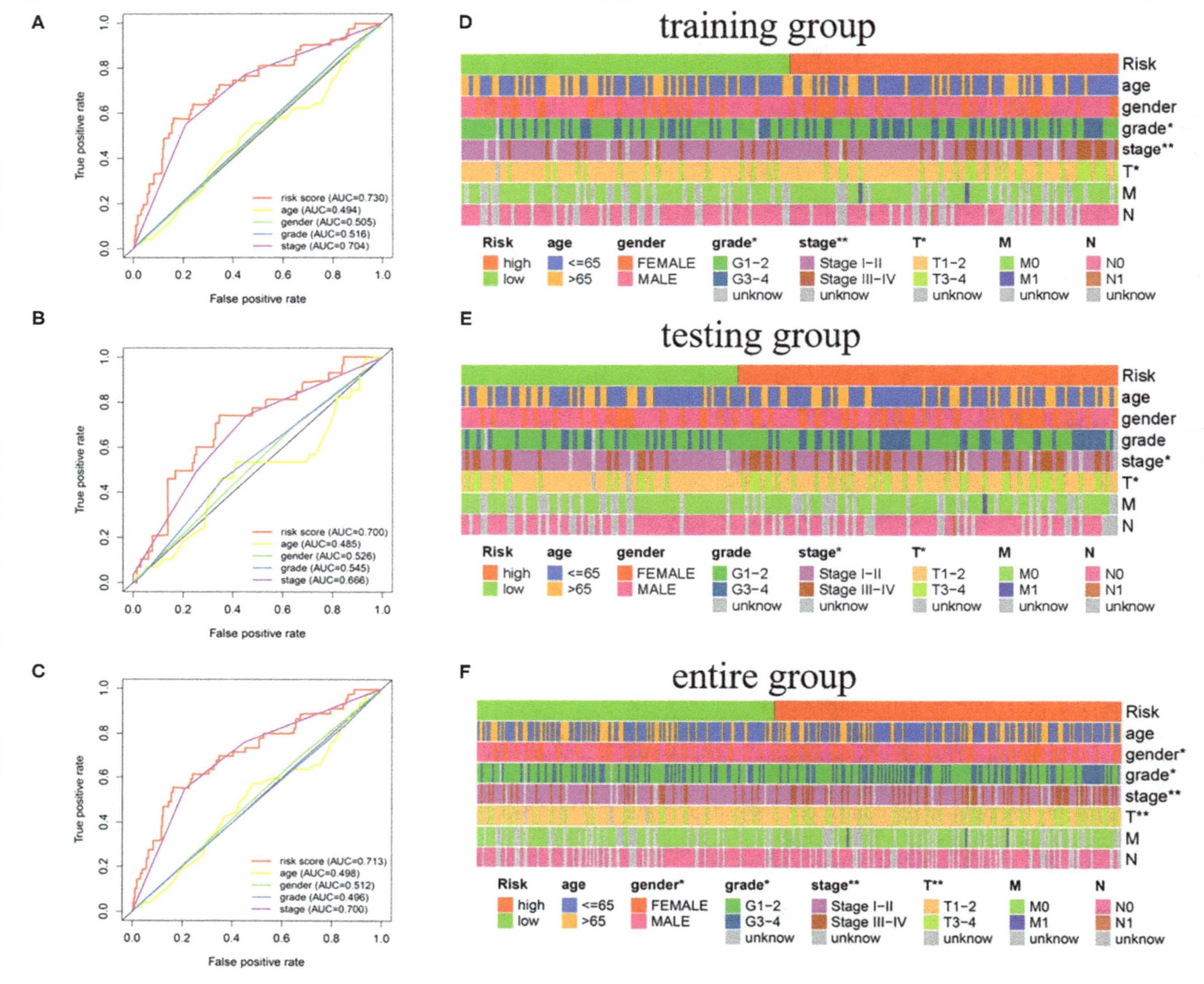

FIGURE 5 | The association of GILncSig and clinical features. **(A–C)** ROC curve analysis of the training group, the testing group, and the entire group. **(D–F)** Differential analysis between GILncSig and clinicopathological features. *$p < 0.05$; **$p < 0.01$.

the training group. The outcomes of the C-index and time-dependent ROC curves illustrated satisfactory discrimination capacity. The calibration curves showed that the prognosis for the patients with HCC could be predicted by the nomogram with satisfactory performance. Therefore, GILncSig is a promising biomarker for forecasting outcomes in patients with liver cancer.

Specific genes can regulate immune pathways and interactions between immune cells, leading to changes in the microenvironment, allowing tumors to evade immune checkpoints. For instance, a recent study revealed that a specific lncRNA, ALAL-1, associated with genomic instability, mediates evasion of the immune system in the lung cancer cells (32). Here, the relationship between the genomic instability-associated risk model and the main immune system-associated factors was estimated using the ssGSEA analysis. A total of 21 out of 29 patients were significantly altered between patients with low- and high-risk. The terms associated with immune checkpoints, APC co-inhibition and co-stimulation, HLA expression, and Tregs were of particular interest. HLA is a gene cluster encoding the human major histocompatibility complex (MHC) (33). If the peptides provided by HLA proteins are altered due to diseases, they can act as autoantigens that target cellular immune rejection. As shown in **Figure 8C**, most HLA family genes were expressed significantly in high-risk patients with liver cancer than in low-risk patients. Overexpression of HLA proteins in tumor cells could undermine recognition by the immune system, which accounts for these differences in the survival results among these patient groups.

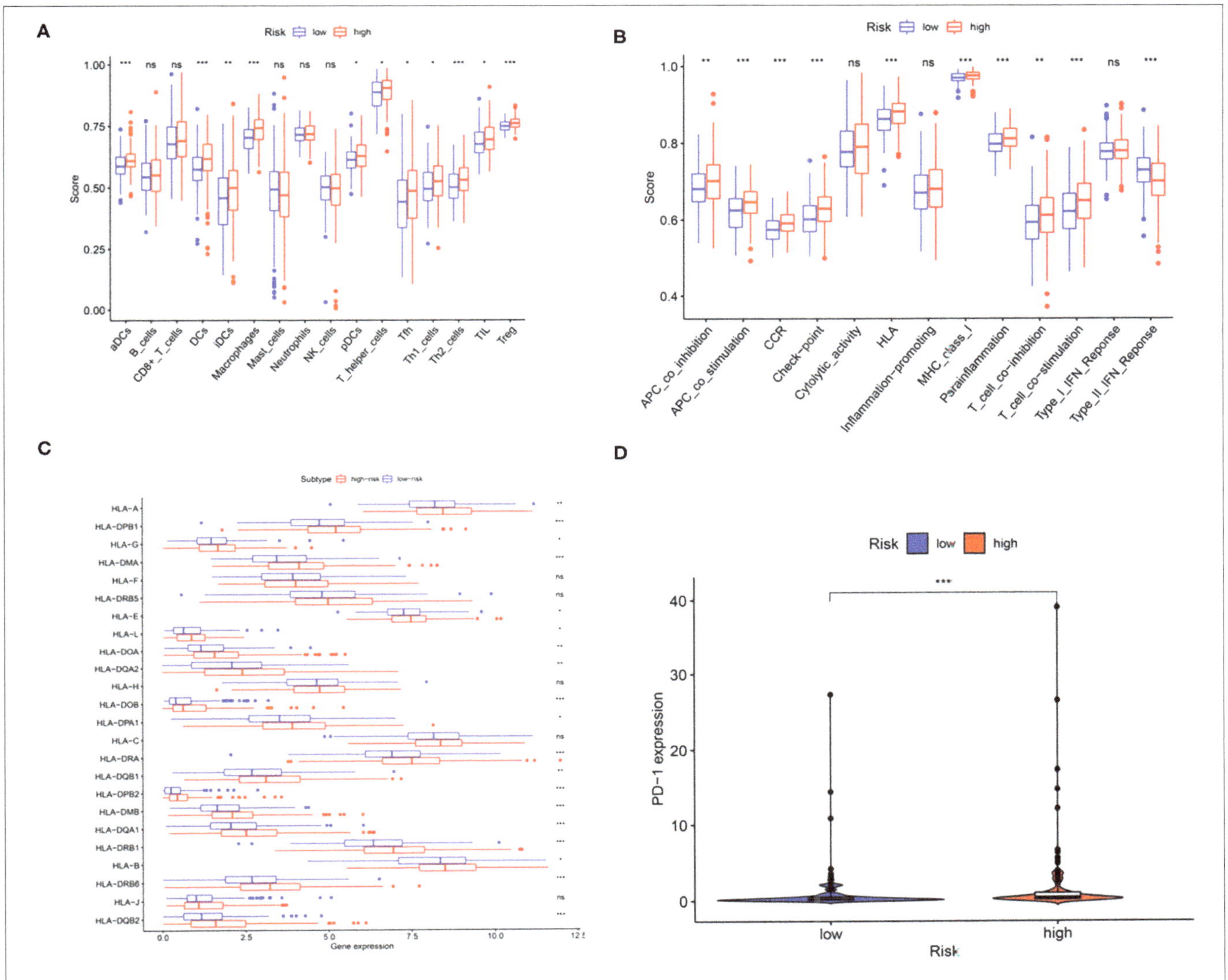

FIGURE 6 | The relationship among the risk scores, immune cell infiltration, and immune functionality in patients with liver cancer. The relative enrichment of immune cell infiltration **(A)** and immune functionality **(B)** in the patients with high- and low-risk liver cancer. HLA family gene **(C)** and PD-1 expression **(D)** in patients with high- and low-risk liver cancer. *$p < 0.05$; **$p < 0.01$; ***$p < 0.001$.

Administration of immune checkpoint inhibitors (ICIs) is by far the most promising immunotherapeutic strategy (34). Immune checkpoint proteins act as biomarkers that could identify whether patients with liver cancer are suitable for immunotherapy (34). Typically, immune checkpoint molecules can suppress immune responses (35). However, many patients with cancer cannot benefit from immune checkpoint suppression due to abnormal immune checkpoint protein expression (36). The expression of immune checkpoint proteins was significantly higher among patients with high-risk than low-risk patients. The immune response may be suppressed if the immune checkpoint proteins are overexpressed. At the same time, insufficient expression of immune checkpoint inhibitors may result in unconstrained harmful immune responses (37, 38).

More importantly, the increase in the expression of PD-1 in tumor-infiltrating lymphocytes is always associated with poor prognosis among patients with HCC (37, 38). PD-1 is a potential biomarker that aids in determining the suitability of immunochemical checkpoint therapy for patients (39). Recent evidence suggests that PD-(L)1 overexpression and genomic instability in tumors are associated with immune checkpoint inhibitor responses (40–42). In the study, the findings demonstrate the promising potential of immunotherapy for patients with HCC.

The current analysis had some limitations. On the one hand, all the data supplied in this research were derived from

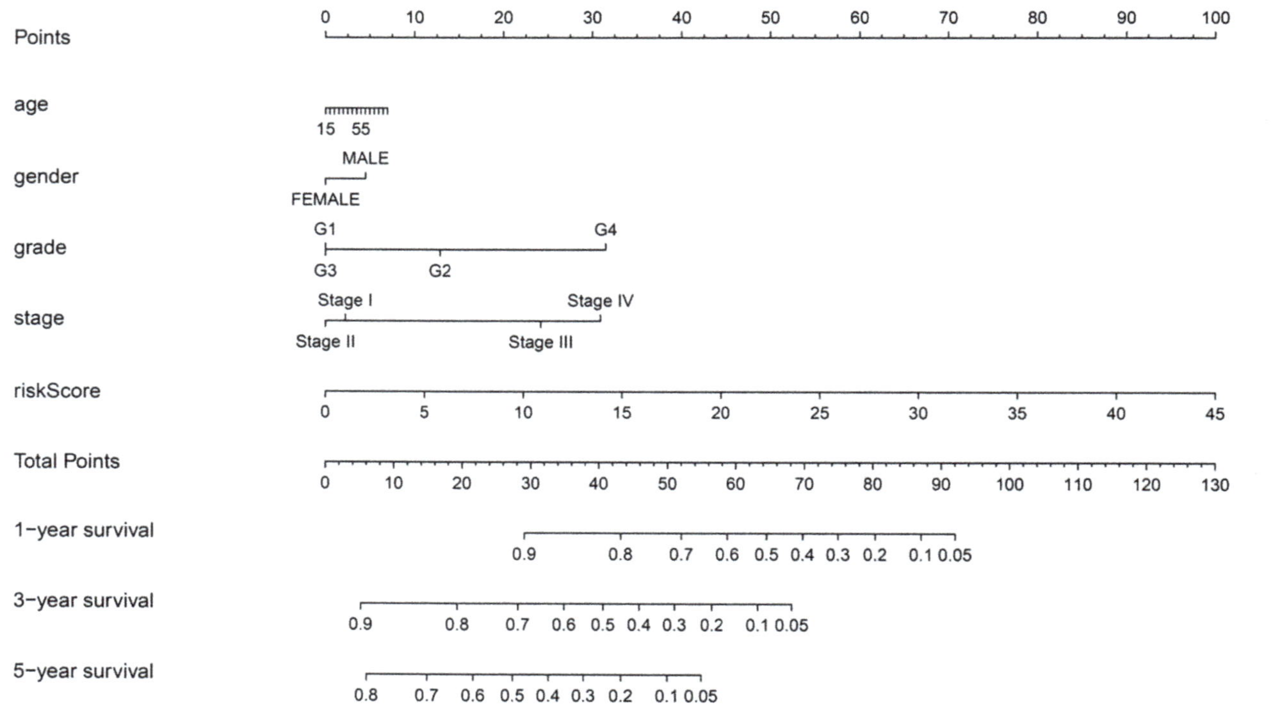

FIGURE 7 | A predictive nomogram for OS in the training group.

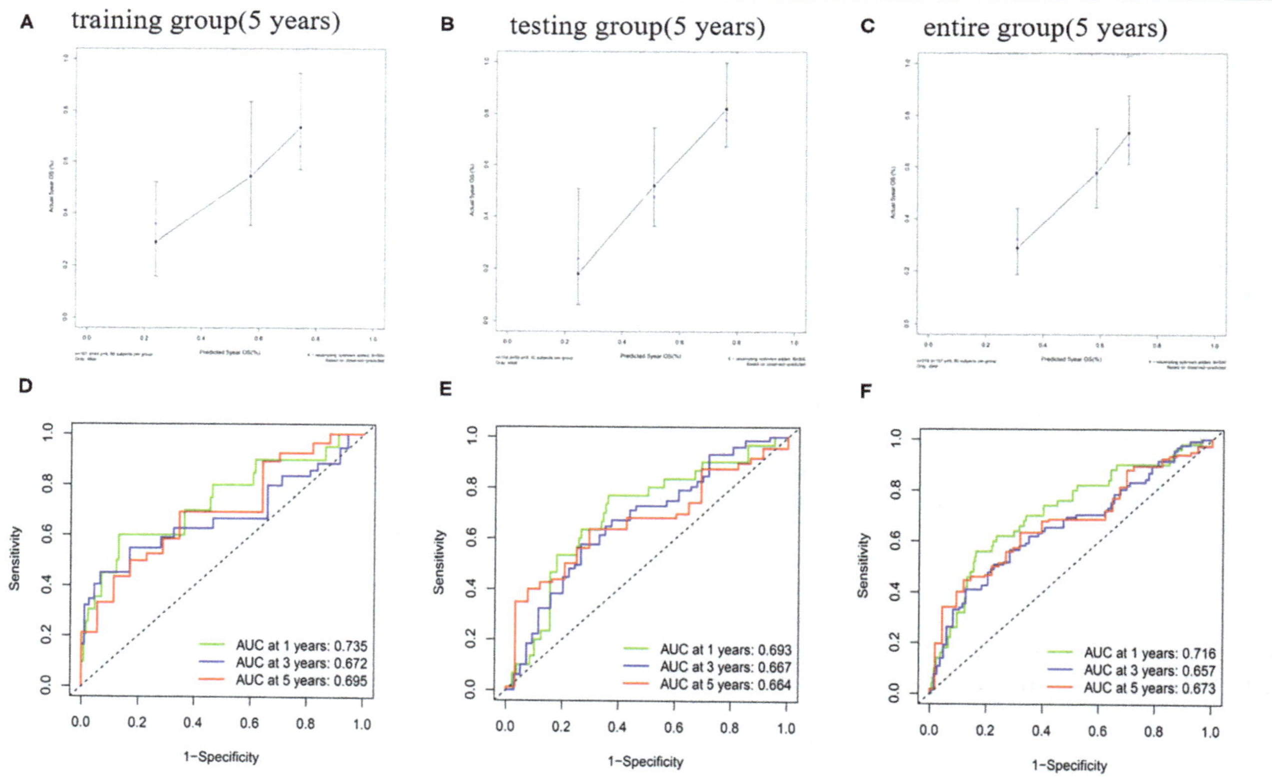

FIGURE 8 | The calibration curve of OS and ROC curve in the training group **(A,D)**, testing group **(B,E)**, and entire group **(C,F)**.

the TCGA database; on the other hand, although patients were randomly divided into training and testing queues, the contribution of this internal verification method is limited. Further external validation is critical to identify and extend these outcomes as a potential method for developing clinically valuable prognostic signatures.

CONCLUSIONS

In summary, GILncSig showed satisfactory efficiency for HCC prognosis. Furthermore, the association between the risk model and immune infiltration was explored. The data suggest that this predictive model may provide effective markers for evaluating patients with HCC and immunotherapeutic strategies.

AUTHOR CONTRIBUTIONS

CG, JZha, and ZhiW designed the study. CG, BM, BJ, YG, ZheW, WW, and RW complicated and analyzed data. CG and JZho wrote this manuscript.

ACKNOWLEDGMENTS

I would like to thank Mrs. Xu, my beloved, for her long-term company and encouragement. We thank Dr. Jianming Zeng (University of Macau), and all the members of his bioinformatics team, biotrainee, for generously sharing their experience and codes. In addition, we would like to thank Editage for English language editing.

REFERENCES

1. Longo DL, Villanueva A. Hepatocellular carcinoma. *N Engl J Med.* (2019) 380:1450–62. doi: 10.1056/NEJMra1713263
2. Pugh RN. Sorafenib in advanced hepatocellular carcinoma. *N Engl J Med.* (2008) 359:2497–8. doi: 10.1056/NEJMc081780
3. Sonbol B, Riaz IB, Naqvi SAA, Almquist DR, Bekaii-Saab T. Systemic therapy and sequencing options in advanced hepatocellular carcinoma: a systematic review and network meta-analysis. *JAMA Oncol.* (2020) 6:e204930. doi: 10.1001/jamaoncol.2020.4930
4. Allaire M, Nault JC. Advances in management of hepatocellular carcinoma. *Curr Opin Oncol.* (2017) 29:288–95. doi: 10.1097/CCO.0000000000000378
5. Kamarajah SK, Frankel TL, Sonnenday C, Cho CS, Nathan H. Critical evaluation of the American Joint Commission on Cancer (AJCC) 8th edition staging system for patients with Hepatocellular Carcinoma (HCC): A Surveillance, Epidemiology, End Results (SEER) analysis. *J Surg Oncol.* (2017) 117:644–50. doi: 10.1002/jso.24908
6. Negrini S, Gorgoulis VG, Halazonetis TD. Genomic instability—an evolving hallmark of cancer. *Nat Rev Mol Cell Biol. Nat Rev Mol Cell Bio.* (2010) 11:220–8. doi: 10.1038/nrm2858
7. Rao CV, Asch AS, Yamada HY. Frequently mutated genes/pathways and genomic instability as prevention targets in liver cancer. *Carcinogenesis.* (2017) 38:2–11. doi: 10.1093/carcin/bgw118
8. Calvisi DF, Simile MM, Ladu S, Pellegrino R, Feo F. Altered methionine metabolism and global DNA methylation in liver cancer: relationship with genomic instability and prognosis. *Int J Cancer.* (2007) 121:2410–20. doi: 10.1002/ijc.22940
9. Seneviratne D, Ma J, Tan X, Kwon YK, Muhammad E, Melhem M, et al. Genomic instability causes HGF gene activation in colon cancer cells, promoting their resistance to necroptosis. *Gastroenterology.* (2015) 148:181–91. doi: 10.1053/j.gastro.2014.09.019
10. Suzuki K, Ohnami S, Tanabe S, Sasaki H, Yasuda J, Katai H, et al.The genomic damage estimated by arbitrarily primed PCR DNA fingerprinting is useful for the prognosis of gastric cancer. *Gastroenterology.* (2003) 125:1330–40. doi: 10.1016/j.gastro.2003.07.006
11. Gómez-González B, Aguilera A. Transcription-mediated replication hindrance: a major driver of genomic instability. *Gene Dev.* (2019) 33:1008–36. doi: 10.1101/gad.324517.119
12. Guttman M, Rinn JL. Modular regulatory principles of large non-coding RNAs. *Nature.* (2012) 482:339–46. doi: 10.1038/nature10887
13. DiStefano JK. Long noncoding RNAs in the initiation, progression, and metastasis of hepatocellular carcinoma. *Non Coding RNA Res.* (2017):129–36. doi: 10.1016/j.ncrna.2017.11.001
14. Liu H, Biology BM, SOM TU. Linking lncRNA to genomic stability. *Sci China.* (2016) 59:328–9. doi: 10.1007/s11427-016-5009-6
15. Lee S, Kopp F, Chang TC, Sataluri A, Chen B, Sivakumar S, et al. Noncoding RNA NORAD regulates genomic stability by sequestering PUMILIO proteins. *Cell.* (2016):69–80. doi: 10.1016/j.cell.2015.12.017
16. Elguindy MM, Kopp F, Goodarzi M, Rehfeld F, Thomas A, Chang TC, et al. NORADPUMILIO, but not RBMX, binding is required for regulation of genomic stability by noncoding RNA. *Elife.* (2019) 8:e48625. doi: 10.7554/eLife.48625
17. Munschauer M, Nguyen CT, Sirckman K, Hartigan CR, Hogstrom L, Engreeitz JM, et al. The NORAD lncRNA assembles a topoisomerase complex critical for genomic stability. *Nature.* (2018) 561:132–6. doi: 10.1038/s41586-018-0453-z
18. Bao S, Zhao H, Yuan J, Fan D, Zhou M. Computational identification of mutator-derived lncRNA signatures of genomic instability for improving the clinical outcome of cancers: a case study in breast cancer. *Brief Bioinform.* (2019) 21:1742–55. doi: 10.1093/bib/bbz118
19. Hänzelmann S, Castelo, R, Guinney J. GSVA: gene set variation analysis for microarray and RNA-Seq data. *BMC Bioinformatics.* (2013) 4:7. doi: 10.1186/1471-2105-14-7
20. Adler D. vioplot: Violin Plot. *R package v. 0.3.5.* (2005). Available online at: https://github.com/TomKellyGenetics/vioplot
21. Steyerberg EW. Regression modeling strategies: with applications, to linear models, logistic and ordinal regression, and survival analysis. *Biometrics.* (2016) 72:1006–7. doi: 10.1111/biom.12569
22. Heagerty PJ, Lumley T, Pepe MS. Time-dependent ROC curves for censored survival data and a diagnostic marker. *Biometrics.* (2000) 56:337–44. doi: 10.1111/j.0006-341X.2000.00337.x
23. Kanda M, Sugimoto H, Kodera Y. Genetic and epigenetic aspects of initiation and progression of hepatocellular carcinoma. *World J Gastroenterol.* (2015) 21:10584–97. doi: 10.3748/wjg.v21.i37.10584
24. Jeng K-S, Chang C-F, Jeng W-J, Sheen I-S, Jeng C-J. Heterogeneity of hepatocellular carcinoma contributes to cancer progression. *Crit Rev Oncol Hematol.* (2015) 94:337–47. doi: 10.1016/j.critrevonc.2015.01.009
25. Weyburne E, Bosco G. Cancer-associated mutations in the condensin II subunit CAPH2 cause genomic instability through telomere dysfunction and anaphase chromosome bridges. *J Cell Physiol.* (2020) 236(5):3579–98. doi: 10.1002/jcp.30113
26. Ivanova E, Ward A, Wiegmans AP, Richard DJ. Circulating tumor cells in metastatic breast cancer: from genomic instability to metastasis. *Front Mol Biosci.* (2020) 7:134. doi: 10.3389/fmolb.2020.00134
27. Mardis ER. Neoantigens and genomic instability: Impact on immunogenomic phenotypes and immunotherapy response. *Genomic Med.* (2019) 11:71. doi: 10.1186/s13073-019-0684-0
28. Carloni V, Lulli M, Madiai S, Mello T, Hall A, Luong TV, et al. CHK2 overexpression and mislocalisation within mitotic structures enhances chromosomal instability and hepatocellular carcinoma progression. *Gut.* (2018) 67:348–61. doi: 10.1136/gutjnl-2016-313114
29. Ferguson LR, Chen H, Collins AR, Connell M, Damia G, Dasgupta S, et al. Genomic instability in human cancer: molecular insights and opportunities for therapeutic attack and prevention through diet and nutrition. *Semin Cancer Biol.* (2015) 35:S5–24. doi: 10.1016/j.semcancer.2015.03.005

30. Lim LJ, Wong SYS, Huang F, Lim S, Lee CG. Roles and regulation of long non-coding RNAs in hepatocellular carcinoma. *Cancer Res.* (2019) 79:5131–9. doi: 10.1158/0008-5472.CAN-19-0255
31. Gao Q, Zhu H, Dong L, Shi W, Fan J. Integrated proteogenomic characterization of HBV-related hepatocellular carcinoma. *Cell.* (2019) 179:1240. doi: 10.1016/j.cell.2019.10.038
32. Athei A, Marchese FP, González J, Lozano T, Raimondi I, Juvvuna PK, et al. Analysis of copy number alterations reveals the lncRNA ALAL-1 as a regulator of lung cancer immune evasion. *J Cell Biol.* (2020) 219:e201908078. doi: 10.1083/jcb.201908078
33. Enito MA, Freund C. Revisiting nonclassical HLA II functions in antigen presentation: peptide editing and its modulation. *HLA.* (2020) 96:415–29. doi: 10.1111/tan.14007
34. Crusz SM, Miller RE. Targeted therapies in gynaecological cancers. *Histopathology.* (2020) 76:157–70. doi: 10.1111/his.14009
35. Wakeley ME, Gray CC, Monaghan SF, Heffernan DS, Ayala A. Check point inhibitors and their role in immunosuppression in sepsis. *Crit Care Clin.* (2019) 36:69–88. doi: 10.1016/j.ccc.2019.08.006
36. Albarel F, Castinetti F, Brue T. Management of endocrine disease immune check point inhibitors-induced hypophysitis. *Eur J Endocrinol.* (2019) 181:R107–18. doi: 10.1530/EJE-19-0169
37. Elsegood CL, Tirnitz-Parker JE, Olynyk JK, Yeoh GC. Immune checkpoint inhibition: prospects for prevention and therapy of hepatocellular carcinoma. *Clin Transl Immunol.* (2017) 6:e161. doi: 10.1038/cti.2017.47
38. Zhang Q, Chen Y, Bai X, Liang T. Immune checkpoint blockade therapy for hepatocellular carcinoma: clinical challenges and considerations. *Front Oncol.* (2020) 10:590058. doi: 10.3389/fonc.2020.590058
39. Moral JA, Leung J, Rojas LA, Ruan J, Zhao J, Sethna Z, et al. ILC2s amplify PD-1 blockade by activating tissue-specific cancer immunity. *Nature.* (2020) 579:130–5. doi: 10.1038/s41586-020-2015-4
40. Miao D, Margolis CA, Gao W, Voss MH, Li W, Martini DJ, et al. Genomic correlates of response to immune checkpoint therapies in clear cell renal cell carcinoma. *Science.* (2018) 359:801–6. doi: 10.1126/science.aan5951
41. Le DT, Durham JN, Smith KN, Wang H, Bartlett BR, Aulakh LK, et al. Mismatch repair deficiency predicts response of solid tumors to PD-1 blockade. *Science.* (2017) 357:409–13. doi: 10.1126/science.aan6733
42. Rosenberg JE, Hoffman-Censits J, Powles T, van der Heijden MS, Balar AV, Necchi A, et al. Atezolizumab in patients with locally advanced and metastatic urothelial carcinoma who have progressed following treatment with platinum-based chemotherapy: a single-arm, multicentre, phase 2 trial. *Lancet.* (2016) 387:1909–20. doi: 10.1016/S0140-6736(16)00561-4

3

Nomogram Based on Systemic Immune Inflammation Index and Prognostic Nutrition Index Predicts Recurrence of Hepatocellular Carcinoma After Surgery

*Junsheng Yang, Yongjin Bao, Weibo Chen, Yunfei Duan and Donglin Sun**

Department of Hepatopancreatobiliary Surgery, The Third Affiliated Hospital of Soochow University, Changzhou, China

Correspondence:
Donglin Sun
czyysdl@163.com

Background: Surgery is a potential cure for hepatocellular carcinoma (HCC), but its postoperative recurrence rate is high, its prognosis is poor, and reliable predictive indicators are lacking. This study was conducted to develop a simple, practical, and effective predictive model.

Materials and Methods: Preoperative clinical and postoperative pathological data on patients with HCC undergoing partial hepatectomies at the Third Affiliated Hospital of Soochow University from January 2010 to December 2015 were retrospectively analyzed, and a nomogram was constructed. The model performance was evaluated using C-indexes, receiver operating characteristic curves, and calibration curves. The results were verified from validation cohort data collected at the same center from January 2016 to January 2017 and compared with the traditional staging systems.

Results: Three hundred three patients were enrolled in this study: 238 in the training cohort and 65 in the validation cohort. From the univariate and multivariate Cox regression analyses in the training cohort, six independent risk factors, i.e., age, alpha-fetoprotein (AFP), tumor size, satellite nodules, systemic immune inflammation index (SII), and prognostic nutritional index (PNI), were filtered and included in the nomogram. The C-index was 0.701 [95% confidence interval (CI): 0.654–0.748] in the training cohort and 0.705 (95% CI: 0.619–0.791) in the validation cohort. The areas under the curve for the 1- and 3-year recurrence-free survival were 0.706 and 0.716 in the training cohort and 0.686 and 0.743 in the validation cohort, respectively. The calibration curves showed good agreement. Compared with traditional American Joint Committee on Cancer 8th edition (AJCC8th) and Barcelona Clinic Liver Cancer (BCLC) staging systems, our nomogram showed better predictive ability.

Conclusion: Our nomogram is simple, practical, and reliable. According to our nomogram, predicting the risk of recurrence and stratifying HCC patient management will yield the greatest survival benefit for patients.

Keywords: hepatocellular carcinoma, recurrence, nomogram, SII, PNI

INTRODUCTION

Hepatocellular carcinoma (HCC) is the sixth most common cancer and the fourth leading cause of cancer-related death worldwide. Approximately 841,000 new cases and 782,000 deaths occur annually, presenting a public health burden (1). Surgery is a potential cure for HCC. However, the recurrence rate can reach 70% at 5 years postsurgery, and two-thirds of recurrences occur within 2 years (2). Traditional staging systems, such as the American Joint Committee on Cancer 8th edition (AJCC8th) and the Barcelona Clinic Liver Cancer (BCLC) staging systems, cannot satisfactorily predict postoperative prognosis (3). As a new clinical prognostic model, nomograms have been explored in several carcinomas (4–6). However, scholars have not reached a unified standard or consensus for a clinical prognosis model of an HCC nomogram. Therefore, a pragmatic and powerful standardized nomogram based on objective measures is needed to predict HCC prognoses.

Nomograms are based on multiple independent risk factors. Previous studies on tumor prognosis have been based primarily on demographic and clinicopathological data. Increasing attention is being given to the relationship between conventional serological indicators and tumor prognosis, including indicators of serum inflammation, serum nutrition, liver function, and coagulation function. Gan et al. (7) reported that fibrinogen and C-reactive protein scores were good prognostic indicators for postoperative patients with HCC. Ho et al. (8) showed that the albumin-bilirubin grade could predict HCC recurrence in patients after surgery.

Here, we constructed a practical and effective nomogram based on conventional prognostic indicators combined with multiple serological indicators to predict the postoperative recurrence of HCC.

MATERIALS AND METHODS

Patients and Study Design

We retrospectively collected and analyzed preoperative clinical and postoperative pathological data for patients diagnosed with HCC who underwent partial hepatectomies at the Third Affiliated Hospital of Soochow University between January 2010 and January 2017. All data were collected in our hospital, and all serum indicators were obtained within 1 week before surgery. The inclusion criteria were (I) aged 20–85 years; (II) histopathologically proven HCC; and (III) initial diagnosis rather than recurrent tumors. Exclusion criteria were (I) acute tumor rupture with hemoperitoneum; (II) distant metastasis; (III) positive surgical margins; (IV) mixed cholangiocarcinoma; (V) other concomitant malignant diseases; (VI) perioperative death (A death occurred within 90 days after surgery) or death from other diseases during follow-up; (VII) incomplete data; and (VIII) lost to follow-up. Patients who were included from January 2010 to December 2015 were defined as the training cohort; patients who were included from January 2016 to January 2017 were defined as the validation cohort. The institutional review board of the Third Affiliated Hospital of Soochow University approved the study.

The model indices were calculated as follows. Body mass index was calculated by dividing the weight by the height squared (kg/m^2). The neutrophil-to-lymphocyte ratio (NLR) was calculated by dividing the neutrophil count by the lymphocyte count. The lymphocyte-to-monocyte ratio was calculated by dividing the lymphocyte count by the monocyte count. The platelet-to-lymphocyte ratio (PLR) was calculated by dividing the platelet count by the lymphocyte count. The systemic immune inflammation index (SII) was calculated as platelet count × neutrophil count/lymphocyte count (10^9/L). The systemic inflammatory response index (SIRI) was calculated as monocyte count × neutrophil count/lymphocyte count (10^9/L). The prognostic nutritional index (PNI) was the sum of serum albumin (g/L) and 5 × lymphocyte count (10^9/L).

Follow-Up

All patients were advised to receive regular follow-up according to clinical guidelines after surgery. The outpatient review was conducted every 3 months for the first 2 postoperative years, then every 6 months thereafter if no recurrence or metastasis occurred. Serum AFP, liver function, routine blood, and abdominal ultrasound examinations were performed at each follow-up visit. If signs of recurrence were noted, further computed tomography (CT) examinations were conducted; otherwise, CT examinations were performed once every 6 months. The event endpoint was tumor recurrence. All tumor recurrences were diagnosed via CT images. Recurrence-free survival (RFS) was defined as the time interval between the date of surgery and the date that recurrence was diagnosed. The follow-up deadline was January 31, 2020.

Statistical Analysis

Statistical analysis was performed using SPSS 19.0 (IBM Corp). Continuous variables were compared using the Mann–Whitney *U*-test; categorical variables were compared using chi-square tests. Continuous variables tested in the laboratory were divided into binary variables according to critical values. The cutoff values for age and model indices were obtained via receiver operating characteristic (ROC) curve analysis, and then these continuous variables were converted into binary variables according to cutoff values. Univariate and multivariate Cox regression analyses were used to identify independent risk factors for HCC recurrence in the training cohort. $P < 0.05$ was considered statistically significant.

A nomogram was constructed based on the multivariate Cox regression analysis results. The concordance index (C-index), ROC curves, and calibration curves were constructed to evaluate the model performance in the training cohort and verify it in the validation cohort. The risk score for recurrence was determined from the nomogram. The median score of the patients in the training cohort was defined as the cutoff value. Patients with values below the cutoff value were considered the low-risk group; patients with values above the cutoff value were considered the high-risk group. RFS was analyzed using the Kaplan–Meier method. The above steps were analyzed in R, version 3.6.0. The main R packages used included "rms," "foreign," "survival," and " survivalROC."

RESULTS

Demographic and Clinical Characteristics

Three hundred three patients were enrolled in this study: 238 in the training cohort and 65 in the validation cohort. **Table 1** lists the detailed demographics, serum indices, pathological characteristics, AJCC8th stage, and BCLC stage of the patients in the two cohorts.

In the training cohort, the average age of the patients was (59.1 ± 11.3) years, 195 (81.9%) cases were male patients, most of them were infected with hepatitis B virus (182 cases, account for 76.5%), the average diameter of the tumors was (5.0 ± 3.0) cm, and 225 (94.5%) patients had a single tumor. Pathology showed that 93.3% of the tumors were low and middle differentiation, 21.4% of them had vascular invasion, and 11.3% of them had satellite nodules. According to the AJCC8th and BCLC stage, early-stage patients accounted for 94.1% (stage I and II) and 53.8% (stage 0 and A), respectively.

In the validation cohort, the average age of the patients was (60.4 ± 11.6) years, and 56 (86.2%) cases were male patients. Similarly, 73.8% of patients were infected with the hepatitis B virus. The average diameter of the tumors was (5.6 ± 3.7) cm, and 61 (93.8%) patients had a single tumor. Pathology showed that 96.9% of the tumors were low and middle differentiation, 13.8% of them had vascular invasion, and 24.6% of them had satellite nodules. According to the AJCC8th and BCLC stage, early-stage patients accounted for 92.3 and 58.5%, respectively.

Compared with the validation cohort, the serum bilirubin (11.4 ± 5.0 vs.14.1 ± 7.7 μmol/L, P = 0.009), albumin (38.3 ± 5.1 vs. 40.2 ± 4.3 g/L, P = 0.008), neutrophil counts (3.5 ± 1.8 vs. 4.1 ± 2.2 × 10^9/L, P = 0.014), and tumor satellite nodules (11.3% vs. 24.6%, P = 0.007) in the training cohort were significantly lower. There was no significant difference in age, sex, BMI, hepatitis B virus infection, serum AFP, alanine aminotransferase (ALT), leukocyte count, lymphocyte count, monocyte count, platelet count, and the size, number, differentiation, vascular invasion, AJCC8th, and BCLC stage of tumors between the two groups.

TABLE 1 | Demographic and clinical characteristics.

Variable	Training cohort (n = 238)	Validation cohort (n = 65)	P-value
Age (years)	59.1 ± 11.3	60.4 ± 11.6	0.429
Sex			0.425
Male	195	56	
Female	43	9	
BMI (kg/m^2)	22.9 ± 3.0	23.5 ± 3.0	0.190
HBsAg			0.662
Positive	182	48	
Negative	56	17	
AFP (ng/ml)	323.2 ± 493.3	247.5 ± 438.6	0.263
ALT (U/L)	43.3 ± 35.9	37.4 ± 27.0	0.222
Bilirubin (μmol/L)	11.4 ± 5.0	14.1 ± 7.7	0.009*
Albumin (g/L)	38.3 ± 5.1	40.2 ± 4.3	0.008*
Leukocyte count (×10^9/L)	5.5 ± 2.2	6.1 ± 2.5	0.068
Neutrophil count (×10^9/L)	3.5 ± 1.8	4.1 ± 2.2	0.014*
Lymphocyte count (×10^9/L)	1.4 ± 0.7	1.5 ± 0.6	0.751
Monocyte count (×10^9/L)	0.4 ± 0.2	0.4 ± 0.1	0.164
Platelet count (×10^9/L)	155.2 ± 74.8	163.0 ± 78.4	0.462
Tumor size (cm)	5.0 ± 3.0	5.6 ± 3.7	0.161
Tumor number			0.830
Single	225	61	
Multiple	13	4	
Differentiation			0.293
Low	80	18	
Middle	142	45	
High	16	2	
Vascular invasion			0.175
Yes	51	9	
No	187	56	
Satellite nodules			0.007*
Yes	27	16	
No	211	49	
AJCC8th			0.158
Stage I	175	52	
Stage II	49	8	
Stage III	9	5	
Stage IV	5	0	
BCLC			0.189
Stage 0	21	3	
Stage A	107	35	
Stage B	54	18	
Stage C	56	9	

P-value < 0.05.

Tumor RFS in the Training and Validation Cohorts

In the training cohort, the median follow-up time was 36.9 months (range, 0.9–120.8 months), and the postoperative 1- and 3-year RFS were 70.6 and 50.8%, respectively. In the validation cohort, the median follow-up time was 36.4 months (range, 1.3–48.6 months), and the postoperative 1- and 3-year RFS were 66.2 and 53.8%, respectively. **Figure 1** shows the RFS curves for both groups.

Independent Risk Factors in the Training Cohort

In the training cohort, the optimal cutoff values for age, NLR, MLR, PLR, SII, SIRI, PNI, and tumor size were determined to be 67 years and 2.71, 0.26, 78.24, 279.29, 0.93, 48.05, and 6.5 cm, respectively, as per the ROC curves. All variables were then divided into categorical variables and analyzed via univariate and multivariate Cox regression analysis. **Table 2** shows the univariate and multivariate Cox regression analysis results. Univariate analyses revealed that age (P = 0.006), AFP (P = 0.002), SII (P = 0.03), PNI (P = 0.015), tumor size (P = 0.003), and satellite nodules (P = 0.003) were identified as significant prognostic

TABLE 2 | Cox proportional hazards regression analyses of recurrence in the training cohort.

Variable	Cases	Univariate analysis		Multivariate analysis	
		HR (95% CI)	*P*-value	HR (95% CI)	*P*-value
Age (years)		1.878 (1.198–2.944)	0.006*	1.710 (1.083–2.702)	0.021*
≤67	183				
>67	55				
Gender		0.801 (0.507–1.266)	0.342		
Male	195				
Female	43				
BMI (kg/m^2)		1.392 (0.961–2.018)	0.080		
<25	177				
≥25	61				
HBsAg		1.434 (0.927–2.217)	0.105		
Positive	182				
Negative	56				
AFP (ng/ml)		1.743 (1.219–2.492)	0.002*	1.498 (1.041–2.156)	0.030*
≤8	100				
>8	138				
ALT (U/L)		1.214 (0.862–1.710)	0.267		
≤40	145				
>40	93				
Bilirubin (μmol/L)		0.955 (0.390–2.334)	0.919		
≤20.5	228				
>20.5	10				
NLR		1.262 (0.880–1.812)	0.206		
≤2.71	147				
>2.71	91				
MLR		1.292 (0.913–1.828)	0.148		
≤0.26	105				
>0.26	133				
PLR		1.308 (0.915–1.869)	0.140		
≤78.24	70				
>78.24	168				
SII		1.455 (1.036–2.042)	0.030*	1.456 (1.034–2.051)	0.031*
≤279.29	102				
>279.29	136				
SIRI		1.360 (0.958–1.931)	0.085		
≤0.93	136				
>0.93	102				
PNI		1.615 (1.098–2.375)	0.015*	1.503 (1.016–2.223)	0.041*
≤48.05	157				
>48.05	81				
Tumor size (cm)		1.753 (1.205–2.550)	0.003*	1.621 (1.109–2.369)	0.013*
≤6.5	183				
>6.5	55				
Differentiation		1.993 (0.947–4.198)	0.069		
Low	80				
Middle	142				
High	16				
Vascular invasion		1.321 (0.891–1.958)	0.165		
Yes	51				
No	187				
Satellite nodules		2.046 (1.281–3.268)	0.003*	1.829 (1.140–2.933)	0.012*
Yes	27				
No	211				

**P-value < 0.05.*

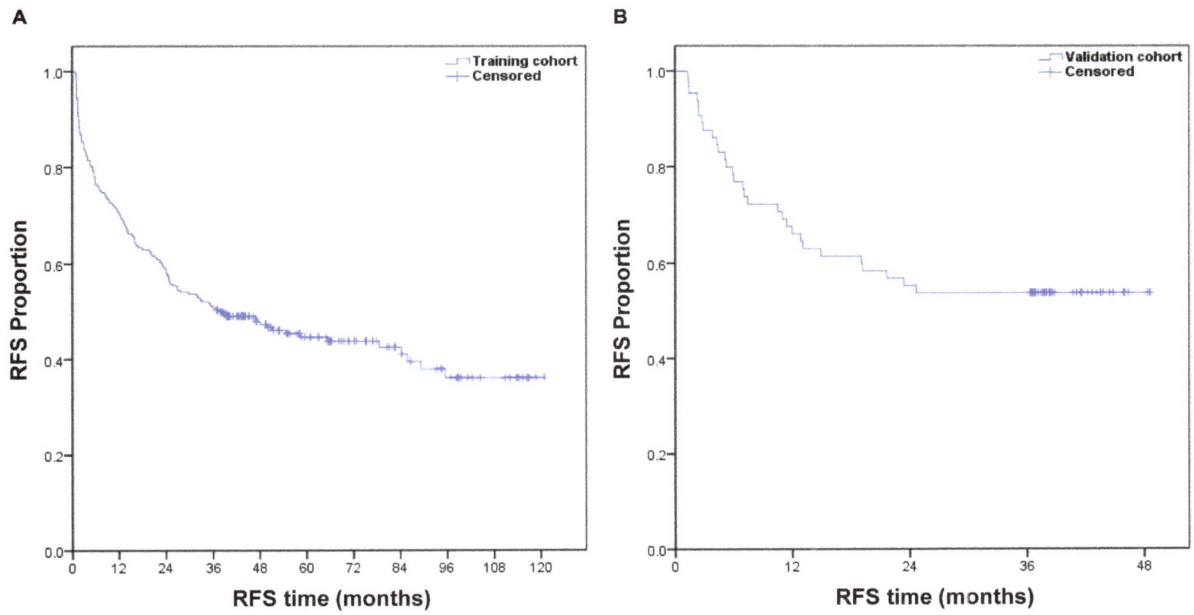

FIGURE 1 | Kaplan–Meier estimate of the postoperative RFS of patients with HCC in the training cohort **(A)** and validation cohort **(B)**.

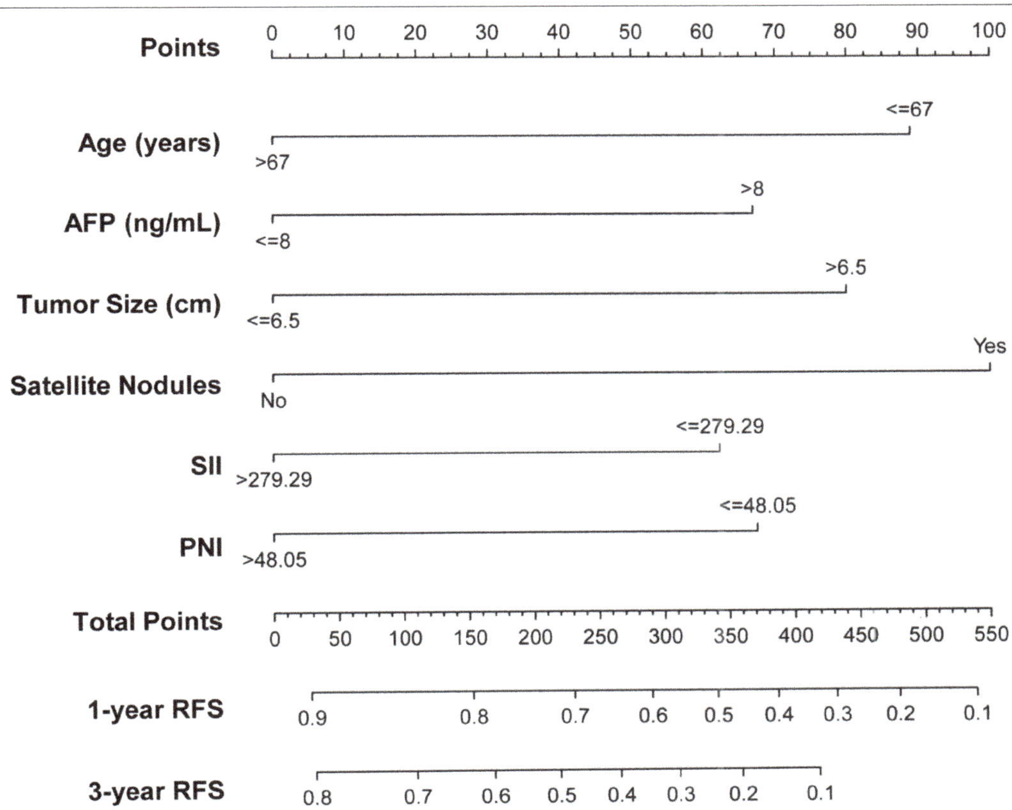

FIGURE 2 | Nomogram predicting 1- and 3-year RFS probabilities of patients with HCC. Each risk factor was assigned a point according to the nomogram. The exact values of each factor are age (0, 89 points), AFP (0, 67 points), tumor size (0, 80 points), satellite nodules (0, 100 points), SII (0, 62 points), and PNI (0, 68 points). The total points were obtained by adding the points of all risk factors. Then, the 1- and 3-year RFS could be predicted based on the total points.

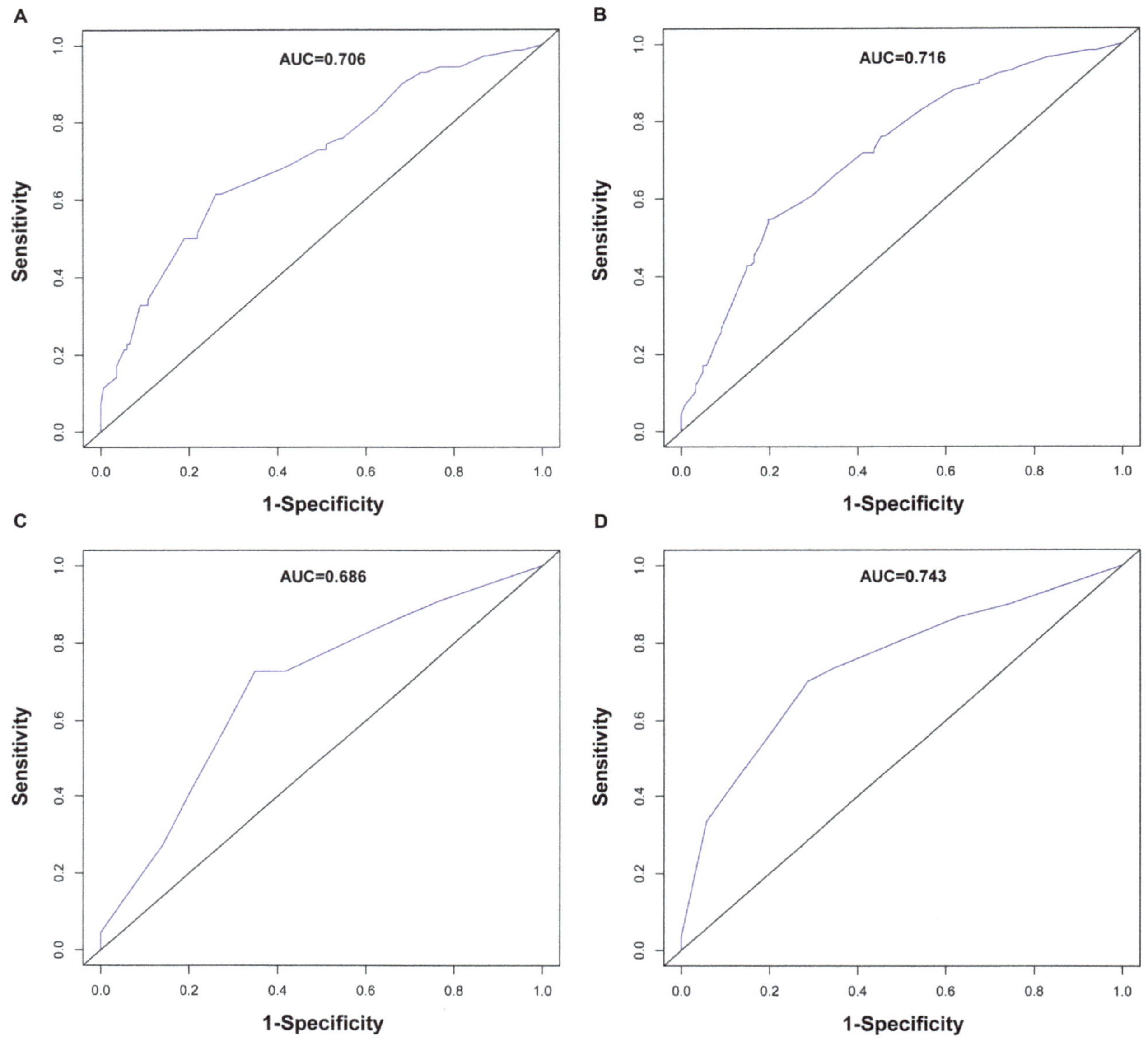

FIGURE 3 | ROC curve evaluating predictive performance of the nomogram for 1-year RFS **(A)** and 3-year RFS **(B)** in the training cohort and 1-year RFS **(C)** and 3-year RFS **(D)** in the validation cohort.

factors for HCC recurrence. In multivariate analysis, age [hazard ratio (HR): 1.710; 95% confidence interval (CI): 1.083–2.702; P = 0.021], AFP (HR: 1.498; 95% CI: 1.041–2.156; P = 0.03), SII (HR: 1.456; 95% CI: 1.034–2.051; P = 0.031), PNI (HR: 1.503; 95% CI: 1.016–2.223; P = 0.041), tumor size (HR: 1.621; 95% CI: 1.109–2.369; P = 0.013), and satellite nodules (HR: 1.829; 95% CI: 1.140–2.933; P = 0.012) were identified as independent risk factors for HCC recurrence.

Construction and Verification of the RFS Nomogram

From the multivariate Cox regression analysis results, age, AFP, tumor size, satellite nodules, SII, and PNI were integrated and used to construct the nomogram (**Figure 2**), which showed that satellite nodules had the greatest impact on HCC recurrence, followed by age, tumor size, PNI, AFP, and SII. The total scores of these six prognostic factors can be used to determine the probabilities of 1- and 3-year RFS.

The performance of the nomogram in the training cohort was evaluated using the C-index, ROC curves, and calibration curves. The C-index for RFS prediction was 0.701 (95% CI: 0.654–0.748). The areas under the ROC curve (AUCs) for the 1- and 3-year RFS were 0.706 and 0.716, respectively (**Figures 3A,B**). The calibration curves for the probability of 1- and 3-year RFS after surgery showed good probability consistencies between the nomogram prediction and actual observation (**Figures 4A,B**).

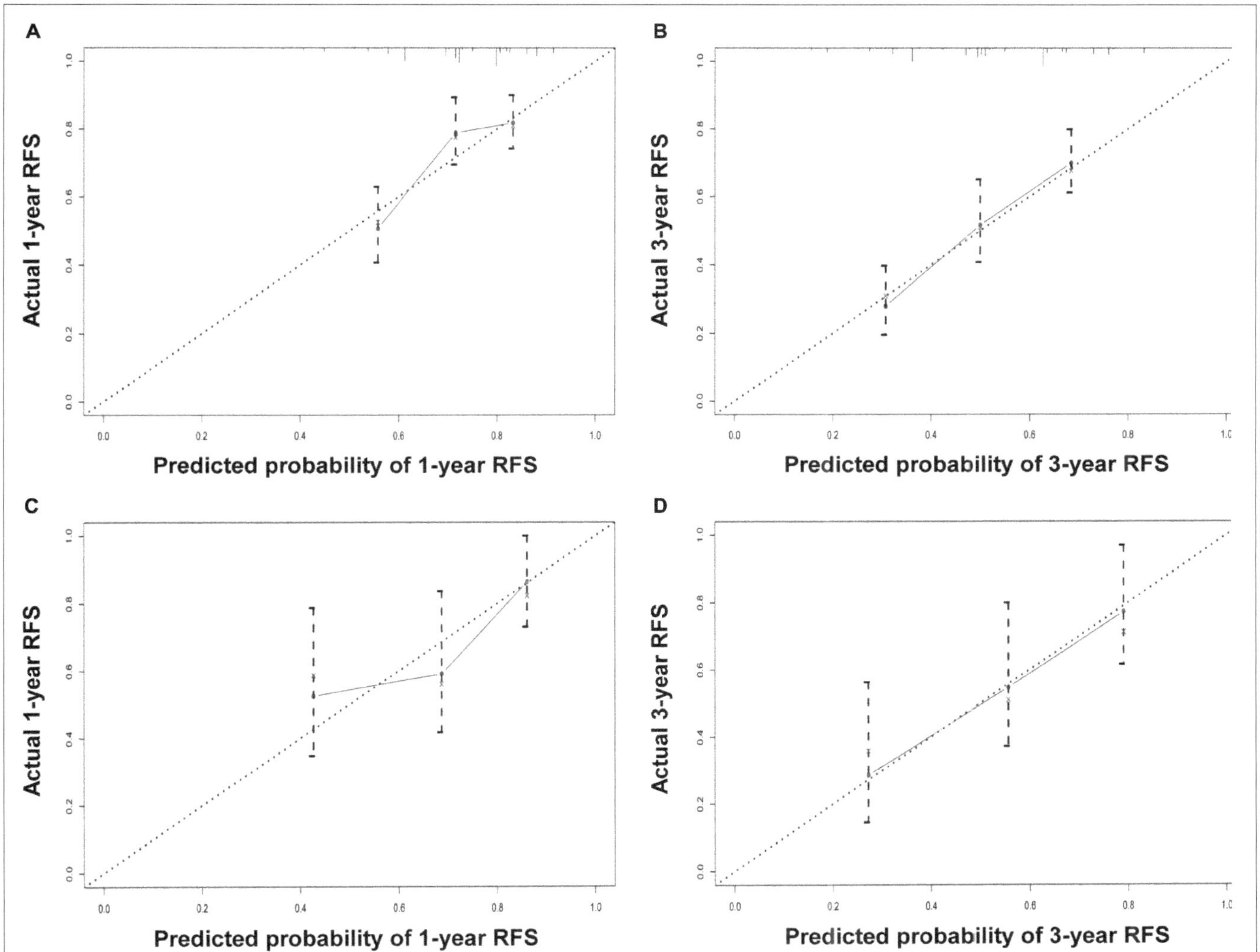

FIGURE 4 | Calibration curve for predicting 1-year RFS **(A)** and 3-year RFS **(B)** in the training cohort and 1-year RFS **(C)** and 3-year RFS **(D)** in the validation cohort. The nomogram-predicted probability of RFS is plotted on the *x*-axis; the actual RFS is plotted on the *y*-axis.

Using the same method, we verified the predictive ability of the nomogram in the validation cohort. The results showed that the C-index was 0.705 (95% CI: 0.619–0.791). The AUCs of the 1- and 3-year RFS were 0.686 and 0.743, respectively (**Figures 3C,D**). The calibration curves also had good prediction consistency (**Figures 4C,D**).

Comparison of Predictive Ability of RFS in HCC Patients Between the Nomogram and Traditional Staging Systems

First, we divided the patients into the low-risk and high-risk groups based on the median nomogram score (218.5 points) for the training cohort. The RFS was then analyzed using the Kaplan–Meier method. The RFS survival probability of the high-risk group was significantly lower than that of the low-risk group in both the training and validation cohorts (**Figures 5A,D**). RFS analysis was performed using the same method based on the AJCC8th and BCLC staging systems. RFS survival probability differed significantly between stages according to the AJCC8th and BCLC staging systems in the validation cohort (**Figures 5E,F**) but not in the training cohort (**Figures 5B,C**). Their predictive abilities were compared by calculating the C-index (**Table 3**). In the training cohort, the C-index of the nomogram (0.701; 95% CI: 0.654–0.748) was higher than that of the AJCC8th (0.533) and BCLC (0.548) staging systems. In the validation cohort, the nomogram performance (C-index: 0.705; 95% CI: 0.619–0.791) was also superior to the AJCC8th (0.672) and BCLC (0.684) staging systems. Therefore, our nomogram better predicted the RFS for HCC patients.

DISCUSSION

For resectable HCC, surgery is the best treatment option. However, high recurrence rates after hepatectomies greatly

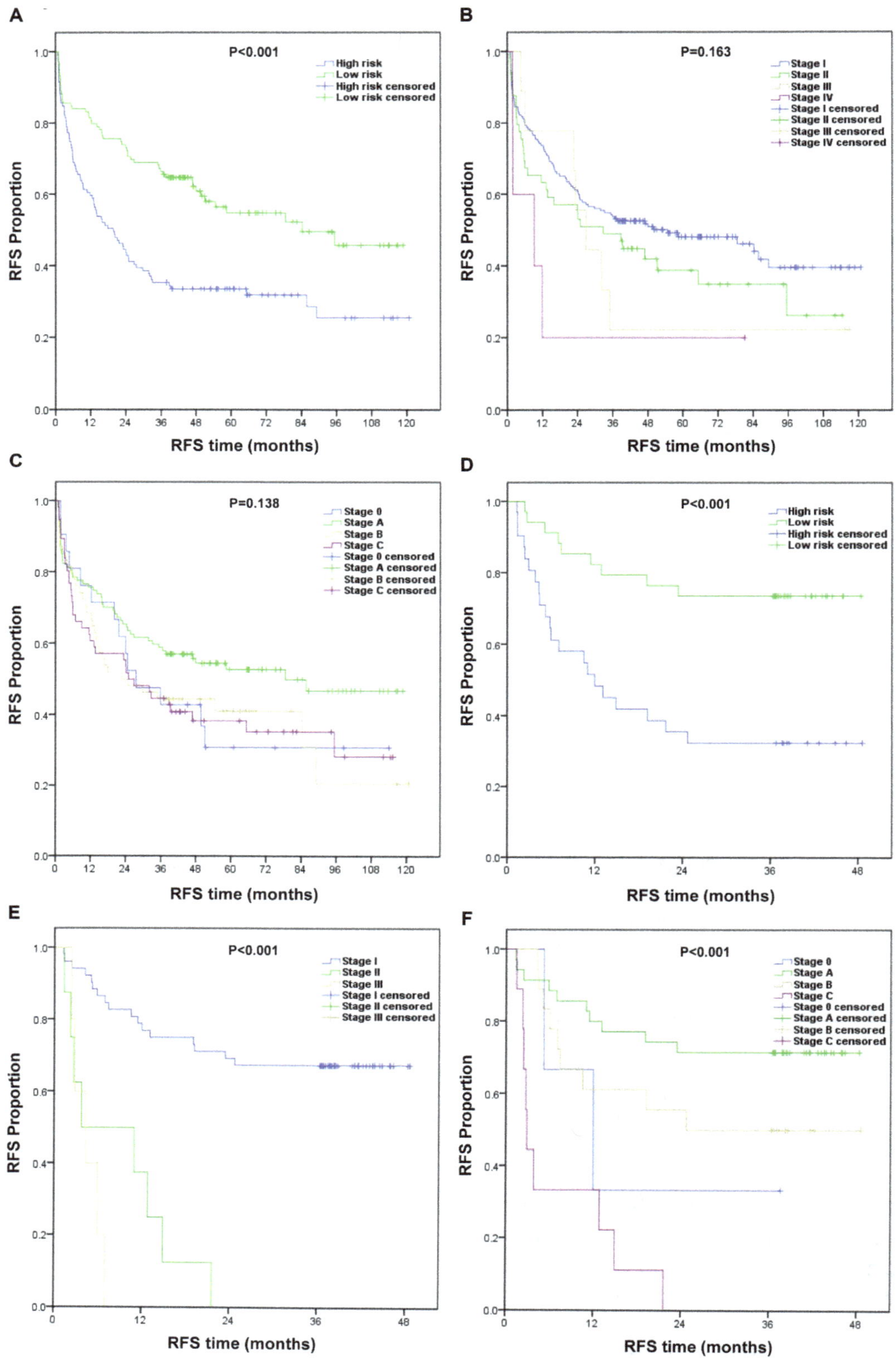

FIGURE 5 | Kaplan–Meier survival curves of RFS for different models. **(A–C)** Training cohort: **(A)** nomogram, **(B)** AJCC8th staging system, and **(C)** BCLC staging system. **(D–F)** Validation cohort: **(D)** nomogram, **(E)** AJCC8th staging system, and **(F)** BCLC staging system.

TABLE 3 | Comparison of the predictive ability of models.

Model	Training cohort			Validation cohort		
	C-index	95% CI	*P*-value	C-index	95% CI	*P*-value
Nomogram	0.701	0.654–0.748	<0.001	0.705	0.619–0.791	<0.001
AJCC8th	0.533	0.494–0.572	0.163	0.672	0.599–0.745	<0.001
BCLC	0.548	0.499–0.597	0.138	0.684	0.588–0.780	<0.001

reduce patients' long-term survival benefit. In the training cohort of this study, the 1- and 3-year HCC recurrence rates were 29.4 and 49.2%, respectively. Therefore, the risk of postoperative HCC recurrence must be predicted and stratified to allow early intervention for high-risk patients. At present, the internationally recognized and widely used systems include the AJCC, BCLC, Italian Liver Cancer Program, and Okuda staging systems. However, these traditional liver cancer staging systems have not achieved satisfactory results in predicting the prognosis (3, 9). The nomogram is a prognostic prediction map based on multiple independent risk factors. It has been researched in a variety of tumors, and several studies have reported that its prediction performance is better than that of traditional liver cancer staging systems (10, 11).

In this study, we established a nomogram based on SII and PNI. The nomogram showed good performance for predicting prognoses as per C-index, ROC curve, calibration curve, and internal cohort verification. The nomogram also exhibited better prognostic predictive ability compared with the traditional AJCC and BCLC staging systems.

Studies have shown that systemic immune inflammatory responses are significantly correlated with cancers (12, 13). Neutrophils in the peripheral blood or tumor microenvironment can produce angiogenic factors that stimulate tumor development and progression (14). Lymphocytes reflect the host immunity status and can inhibit tumor progression (15). Therefore, cancer-related inflammation is considered the seventh hallmark of cancer (16). Recent studies have mainly focused on the inflammation index converted from multiple serum inflammatory indicators, such as the NLR, MLR, PLR, SII, and SIRI, modified Glasgow prognostic score (mGPS), and C-reactive protein/albumin ratio (CAR). Nomogram clinical models based on inflammatory indicators such as NLR, PLR, hypersensitive C-reactive protein (hs-CRP), and FC-score composed of fibrinogen and C-reactive protein are reported to have good predictive prognostic performances for HCC (7, 17–19). In this study, several easily available inflammatory indicators were analyzed, including NLR, PLR, MLR, SIRI, and SII. Although the prognostic ability of CAR in HCC is reportedly better than that of other inflammatory indexes (10), C-reactive protein is not used in routine preoperative examinations in our center; thus, it was excluded from the study, as was the mGPS. Our results indicated that only the inflammatory index SII was an independent risk factor for postoperative HCC recurrence. Fu et al. (20) reported that preoperative SII was a powerful prognostic biomarker in HCC patients who undergo liver transplantation, and it was superior to PLR, NLR, and MLR for prediction of overall survival. Jomrich et al. (21) also showed that SII was superior to PLR and NLR for predicting overall survival in pancreatic ductal adenocarcinoma patients. Therefore, SII was a convenient, low-cost, and effective inflammatory indicator to predict the prognosis of tumors. Previous studies have only reported the use of SII in nomograms for gastric and tongue cancer (22, 23). Here, we report for the first time that nomograms based on SII can effectively predict postoperative HCC recurrence.

Relationships between nutritional status and cancer prognosis have gained attention from researchers over the last decade. Studies have shown that malnutrition often leads to poor tumor prognosis (24). In studying the HCC clinical nomogram model, albumin-based nutritional indexes, including the albumin-bilirubin grade and lactic dehydrogenase/albumin ratio, showed good prognostic predictive performance (25, 26). In this study, we explored the albumin-based PNI. The PNI was originally designed to assess the nutritional status of patients undergoing gastrointestinal surgery (27). Pinato et al. (28) found for the first time that the PNI independently predicted overall survival of HCC patients. Our results also indicated that low PNI ($\leq$48.05) was an independent risk factor for postoperative HCC recurrence, and our PNI-based nomogram showed good prediction performance. Cancer cachexia is reportedly driven by a sustained inflammatory response (29). Therefore, we believe that inflammation and malnutrition jointly promote tumor progression; thus, our nomogram comprehensively includes both inflammation and nutrition indexes.

Our nomogram also included four common factors: age, serum AFP, tumor size, and satellite nodules; for these, we included demographic characteristics, serum indicators, and clinicopathological data to optimize the overall predictive ability.

At present, there was no uniform standard for predicting the prognosis of HCC. The AJCC and BCLC staging systems were the most common staging systems for liver cancer and were primarily meant to formulate patient's treatment plans in oncology settings. In recent studies, Kee and Chun et al. (9, 30) reported that the AJCC staging system had a predictive ability for the prognosis of HCC. Grieco et al. (31) reported that the BCLC staging system gave a better prediction of prognosis in patients with HCC at a very early stage. Kim et al. (32) also found that the BCLC staging system was the best long-term prognostic model for treatment-naive HCC in a large scale Korean cohort. These reports indicated that AJCC and BCLC staging systems had predictive value for the prognosis of HCC. So, we compared the AJCC8th and BCLC staging systems with our nomogram model in our study. Combining the above six independent risk factors, our nomogram model showed a better predictive ability for postoperative recurrence of HCC than the AJCC8th and BCLC staging systems.

According to our nomogram, we can assess the risk of recurrence of HCC after surgery and conduct early individualized interventions for high-risk patients. We think that early interventions mainly include the following aspects: First, etiological interventions are critical, such as anti-hepatitis B virus, alcohol withdrawal, etc. Second, early postoperative transarterial chemoembolization (TACE) may play a role in preventing tumor recurrence, especially for patients with large and multiple lesions. Third, early postoperative immunoregulatory therapy may be a strategy, such as programmed cell death protein 1 (PD-1) inhibitor, thymosin, interferon, etc. Fourth, the detection of gene targets should be conducted after surgery, and targeted therapy may bring survival benefits to suitable patients. The early implementation of these methods may reduce the risk of tumor recurrence to a certain extent.

This study also had several limitations. First, this was a retrospective study. Second, our nomogram performance was verified with an internal cohort, without external or multicenter verification. Third, the number of patients enrolled in the model was relatively small. Therefore, further large-sample, multicenter, and prospective verification studies are needed. Besides, the exclusion of patients who were lost to follow-up was the main bias in this study.

In conclusion, our nomogram based on SII and PNI is simple, practical, and reliable. It has a good predictive ability for postoperative HCC recurrence. Our nomogram suggests that predicting the risk of recurrence and stratifying the management of HCC patients will yield the greatest survival benefit for patients.

AUTHOR CONTRIBUTIONS

DS conceived and designed the study. JY collected the data and wrote the manuscript. YB analyzed the data. YD and WC modified the manuscript. All co-authors have reviewed and approved this version of the manuscript. All authors contributed to the article and approved the submitted version.

ACKNOWLEDGMENTS

All authors are grateful to all the patients who contributed data to this study.

REFERENCES

1. Bray F, Ferlay J, Soerjomataram I, Siegel RL, Torre LA, Jemal A. Global cancer statistics 2018: GLOBOCAN estimates of incidence and mortality worldwide for 36 cancers in 185 countries. *CA Cancer J Clin.* (2018) 68:394–424. doi: 10.3322/caac.21492
2. Kulik L, El-Serag HB. Epidemiology and management of hepatocellular carcinoma. *Gastroenterology.* (2019) 156:477–491.e471. doi: 10.1053/j.gastro.2018.08.065
3. Huitzil-Melendez FD, Capanu M, O'reilly EM, Duffy A, Gansukh B, Saltz LL, et al. Advanced hepatocellular carcinoma: which staging systems best predict prognosis? *J Clin Oncol.* (2010) 28:2889–95. doi: 10.1200/JCO.2009.25.9895
4. Chen SH, Wan QS, Zhou D, Wang T, Hu J, He YT, et al. A simple-to-use nomogram for predicting the survival of early hepatocellular carcinoma patients. *Front Oncol.* (2019) 9:584. doi: 10.3389/fonc.2019.00584
5. Chen M, Cao J, Zhang B, Pan L, Cai X. A nomogram for prediction of overall survival in patients with node-negative gallbladder cancer. *J Cancer.* (2019) 10:3246–52. doi: 10.7150/jca.30046
6. Yu C, Zhang Y. Development and validation of prognostic nomogram for young patients with gastric cancer. *Ann Transl Med.* (2019) 7:641. doi: 10.21037/atm.2019.10.77
7. Gan W, Yi Y, Fu Y, Huang J, Lu Z, Jing C, et al. Fibrinogen and C-reactive protein score is a prognostic index for patients with hepatocellular carcinoma undergoing curative resection: a prognostic nomogram study. *J Cancer.* (2018) 9:148–56. doi: 10.7150/jca.22246
8. Ho SY, Hsu CY, Liu PH, Hsia CY, Su CW, Huang YH, et al. Albumin-bilirubin (ALBI) grade-based nomogram to predict tumor recurrence in patients with hepatocellular carcinoma. *Eur J Surg Oncol.* (2019) 45:776–81. doi: 10.1016/j.ejso.2018.10.541
9. Chun YH, Kim SU, Park JY, Kim DY, Han KH, Chon CY, et al. Prognostic value of the 7th edition of the AJCC staging system as a clinical staging system in patients with hepatocellular carcinoma. *Eur J Cancer.* (2011) 47:2568–75. doi: 10.1016/j.ejca.2011.07.002
10. Chen J, Fang A, Chen M, Tuoheti Y, Zhou Z, Xu L, et al. A novel inflammation-based nomogram system to predict survival of patients with hepatocellular carcinoma. *Cancer Med.* (2018) 7:5027–35. doi: 10.1002/cam4.1787
11. Xu L, Peng ZW, Chen MS, Shi M, Zhang YJ, Guo RP, et al. Prognostic nomogram for patients with unresectable hepatocellular carcinoma after transcatheter arterial chemoembolization. *J Hepatol.* (2015) 63:122–30. doi: 10.1016/j.jhep.2015.02.034
12. Ringelhan M, Pfister D, O'connor T, Pikarsky E, Heikenwalder M. The immunology of hepatocellular carcinoma. *Nat Immunol.* (2018) 19:222–32. doi: 10.1038/s41590-018-0044-z
13. Diakos CI, Charles KA, Mcmillan DC, Clarke SJ. Cancer-related inflammation and treatment effectiveness. *Lancet Oncol.* (2014) 15:e493–503. doi: 10.1016/S1470-2045(14)70263-3
14. Dings RP, Nesmelova I, Griffioen AW, Mayo KH. Discovery and development of anti-angiogenic peptides: a structural link. *Angiogenesis.* (2003) 6:83–91. doi: 10.1023/B:AGEN.0000011730.94233.06
15. Dunn GP, Old LJ, Schreiber RD. The immunobiology of cancer immunosurveillance and immunoediting. *Immunity.* (2004) 21:137–48. doi: 10.1016/j.immuni.2004.07.017
16. Hanahan D, Weinberg RA. Hallmarks of cancer: the next generation. *Cell.* (2011) 144:646–74. doi: 10.1016/j.cell.2011.02.013
17. Chon YE, Park H, Hyun HK, Ha Y, Kim MN, Kim BK, et al. Development of a new nomogram including neutrophil-to-lymphocyte ratio to predict survival in patients with hepatocellular carcinoma undergoing transarterial chemoembolization. *Cancers (Basel).* (2019) 11:509. doi: 10.3390/cancers11040509
18. Li X, Huang H, Yu X, Chen P, Ouyang J, Huang B. A novel prognostic nomogram based on microvascular invasion and hematological biomarkers to predict survival outcome for hepatocellular carcinoma patients. *Surg Oncol.* (2020) 33:51–7. doi: 10.1016/j.suronc.2020.01.006
19. Jing CY, Fu YP, Zheng SS, Yi Y, Shen HJ, Huang JL, et al. Prognostic nomogram for patients with hepatocellular carcinoma underwent adjuvant transarterial

chemoembolization following curative resection. *Medicine (Baltimore)*. (2017) 96:e6140. doi: 10.1097/MD.0000000000006140

20. Fu H, Zheng J, Cai J, Zeng K, Yao J, Chen L, et al. Systemic immune-inflammation index (SII) is useful to predict survival outcomes in patients after liver transplantation for hepatocellular carcinoma within hangzhou criteria. *Cell Physiol Biochem*. (2018) 47:293–301. doi: 10.1159/000489807
21. Jomrich G, Gruber E, Winkler D, Hollenstein M, Gnant M, Sahora K, et al. Systemic immune-inflammation index (SII) predicts poor survival in pancreatic cancer patients undergoing resection. *J Gastroint Surgery*. (2020) 24:610–8. doi: 10.1007/s11605-019-04187-z
22. Shi H, Jiang Y, Cao H, Zhu H, Chen B, Ji W. Nomogram based on systemic immune-inflammation index to predict overall survival in gastric cancer patients. *Dis Markers*. (2018) 2018:1787424. doi: 10.1155/2018/1787424
23. Lu Z, Yan W, Liang J, Yu M, Liu J, Hao J, et al. Nomogram based on systemic immune-inflammation index to predict survival of tongue cancer patients who underwent cervical dissection. *Front Oncol*. (2020) 10:341. doi: 10.3389/fonc.2020.00341
24. Wu N, Chen G, Hu H, Pang L, Chen Z. Low pretherapeutic serum albumin as a risk factor for poor outcome in esophageal squamous cell carcinomas. *Nutr Cancer*. (2015) 67:481–5. doi: 10.1080/01635581.2015.1004726
25. He W, Peng B, Tang Y, Yang J, Zheng Y, Qiu J, et al. Nomogram to predict survival of patients with recurrence of hepatocellular carcinoma after surgery. *Clin Gastroenterol Hepatol*. (2018) 16:756–64. doi: 10.1016/j.cgh.2017.12.002
26. Gan W, Zhang MX, Wang JX, Fu YP, Huang JL, Yi Y, et al. Prognostic impact of lactic dehydrogenase to albumin ratio in hepatocellular carcinoma patients with Child-Pugh I who underwent curative resection: a prognostic nomogram study. *Cancer Manag Res*. (2018) 10:5383–94. doi: 10.2147/CMAR.S176317
27. Nozoe T, Kimura Y, Ishida M, Saeki H, Korenaga D, Sugimachi K. Correlation of pre-operative nutritional condition with post-operative complications in surgical treatment for oesophageal carcinoma. *Eur J Surg Oncol*. (2002) 28:396–400. doi: 10.1053/ejso.2002.1257
28. Pinato DJ, North BV, Sharma R. A novel, externally validated inflammation-based prognostic algorithm in hepatocellular carcinoma: the prognostic nutritional index (PNI). *Br J Cancer*. (2012) 106:1439–45. doi: 10.1038/bjc.2012.92
29. Esper DH, Harb WA. The cancer cachexia syndrome: a review of metabolic and clinical manifestations. *Nutr Clin Pract*. (2005) 20:369–76. doi: 10.1177/0115426505020004369
30. Kee K, Wang J, Lee C, Chen C, Changchien C, Hu T, et al. Validation of clinical AJCC/UICC TNM staging system for hepatocellular carcinoma: analysis of 5,613 cases from a medical center in southern Taiwan. *Int J Cancer*. (2007) 120:2650–5. doi: 10.1002/ijc.22616
31. Grieco A, Pompili M, Caminiti G, Miele L, Covino M, Alfei B, et al. Prognostic factors for survival in patients with early-intermediate hepatocellular carcinoma undergoing non-surgical therapy: comparison of Okuda, CLIP, and BCLC staging systems in a single Italian centre. *Gut*. (2005) 54:411–8. doi: 10.1136/gut.2004.048124
32. Kim B, Kim S, Park J, Kim D, Ahn S, Park M, et al. Applicability of BCLC stage for prognostic stratification in comparison with other staging systems: single centre experience from long-term clinical outcomes of 1717 treatment-naïve patients with hepatocellular carcinoma. *Liver Int*. (2012) 32:1120–7. doi: 10.1111/j.1478-3231.2012.02811.x

4

A Novel Nomogram to Predict Prolonged Survival After Hepatectomy in Repeat Recurrent Hepatocellular Carcinoma

Qiongxuan Fang[1], Ruifeng Yang[1], Dongbo Chen[1], Ran Fei[1], Pu Chen[2], Kangjian Deng[2], Jie Gao[3], Weijia Liao[2]* and Hongsong Chen[1]**

[1] Beijing Key Laboratory of Hepatitis C and Immunotherapy for Liver Diseases, Peking University Hepatology Institute, Peking University People's Hospital, Beijing, China, [2] Laboratory of Hepatobiliary and Pancreatic Surgery, Affiliated Hospital of Guilin Medical University, Guilin, China, [3] Department of Hepatobiliary Surgery, Peking University People's Hospital, Beijing, China

***Correspondence:**
Hongsong Chen
chenhongsong2999@163.com
Weijia Liao
liaoweijia288@163.com
Jie Gao
gaojie_1131@163.com

Background: Repeat hepatectomy is an important treatment for patients with repeat recurrent hepatocellular carcinoma (HCC).

Methods: This study was a multicenter retrospective analysis of 1,135 patients who underwent primary curative liver resection for HCC. One hundred recurrent patients with second hepatectomy were included to develop a nomogram to predict the risk of post-recurrence survival (PRS). Thirty-eight patients in another institution were used to externally validate the nomogram. Univariate and multivariate Cox regression analyses were used to identify independent risk factors of PRS. Discrimination, calibration, and the Kaplan–Meier curves were used to evaluate the model performance.

Results: The nomogram was based on variables associated with PRS after HCC recurrence, including the tumor, node, and metastasis (TNM) stage; albumin and aspartate aminotransferase levels at recurrence; tumor size, site, differentiation of recurrences; and time to recurrence (TTR). The discriminative ability of the nomogram, as indicated by the C statistics (0.758 and 0.811 for training cohort and external validation cohorts, respectively), was shown, which was better than that of the TNM staging system (0.609 and 0.609, respectively). The calibration curves showed ideal agreement between the prediction and the real observations. The area under the curves (AUCs) of the training cohort and external validation cohorts were 0.843 and 0.890, respectively. The Kaplan–Meier curve of the established nomogram also performed better than those of both the TNM and the BCLC staging systems.

Conclusions: We constructed a nomogram to predict PRS in patients with repeat hepatectomy (RH) after repeat recurrence of HCC.

Keywords: nomogram, post-recurrence survival, prognosis, TNM stage, BCLC stage

INTRODUCTION

Hepatocellular carcinoma (HCC) recurrence is a common phenomenon after resection in patients with preserved liver function reserve. The 5-year HCC recurrence rate after curative resection is over 50% (1, 2); and, of all recurrence patterns, the most frequent is intrahepatic recurrence (3, 4). However, there is little agreement on the criteria for a standardized treatment strategy for recurrent HCC. Repeated hepatectomy (RH) is one of the important treatments for repeat recurrence HCC. Aggressive treatment of HCC recurrence after liver resection is related to prolonged overall survival (OS) (5, 6). Faber et al. (7) retrospectively studied 27 patients to clarify the safety and effectiveness of RH as a curative option for intrahepatic HCC recurrence. Chan et al. (8) evaluated the efficacy of salvage liver transplantation (SLT), RH, and repeated radiofrequency ablation (rRFA) in patients with post-operative HCC recurrence and found that SLT and RH led to comparable survival outcomes and that both treatments were better than rRFA.

However, RH is not indicated for patients with impaired liver function and multifocal intrahepatic or extrahepatic recurrence. A previous study reported the use of a nomogram to predict prognosis after the second hepatectomy (9). Given that the nomogram did not include factors related to impaired liver function, clinical physicians had to further consider these factors, but they could not determine the relative importance of these factors in prognosis. Moreover, there were no external validation cohorts to validate the nomogram.

Post-recurrence survival (PRS) of patients with HCC is greatly impacted by features of recurrence rather than by features of the primary tumors, and it could also be convenient for clinical physicians to evaluate the survival time for patients who received the second operation. The purpose of this study was to identify the clinical and pathological characteristics associated with PRS after RH in patients with HCC. For patients from the Affiliated Hospital of Guilin Medical College (Guilin cohort), we first used the information of 100 patients who underwent a second hepatectomy for recurrent HCC to construct a nomogram to predict the individual risk of PRS after initial recurrence. We validated the nomogram with 38 patients who underwent a second hepatectomy for recurrent HCC from the external Peking University People's Hospital (PKUPH) cohort.

MATERIALS AND METHODS

Patient Population and Data Collection

Between September 27, 1995 and December 31, 2016, data on consecutive patients with primary HCC who underwent curative liver resection were prospectively collected at the Affiliated Hospital of Guilin Medical University, China. Between December 2005 and December 2019, data on consecutive patients with primary HCC who underwent curative liver resection were prospectively collected at PKUPH, China. The Institutional Ethics Committee of the Affiliated Hospital of Guilin Medical College and PKUPH approved this study, which follows the ethical guidelines of the 2013 Declaration of Helsinki. Due to the long-term of the study, we proceeded to inform the patients before the surgical treatment and provided them with the informed consent form to sign.

The inclusion criteria were as follows: (1) Patients who underwent R0 liver resection; (2) patients with no evidence of extrahepatic metastasis or macroscopic tumor thrombus in the major portal/hepatic vein and biliary tract before the primary and repeat hepatectomies; (3) patients who were not receiving adjuvant treatment; and (4) patients with Child-Pugh A or B liver function. The exclusion criteria were as follows: (1) Patients who had received any preoperative or post-operative anticancer treatments; (2) patients who had a history of other cancers or had incomplete clinical data; and (3) patients who died within 30 days of operation (to avoid the inclusion of deaths due to post-operative complications). We used the data from patients at PKUPH ($n = 362$) between 2005 and 2019 as an external validation cohort using the same inclusion and exclusion criteria.

Demographic and clinicopathological data of the patients with primary recurrences were collected, including age, sex, family history, alcohol history, liver function, blood routine examination, and serum a-fetoprotein (AFP) tests, lymph node metastasis, tumor size, tumor number, tumor site (caudate lobe, left, or right), tumor differentiation (i.e., low, median or high), time to recurrence (TTR), and the TNM stage of the disease. Tumor size was defined as the sum of the diameters of all the resected tumors. The final pathological outcomes were used to evaluate the resection margin status (negative [R0]) and the lymph node status (no metastasis[N0] or lymph node metastasis [N1]). The primary outcomes of interest were PRS.

Follow-Up

After curative liver resection, patients received regular medical follow-ups every 2 months for the first 2 years and every 3–6 months thereafter. At each follow-up visit, patients had a routine examination of the physical checkup, determination of serum AFP levels, liver function tests, and at least one imaging examination, including abdominal ultrasound, contrast-enhanced CT scan, or MRI. For patients who were suspected of having HCC recurrence based on liver ultrasound or dynamically elevated AFP levels, either a contrast-enhanced CT scan or MRI was carried out to confirm or exclude the diagnosis. Chest CT was annually performed to exclude lung metastasis. Each recurrence time was defined as the date of the first positive imaging examination result. PRS was defined as the interval from the time of the primary recurrence to the final follow-up date or the time of patient death.

Statistical Analysis

Categorical variables were presented as whole numbers and proportions and were compared using the χ^2 test. Continuous variables were presented as medians with interquartile ranges (IQRs) and compared using an unpaired, two-tailed t-test or the Mann–Whitney test. The Mann–Whitney test was used when normal distribution and homogeneity of variance could not meet the requirements of the t-test. Survival curves were

Abbreviations: PRS, post-recurrence survival; RH, repeat hepatectomy; TTR, time to recurrence; HCC, hepatocellular carcinoma.

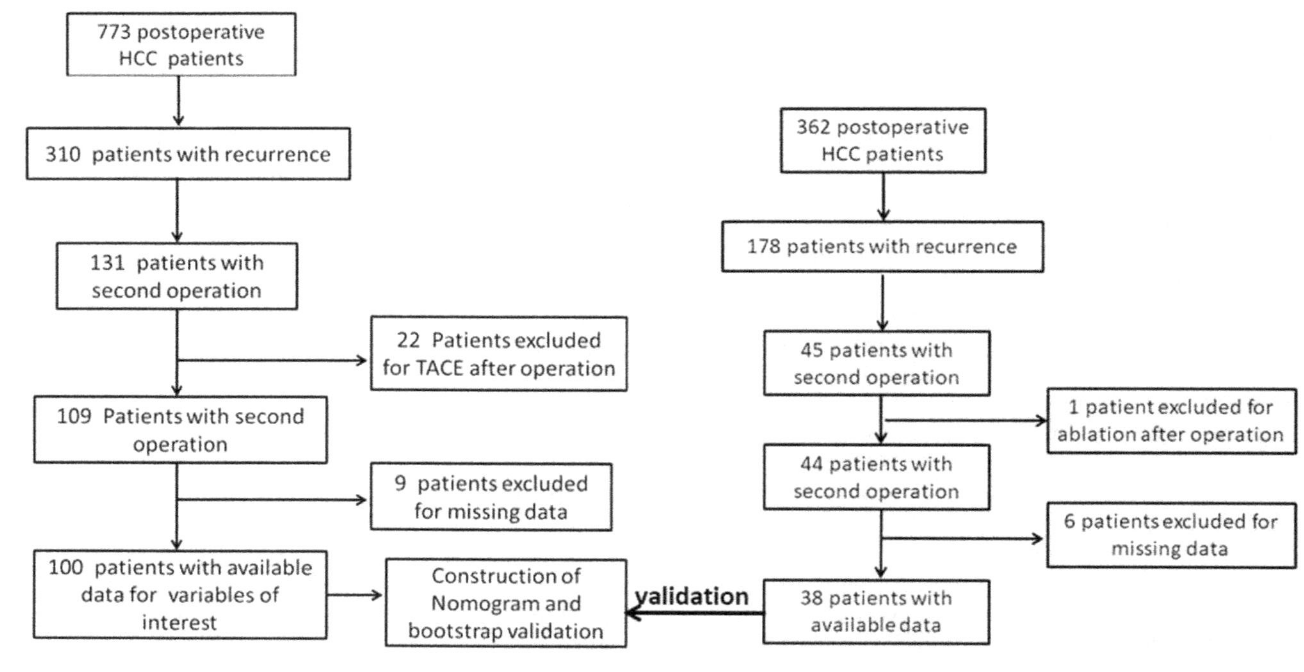

FIGURE 1 | Flowchart of this study.

TABLE 1 | Cox proportional hazards regression model showing the association of variables with post-recurrence survival.

	Guilin cohort (*n* = 100)			
	Univariable		**Multivariable**	
Variable	**HR (95% CI)**	***P*-value**	**HR (95% CI)**	***P*-value**
Factors selected				
TNM stage				
I	1 [Reference]		1 [Reference]	
II	2.22 (1.13–4.36)	0.02	2.82 (1.17–6.77)	0.02
III	3.93 (1.86–8.32)	<0.001	2.76 (1.08–7.04)	0.03
Differentiation				
Low	1 [Reference]		1 [Reference]	
High	0.24 (0.08–0.67)	<0.01	0.19 (0.06–0.61)	<0.01
Median	0.59 (0.23–1.09)	0.09	0.35 (0.17–0.73)	<0.01
Tumor site				
Caudate lobe	1 [Reference]		1 [Reference]	
Left	0.35 (0.08–1.53)	0.16	0.14 (0.03–0.74)	0.02
Right	0.21 (0.05–0.91)	0.03	0.05 (0.01–0.31)	<0.001
Diameter, cm				
<=5	1 [Reference]		1 [Reference]	
>5	2.68 (1.45–4.97)	<0.01	1.39 (0.66–2.91)	0.05
ALB (g/L)				
<28	1 [Reference]		1 [Reference]	
(28, 35)	0.008 (0.0004–0.15)	<0.01	0.003 (0.0002–0.07)	<0.001
>=35	0.007 (0.0004–0.11)	<0.001	0.002 (0.0001–0.04)	<0.001
AST (IU/L)				
<=40	1 [Reference]		1 [Reference]	
>40	2.36 (1.36–4.11)	<0.01	2.26 (1.07–4.77)	0.03
TTR (month)				
<=12	1 [Reference]		1 [Reference]	
>12	0.447 (0.26–0.76)	<0.01	0.38 (0.21–0.68)	<0.01

compared using the Kaplan–Meier method and the log-rank test. Clinicopathological variables were considered discrete and were converted to categorical variables based on the clinical importance and were identified predictors according to previously published studies (9, 10).

We performed univariate and multivariate Cox regression analyses to confirm independent prognostic factors of PRS. Variables with statistically significant *P*-values on univariate analysis were selected into the multivariate Cox proportional hazard regression model. Backward stepwise selection with the Akaike information criterion (AIC) was applied to select the independent significant variables used in the development of the nomogram. The variation inflation factor was used to evaluate multicollinearity, and no significant interaction was found. Hazard ratios (HRs) of the variables were shown with their 95% CIS (11). The model performance was evaluated internally and externally by discrimination and calibration *via* the Harrell's concordance index (C-index) (12). Finally, the Kaplan–Meier curves were plotted with the tertiles of patients layered on the scores predicted by the established nomogram to further evaluate calibration. The model was validated by bootstrapping with a resampling of 1,000 to quantify any overfitting of the modeling strategy. All the statistical analyses were performed using the R software version 3.6.1 (www.r-project.org). *P*-values lower than 0.05 were considered statistically significant, and all tests were two-sided.

RESULTS

Clinicopathological Characteristics

The flowchart of patient recruitment is shown in **Figure 1**. In the Guilin cohort, 773 post-operative patients were enrolled for follow-up; of these, 294 patients recurred after the primary surgery, 131 recurrent patients received the second hepatectomy, 22 patients were excluded because they received transarterial chemoembolization (TACE) treatment after hepatectomy, nine patients were lost to follow-up, and finally 100 patients were identified as training cohort; In the PKUPH cohort, 362 post-operative patients were enrolled for follow-up; of these, 178 patients recurred after the primary surgery, 45 recurrent patients received the second hepatectomy, 1 patient was excluded because they received the ablation treatment after hepatectomy, 6 patients were lost to follow-up, and finally 38 patients were identified as the external validation cohort. The clinical and pathological characteristics of patients with HCC in the training cohort ($n = 100$) and external validation cohort are summarized in (**Supplementary Table 1**). There were no differences in baseline indicators between the training cohort and the external validation cohorts, except in factors such as age, WBC count, LYMPH count, NEUT count, ALT and AST level, tumor difference, and HBsAg level. For the Guilin cohort, the median follow-up time was 34.2 months (range 19.7–56.5). About 38.1% (294 of 773) of the patients had a first recurrence of the disease, and 26% (26 of 100) of the patients had re-recurrence. The 2- and 5-year PRS rates were 57 and 15%, respectively, and the median PRS was 27.5 months.

Independent Prognostic Factors in the Training Cohort

All variables listed in **Supplementary Table 1** were used for univariate analysis, which was shown in **Table 1** and **Supplementary Table 2**. Variables with $P < 0.05$ were used in the multivariate Cox regression analysis. Multivariate analysis revealed that the TNM stage, tumor site, tumor size, tumor differentiation, albumin (ALB) and aspartate aminotransferase (AST) levels, and TTR time were the seven independent prognostic factors for PRS ($P < 0.05$) (**Table 1**).

Prognostic Nomogram for PRS

The prognostic nomogram for predicting PRS of the recurrent patients after RH is shown in **Figure 2A**. The nomogram was constructed based upon the following seven independent prognostic factors identified in the Cox model: TNM stage (I, II, or III), tumor site (caudate lobe, left, or right), tumor size (≤5 or >5 cm), tumor differentiation (low, high, or median), ALB (<28, 28–35 or ≥35 g/L), AST (≤40 or >40 IU/L), and TTR (≤ 12 or >12 months). The nomogram was then used to predict 3- and 5-year PRS rates for recurrent patients after RH of HCC (**Figure 2A**). Each individual can be assigned a mortality risk by adding seven individual scores identified in the nomogram; the higher total scores are associated with a worse prognosis.

Discriminative Ability of the Prognostic Nomogram

The discriminative ability of the PRS prediction model by C statistics was 0.758 (95% CI, 0.685–0.831), which is better than the TNM staging system of recurrence (0.609, 95% CI, 0.535–0.683, $P < 0.01$). The prediction of the 1-, 2-, 3-, and 5-year PRS rates by the 33-sample bootstrapped calibration plot are shown in **Figures 2B–E**, demonstrating an ideal agreement between nomogram prediction and real observations. The generated model was internally validated by the bootstrap validation method with 1,000 resamplings (the C statistics was 0.703). For the external validation cohort, the C statistics was 0.811 (95% CI, 0.762–0.860), which is better than the TNM staging system of recurrence (0.609, 95% CI, 0.546–0.672, $P < 0.01$). The prediction of the 1-, 2-, 3-, and 5-year PRS rates by the 12-sample bootstrapped calibration plot were shown in **Figures 3A–D**, demonstrating an ideal agreement between nomogram prediction and real observations. The AUCs of the training cohort and external validation cohorts were 0.843 and 0.890, respectively, which were better than those of the TNM and BCLC stage systems as shown in **Figures 2F–H** and **Figures 3E–G**.

The Kaplan–Meier curves were plotted to further verify the power of the nomogram in predicting PRS (**Figures 4A,D**). In the training cohort, the nomogram stratified patients into low- (total score ≤ 27), medium- (total score 27–47), and

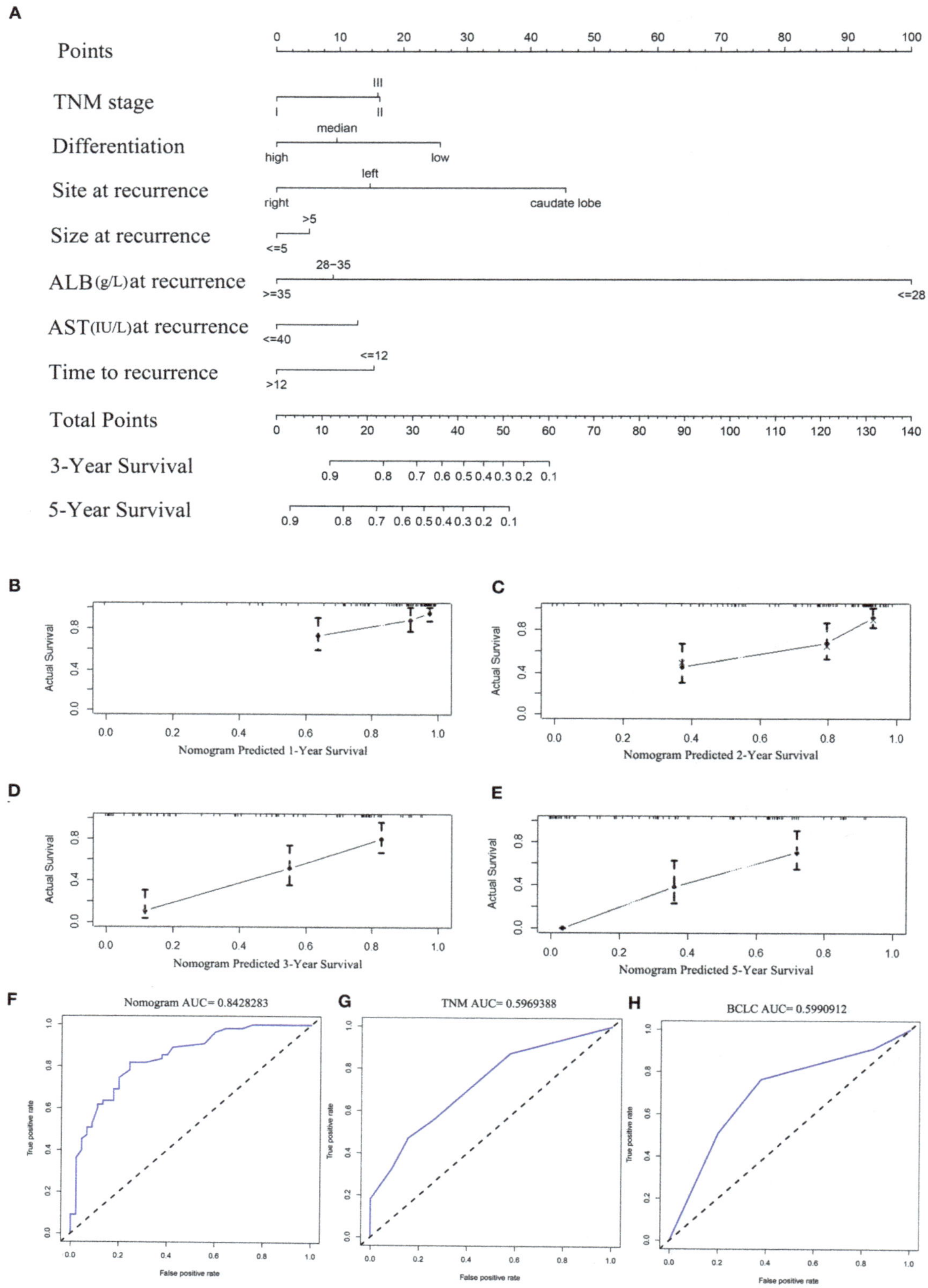

FIGURE 2 | (A) Nomogram for predicting the 3- and 5-year post-recurrence survival rates in patients with repeat hepatectomy (RH) of hepatocellular carcinoma (HCC). The calibration curve for predicting the 1-, 2-, 3-, and 5- year post-recurrence survival in the training **(B–E)** cohort; nomogram-predicted probability of PRS is plotted on the x-axis; actual PRS is plotted on the y-axis. The area under the curve (AUC) of the nomogram, and the tumor, node, and metastasis (TNM) and BCLC stage systems in the training cohort **(F–H)**.

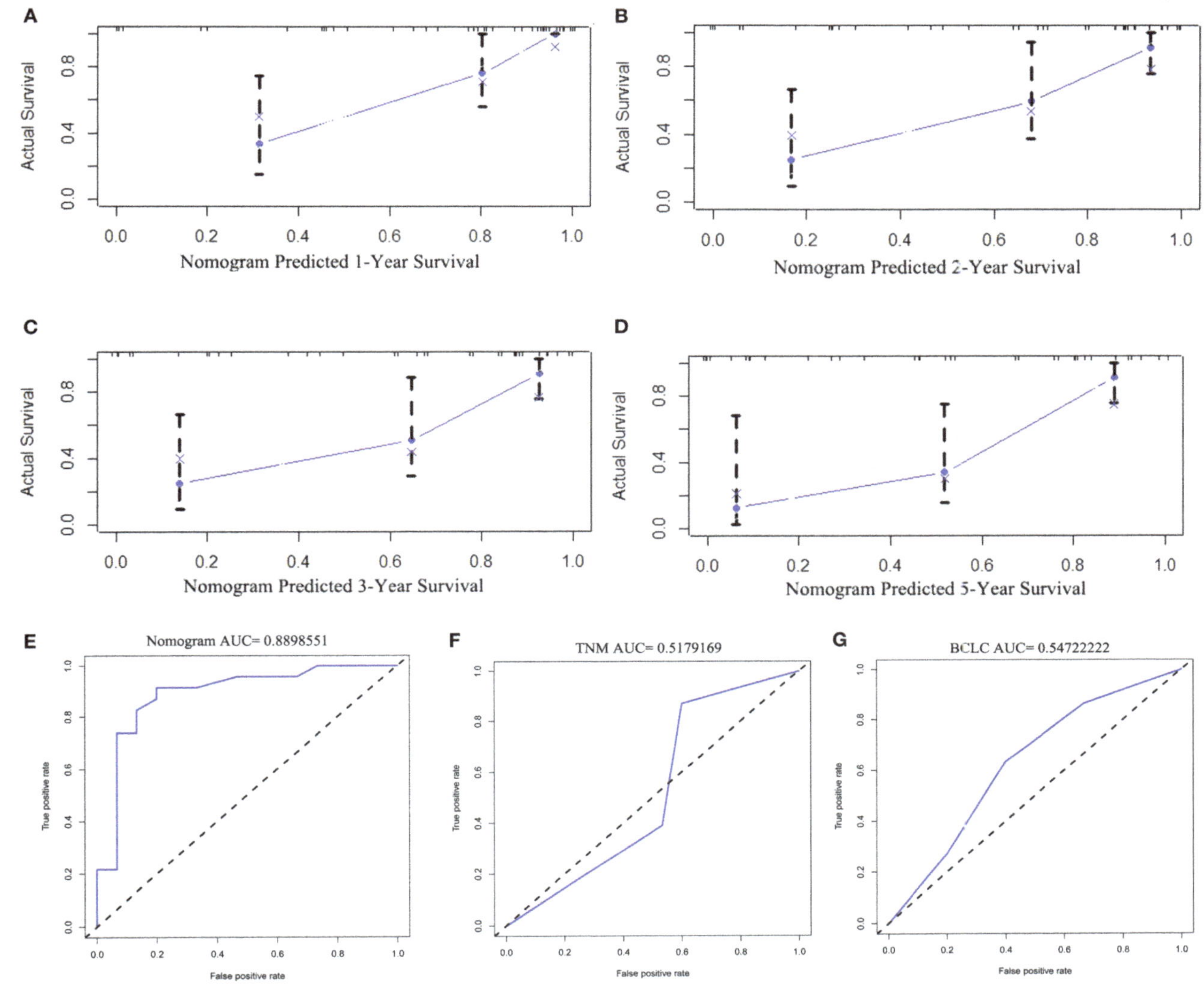

FIGURE 3 | The calibration curve for predicting the 1-, 2-, 3-, and 5- year post-recurrence survival in the training **(A–D)** cohort; nomogram-predicted probability of PRS is plotted on the x-axis; actual PRS is plotted on the y-axis. The AUC of the nomogram, and the TNM and BCLC stage systems in external validation cohorts **(E–G)**.

high-risk (total score > 47) subgroups. Patients in the high-risk group (tertile 3) had a worse outcome (0% 5-year PRS) in comparison with patients in the low-risk group (tertile 1) and the median-risk group (tertile 2) (69.6 and 39.5% 5-year PRS, respectively) ($P < 0.001$), meanwhile, the predicted 2-year PRS rates in low-, median-, and high-risk groups were 87.2, 68.6, and 45.4%, respectively ($P < 0.001$) (**Figure 4A**). The Kaplan–Meier curves were also constructed for the TNM and BCLC staging systems of both the training and validation groups (**Figures 4B,C,E,F**). There was an overlap of curves for patients in TNM stage I, II, and III of the training cohort during the first 2 years of survival (**Figure 4B**), and patients in the BCLC stage had a similar result (**Figure 4C**). In the external validation cohort, the Kaplan–Meier curve of the established nomogram (**Figure 4D**) also performed better than those of both the TNM (**Figure 4E**) and BCLC (**Figure 4F**) staging system.

DISCUSSION

In the current study, we constructed a novel nomogram to predict PRS in recurrent patients after RH in HCC and then externally validated patients in the PKUPH cohort. This clinical context occurs in patients treated with RH without other treatments.

Repeat hepatectomy is reported to prolong the OS time for patients with recurrent HCC after liver resection (5, 13–15). A previous study established a nomogram to predict the survival of patients with recurrence of HCC after the primary operation and identified repeat resection as an independent prognostic factor associated with prolonged survival, but it also included

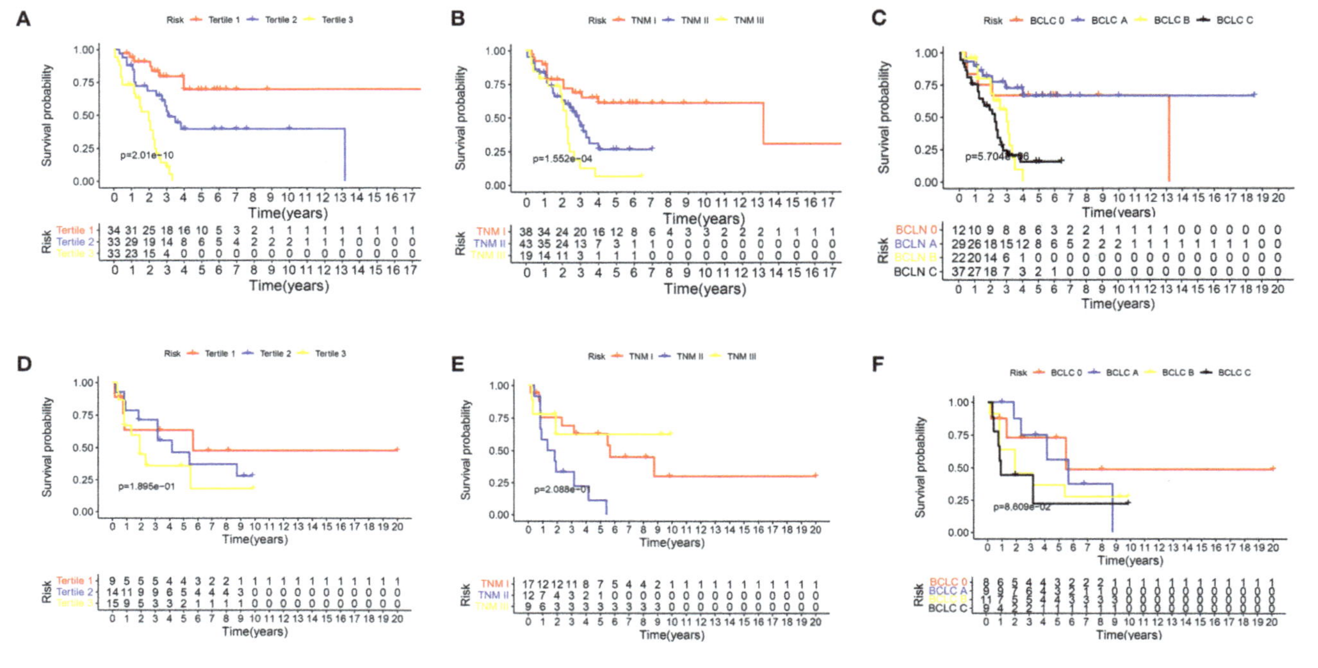

FIGURE 4 | The Kaplan–Meier curves for subgroups of patients. Patients were stratified by the prognostic score **(A)**, TNM stage **(B)**, and BCLC stage **(C)** in the training cohort. Patients were stratified by the prognostic score **(D)**, TNM stage **(E)**, and BCLC stage **(F)** in the external validation cohorts.

patients managed with other treatments, including molecular targeted therapy, systematic chemotherapy, radiotherapy, and supportive care (10), so this nomogram is not particularly helpful. For example, RH treatment is scored zero in the nomogram, which means patients who select RH have a better prognosis than those who select other treatments. However, RH is not fit for all recurrent patients. In our opinion, all treatments should have their own standards for evaluation. Clinical physicians could compare the outcomes based on these standards and select the optimal treatment for patients with recurrent HCC.

Another particular strength of this study is that the nomogram included a wide array of variables (TNM stage, liver function, tumor characteristics, and TTR) identified in previous publications as being related to prognosis after liver resection of the HCC (10, 13, 14, 16). Zou et al. (9) previously developed a nomogram among patients with RH of HCC that incorporated TTR, HBV-DNA level, and tumor characteristics at the initial surgery in the model, having identified TTR as the most effective predictive factor for mortality. The inclusion of risk factors without liver function is problematic because it is self-explanatory that liver function is closely related to prognosis (17). Our study incorporated all the variables collected at recurrences, and both serum AST and ALB are included in the liver function tests, which implies that the liver function has been taken into account in our model. It is worth mentioning that serum ALB levels occupy the most important position in the nomogram. Some studies (18–20) have reported that tumor differentiation and tumor size are associated with disease-free survival and/or OS after the initial surgery. In contrast, other researchers have put forward that there is no correlation between these tumor characteristics and disease-free survival and/or OS (21). In the present study, we found a significant association not only between tumor differentiation and tumor size but also proved that tumor site (left, right, or caudate lobe) is correlated with PRS, the hazard ratio being shown in **Table 1**. Because of a specific anatomical characteristic, tumors on the caudate lobe are difficult to completely resect (22), which was first identified as the independent risk factor in predicting PRS in this study. Furthermore, we also noted that TTR is strongly linked to outcomes. A previous study has identified 2 years after resection as the optimal cutoff value to distinguish late recurrence from early recurrence (23), while this study implies that < 2 year from repeat resection to recurrence has a close correlation with PRS, which is in accordance with nomograms in other studies (9, 10).

Accurate risk stratification of the patients with post-operative recurrence in HCC is essential because the prognosis of patients may vary (24). However, the TNM staging system was less useful than the nomogram developed in this study for PRS prediction in both the training cohorty and external validation cohorts (C-index, 0.758 vs. 0.609, 0.811 vs. 0.609, respectively), which suggests that our nomogram has the ability to predict post-operative survival after recurrence. Indeed, when stratified into tertiles in the survival analysis, the established nomogram could identify subgroups of patients who were at different risks of death in both the training cohort and validation cohorts.

In conclusion, we constructed a nomogram to predict PRS in patients with RH after the recurrence of HCC. The nomogram performed well on external validation cohort. This study also has limitations. The number of patients who accepted a second radical surgery is small, although the clinical and pathological data were collected in two centers. The sample size is still small, and more studies are needed to externally validate the established nomogram. In addition, imaging data were not collected; therefore, the nomogram could not evaluate its effect.

AUTHOR CONTRIBUTIONS

HC, QF, WL, and JG designed the study. QF analyzed the data and wrote the manuscript. RY, DC, and RF provided technical expertise and support. PC and KD collected the clinical information and scheduled the follow-up plan. All authors contributed to the article and approved the submitted version.

ACKNOWLEDGMENTS

We sincerely thank the researchers and study participants for their contributions toward this study.

REFERENCES

1. Inoue K, Takayama T, Higaki T, Watanabe Y, Makuuchi M. Clinical significance of early hepatocellular carcinoma. *Liver Transpl.* (2004) 10:S16–9. doi: 10.1002/lt.20049
2. Grazi GL, Cescon M, Ravaioli M, Ercolani G, Gardini A, Del Gaudio M, et al. Liver resection for hepatocellular carcinoma in cirrhotics and noncirrhotics. Evaluation of clinicopathologic features and comparison of risk factors for long-term survival and tumour recurrence in a single centre. *Aliment Pharmacol Ther.* (2003) 17:119–29. doi: 10.1046/j.1365-2036.17.s2.9.x
3. Hanazaki K, Kajikawa S, Shimozawa N, Mihara M, Shimada K, Hiraguri M, et al. Survival and recurrence after hepatic resection of 386 consecutive patients with hepatocellular carcinoma. *J Am Coll Surg.* (2000) 191:381–8. doi: 10.1016/S1072-7515(00)00700-6
4. Fan ST, Poon RT, Yeung C, Lam CM, Lo CM, Yuen WK, et al. Outcome after partial hepatectomy for hepatocellular cancer within the Milan criteria. *Br J Surg.* (2011) 98:1292–300. doi: 10.1002/bjs.7583
5. Itamoto T, Nakahara H, Amano H, Kohashi T, Ohdan H, Tashiro H, et al. Repeat hepatectomy for recurrent hepatocellular carcinoma. *Surgery.* (2007) 141:589–97. doi: 10.1016/j.surg.2006.12.014
6. Tralhão JG, Dagher I, Lino T, Roudié J, Franco D. Treatment of tumour recurrence after resection of hepatocellular carcinoma. Analysis of 97 consecutive patients. *Eur J Surg Oncol.* (2007) 33:746–51. doi: 10.1016/j.ejso.2006.11.015
7. Faber W, Seehofer D, Neuhaus P, Stockmann M, Denecke T, Kalmuk S, et al. Repeated liver resection for recurrent hepatocellular carcinoma. *J Gastroenterol Hepatol.* (2011) 26:1189–94. doi: 10.1111/j.1440-1746.2011.06721.x
8. Chan AC, Chan SC, Chok KS, Cheung TT, Chiu DW, Poon RT, et al. Treatment strategy for recurrent hepatocellular carcinoma: salvage transplantation, repeated resection, or radiofrequency ablation? *Liver Transpl.* (2013) 19:411–9. doi: 10.1002/lt.23605
9. Zou Q, Li J, Wu D, Yan Z, Wan X, Wang K, et al. Nomograms for pre-operative and post-operative prediction of long-term survival of patients who underwent repeat hepatectomy for recurrent hepatocellular carcinoma. *Ann Surg Oncol.* (2016) 23:2618–26. doi: 10.1245/s10434-016-5136-0
10. He W, Peng B, Tang Y, Yang J, Zheng Y, Qiu J, et al. Nomogram to predict survival of patients with recurrence of hepatocellular carcinoma after surgery. *Clin Gastroenterol Hepatol.* (2018) 16:756–64.e710. doi: 10.1016/j.cgh.2017.12.002
11. Simon R. Confidence intervals for reporting results of clinical trials. *Ann Intern Med.* (1986) 105:429–35. doi: 10.7326/0003-4819-105-3-429
12. Harrell FE Jr, Califf RM, Pryor DB, Lee KL, Rosati RA. Evaluating the yield of medical tests. *JAMA.* (1982) 247:2543–6. doi: 10.1001/jama.1982.03320430047030
13. Tsujita E, Yamashita Y, Takeishi K, Matsuyama A, Tsutsui S, Matsuda H, et al. Poor prognostic factors after repeat hepatectomy for recurrent hepatocellular carcinoma in the modern era. *Am Surg.* (2012) 78:419–25. doi: 10.1177/000313481207800431
14. Poon RT, Fan ST, Lo CM, Liu CL, Wong J. Intrahepatic recurrence after curative resection of hepatocellular carcinoma: long-term results of treatment and prognostic factors. *Ann Surg.* (1999) 229:216–22. doi: 10.1097/00000658-199902000-00009
15. Sugimachi K, Maehara S, Tanaka S, Shimada M, Sugimachi K. Repeat hepatectomy is the most useful treatment for recurrent hepatocellular carcinoma. *J Hepatobiliary Pancreat Surg.* (2001) 8:410–6. doi: 10.1007/s005340100002
16. Huang ZY, Liang BY, Xiong M, Zhan DQ, Wei S, Wang GP, et al. Long-term outcomes of repeat hepatic resection in patients with recurrent hepatocellular carcinoma and analysis of recurrent types and their prognosis: a single-center experience in China. *Ann Surg Oncol.* (2012) 19:2515–25. doi: 10.1245/s10434-012-2269-7
17. Johnson PJ, Berhane S, Kagebayashi C, Satomura S, Teng M, Reeves HL, et al. Assessment of liver function in patients with hepatocellular carcinoma: a new evidence-based approach-the ALBI grade. *J Clin Oncol.* (2015) 33:550–8. doi: 10.1200/JCO.2014.57.9151
18. Torzilli G, Donadon M, Belghiti J, Kokudo N, Takayama T, Ferrero A, et al. Predicting individual survival after hepatectomy for hepatocellular carcinoma: a novel nomogram from the "HCC East & West Study Group". *J Gastrointest Surg.* (2016) 20:1154–62. doi: 10.1007/s11605-016-3132-0
19. Zhang W, Tan Y, Shen S, Jiang L, Yan L, Yang J, et al. Prognostic nomogram for hepatocellular carcinoma in adolescent and young adult patients after hepatectomy. *Oncotarget.* (2017) 8:106393–404. doi: 10.18632/oncotarget.18192
20. Pan YX, Chen JC, Fang AP, Wang XH, Chen JB, Wang JC, et al. A nomogram predicting the recurrence of hepatocellular carcinoma in patients after laparoscopic hepatectomy. *Cancer Commun.* (2019) 39:55. doi: 10.1186/s40880-019-0404-6
21. Ma KW, She WH, Cheung TT, Chan ACY, Dai WC, Fung JYY, et al. Validated nomogram for the prediction of disease-free survival after hepatectomy for hepatocellular carcinoma within the Milan criteria: individualizing a surveillance strategy. *Surg Today.* (2019) 49:521–8. doi: 10.1007/s00595-019-1764-x
22. Clavien PA, Petrowsky H, DeOliveira ML, Graf R. Strategies for safer liver surgery and partial liver transplantation. *N Engl J Med.* (2007) 356:1545–59. doi: 10.1056/NEJMra065156
23. Portolani N, Coniglio A, Ghidoni S, Giovanelli M, Benetti A, Tiberio GA, et al. Early and late recurrence after liver resection for hepatocellular carcinoma: prognostic and therapeutic implications. *Ann Surg.* (2006) 243:229–35. doi: 10.1097/01.sla.0000197706.21803.a1
24. Jang TY, Huang CI, Yeh ML, Lin ZY, Chen SC, Chuang WL. The prognosis of bulky hepatocellular carcinoma with nonmajor branch portal vein tumor thrombosis. *Medicine.* (2019) 98:e15066. doi: 10.1097/MD.00000000000 15066

5

A Starvation-Based 9-mRNA Signature Correlates with Prognosis in Patients with Hepatocellular Carcinoma

Dengliang Lei[1], Yue Chen[2], Yang Zhou[1], Gangli Hu[1] and Fang Luo[1]*

[1] Department of Hepatobiliary Surgery, The First Affiliated Hospital of Chongqing Medical University, Chongqing, China,
[2] Central Laboratory, The First Affiliated Hospital of Chongqing Medical University, Chongqing, China

***Correspondence:**
Fang Luo
luofang@hospital.cqmu.edu.cn*

Background: Hepatocellular carcinoma (HCC) is one of the world's most prevalent and lethal cancers. Notably, the microenvironment of tumor starvation is closely related to cancer malignancy. Our study constructed a signature of starvation-related genes to predict the prognosis of liver cancer patients.

Methods: The mRNA expression matrix and corresponding clinical information of HCC patients were obtained from the International Cancer Genome Consortium (ICGC) and The Cancer Genome Atlas (TCGA). Gene set enrichment analysis (GSEA) was used to distinguish different genes in the hunger metabolism gene in liver cancer and adjacent tissues. Gene Set Enrichment Analysis (GSEA) was used to identify biological differences between high- and low-risk samples. Univariate and multivariate analyses were used to construct prognostic models for hunger-related genes. Kaplan-Meier (KM) and receiver-operating characteristic (ROC) were used to assess the model accuracy. The model and relevant clinical information were used to construct a nomogram, protein expression was detected by western blot (WB), and transwell assay was used to evaluate the invasive and metastatic ability of cells.

Results: First, we used univariate analysis to identify 35 prognostic genes, which were further demonstrated to be associated with starvation metabolism through Kyoto Encyclopedia of Genes and Genomes (KEGG) and Gene Ontology (GO). We then used multivariate analysis to build a model with nine genes. Finally, we divided the sample into low- and high-risk groups according to the median of the risk score. KM can be used to conclude that the prognosis of high- and low-risk samples is significantly different, and the prognosis of high-risk samples is worse. The prognostic accuracy of the 9-mRNA signature was also tested in the validation data set. GSEA was used to identify typical pathways and biological processes related to 9-mRNA, cell cycle, hypoxia, p53 pathway, and PI3K/AKT/mTOR pathway, as well as biological processes related to the model. As evidenced by WB, EIF2S1 expression was increased after starvation. Overall, EIF2S1 plays an important role in the invasion and metastasis of liver cancer.

Conclusions: The 9-mRNA model can serve as an accurate signature to predict the prognosis of liver cancer patients. However, its mechanism of action warrants further investigation.

Keywords: starvation, gene set enrichment analysis, hepatocellular carcinoma, mRNA signature, EIF2S1

INTRODUCTION

Liver cancer is a type of cancer with the highest incidence worldwide, and hepatocellular carcinoma (HCC) accounts for 80% of liver cancer cases (1). Despite advances in treatments such as surgery, ablation, and liver transplantation (2), liver cancer remains one of the leading causes of death among all cancers (3, 4). Furthermore, increases in non-alcoholic fatty liver disease (NAFLD), metabolic syndrome, and obesity elevated the risk of liver disease (5).

Therefore, the identification of new biological molecular predictors to improve the prognosis of HCC is urgent.

The tumor microenvironment is mainly composed of hematopoietic and mesenchymal cells, as well as non-cellular components (6). it is closely associated with disease progression, local resistance, immune escape, and metastasis (7). Malnutrition is one of the most common conditions in tumor microenvironments due to increased nutrient depletion in cancer cells and inadequate vascular supply (8, 9). Starvation is reportedly associated with epithelial-mesenchymal transition (EMT), angiogenesis, and autophagy (10–12). For instance, in bladder cancer, starvation can induce autophagy in cancer cells, thereby enhancing the EMT of bladder cancer through the TGF pathway (13). Studies have reported that starvation can induce invasion and metastasis of HCC cells (14). However, studies on the characteristics of starvation-related malignancies in HCC survival are still lacking.

In this study, we first established a hunger-related 9-mRNA independent prognostic model using TCGA and verified the model accuracy in the ICGC database. In addition, we constructed a nomogram to assess clinical significance using risk scores and clinical factors. We then analyzed the typical pathways and biological processes associated with the 9-mRNA model through GSEA. Finally, we found that the expression and phosphorylation of the core model gene EIF2S1 were increased under starvation induction, which induced autophagy to increase EMT in HCC.

METHODS

Data Collection

RNA expression data and related clinical information were obtained from TCGA (https://cancergenome.nih.gov/). A total of 424 samples in TCGA-LIHC were used in the following study as a training cohort (**Supplementary File 1**). In addition, data from 231 HCC patients from ICGA-LIRI-JP (https://dcc.icgc.org/) were downloaded as an independent, external validation cohort (**Supplementary File 2**). This research strictly follows TCGA and ICGC access rules and publication guidelines. Detailed information is shown in **Table 1**. The starvation-related gene set was obtained from Gene Set Enrichment Analysis (GSEA) 'GOBP RESPONSE TO STARVATION ' in The Molecular Signatures Database(https://broadinstitute.org/gsea/msigdb/). It contained 196 genes responsible for the changes in the state/activity of a cell/organism as a result of a starvation stimulus (**Supplementary File 3**).

Construction and Validation of a Signature

In the training set, we first identified 142 differentially expressed genes associated with starvation metabolism in 374 samples using R ($P < 0.05$) (**Supplementary File 4**). Univariate Cox regression analysis ($P < 0.05$) was used to obtain 39 genes associated with prognosis. Finally, multivariate Cox regression analysis was used to construct a signature containing nine genes, detailed in **Table 2**. The risk score for each patient was calculated using the following equation: risk score = ($\beta 1 \times$ expression of gene1) + ($\beta 2 \times$ expression of gene2) + … + ($\beta 9 \times$ expression of gene9). All patients were divided into high- and low-risk groups based on the median risk score. Kaplan-Meier survival curve and two-sided log-rank test were used to compare the overall survival (OS) of the high- and low-risk group patients. Receiver-operating characteristic (ROC) curves were applied to assess the diagnostic efficacy of each clinicopathological characteristic and the prognostic signature. Stratified survival analysis was performed to examine the accuracy of the prognostic signature in

TABLE 1 | Summary of baseline clinical pathological parameters of patients with HCC in the two datasets.

Characteristic	train	test
Age (years)		
≤ 65	227	98
> 65	122	162
Gender		
Male	239	192
Female	110	68
Grade		
1	45	N/A
2	171	N/A
3	120	N/A
4	13	N/A
Stage		
I	173	40
II	85	117
III	86	80
IV	5	23
Survival status		
Alive	236	214
Deceased	113	56

HCC, hepatocellular carcinoma; N/A, not applicable.

TABLE 2 | The information of nine mRNAs associated with overall survival in patients with HCC.

mRNA	Coef	HR	p-value	Risk
EHMT2	-0.039384857	0.961380644	P=0.005	Low
HNRNPL	-0.054911705	0.946568721	P<0.001	Low
EIF2S1	0.119336909	1.126749466	P<0.001	High
PPARGC1A	-0.058903674	0.942797581	P=0.004	Low
RRP8	0.401757994	1.494449623	P<0.001	High
FOXK1	0.270963075	1.311226652	P<0.001	High
CAD	0.160686777	1.174317088	P<0.001	High
FOXK2	0.101894034	1.107266133	P<0.001	High
MYBBP1A	-0.089665498	0.914236948	P=0.002	Low

HCC, hepatocellular carcinoma.

predicting patient survival outcomes. Furthermore, we performed univariate and multivariate Cox regression analyses to evaluate whether the risk score was independent in determining the prognosis of the HCC patients. The M and N stages were not analyzed because data were missing for several patients. $P < 0.05$ was considered statistically significant.

The mRNA expression profile matrix of 231 HCC patients from ICGC was used as an external independent validation cohort to validate the accuracy of the 9 gene signature.

Functional Enrichment Analysis

The biological processes, molecular functions, and cell component Gene Ontology (GO) of mRNAs associated with survival were identified using GO enrichment analysis. The main signaling pathways of mRNA regulation were identified using the Kyoto Encyclopedia of Genes and Genomes (KEGG) pathway analysis.

Establishment and Assessment of the Nomogram

We constructed a nomogram by integrating clinicopathologic characteristics, such as age, stage, sex, and grade, as well as the risk score derived from the prognostic signature to analyze the probable 3-year and 5-year OS of the patients with HCC. Calibration charts were used to evaluate the performance of the Nomogram.

GSEA

GSEA software 4.0.1 was used to identify starvation-related gene sets in 50 HCC tissues and their adjacent tissues. Patients with HCC were divided into low- and high-risk groups based on the median risk value. GSEA was used to further analyze gene expression differences between the high- and the low-risk resistance groups. The Hallmark gene sets (h.all.v7.4.symbols.gmt), KEGG gene sets (c2.cp.kegg.v7.4.symbols.gmt) and GO gene sets (c5.go.v7.4.symbols.gmt) were downloaded from the Molecular Signatures Database (https://www.gsea-msigdb.org/gsea/msigdb/genesets.jsp). The gene sets were filtered using the maximum and minimum gene set sizes of 500 and 15 genes, respectively. The enriched gene sets were obtained based on a P-value < 0.05 and a false discovery rate (FDR) < 0.25 after performing 1,000 permutations.

Cell Culture

Liver cancer cells (Hep-3B and Huh-7) were obtained from the Institute of Chinese Academy of Sciences. Hep-3B and Huh-7 cell lines were cultured in DMEM (Corning Incorporated, Corning, NY, USA) supplemented with 10% fetal bovine serum (FBS, Gibco, Thermo Scientific, Waltham, MA, USA). All cells were cultured in an incubator with an atmosphere of 95% O_2 and 5% CO_2 at 37°C.

Western Blot

Total protein was extracted with RIPA lysis buffer (Beyotime Institute of Biotechnology, Jiangsu, China) containing protease and phosphatase inhibitors. The protein concentration was detected using a BCA protein detection kit (Jiangsu Beyotime Biotechnology Research Institute). Equivalent proteins were separated on 10% SDS-PAGE gels and then transferred to polyvinylidene fluoride (PVDF) membranes. After blocking with skimmed milk (dissolved in TBST) for 2 h, the membranes were subsequently probed using antibodies against B-actin (Cell Signaling Technology, USA, 1:10000), EIF2S1 (Cell Signaling Technology, USA, 1:1000),p-EIF2S1 (Cell Signaling Technology, USA, 1:1000), Vimentin(Cell Signaling Technology, USA, 1:1000) and E-cadherin(Cell Signaling Technology, USA, 1:1000) overnight at 4°C. The membranes were then washed with Tris-buffered saline containing Tween and incubated with an HRP-conjugated anti-rabbit antibody at 37°C for 1 h. Finally, the protein bands on the membranes were observed with an Odyssey Scanning System.

Small Interfering RNA Transfection

Small interfering RNA (siRNA) was purchased from GenePharma Biological Technology (Shanghai, China). Lipofectamine 2000 was transfected according to the manufacturer's protocol. Cells were transfected with EIF2S1 siRNAs (siRNA-1: sense, GCCAUAAUCGUCCUCACCA; siRNA-2: sense, CCAUAAUCGUCCUCACCAA, siRNA-2: sense, CCAUAAUCGUCCUCACCAA) at a concentration of 50 nM for 6 h. After 48 h, the treated cells were collected for subsequent experiments.

Immunofluorescence (IF)

The cells were immobilized with 4% paraformaldehyde, planted evenly on a slide, infiltrated with TRITON, then sealed with goat serum. The primary and fluorescent secondary antibodies were incubated overnight. Finally, nuclei were counterstained with DAPI.

Transwell Assay

The ability of cells to migrate and invade was analyzed using a transwell chamber. A total of 8×104 cells were directly and uniformly distributed in the wells in serum-free medium for the migration experiment. Similarly, the invasion test was performed almost identically to the migration test, except that the upper chamber was first coatedwith the matrix according to the manufacturer's instructions. For both tests, medium containing 15% FBS was added to the lower chamber as a chemical attractant. Cells were incubated in 5% CO_2 for 8 h (migration) or 12 h (invasion). The membrane was wiped with a cotton swab; cells were removed from the upper surface of the cavity, fixed with 4% formaldehyde, and stained with 0.5% crystal violet.

Statistical Analysis

Statistical analyses were conducted using GraphPad Prism 5.0 (San Diego, CA). The data were processed using the PERL programming language (version 5.30.2, http://www.perl.org). All statistical analyses were performed using R (version 3.6.2, https://www.r-project.org/). $P < 0.05$ was regarded as statistically significant.

RESULTS

Identification of Starvation-Related Genes

GSEA was used to determine whether there were significant differences in the starvation-related gene set between HCC samples and paired adjacent normal samples. The results suggested that the starvation-related gene set was significantly enriched in HCC samples (NES = 1.64, nominal $P < 0.001$, FDR < 0.001) (**Figure 1A**). A total of 195 starvation-related genes were used in the following study (**Figure 1B**).

Identification of Differential Starvation-Related Genes Associated With Prognosis in Patients with HCC

In TCGA database, we first identified differentially expressed genes related to hunger ($P < 0.05$). As shown in **Figures 2A, B**, 32 of the 142 differentially expressed genes were downregulated, and

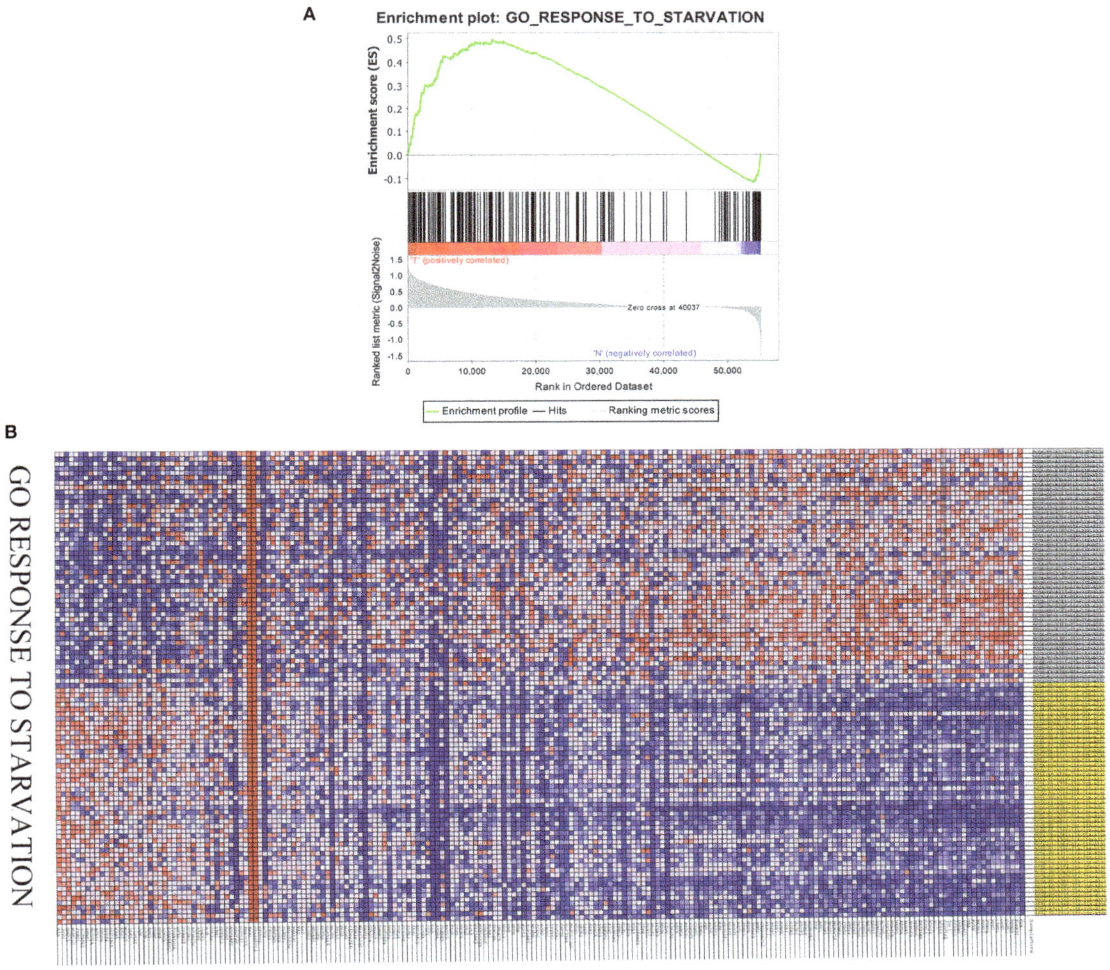

FIGURE 1 | GSEA of starvation-related gene sets. **(A)** Enrichment map of one starvation-related gene set between liver cancer and paired adjacent tissues identified by GSEA. **(B)** Heat map of 196 genes in liver cancer and normal tissue response to starvation gene sets.

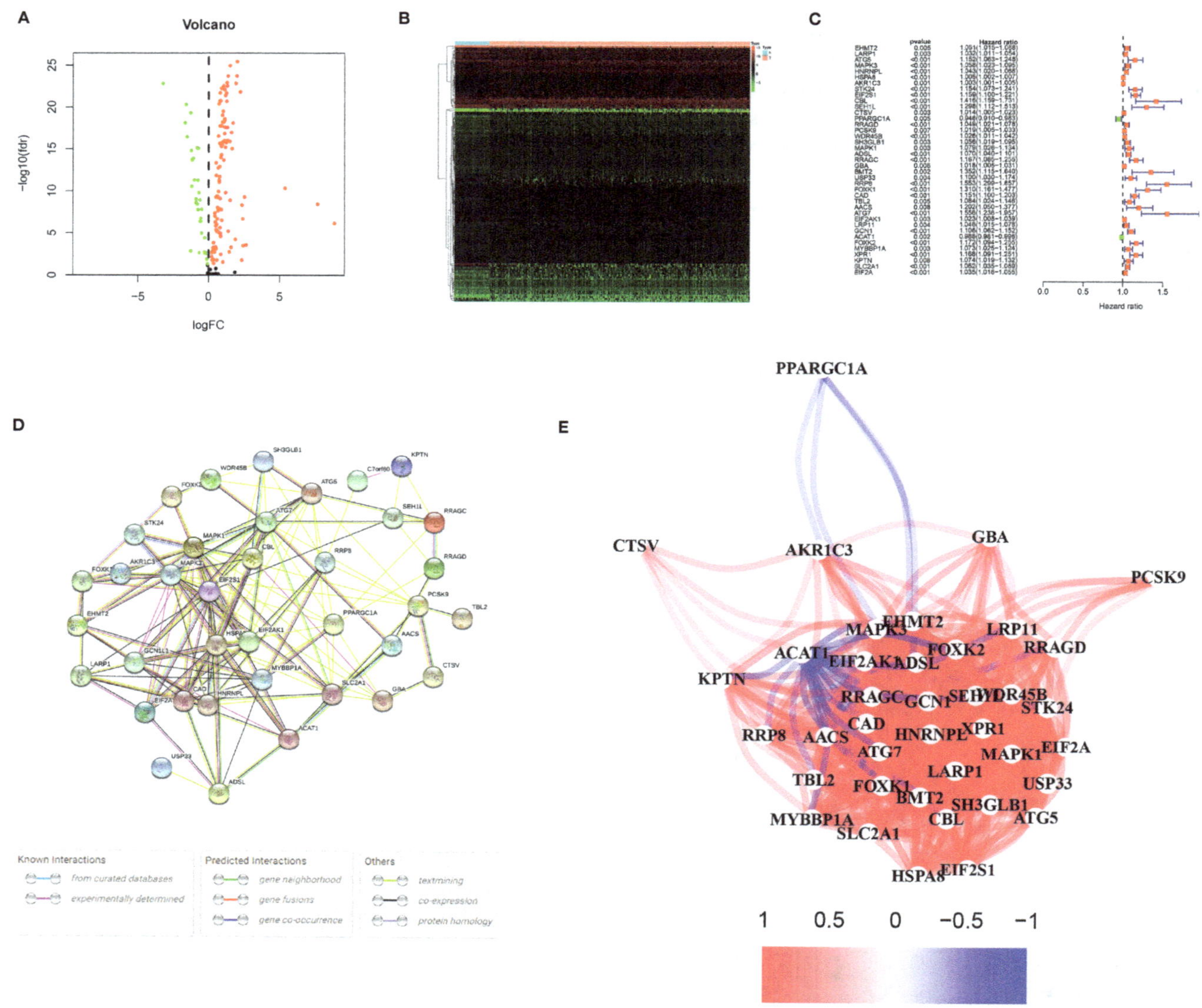

FIGURE 2 | Identification of prognostic mRNAs. **(A, B)** Volcanic and heat maps of starvation-related differential genes in TCGA. $P < 0.05$. **(C)** Thirty-nine genes associated with patient prognosis. **(D, E)** Interaction between 39 patient prognosis-related genes.

110 were upregulated. Then, we identified 39 prognostic differential genes using the univariate Cox regression analysis, among which 37 had a positive and 2 had a negative correlation with risk (**Figure 2C**). It can be seen from the hunger-related prognostic gene protein interaction network in **Figure 2D** that EIF2S1 is at the core-site. The correlation of hunger-related prognostic genes is shown in **Figure 2E**.

KEGG and GO Analysis

GO analysis and KEGG pathway enrichment analysis were used to verify whether the genes screened were involved in hunger-related energy metabolism. As shown in **Figures 3A, B**, the most notable correlation in GO is related to starvation metabolism. The same conclusion was obtained by KEGG pathway enrichment analysis (**Figures 3C, D**). GO analysis and KEGG enrichment analysis further verified that our candidate genes were closely related to hunger metabolism.

Construction and Validation of a Starvation-Related Gene Prognostic Signature

We carried out a multivariate analysis of the 39 genes obtained above and obtained 9 genes: EHMT2, HNRNPL, EIF2S1, PPARGC1A, RRP8, FOXK1, CAD FOXK2, and MYBBP1A. Among these genes were four protective genes, those with HR < 1, and five potentially harmful genes, those with HR > 1 (**Table 2**). We built a signature based on these nine genes and calculated the risk score for each patient based on the resulting model. Based on the median risk score,

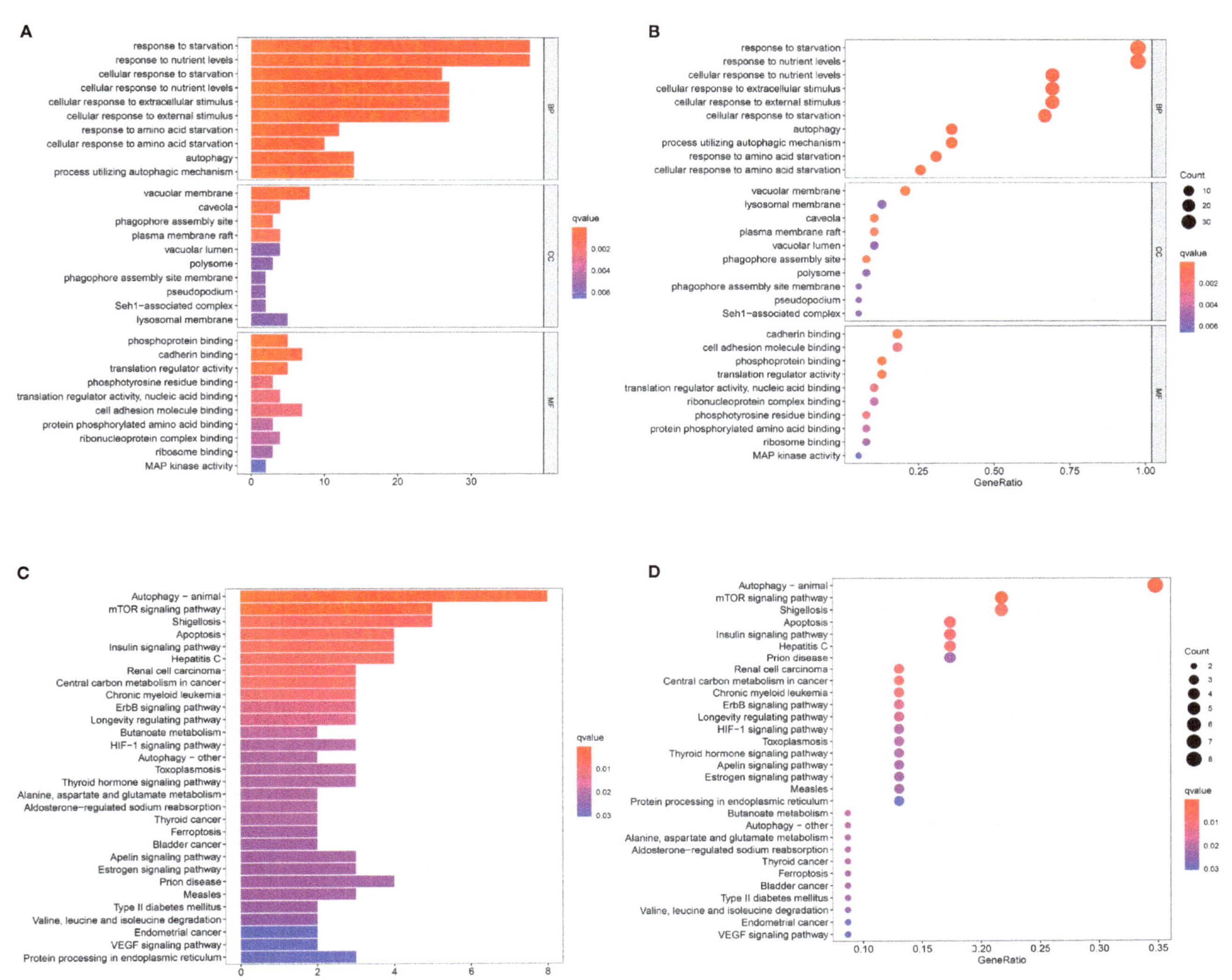

FIGURE 3 | Functional enrichment analyses. **(A–D)** Gene Ontology (GO) analysis and Kyoto Encyclopedia of Genes and Genomes (KEGG) pathway analysis results showing the functions and enriched signaling pathways associated with the starvation-related mRNAs.

we divided the patients into low- and high-risk groups (**Figure 4A**). According to the graph, the number of patient deaths increases with increased risk values in the training and validation sets (**Figure 4B**). As can be seen from the training and validation sets, there were significant differences in OS between the high- and the low-risk groups ($P < 0.001$ and $P < 0.001$, respectively), indicating a higher mortality rate in the high-risk group (**Figure 4C**). ROC was used to validate the model; the AUC values for 5-year survival for the training and validation cohorts were 0.73 and 0.76, respectively, demonstrating the high accuracy of this model (**Figure 4D**).

Starvation-Related mRNA Signature as an Independent Predictor of Survival in HCC Patients

Univariate and multivariate analyses were used to determine whether our hunger-related gene model could be an independent prognostic factor. In TCGA, risk scores and sex, age, grade, and stage of starvation-related gene-building models were used for univariate and multivariate analyses. In the univariate analysis, stage (HR = 2.479, 95% CI 1.698–3.619, $P < 0.001$) and risk score (HR = 1.243, 95% CI 1.182–1.307, $P < 0.001$) were associated with OS. In the multivariate analysis, stage (HR = 2.047, 95% CI 1.374–3.049, $P < 0.001$) and risk score (HR = 1.208, 95% CI 1.146–1.273, $P < 0.001$) were associated with OS (**Figure 5A**). In the ICGC, the risk scores of the starvation-related gene-building prognostic models and clinical characteristics such as age, sex, and stage were also analyzed by univariate and multivariate analyses. The results of the univariate analysis showed that gender, stage, and risk scores were associated with OS. The results of the multivariate analysis showed that gender, stage, and risk scores were also associated with OS (**Figure 5B**).

In the training and validation cohorts, it is evident that the starvation-related gene prognostic model we constructed can act as an independent prognostic factor in patients with liver cancer. areas under the curve (AUC) values in the training and validation sets

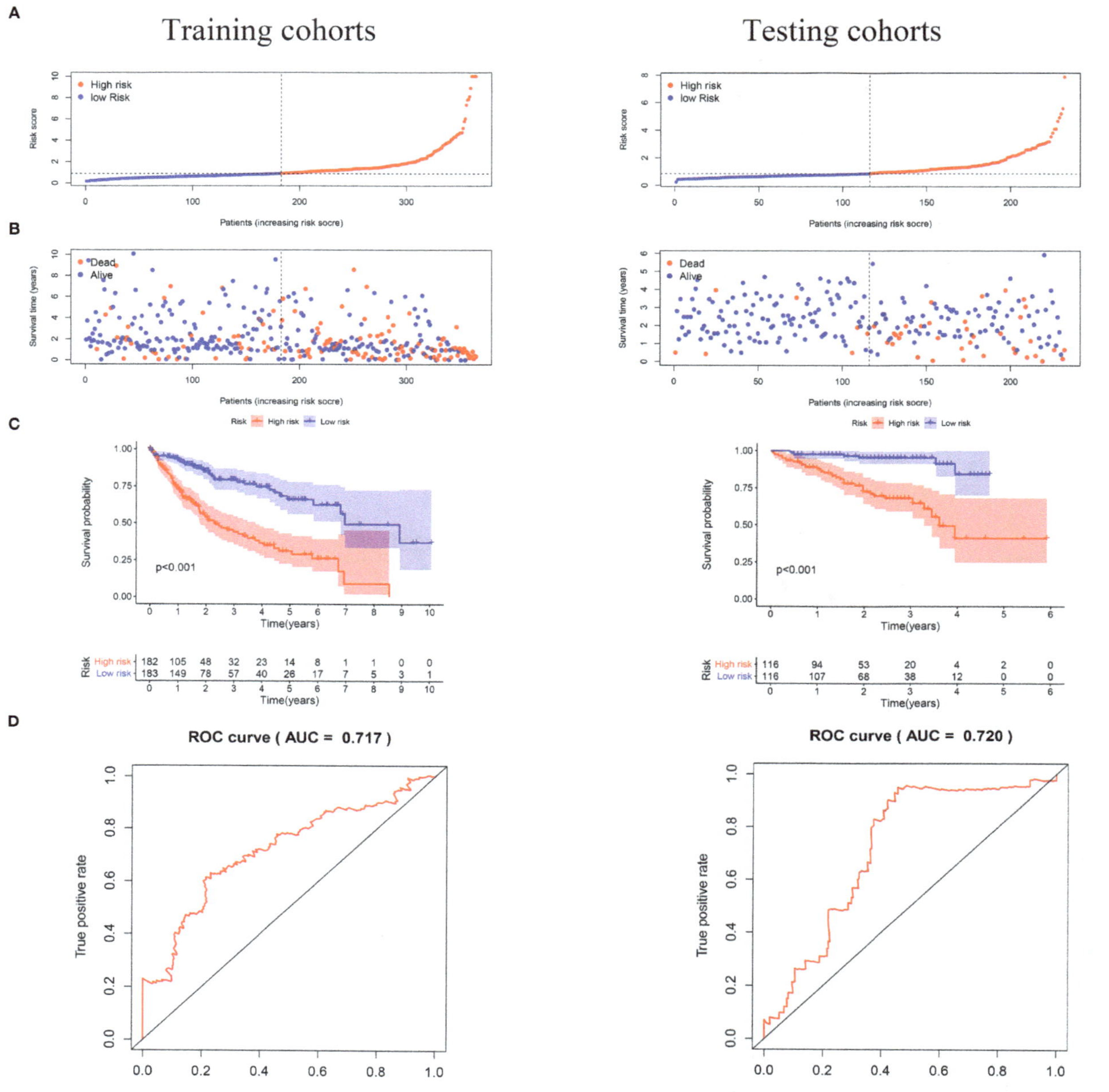

FIGURE 4 | In the training and validation cohorts, the risk score based on the 9-mRNA signature predicted the OS of patients with liver cancer. **(A, B)** Risk distribution and survival status of each patient according to the 9-mRNA signature. **(C)** In the training and validation cohort, Kaplan-Meier curves showed survival outcomes for the high- and low-risk groups. **(D)** Time-dependent ROC curve of the 5 years OS was predicted with the 9-mRNA signature in the training and validation sets.

were 0.745 and 0.731, respectively, indicating high accuracy of the risk score as an independent prognostic factor (**Figure 5C**).

Identification of Differential Starvation-Related Genes Associated With Prognosis in Patients With HCC

We further analyzed the relationship between the model of genes related to starvation and clinical characteristics. It is evident that the model is not related to age and gender (**Figures 6A, B**) but is closely related to the liver cancer grade and liver cancer stage (**Figures 6C, D**). The higher the stage and grade of the patients with increased risk value, the higher the model of hunger-related gene construction and HCC progression were closely related.

Stratified Analysis

We conducted a stratified analysis of age, sex, staging, and grading to verify the accuracy of our model. We divided the patients into low- and high-risk groups based on the median risk

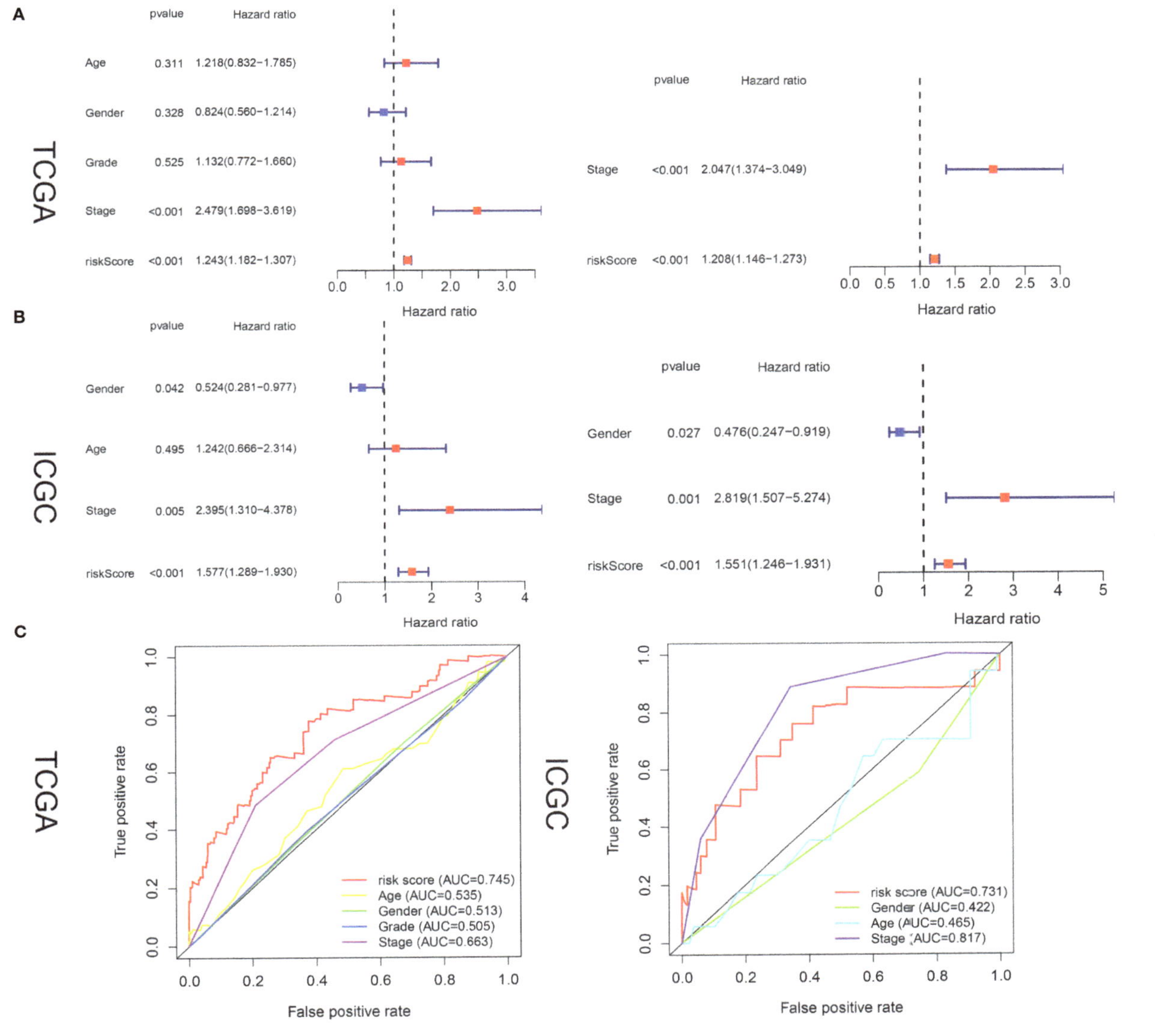

FIGURE 5 | Estimated prognostic accuracy of the starvation-related mRNAs prognostic signature and other clinicopathological variables in HCC patients in the training and validation cohorts. **(A, B)** In the training and validation cohorts, univariate and multivariate analyses were performed for risk scores and each clinical feature. **(C)** Time-dependent ROC curve of risk scores and clinical features were predicted in the training and validation sets at 5 years.

score. The results showed that our model had excellent predictive significance at ages > 65 years and < 65 years for both males and females, grade 1–2 and grade 3–4, stage 1–2 and levels 3-4 (**Figures 7A–D**).

Establishment of a Nomogram Based on Starvation-Related Genes

To provide clinicians with a practical clinical tool for predicting 3-year and 5-year OS incidence in liver cancer patients, we constructed a nomogram based on clinicopathological characteristics (age, sex, grade, stage) and risk score based on the 9-mRNA signature (**Figure 8A**). The 3-year and 5-year overall survival (OS) calibration curve is a better predictor than the ideal model (**Figures 8B, C**).

Analysis of Biological Processes Associated With Starvation-Related Genes

The expression level of EHMT2, HNRNPL, EIF2S1, RRP8, FOXK1, CAD FOXK2, and MYBBP1A increased with an increase in the risk coefficient of the patient, while the expression level of PPARGC1A decreases with an increase in the risk coefficient (**Figure 9A**). The expression level of EHMT2, HNRNPL, EIF2S1, RRP8, FOXK1, CAD FOXK2, and MYBBP1A was significantly higher in cancer, while the expression of PPARGC1A was lower in liver cancer (**Figure 9B**). **Figure 9C**

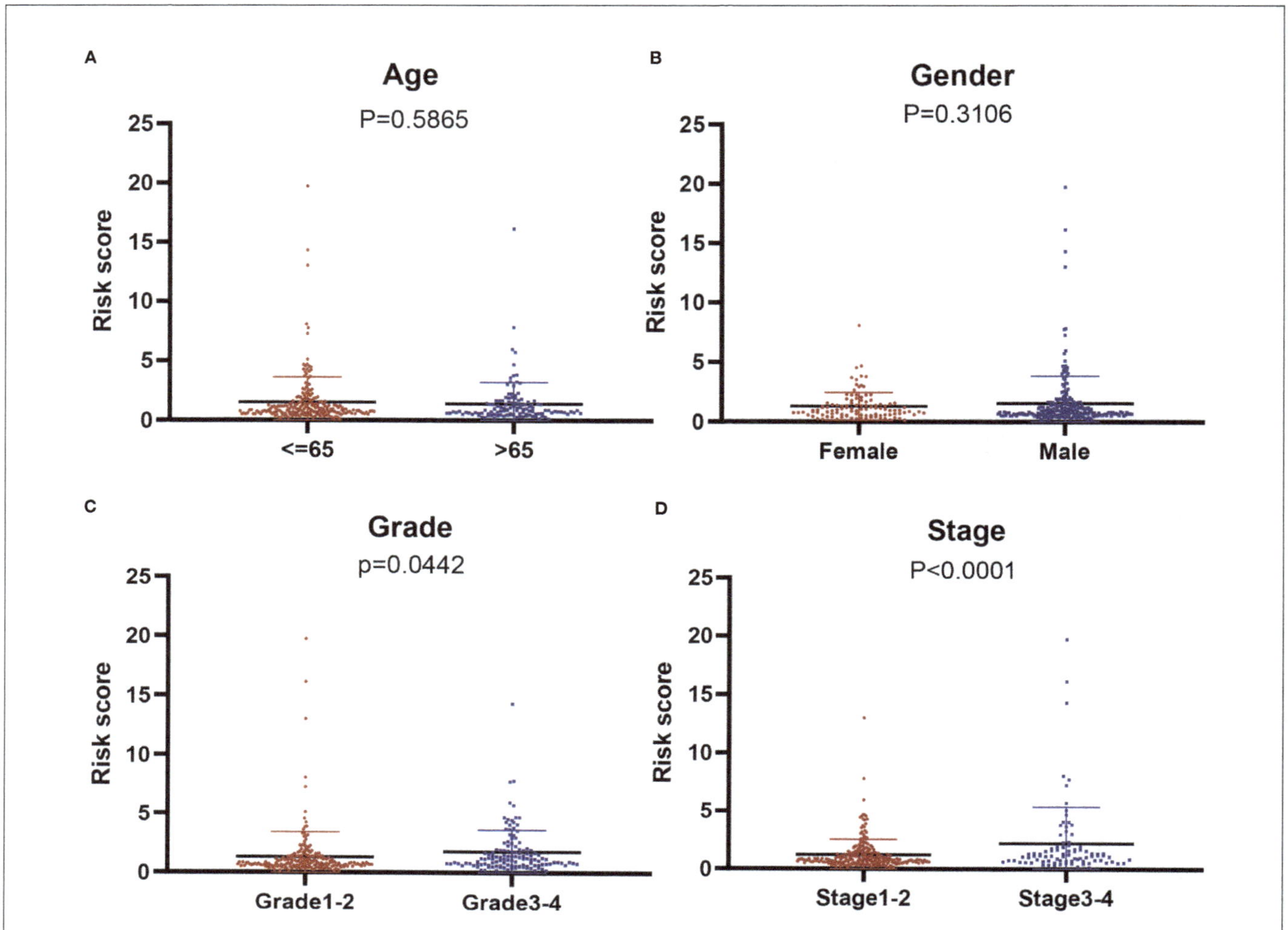

FIGURE 6 | The correlation of our signature with the clinicopathological characters of HCC. **(A)** Age (≥ 65 *vs.* < 6 5 years; P = 0,5865), **(B)** gender (male *vs.* female; P = 0.3106), **(C)** tumor grade (grade 1-2 *vs.* 3-4; P = 0.0442) **(D)** tumor stage (stage 3-4 *vs.* 1-2; P < 0.001).

shows the correlation of genes in the nine models. CAD and HNRNPL had the strongest positive correlation, while PPARGC1A and EHMT2 had the strongest negative correlation. GSEA was conducted to identify starvation-related biological processes and carcinogenic signaling pathways. The results revealed that "Hallmark analysis" gene sets involving cell cycle signals, PI3K/AKT/mTOR pathway, glycolysis, and p53 pathways related to cancer biological processes were enriched in the high-risk group. In addition, several typical pathways from the GO and KEGG genomes, including cell cycle pathways, mTOR signaling pathways, and apoptotic responses, were highly enriched in high-risk phenotypes (**Figures 9D–F**).

Knockdown of EIF2S1 Inhibits Cell Invasion and Migration in HCC

As shown in **Figures 10A, B**, EIF2S1 expression level in liver cancer is increased and is closely related to the degree of malignancy and prognosis of the disease. Thehigher the expression level of EIF2S1, the worse the prognosis of patients. It can be seen from **Figures 10C, D** that EIF2S1 expression levels were higher in HCC patients with high stage or grade HCC. EIF2S1 expression and phosphorylation levels were higher when HCC cells 3B and Huh-7 were in the starvation state (**Figures 10E, F**). **Figure 10G** further demonstrated that starvation could increase EIF2S1 expression in HCC cells Huh-7. Hunger and false hunger can induce cancer metastasis (10). We knocked down the expression levels of EIF2S1 in HCC cells 3B and Huh-7 (**Figure 10H**). EIF2S1 knockdown can reduce the invasive and metastatic ability of HCC cells 3B and Huh-7, both under starvation and normal conditions (**Figure 10I**). In addition, upon EIF2S1 knockdown in Huh-7 cells, the protein expression of E-cadherin increased while that of Vimentin decreased, suggesting that EIF2S1 may affect the invasion and metastasis ability of HCC cells through EMT (**Figure 10J**).

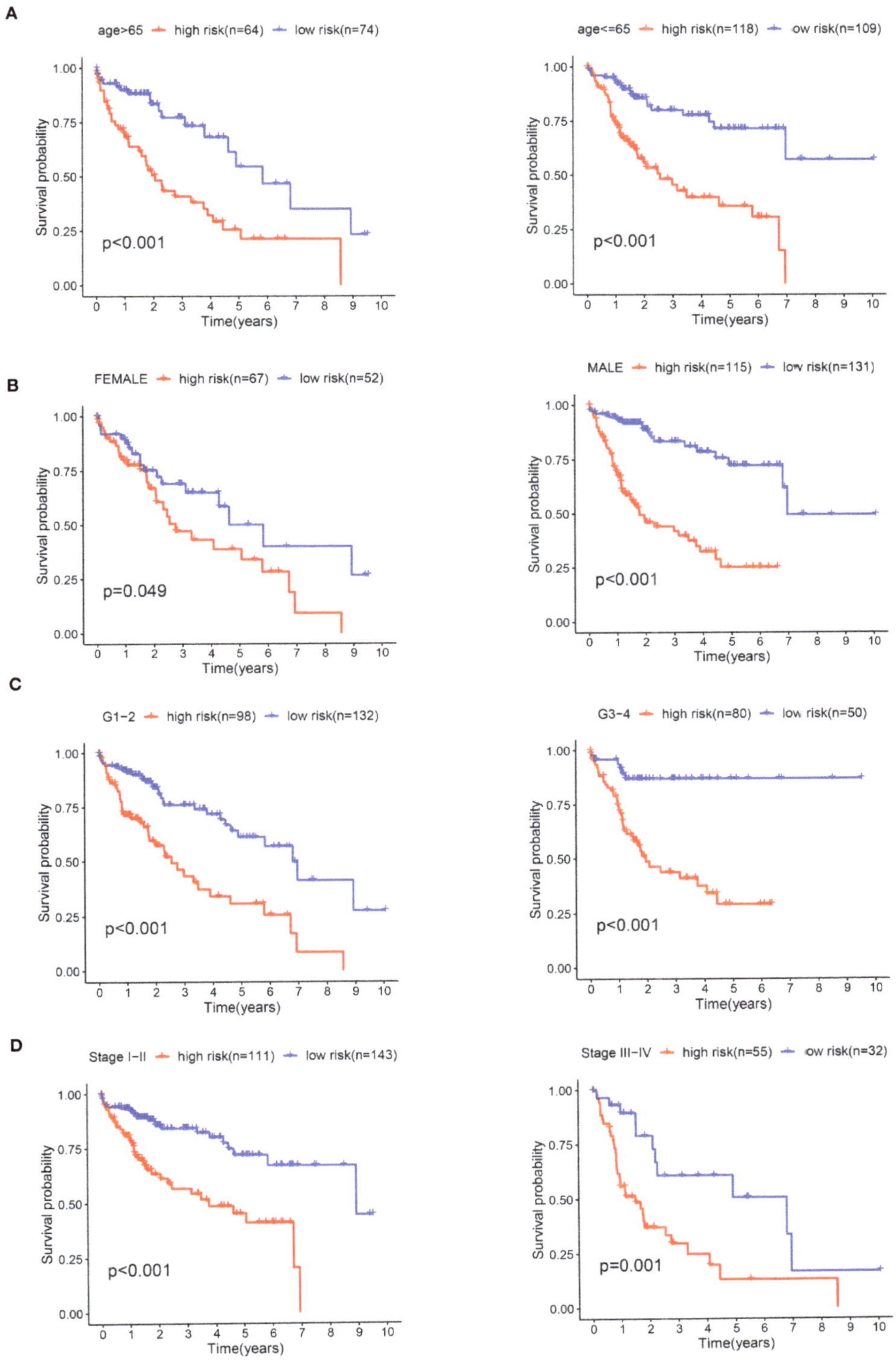

FIGURE 7 | The survival rates of high- and low-risk HCC patients stratified by different clinicopathological characteristics. Kaplan-Meier survival curve analysis shows overall survival (OS) rates of high- and low-risk HCC patients from the TCGA database stratified by age (≤ 65 *vs.* > 65) **(A)**, gender (male *vs.* female) **(B)**, tumor grades (high grade *vs.* low grade) **(C)**, stages (stages I and II *vs.* stages III and IV) **(D)**.

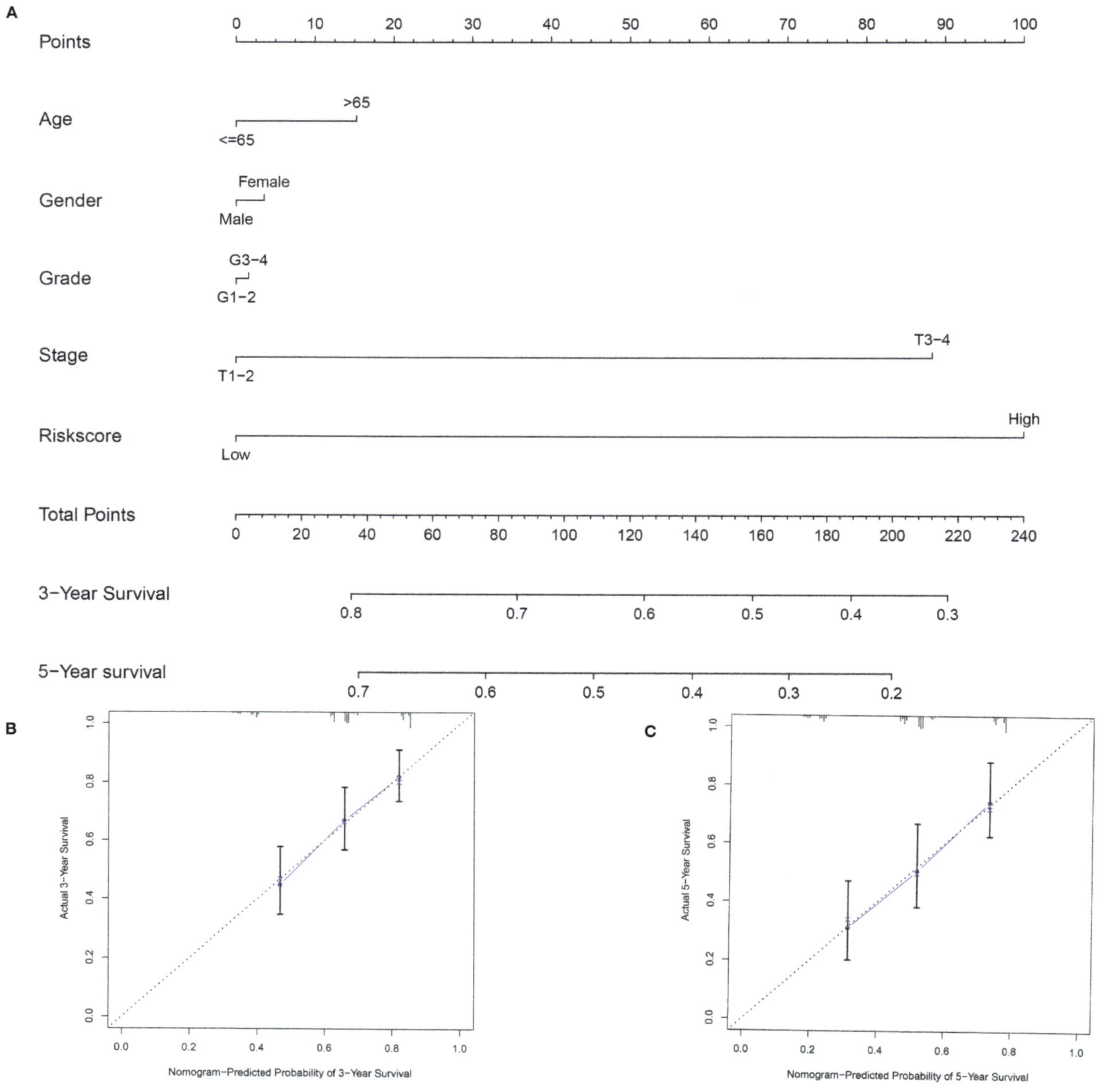

FIGURE 8 | An established nomogram for predicting OS. **(A)** Construction and validation of the prognostic nomogram with starvation-related mRNA prognostic signature risk score as one of the parameters in TCGA. Calibration curve of the nomogram for the prediction of 3- **(B)** and 5-year OS **(C)**.

DISCUSSION

An increasing amount of evidence indicates that the interaction between the tumor microenvironment and tumor cells is closely related to the occurrence and development of tumors (15). Wang et al. reported that stromal components of liver cancer contribute to the malignant progression of cancer by stimulating proliferation, migration, and invasion of cancer cells and activating angiogenesis (16). Due to dysregulation of cancer growth metabolism and inadequate nutrient supply, especially glucose deficiency, nutritional deprivation in cancer is a common condition in the tumor microenvironment (17). In bladder cancer, hunger leads to autophagy, increasing cancer cell invasive and metastatic potentials (13). In oral squamous cell carcinoma (OSCC), the expression of the glycolytic enzyme phosphofructokinase-platelets (PFKP) is significantly elevated under starvation conditions, and PFKP

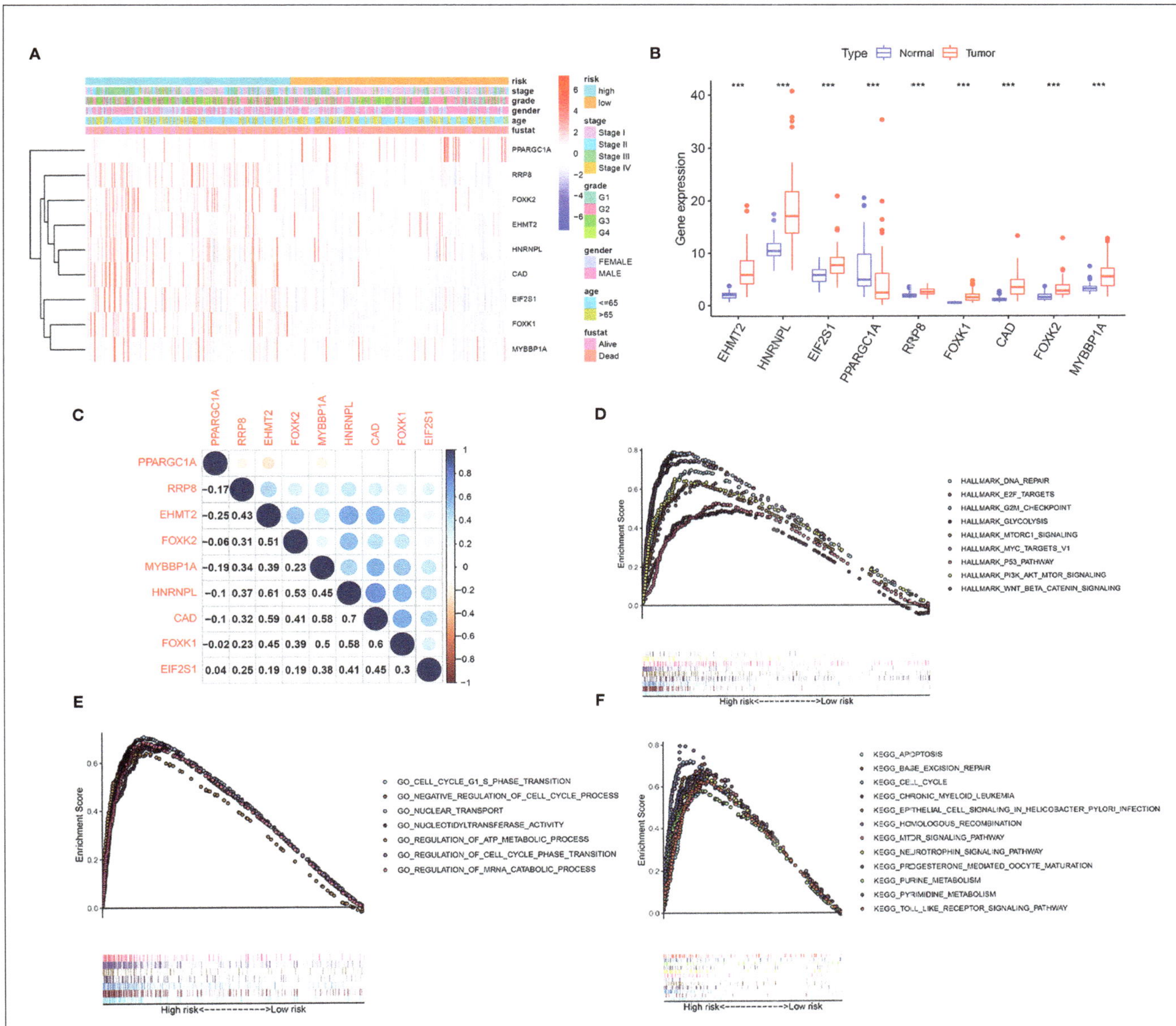

FIGURE 9 | Identification of the 9 starvation-related genes. **(A)** Risk factor score, clinical features, and expression of 9 mRNAs in each patient. **(B)** Expression of 9 mRNAs in hepatocellular carcinoma and its adjacent tissues. ***P < 0.001 vs adjacent tissues. **(C)** Correlation between 9 mRNAs. **(D)** Hallmark, **(E)** GO, and **(F)** KEGG associated with signature-based risk score were performed by GSEA with nominal P-value < 0.05.

knockdown inhibits starvation-mediated glycolysis, autophagy, and EMT in OSCC cells, thus promoting the malignant progression of OSCC (18). Glucose starvation can promote apoptosis of the TNBC cell line MDA-MB-231 and reduce its migration potential, therefore, suggesting a role for nutritional restriction in carcinogenesis (19). Starvation induces autophagy to capture and degrade intracellular proteins and organelles in lysosomes, recycling intracellular components to fuel metabolism and survival (20). Autophagy is closely related to drug resistance, stem cell resistance, and EMT in cancer (21–23). Increasing evidence shows that hunger is closely related to the occurrence and development of cancer.

With the limitation of a single gene as a prognostic factor, an increasing number of studies have shown that mRNA-constructed models can be a good independent prognostic factor for cancer. In pancreatic ductal adenocarcinoma, the model constructed using 6-mRNAs can be an independent prognostic factor and is closely related to the grade of pancreatic ductal adenocarcinoma (24). In HCC, Xie et al. described a new model comprising seven gene compositions closely related to patient prognosis (25). Another

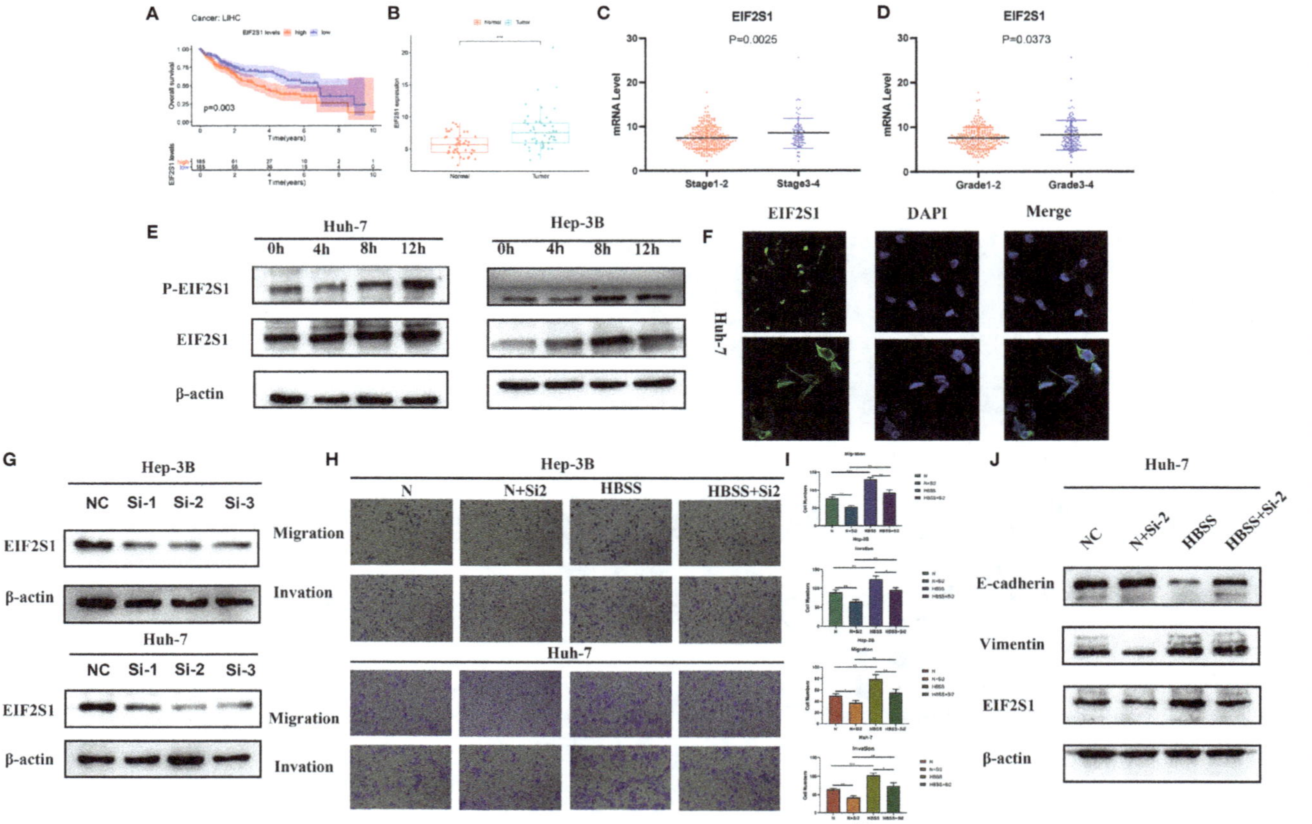

FIGURE 10 | Effect of EIF2S1 on cell migration and invasion in HCC cells. **(A)** Kaplan-Meier curves show survival outcomes in patients with high and low EIF2S1 expression. **(B)** EIF2S1 expression in hepatocellular carcinoma and its adjacent tissues. **(C, D)** EIF2S1 expression in early and advanced HCC. **(E, F)** EIF2S1 expression in 3B and Huh-7 cells was induced by starvation. **(G)** Western blotting was used to detect the expression of EIF2S1 in siRNA-transfected huh-7 and 3B cells. **(H, I)** Transwell assay was used to assess the starvation-induced migration and invasion of hepatocellular carcinoma cells after EIF2S1 transfection (100x magnification). *P < 0.05, **P < 0.01 and ***P < 0.001 *vs* NC (Huh-7) or NC (Hep-3B). **(J)** Western blots showing the levels of the EIF2S1, E-cadherin, and vimentin proteins.

four-gene model is a good predictor of survival in patients with lung adenocarcinoma with lymph node metastasis (26). Xie et al. identifiedfour models of metastasis-related gene composition as good prognostic factors for breast cancer patients (27). Wu et al. constructed a model of nine genes in renal cell carcinoma that could predict the prognosis of stage III clear cell renal cell carcinoma (28).

Furthermore, cancer cells reprogram their metabolism to sustain their rapid growth; Zhang et al. analyzed the mechanisms underlying dysregulated glucose metabolite-related pathways in HCC to identify diagnostic, prognostic, or therapeutic targets for HCC (29). Therefore, a starvation-related mRNA signature may be a new marker for liver cancer malignancy and a potential indicator of prognosis in liver cancer patients.

Here, we first constructed a model with nine hunger-related genes and verified the model accuracy through an external cohort. Our study shows that our model is associated with the malignant progression of HCC and can act as an independent prognostic factor. We constructed a nomogram composed of models and clinical features to predict the prognosis of patients and verified the accuracy of the nomogram prediction. We further analyzed the core gene EIF2S2 for protein interaction in the nine modeled genes. *In vitro* experiments showed that the expression and phosphorylation of EIF2S1 were significantly increased following starvation induction. After EIF2S1 expression was inhibited, the invasion, and metastatic ability of HCC cells were lower under starvation.

We divided patients into high- and low-risk groups according to the median risk value. Through GSEA, we found that the MTORC1 and cell cycle-related pathways were significantly enriched in high-risk patients. The MORTC1 signal pathway is closely related to cell metabolism, growth, and autophagy (30). MTORC1 can promote the transport, processing, and synthesis of SREBPs (a family of important transcription factors for lipid synthesis), thus playing an important role in promoting fat formation (31). Rapamycin complex 1 (mTORC1) maintains cell homeostasis by linking environmental cues, including the use of nutrients in glioblastoma; hunger induces autophagy that forces tumor cells in the G1 phase, leaving them in a resting state. These factors enhance glioblastoma cell survival and chemical resistance (32). We speculate that a similar mechanism might be at play in HCC; however, this must be verified experimentally.

Growth factors and metabolic process-related stress might further amplify the perceived fluctuations in extracellular and intracellular nutrients, thereby regulating cell growth, metabolism, and survival (33). Of note, EIF2S1 plays an important role in protein translation initiation (10), and its expression is significantly increased after chemotherapy in breast cancer patients. It can promote the survival of breast cancer cells during chemotherapy (34). EIF2S1 interacts with TOR signaling modulator-like (TIPRL) proteins to induce autophagy and enhance lung cancer malignancy (35). In our study, we found that starvation induction can promote the expression of EIF2S1 and P-EIF2s1 in HCC. EIF2S1 can affect the invasion and metastasis ability of liver cancer.

In conclusion, a nine starvation-related mRNA signature correlated with HCC progression and prognosis and could be used as independent prognostic molecular biomarkers for predicting HCC survival.

AUTHOR CONTRIBUTIONS

DL developed the study concept and design, performed data acquisition and analysis, and drafted the manuscript. YC performed the bioinformatics and statistical data analyses. YZ and GH constructed the figures and tables. FL was responsible for the integrity of the entire study and manuscript review. All authors contributed to the article and approved the submitted version.

ACKNOWLEDGMENTS

We appreciated TCGA database and ICGC for providing the original data.

REFERENCES

1. Siegel RL, Miller KD, Jemal A. Cancer Statistics, 2020. *CA Cancer J Clin* (2020) 70:7–30. doi: 10.3322/caac.21590
2. Yang JD, Hainaut P, Gores GJ, Amadou A, Plymoth A, Roberts LR. A Global 391 View of Hepatocellular Carcinoma: Trends, Risk, Prevention and Management. *Nat Rev Gastroenterol Hepatol* (2019) 16:589–604. doi: 10.1038/s41575-019-0186-y
3. Bray F, Ferlay J, Soerjomataram I, Siegel RL, Torre LA, Jemal A. Global Cancer Statistics 2018: GLOBOCAN Estimates of Incidence and Mortality Worldwide for 36cancers in 185 Countries. *CA Cancer J Clin* (2018) 68:394–424. doi: 10.3322/caac.21492
4. Younossi Z, Stepanova M, Ong JP, Jacobson IM, Bugianesi E, Duseja A, et al. Nonalcoholic Steatohepatitis Is the Fastest Growing Cause of Hepatocellula Carcinoma in Liver Transplant Candidates. *Clin Gastroenterol Hepatol* (2019) 17:748–55.e3. doi: 10.1016/j.cgh.2018.05.057
5. Mizushima N. Autophagy: Process and Function. *Genes Dev* (2007) 21:2861–73. doi: 10.1101/gad.1599207
6. Pattabiraman DR, Weinberg RA. Tackling the Cancer Stem Cells - What Hallenges Do They Pose. *Nat Rev Drug Discov* (2014) 13:497–512. doi: 10.1038/nrd4253402
7. Butturini E, Carcereri de Prati A, Boriero D, Mariotto S. Tumor Dormancy and Interplay With Hypoxic Tumor Microenvironment. *Int J Mol Sci* (2019) 20:4305. doi: 10.3390/ijms20174305
8. Vaupel P, Kallinowski F, Okunieff P. Blood Flow, Oxygen and Nutrient Supply, and Metabolic Microenvironment of Human Tumors: A Review. *Cancer Res* (1989) 49:6449–65.
9. Pavlova NN, Thompson CB. The Emerging Hallmarks of Cancer Metabolism. *Cell Metab* (2016) 23:27–47. doi: 10.1016/j.cmet.2015.12.006
10. García-Jiménez C, Goding CR. Starvation and Pseudo-Starvation as Drivers of Cancer Metastasis Through Translation Reprogramming. *Cell Metab* (2019) 29:254–67. doi: 10.1016/j.cmet.2018.11.018
11. Kardideh B, Samimi Z, Norooznezhad F, Kiani S, Mansouri K. Autophagy, Cancer and Angiogenesis: Where is the Link. *Cell Biosci* (2019) 9:65. doi: 10.1186/s13578-019-0327-6
12. White E, Mehnert JM, Chan CS. Autophagy, Metabolism, and Cancer. *Clin Cancer Res* (2015) 21:5037–46. doi: 10.1158/1078-0432.CCR-15-0490
13. Tong H, Yin H, Hossain MA, Wang Y, Wu F, Dong X, et al. Starvation-Nduced Autophagy Promotes the Invasion and Migration of Human Bladder Cancer Cells via TGF-β1/Smad3-Mediated Epithelial-Mesenchymal Transition Activation. *J Cell Biochem* (2019) 120:5118–27. doi: 10.1002/jcb.27788
14. Li J, Yang B, Zhou Q, Wu Y, Shang D, Guo Y, et al. Autophagy Promotes Hepatocellular Carcinoma Cell Invasion Through Activation of Epithelial-Esenchymal Transition. *Carcinogenesis* (2013) 34:1343–51. doi: 10.1093/carcin/bgt063
15. Hanahan D, Weinberg RA. Hallmarks of Cancer: The Next Generation. *Cell* (2011) 144:646–74. doi: 10.1016/j.cell.2011.02.013
16. Hernandez-Gea V, Toffanin S, Friedman SL, Llovet JM. Role of the Microenvironment in the Pathogenesis and Treatment of Hepatocellular Carcinoma. *Gastroenterology* (2013) 144:512–27. doi: 10.1053/j.gastro.2013.01.002
17. Grasmann G, Smolle E, Olschewski H, Leithner K. Gluconeogenesis in Cancer Cells - Repurposing of a Starvation-Induced Metabolic Pathway. *Biochim Biophys Acta Rev Cancer* (2019) 1872:24–36. doi: 10.1016/j.bbcan.2019.05.006
18. Chen G, Liu H, Zhang Y, Liang J, Zhu Y, Zhang M, et al. Silencing PFKP Inhibits Starvation-Induced Autophagy, Glycolysis, and Epithelial Mesenchymal Transition in Oral Squamous Cell Carcinoma. *Exp Cell Res* (2018) 370:46–57. doi: 10.1016/j.yexcr.2018.06.007
19. Raut GK, Chakrabarti M, Pamarthy D, Bhadra MP. Glucose Starvation-Induced Oxidative Stress Causes Mitochondrial Dysfunction and Apoptosis *via* Prohibitin Upregulation in Human Breast Cancer Cells. *Free Radic Biol Med* (2019) 145:428–41. doi: 10.1016/j.freeradbiomed.2019.09.020
20. Amaravadi R, Kimmelman AC, White E. Recent Insights Into the Function of Autophagy in Cancer. *Genes Dev* (2016) 30:1913–30. doi: 10.1101/gad.287524.116
21. Li YJ, Lei YH, Yao N, Wang CR, Hu N, Ye WC, et al. Autophagy and Ultidrug Resistance in Cancer. *Chin J Cancer* (2017) 36:52. doi: 10.1186/s40880-017-0219-2
22. Smith AG, Macleod KF. Autophagy, Cancer Stem Cells and Drug Resistance. *J Pathol* (2019) 247:708–18. doi: 10.1002/path.5222
23. Chen HT, Liu H, Mao MJ, Tan Y, Mo XQ, Meng XJ, et al. Crosstalk Between Autophagy and Epithelial-Mesenchymal Transition and its Application in Cancer Therapy. *Mol Cancer* (2019) 18:101. doi: 10.1186/s12943-019-1030-2
24. Zhou C, Zhao Y, Yin Y, Hu Z, Atyah M, Chen W, et al. A Robust 6-mRNA Signature for Prognosis Prediction of Pancreatic Ductal Adenocarcinoma. *Int J Biol Sci* (2019) 15:2282–95. doi: 10.7150/ijbs.32899
25. Xie H, Liu S, Zhang Z, Chen P, Tao Y. A Novel Seven-Gene Signature as Prognostic Biomarker in Hepatocellular Carcinoma. *J Cancer* (2020) 11:5768–81. doi: 10.7150/jca.44573
26. Wang Y, Zhang Q, Gao Z, Xin S, Zhao Y, Zhang K, et al. A Novel 4-Gene Signature for Overall Survival Prediction in Lung Adenocarcinoma Patients With Lymph Node Metastasis. *Cancer Cell Int* (2019) 19:100. doi: 10.1186/s12935-019-0822-1
27. Xie X, Wang J, Shi D, Zou Y, Xiong Z, Li X, et al. Identification of a 4-mRNA Metastasis-Related Prognostic Signature for Patients With Breast Cancer. *J Cell Mol Med* (2019) 23:1439–47. doi: 10.1111/jcmm.14049
28. Wu J, Jin S, Gu W, Wan F, Zhang H, Shi G, et al. Construction and Validation of a 9-Gene Signature for Predicting Prognosis in Stage III Clear Cell Renal Cell Carcinoma. *Front Oncol* (2019) 9:152. doi: 10.3389/fonc.2019.00152

29. Zhang X, Li J, Ghoshal K, Fernandez S, Li L. Identification of a Subtype of Hepatocellular Carcinoma With Poor Prognosis Based on Expression of Genes Within the Glucose Metabolic Pathway. *Cancers (Basel)* (2019) 11:2023. doi: 10.3390/cancers11122023
30. Condon KJ, Sabatini DM. Nutrient Regulation of mTORC1 at a Glance. *J Cell Sci* (2019) 132:jcs222570. doi: 10.1242/jcs.222570
31. Han J, Wang Y. mTORC1 Signaling in Hepatic Lipid Metabolism. *Protein Cell* (2018) 9:145–51. doi: 10.1007/s13238-017-0409-3
32. Rabanal-Ruiz Y, Otten EG, Korolchuk VI. mTORC1 as the Main Gateway to Autophagy. *Essays Biochem* (2017) 61:565–84. doi: 10.1042/EBC20170027
33. Wang L, Shang Z, Zhou Y, Hu X, Chen Y, Fan Y, et al. Autophagy Mediates Glucose Starvation-Induced Glioblastoma Cell Quiescence and Chemoresistance Through Coordinating Cell Metabolism, Cell Cycle, and Survival. *Cell Death Dis* (2018) 9:213. doi: 10.1038/s41419-017-0242-x
34. Chen L, He J, Zhou J, Xiao Z, Ding N, Duan Y, et al. EIF2A Promotes Cell Survival During Paclitaxel Treatment *In Vitro* and *In Vivo*. *J Cell Mol Med* (2019) 23:6060–71. doi: 10.1111/jcmm.14469
35. Jeon SJ, Ahn JH, Halder D, Cho HS, Lim JH, Jun SY, et al. TIPRL Potentiates Survival of Lung Cancer by Inducing Autophagy Through the eIF2α-ATF4 Pathway. *Cell Death Dis* (2019) 10:959. doi: 10.1038/s41419-019-2190-0

6

A Novel Post-Operative ALRI Model Accurately Predicts Clinical Outcomes of Resected Hepatocellular Carcinoma Patients

Minjun Liao[1‡], Jiarun Sun[1‡], Qifan Zhang[2‡], Cuirong Tang[1], Yuchen Zhou[2,3], Mingrong Cao[4], Tao Chen[5], Chengguang Hu[1], Junxiong Yu[6], Yangda Song[1], Meng Li[1], Weijia Liao[6†] and Yuanping Zhou[1*†]*

[1] Guangdong Provincial Key Laboratory of Gastroenterology, Department of Gastroenterology and Hepatology Unit, Nanfang Hospital, Southern Medical University, Guangzhou, China, [2] Department of Hepatobiliary Surgery, Nanfang Hospital, Southern Medical University, Guangzhou, China, [3] Department of General Surgery, Integrated Hospital of Traditional Chinese Medicine, Southern Medical University, Guangzhou, China, [4] Department of Hepatobiliary Surgery, the First Affiliated Hospital of Jinan University, Guangzhou, China, [5] Department of Hepatobiliary Surgery, Sun Yat-Sen Memorial Hospital, Sun Yat-Sen University, Guangzhou, China, [6] Laboratory of Hepatobiliary and Pancreatic Surgery, Affiliated Hospital of Guilin Medical University, Guilin, China

***Correspondence:**
Weijia Liao
liaoweijia288@163.com
Yuanping Zhou
yuanpingzhou@163.com*

Background: Hepatocellular carcinoma (HCC) is one of the leading malignant tumors worldwide. Prognosis and long-term survival of HCC remain unsatisfactory, even after radical resection, and many non-invasive predictors have been explored for post-operative patients. Most prognostic prediction models were based on preoperative clinical characteristics and pathological findings. This study aimed to investigate the prognostic value of a newly constructed nomogram, which incorporated post-operative aspartate aminotransferase to lymphocyte ratio index (ALRI).

Methods: A total of 771 HCC patients underwent radical resection from three medical centers were enrolled and grouped into the training cohort (n = 416) and validation cohort (n = 355). Prognostic prediction potential of ALRI was assessed by receiver operating curve (ROC) analysis. The Cox regression model was used to identify independent prognostic factors. Nomograms for overall survival (OS) and disease-free survival (DFS) were constructed and further validated externally.

Results: The ROC analysis ranked ALRI as the most effective prediction marker for resected HCC patients, with the cut-off value determined at 22.6. Higher ALRI level positively correlated with larger tumor size, higher tumor node metastasis (TNM) stage, and inversely with lower albumin level and shorter OS and DFS. Nomograms for OS and DFS were capable of discriminating HCC patients into different risk-groups.

Conclusions: Post-operative ALRI was of prediction value for HCC prognosis. This novel nomogram may categorize HCC patients into different risk groups, and offer individualized surveillance reference for post-operative patients.

Keywords: Hepatocellular carcinoma, ALRI, biomarker, post-operative, prognosis

INTRODUCTION

Hepatocellular carcinoma (HCC) is the sixth most common malignant cancer, and the fourth leading cause of cancer-related death in the world (1). Liver cancer results from multiple factors, chief among them is chronic hepatitis B virus (HBV) infection (2, 3), which is endemic in east-Asian and sub-Saharan African regions (4), where 85% of liver cancer incidence occurred (5). Globally, 248 million people are chronically infected with HBV, and a significant portion of them may develop into cirrhosis and liver cancer in the absence of early detection and effective treatments (6). Liver cancer patients could benefit from several radical treatments including surgical resection, regional ablation, and liver transplantation (7). To date, curative resection remains to be a first choice if cancer lesion deemed resectable. But recurrence or distant metastasis were reported in 60–70% patients within 5 years after surgery (8, 9). It is critical that HCC patients participate in post-operative follow-ups and monitorings.

New tumor biomarkers were identified to detect liver cancer in early-stage (10–12), and various prognostic models that aim to predict post-operative prognosis for liver cancer have been developed, such as aspartate aminotransferase to lymphocyte ratio index (ALRI) reported in our previous study and other studies (13, 14); moreover, systemic immune-inflammation index (SII) and neutrophil to lymphocyte ratio (NLR) were reported frequently in many studies (15–19). However, these models mainly used the preoperative data and few incorporated long-term follow-up results. The importance of long-term follow up data in predicting prognosis lies in the fact that clinical outcome of each patient can be determined through early detection of recurrent cancer or metastasis and new treatment options may be selected during the follow-ups. The prognosis prediction mainly based on preoperative factors is insufficient, while accumulated data and results from postoperative surveillance may indicate how HCC patients generally further develop after surgery. Among the indices mentioned above, which one of them could tell prognosis of patients when applying the post-operative data remains unstudied; and whether we could made more accurate prognosis prediction or not remains a challenging task. In this study, we made further investigation into the ALRI index using hematological examination results obtained 2 months after operation, as well as further evaluation of the underlying prediction potency of the novel nomogram which incorporated post-operative ALRI.

MATERIALS AND METHODS

Patients Enrollment

A total of 1,169 HCC patients were initially retrospectively analyzed, and 648 patients among them underwent hepatic resection in the Nanfang Hospital, Southern Medical University and the First Affiliated Hospital of Jinan University from April 2009 to December 2016, and the remaining 521 patients received hepatic resection in the Affiliated Hospital of Guilin Medical University from October 2008 through March 2017. The exclusion criteria were as follows: 1) non-radical surgery; 2) postoperative pathological diagnosis as non-HCC; 3) not the first primary cancer; 4) IV stage of TNM stage; 5) received liver transplantation; 6) died in 2 months after operation; 7) with clinical evidence of infection, immune-system diseases, or hematological diseases etc.; 8) lost contact in follow-ups. Finally, 771 patients were eligible for final analyses, 416 from Nanfang Hospital of Southern Medical University and the First Affiliated Hospital of Jinan University as training cohort and 355 patients from the Affiliated Hospital of Guilin Medical University as validation cohort. The flowchart of patient selection is shown in **Figure 1**.

Clinicopathologic Characteristics of HCC Patients

HCC patients' baseline information and clinical data were collected, including (1) preoperative demographics and medical history: age, gender, family history, drinking and smoking history, and hepatitis B virus infection history etc.; (2) hematological examination data obtained during follow-up of 2 months after operation: white blood cell (WBC), neutrophil, lymphocyte, and platelet count; albumin, aspartate aminotransferase (AST), alanine aminotransferase (ALT), gamma-glutamyl transpeptidase (GGT), total bilirubin (TBIL), α-fetoprotein (AFP), etc.; (3) the number of tumor, tumor size, Child stage and TNM stage, etc.; (4) pathological lesions of cirrhosis, and recurrence (**Table 1**). We decided to choose hematological examination results of 2 months after operation as the time-point in consideration of the reason that generally this was the first time-point during regular follow-ups. Post-operative ALRI was calculated based on the following formula: (AST value/lymphocyte count) × 10^9/U, and SII = P × N/L, NLR = N/L, where P, N, and L were the peripheral platelet, neutrophil, and lymphocyte counts, respectively. The study was approved by the research ethics committee of the Affiliated Hospital of Guilin Medical University, Nanfang Hospital of Southern Medical University and the First Affiliated Hospital of Jinan University, and conformed to the Declaration of Helsinki. Written informed consents were obtained from all patients.

Follow-Ups

All 771 patients were instructed to attend regular follow-up visits after radical resection. Tumor recurrence was monitored by testing serum AFP, hepatic function, ultrasonography, and chest radiography every 2 months for the first 2 years and every 3–6 months thereafter; and CT enhanced scanning and MRI examination were needed when recurrence were suspected during follow-ups. Average follow-up period was 36.7 months (median, 26.0 months; range, 2.0 to 84.0 months). Disease-free survival (DFS) was defined from date of surgery to date of

Abbreviations: HCC, hepatocellular carcinoma; AST, aspartate aminotransferase; ALRI, aspartate aminotransferase to lymphocyte ratio index; SII, systemic immune-inflammation index; NLR, neutrophil to lymphocyte ratio; ROC, receiver operating characteristic; OS, overall survival; DFS, disease-free survival; TNM, tumor node metastasis; HR, hazard ratios.

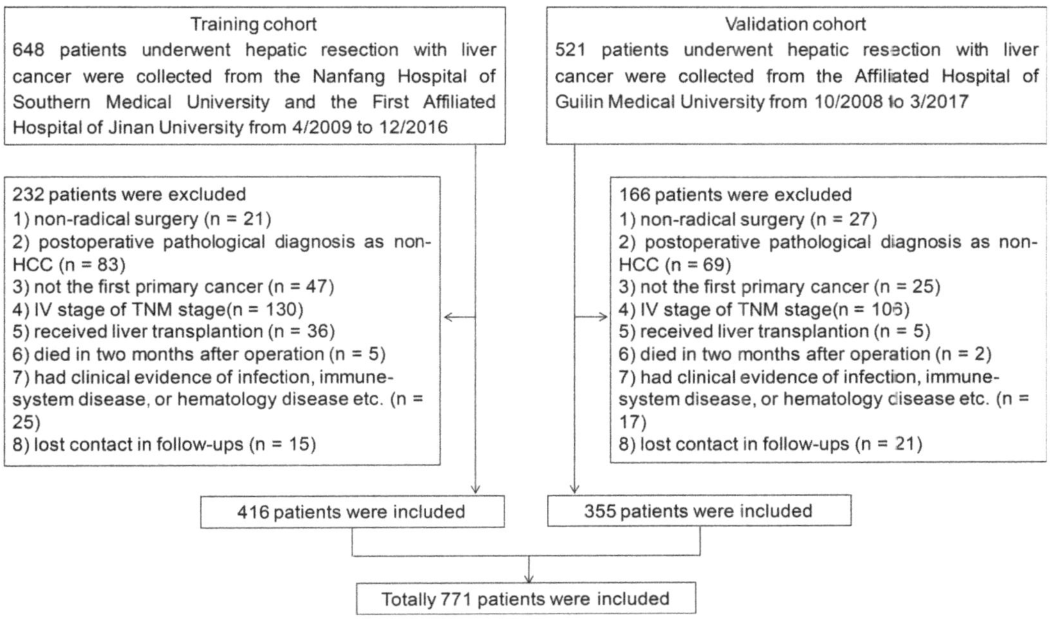

FIGURE 1 | HCC patients' enrollment flowchart.

TABLE 1 | Comparison of clinicopathological characteristics of two groups' patients.

Parameter	Total patients (n = 771)	Training cohort (Guangzhou) (n = 416)	Validation cohort (Guilin) (n = 355)	*p* value
Gender: female/male (n)	101/670	57/359	44/311	0.592
Age (years)	50.07 ± 11.41	50.47 ± 11.15	49.61 ± 11.71	0.297
HBsAg: negative/positive (n)	123/648	63/353	60/295	0.507
Family history: absent/present (n)	687/84	371/45	316/39	0.940
Alcohol abuse: absent/present (n)	420/351	238/178	182/173	0.099
Smoking: absent/present (n)	441/330	250/166	191/164	0.078
Cirrhosis: absent/present (n)	58/713	32/384	26/329	0.847
Tumor size (cm)	8.04 ± 4.53	7.90 ± 4.62	8.22 ± 4.45	0.335
Tumor number: single/multiple (n)	543/228	291/125	252/103	0.754
Child stage: A/B (n)	688/83	369/47	319/36	0.605
TNM stage: I/II/III (n)	113/287/371	66/148/202	47/139/169	0.450
Recurrence: absent/present (n)	430/341	224/192	206/149	0.244
Hematology test value 2 months after operation				
WBC ($\times10^9$/L)	6.91 ± 2.65	7.01 ± 2.63	6.80 ± 2.69	0.275
Platelets ($\times10^9$/L)	194.66 ± 92.33	200.35 ± 98.20	188.57 ± 85.69	0.079
NEUT ($\times10^9$/L)	4.42 ± 2.37	4.51 ± 2.35	4.33 ± 2.41	0.303
LYMPH ($\times10^9$/L)	1.63 ± 0.62	1.63 ± 0.66	1.62 ± 0.60	0.849
Albumin (g/L)	36.01 ± 5.99	35.68 ± 6.01	36.45 ± 5.95	0.074
Globulin (g/L)	33.68 ± 6.50	34.01 ± 6.75	33.30 ± 6.19	0.134
TBIL (μmol/L)	16.20 ± 10.78	16.10 ± 10.56	16.32 ± 11.05	0.772
DBIL (μmol/L)	7.50 ± 7.03	7.43 ± 6.82	7.58 ± 7.27	0.778
ALT (U/L)	47.03 ± 42.43	46.05 ± 42.04	48.19 ± 42.93	0.484
AST (U/L)	49.60 ± 42.03	50.81 ± 44.35	48.06 ± 38.89	0.378
GGT (U/L)	120.80 ± 110.74	117.38 ± 108.16	124.90 ± 113.78	0.361
ALP (U/L)	107.12 ± 76.69	105.80 ± 82.52	108.63 ± 68.78	0.618
AFP (ng/ml): median (IQR)	11.32 (6.31–38.95)	10.98 (5.46–32.36)	13.30 (7.50–47.33)	0.511
NLR level	3.13 ± 2.24	3.19 ± 2.20	3.06 ± 2.28	0.408
SII level	613.98 ± 528.02	630.01 ± 521.10	585.76 ± 530.46	0.172
ALRI level	35.71 ± 33.01	36.18 ± 32.63	35.20 ± 33.26	0.690

n, number of patients; HBsAg, hepatitis B surface antigen; TNM, tumor-node-metastasis; WBC, white blood cell; NEUT, neutrophil count; LYMPH, lymphocyte count; TBIL, total bilirubin; DBIL, direct bilirubin; ALT, alanine aminotransferase; AST, aspartate aminotransferase; GGT, Gamma-glutamyl transpeptidase; ALP, alkaline phosphatase; AFP, alpha-fetoprotein; IQR, interquartile range; NLR, neutrophil to lymphocyte ratio; SII, systemic immune-inflammation index; ALRI, AST to lymphocyte ratio index.

recurrence, metastasis, death, or the last follow-up; and overall survival (OS) was defined from date of surgery to date of death or the last follow-up.

Statistical Analysis

Continuous variables conforming to Gaussian distribution were expressed as mean ± standard deviation (SD) and the differences were compared using independent sample t-test, and classification factors were identified by Pearson chi-square test or Fisher exact test. All statistical analyses were conducted using SPSS 24.0 (SPSS Inc, Chicago, IL, USA) and R version 4.0.3 (https://www.rproject.org/). The ROC curve guided selecting the optimal cut-off value of post-operative ALRI and was plotted *via* timeROC package. Univariate and multivariate analyses were used to identify the independent prognostic factors for DFS and OS; and the nomogram was built *via* rms package, while the calibration curve was established by the rms package. Decision curve analysis (DCA) was based on the rmda package, and Cox proportional hazards regression model was employed to construct the novel nomogram. The performance of the novel model was evaluated by the calibration curves, and discriminatory ability was assessed by AUC of the ROC curve. Survival curve analyses were performed using the Kaplan-Meier method. Hazard ratios (HR) and 95% confidence intervals (95% CI) were calculated. $P < 0.05$ was considered statistically significant.

RESULTS

Baseline and Post-Operative Information of HCC Patients

A total of 771 patients were enrolled in the study. The training cohort and the validation cohort consisted of 416 and 355 patients, respectively. There was no significant difference in HCC patients' clinical and pathological characteristics between the training and the validation cohorts ($P > 0.05$).

Determination of the Optimal Cut-Off Value of Post-Operative ALRI

Receiver operating characteristic (ROC) curve was used to compare post-operative ALRI, SII, and NLR's prediction potential for post-operative HCC patients. ALRI in both training cohort (**Figure 2A**) and validation cohort (**Figure S1A**) had the largest area under the curve (AUC: 0.671, 95% CI: 0.623–0.716). Sensitivity and specificity reached 61.6 and 67.5%, respectively, when the optimal cut-off value set at 22.6. Furthermore, a comparison of patients' post-operative ALRI level was made between patients with different tumor size (≤6 or >6 cm), different TNM stage (I-II or III), and different albumin level (≤34 or >34 g/L), and results showed that advanced tumor (tumor size >6 cm, III stage of TNM stage, or lower albumin ≤34 g/L) had higher ALRI level ($P < 0.05$) (**Figures 2B** and **S1B**), suggesting that high ALRI might be associated with poor physical condition of HCC patients, thus leading to poor clinical outcomes.

Univariate and Multivariate Cox Regression Analyses

In the univariate analysis of training cohort, tumor size (>6 cm), multiple tumor number, TNM stage III, albumin (≤34 g/L), GGT (>45 U/L), ALP (>90 U/L), and ALRI (>22.6) were identified as significant prognostic factors of poor OS and DFS, and their hazard ratio (HR) and 95% confidence interval (95% CI) were shown in **Table 2**. After adjusting other confounding factors, a stepwise multivariate Cox proportional hazards model revealed that tumor size (HR, 1.786; 95% CI, 1.354–2.356; $P < 0.001$), TNM stage (HR, 1.802; 95% CI, 1.420–2.287; $P < 0.001$), albumin (HR, 1.448; 95% CI, 1.126–1.891; $P = 0.004$), and ALRI (HR, 1.872; 95% CI, 1.420–2.467; $P < 0.001$) were identified as independent predictive factors of OS (**Table 2**). Tumor size (HR, 1.479; 95% CI, 1.114–1.965; $P = 0.007$), TNM stage (HR, 1.642; 95% CI, 1.238–2.177; $P = 0.001$), albumin (HR, 1.547; 95%

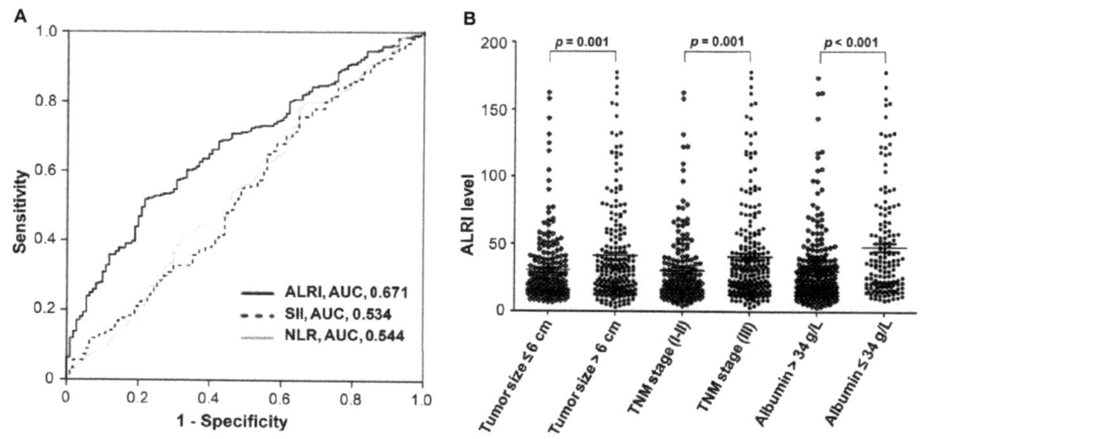

FIGURE 2 | Prognostic prediction value of ALRI for post-operative HCC patients in the training cohort and the comparison of ALRI level in different sub-groups. **(A)** Comparison of prediction performance of ALRI, SII, and NLR using the ROC analyses. **(B)** Comparison of ALRI level in different tumor size, TNM stage, and serum albumin sub-groups.

TABLE 2 | Univariate and multivariate Cox regression analyses of the clinicopathologic characteristics for OS and DFS in training cohort with HCC.

Variable	Univariate analysis			Multivariate analysis		
	HR	95% CI	*p* value	HR	95% CI	*p* value
Overall survival						
Sex (male *vs.* female)	1.134	0.810–1.587	0.463			
Age, yeas (≤55 *vs.* 55)	1.339	0.958–1.692	0.055			
HBsAg (positive *vs.* negative)	1.105	0.805–1.516	0.538			
Tumor size, cm (>6 *vs.* ≤6)	2.393	1.839–3.106	<0.001	1.786	1.354–2.356	<0.001
Tumor number (multiple *vs.* single)	1.430	1.125–1.817	0.003			
TNM stage (III *vs.* I-II)	2.593	2.014–3.230	<0.001	1.802	1.420–2.287	<0.001
Recurrence: absent/present (n)	1.020	0.814–1.278	0.863			
Albumin, g/L (≤34 *vs.* >34)	1.615	1.264–2.065	<0.001	1.448	1.126–1.891	0.004
Globulin, g/L (>33 *vs.* ≤33)	1.032	0.823–1.293	0.785			
ALT, U/L (>38 *vs.* ≤38)	1.196	0.953–1.499	0.122			
GGT, U/L (>45 *vs.* ≤45)	1.779	1.283–2.469	<0.001			
ALP, U/L (>90 *vs.* ≤90)	1.456	1.156–1.833	0.001			
AFP, ng/ml (>20 *vs.* ≤20)	1.011	0.766–1.334	0.938			
ALRI level (>22.6 *vs.* ≤22.6)	1.966	1.574–2.534	<0.001	1.872	1.420–2.467	<0.001
Disease-free survival						
Sex (male *vs.* female)	1.125	0.804–1.575	0.492			
Age, yeas (≤55 *vs.* >55)	1.320	0.944–1.669	0.105			
HBsAg (positive *vs.* negative)	1.137	0.828–1.560	0.428			
Tumor size, cm (>6 *vs.* ≤6)	2.253	1.783–2.470	<0.001	1.479	1.114–1.965	0.007
Tumor number (multiple *vs.* single)	1.503	1.182–1.911	0.001			
TNM stage (III *vs.* I-II)	2.414	1.894–3.077	<0.001	1.642	1.238–2.177	0.001
Albumin, g/L (≤34 *vs.* >34)	1.719	1.344–2.198	<0.001	1.547	1.194–2.003	0.001
Globulin, g/L (>33 *vs.* ≤33)	1.060	0.846–1.328	0.614			
ALT, U/L (>38 *vs.* ≤38)	1.249	0.996–1.566	0.055			
GGT, U/L (>45 *vs.* ≤45)	1.663	1.199–2.308	0.002			
ALP, U/L (>90 *vs.* ≤90)	1.441	1.144–1.815	0.003			
AFP, ng/ml (>20 *vs.* ≤20)	1.006	0.762–1.328	0.967			
ALRI level (>22.6 *vs.* ≤22.6)	2.081	1.657–2.612	<0.001	1.703	1.339–2.166	<0.001

HR, hazard ratio; CI, confidence interval; HBsAg, hepatitis B surface antigen; TNM, tumor-node-metastasis; ALT, alanine aminotransferase; AST, aspartate aminotransferase; GGT, Gamma-glutamyl transpeptidase; ALP, alkaline phosphatase; AFP, alpha-fetoprotein; ALRI, aspartate aminotransferase to lymphocyte ratio index.

CI, 1.194–2.003; $P = 0.001$), and ALRI (HR, 1.703; 95% CI, 1.339–2.166; $P < 0.001$) were identified as independent predictive factors of DFS (**Table 2**).

In validation cohort, the results of the univariate and multivariate analyses were very consistent with the training cohort (**Table S1**). In the multivariate analysis, ALRI remained an independent predictor for OS (HR, 1.933; 95% CI, 1.478–2.527; $P < 0.001$) and DFS (HR, 1.701; 95% CI, 1.305–2.218; $P < 0.001$).

Construction and Evaluations of Prognostic Nomograms for OS and DFS

Tumor size, TNM stage, serum albumin, and ALRI were identified as independent prognostic factors for OS and DFS by univariate and multivariate cox regression analyses mentioned above, and were utilized to construct novel nomograms to predict 1-, 3-, and 5-year OS as well as 1-, 3-, and 5-year DFS for post-operative HCC patients (**Figures 3** and **S2**).

Our nomogram showed potential clinical utility as it predicted post-operative survival with C-index of 0.705 (95% CI: 0.661–0.756) for OS and 0.678 (95% CI: 0.631–0.725) for DFS in the training cohort, while, the C-index in validation cohort was 0.711 (95% CI: 0.667–0.763) for OS and 0.666 (95% CI: 0.619–0.714) for DFS. The calibration curves of 1-, 3-, and 5-year OS and 1-, 3-, and 5-year DFS in the training cohort largely coincided with their standard curves, and similar results were observed in validation cohort (**Figures 4A–C, E–G** and **Figures S3A–C, E–G**). In training cohort, the AUC of ROC curves for 1-, 3-, and 5-year OS were 0.791, 0.763, and 0.794 (**Figure 4D**), respectively; and 0.733, 0.751, and 0.790 for 1-, 3-, and 5-year DFS (**Figure 4H**), respectively, achieving more than 70% prediction accuracy for post-operative HCC patients. The AUC of ROC in validation cohort curves were 0.751, 0.810, and 0.783 for 1-, 3-, and 5-year OS, respectively; and 0.723, 0.763, and 0.764 for 1-, 3-, and 5-year DFS, respectively (**Figures S3D, H**), which further validated the predictive performance of the novel nomograms.

Survival Outcomes

Kaplan-Meier survival analysis showed that a higher post-operative ALRI value (ALRI > 22.6) was associated with shorter OS and DFS in the training cohort ($P < 0.001$) (**Figures 5A, B**), so was it in the validation cohort (**Figures S4A, B**). The post-operative liver cancer patients were further divided into three different risks' groups to predict OS and DFS based on their total risk scores calculated by the novel nomogram (patient of score 0–90, 90–190, >190 into the low-, intermediate-, high-risk groups, respectively). The OS and DFS in different risk groups were further analyzed, revealing significant differences in

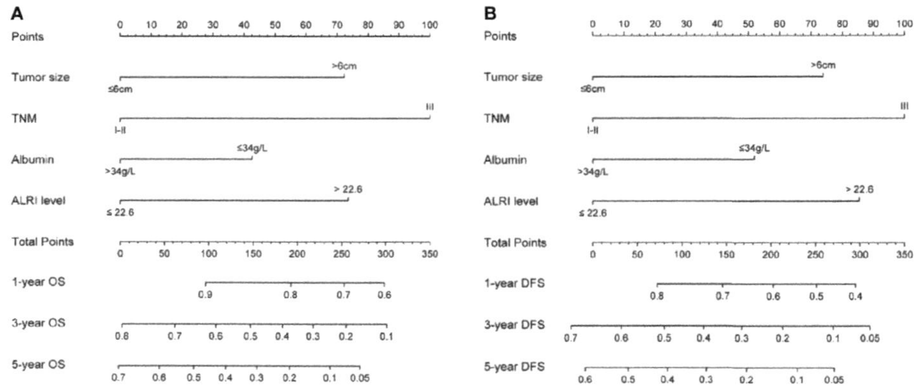

FIGURE 3 | Nomograms for OS and DFS in the training cohort. Sum up the score of each factor, and 1-, 3-, and 5-year OS were determined according to the total score. The 1-, 3-, and 5-year DFS were determined in the same way **(A, B)**.

OS and DFS among different risk groups in both training cohort ($P < 0.001$) (**Figures 5C, D**) and validation cohort ($P < 0.001$) (**Figures S4C, D**).

DISCUSSION

HCC is one of the most aggressive human cancers, which is difficult to cure, as up to 60–70% of HCC patients may experience recurrent cancer and/or metastasis after hepatectomy (8, 9). Recommended management of post-operative HCC patients includes regular monitoring schedule with routine blood and liver function tests, ultrasonography, CT, and MRI examinations. Continuous efforts to identify new tumor biomarkers may help detect early-stage liver cancer, facilitating early intervention and improving clinical outcomes (10–12).

There are several noninvasive and low-cost prognostic predictive models including ALRI (13, 14), NLR, and SII (15–19), which mainly utilize preoperative parameters such as baseline parameters or clinical information collected before surgery, and their performance was relatively satisfactory. However, in order to improve the prediction with those markers, we incorporated the postoperative data to evaluate these predictors in this study.

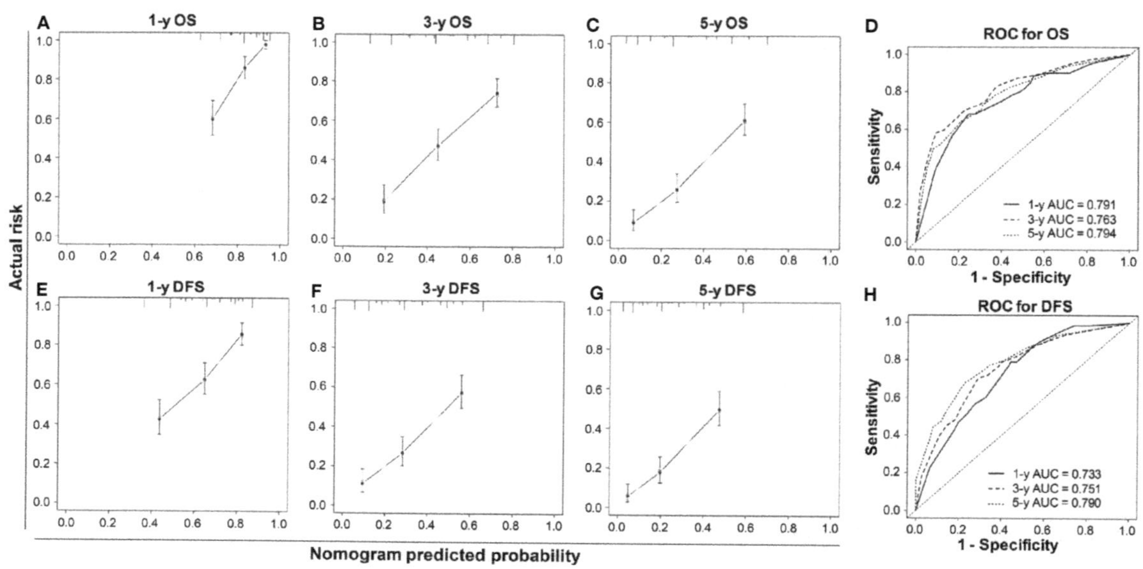

FIGURE 4 | The calibration curves and ROC curves of 1-, 3-, and 5-year OS **(A–D)** and 1-, 3-, and 5-year DFS **(E–H)** in the training cohort. For the calibration curve, the x-axis was the predicted-survival based on the nomogram, and the y-axis was the actual-survival; the more the predicted line coincided with the diagonal line, the more accurate the prognosis nomogram would be.

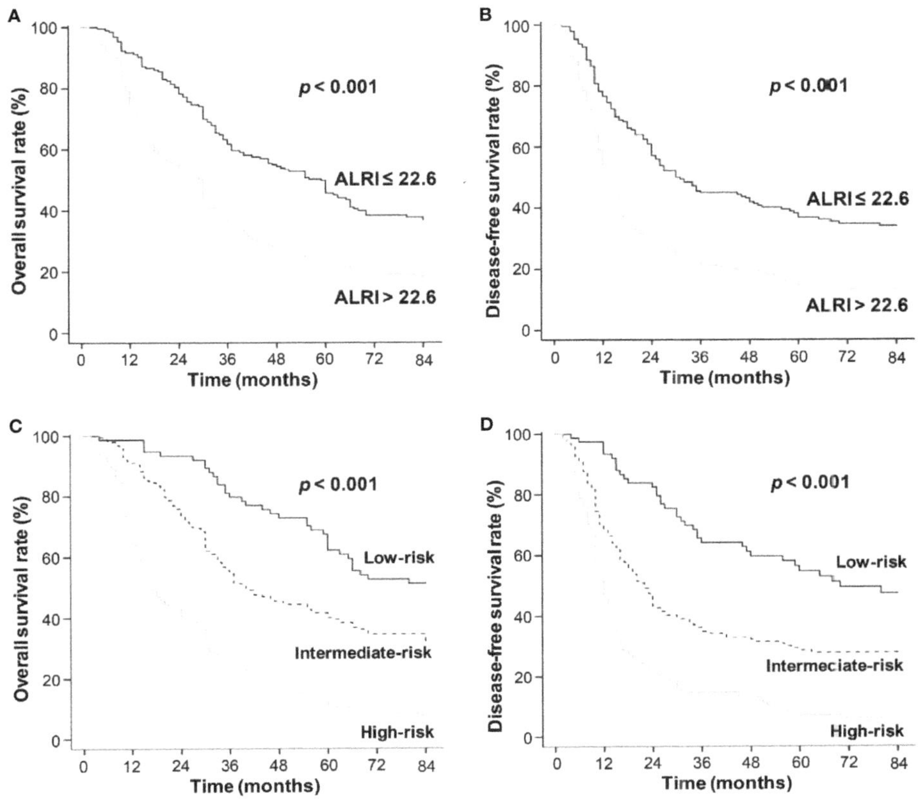

FIGURE 5 | The OS and DFS curves in the training cohort. Kaplan-Meier survival analyses revealed that HCC patients with ALRI > 22.6 had shorter OS and DFS **(A, B)**. The black line refers to ALRI ≤ 22.6 and the gray line refers to ALRI > 22.6. Kaplan-Meier survival analyses of HCC patients in different risk groups **(C, D)**. The black line refers to low-risk group, the dotted line: intermediate-risk group and the gray line: high-risk group.

Distinct outcomes have been clinically noted among HCC patients who shared many similarities including age, gender, tumor size, pathological stage, or laboratory findings. Some patients may achieve up to 10 years of disease-free survival (DFS), while other patients have recurrent cancer 1~2 years after resection, suggesting post-operative conditions likely represent key factors determining different outcomes. We found the study that investigated the influence of post-operative inflammation scores for prognosis in HCC patients after surgery (16). Surprisingly in our pilot study, we found that, NLR and SII based on hematologic findings extracted 2 months after radical resection had unfavorable predictive utility; but ALRI appeared to accurately indicate patients' physical conditions after surgery and provided as a useful measurement that may offer reference to post-operative treatments.

In some studies, the models applying data of a specific time-point after surgery remained to be effective predictors of HCC prognosis, such as ALBI grade at the first year after resection (20), AFP response (change of AFP before and 1 week after hepatectomy) (21), daily decrease of post-operative AFP (22), postoperative serum osteopontin level (23), etc. In this study, we further investigated the postoperative ALRI model using hematologic findings extracted 2 months after radical resection, which more accurately predicted patients' physical condition after surgery.

Systematic inflammation is associated with cancer progression by promoting angiogenesis (24), suppressing cell apoptosis and facilitating cancer invasion (25). Several prognostic models have incorporated inflammatory markers, such as lymphocyte counting and AST level. Lymphocytes are crucial in surveillance and suppression of cancer occurrence, growth, and migration (26). The amount of peripheral and infiltrating lymphocytes reflects the intensity of anti-cancer response a cancer patient can assemble (27). Serum AST, released by destructed hepatocytes, is a sensitive and reliable indicator for the extent of liver injury (28, 29). Therefore, ALRI using lymphocyte count and AST level, as reported, had predictive value of clinical outcomes for post-operative HCC patients (13, 14). In addition, serum albumin level represents the functional capacity of liver. Serum albumin level reduced when an injured liver deteriorated into the decompensated state. Clearly, tumor burden negatively impact post-operative prognosis as larger tumor size and advanced tumor are associated with poorer immunological function of patients (30–32).

Guided by the above reasoning, we constructed the novel survival nomograms for OS and DFS to predict outcomes of post-operative HCC patients. Four independent factors were incorporated in this nomogram: tumor size, TNM stage, post-operative serum albumin level, and post-operative ALRI value. Kaplan-Meier survival analyses showed that the nomograms performed well in categorizing HCC patients into different risk groups, and high-risk group had the worst OS and DFS ($P < 0.001$). This new nomogram containing ALRI also showed satisfactory prediction capacity and may bring reference value to post-operative follow-ups and monitorings.

There are limitations in this study. First, this was a retrospective study that may carry inherent bias in enrollment. Second, we didn't include data beyond 2-month after surgery. Further evaluation of the predictive results of later time-points is required. Third, most of our patients were hepatitis B virus infected. Therefore, future prospective studies that enroll larger sample size of post-operative HCC patients from multiple centers, with different etiologies, may provide further validation of our findings in this study.

AUTHOR CONTRIBUTIONS

YPZ and WJL put forward the ideas of this article. MJL, JRS and QFZ wrote this article. CRT, YDS and ML help revise this manuscript. YCZ, MRC and TC helped the collection of data. CGH and JXY conducted the analysis of data. All authors contributed to the article and approved the submitted version.

REFERENCES

1. Bray F, Ferlay J, Soerjomataram I, Siegel RL, Torre LA, Jemal A. Global Cancer Statistics 2018: GLOBOCAN Estimates of Incidence and Mortality Worldwide for 36 Cancers in 185 Countries. *CA Cancer J Clin* (2018) 68:394–424. doi: 10.3322/caac.21492
2. Yang JD, Gyedu A, Afihene MY, Duduyemi BM, Micah E, Kingham TP, et al. Hepatocellular Carcinoma Occurs at an Earlier Age in Africans, Particularly in Association With Chronic Hepatitis B. *Am J Gastroenterol* (2015) 110:1629–31. doi: 10.1038/ajg.2015.289
3. Yang JD, Mohamed EA, Aziz AO, Shousha HI, Hashem MB, Nabeel MM, et al. Characteristics, Management, and Outcomes of Patients With Hepatocellular Carcinoma in Africa: A Multicountry Observational Study From the Africa Liver Cancer Consortium. *Lancet Gastroenterol Hepatol* (2017) 2:103–11. doi: 10.1016/S2468-1253(16)30161-3
4. Tang A, Hallouch O, Chernyak V, Kamaya A, Sirlin CB. Epidemiology of Hepatocellular Carcinoma: Target Population for Surveillance and Diagnosis. *Abdom Radiol (NY)* (2018) 43:13–25. doi: 10.1007/s00261-017-1209-1
5. El-Serag HB. Epidemiology of Viral Hepatitis and Hepatocellular Carcinoma. *Gastroenterology* (2012) 142:1264–73. doi: 10.1053/j.gastro.2011.12.061
6. Schweitzer A, Horn J, Mikolajczyk RT, Krause G, Ott JJ. Estimations of Worldwide Prevalence of Chronic Hepatitis B Virus Infection: A Systematic Review of Data Published Between 1965 and 2013. *Lancet* (2015) 386:1546–55. doi: 10.1016/S0140-6736(15)61412-X
7. Vitale A, Peck-Radosavljevic M, Giannini EG, Vibert E, Sieghart W, Van Poucke S, et al. Personalized Treatment of Patients With Very Early Hepatocellular Carcinoma. *J Hepatol* (2017) 66:412–23. doi: 10.1016/j.jhep.2016.09.012
8. Nakagawa S, Wei L, Song WM, Higashi T, Ghoshal S, Kim RS, et al. Molecular Liver Cancer Prevention in Cirrhosis by Organ Transcriptome Analysis and Lysophosphatidic Acid Pathway Inhibition. *Cancer Cell* (2016) 30:879–90. doi: 10.1016/j.ccell.2016.11.004
9. Cha C, Fong Y, Jarnagin WR, Blumgart LH, DeMatteo RP. Predictors and Patterns of Recurrence After Resection of Hepatocellular Carcinoma. *J Am Coll Surg* (2003) 197:753–8. doi: 10.1016/j.jamcollsurg.2003.07.003
10. Luo P, Yin P, Hua R, Tan Y, Li Z, Qiu G, et al. A Large-Scale, Multicenter Serum Metabolite Biomarker Identification Study for the Early Detection of Hepatocellular Carcinoma. *Hepatology* (2018) 67:662–75. doi: 10.1002/hep.29561
11. Xie Z, Zhou F, Yang Y, Li L, Lei Y, Lin X, et al. Lnc-PCDH9-13:1 Is a Hypersensitive and Specific Biomarker for Early Hepatocellular Carcinoma. *EBioMedicine* (2018) 33:57–67. doi: 10.1016/j.ebiom.2018.06.026
12. Hlady RA, Zhao X, Pan X, Yang JD, Ahmed F, Antwi SO, et al. Genome-Wide Discovery and Validation of Diagnostic DNA Methylation-Based Biomarkers for Hepatocellular Cancer Detection in Circulating Cell Free DNA. *Theranostics* (2019) 9:7239–50. doi: 10.7150/thno.35573.eCollection2019
13. Jin J, Zhu P, Liao Y, Li J, Liao W, He S. Elevated Preoperative Aspartate Aminotransferase to Lymphocyte Ratio Index as an Independent Prognostic Factor for Patients With Hepatocellular Carcinoma After Hepatic Resection. *Oncotarget* (2015) 6:19217–27. doi: 10.18632/oncotarget.4265
14. Zhao LY, Yang DD, Ma XK, Liu MM, Wu DH, Zhang XP, et al. The Prognostic Value of Aspartate Aminotransferase to Lymphocyte Ratio and Systemic Immune-Inflammation Index for Overall Survival of Hepatocellular Carcinoma Patients Treated With Palliative Treatments. *J Cancer* (2019) 10:2299–311. doi: 10.7150/jca.30663.eCollection2019
15. Hu B, Yang XR, Xu Y, Sun YF, Sun C, Guo W, et al. Systemic Immune-Inflammation Index Predicts Prognosis of Patients After Curative Resection for Hepatocellular Carcinoma. *Clin Cancer Res* (2014) 20:6212–22. doi: 10.1158/1078-0432.CCR-14-0442
16. Wang BL, Tian L, Gao XH, Ma XL, Wu J, Zhang CY, et al. Dynamic Change of the Systemic Immune Inflammation Index Predicts the Prognosis of Patients With Hepatocellular Carcinoma After Curative Resection. *Clin Chem Lab Med* (2016) 54:1963–9. doi: 10.1515/cclm-2015-1191
17. Wang C, He W, Yuan Y, Zhang Y, Li K, Zou R, et al. Comparison of the Prognostic Value of Inflammation-Based Scores in Early Recurrent Hepatocellular Carcinoma After Hepatectomy. *Liver Int* (2020) 40:229–39. doi: 10.1111/liv.14281
18. Halazun KJ, Hardy MA, Rana AA, Woodland DC, Luyten EJ, Mahadev S, et al. Negative Impact of Neutrophil-Lymphocyte Ratio on Outcome After Liver Transplantation for Hepatocellular Carcinoma. *Ann Surg* (2009) 250:141–51. doi: 10.1097/SLA.0b013e3181a77e59
19. Wang D, Bai N, Hu X, OuYang XW, Yao L, Tao Y, et al. Preoperative Inflammatory Markers of NLR and PLR as Indicators of Poor Prognosis in Resectable HCC. *PeerJ* (2019) 7:e7132. doi: 10.7717/peerj.7132.eCollection2019
20. Cho WR, Hung CH, Chen CH, Lin CC, Wang CC, Liu YW, et al. Ability of the Post-Operative ALBI Grade to Predict the Outcomes of Hepatocellular Carcinoma After Curative Surgery. *Sci Rep* (2020) 10:7290. doi: 10.1038/s41598-020-64354-0
21. Li XL, Zhu XD, Cai H, Li Y, Zhou J, Fan J, et al. Postoperative α-Fetoprotein Response Predicts Tumor Recurrence and Survival After Hepatectomy for Hepatocellular Carcinoma: A Propensity Score Matching Analysis. *Surgery* (2019) 165:1161–7. doi: 10.1016/j.surg.2019.01.009
22. Zhou PY, Yang CP, Tang Z, Yi Y, Liu WR, Tian MX, et al. Daily Decrease of Post-Operative Alpha-Fetoprotein by 9% Discriminates Prognosis of HCC: A Multicenter Retrospective Study. *Aging (Albany NY)* (2019) 11:11111–23. doi: 10.18632/aging.102513
23. Zhou C, Zhou HJ, Zhang XF, Lou LL, Ye QH, Zheng Y, et al. Postoperative Serum Osteopontin Level is a Novel Monitor for Treatment Response and Tumor Recurrence After Resection of Hepatitis B-Related Hepatocellular Carcinoma. *Ann Surg Oncol* (2013) 20:929–37. doi: 10.1245/s10434-012-2749-9
24. Mantovani A, Allavena P, Sica A, Balkwill F. Cancer-Related Inflammation. *Nature* (2008) 454:436–44. doi: 10.1038/nature07205
25. Pinato DJ, North BV, Sharma R. A Novel, Externally Validated Inflammation-Based Prognostic Algorithm in Hepatocellular Carcinoma: The Prognostic Nutritional Index (PNI). *Br J Cancer* (2012) 106:1439–45. doi: 10.1038/bjc.2012.92
26. Lin ZX, Ruan DY, Li Y, Wu DH, Ma XK, Chen J, et al. Lymphocyte-to-Monocyte Ratio Predicts Survival of Patients With Hepatocellular Carcinoma

After Curative Resection. *World J Gastroenterol* (2015) 21:10898–906. doi: 10.3748/wjg.v21.i38.10898

27. Pagès F, Galon J, Dieu-Nosjean MC, Tartour E, Sautès-Fridman C, Fridman WH. Immune Infiltration in Human Tumors: A Prognostic Factor That Should Not be Ignored. *Oncogene* (2010) 29:1093–102. doi: 10.1038/onc.2009.416
28. Aleksandrova K, Bamia C, Drogan D, Lagiou P, Trichopoulou A, Jenab M, et al. The Association of Coffee Intake With Liver Cancer Risk Is Mediated by Biomarkers of Inflammation and Hepatocellular Injury: Data From the European Prospective Investigation Into Cancer and Nutrition. *Am J Clin Nutr* (2015) 102:1498–508. doi: 10.3945/ajcn.115.116095
29. Takeishi K, Maeda T, Shirabe K, Tsujita E, Yamashita Y, Harimoto N, et al. Clinicopathologic Features and Outcomes of Non-B, Non-C Hepatocellular Carcinoma After Hepatectomy. *Ann Surg Oncol* (2015) 22(Suppl 3):S1116–24. doi: 10.1245/s10434-015-4728-4
30. Levi Sandri GB, Spoletini G, Vennarecci G, Francone E, Abu Hilal M, Ettorre GM. Laparoscopic Liver Resection for Large HCC: Short- and Long-Term Outcomes in Relation to Tumor Size. *Surg Endosc* (2018) 32:4772–9. doi: 10.1007/s00464-018-6225-x
31. Liu S, Li H, Guo L, Zhang B, Zhou B, Zhang W, et al. Tumor Size Affects Efficacy of Adjuvant Transarterial Chemoembolization in Patients With Hepatocellular Carcinoma and Microvascular Invasion. *Oncologist* (2019) 24:513–20. doi: 10.1634/theoncologist.2018-0305
32. Chan AWH, Zhong J, Berhane S, Toyoda H, Cucchetti A, Shi K, et al. Development of Pre and Post-Operative Models to Predict Early Recurrence of Hepatocellular Carcinoma After Surgical Resection. *J Hepatol* (2018) 69:1284–93. doi: 10.1016/j.jhep.2018.08.027

7

A Pre-Operative Prognostic Score for Patients with Advanced Hepatocellular Carcinoma Who Underwent Resection

Han Xiao[1†], Jia-Li Li[2†], Shu-Ling Chen[1†], Mi-Mi Tang[3], Qian Zhou[4], Ting-Fan Wu[5], Xin Li[6], Zhen-Wei Peng[4,7], Shi-Ting Feng[3], Sui Peng[4,8] and Ming Kuang[1,9*]*

[1] Division of Interventional Ultrasound, The First Affiliated Hospital of Sun Yat-sen University, Guangzhou, China, [2] Department of Liver Surgery, Dongguan People's Hospital, Dongguan, China, [3] Department of Medical Imaging, The First Affiliated Hospital of Sun Yat-sen University, Guangzhou, China, [4] Clinical Trials Unit, The First Affiliated Hospital of Sun Yat-sen University, Guangzhou, China, [5] Clinical Education Team, GE Healthcare, Beijing, China, [6] Global Research, GE Healthcare, Beijing, China, [7] Department of Radiotherapy, The First Affiliated Hospital of Sun Yat-sen University, Guangzhou, China, [8] Department of Gastroenterology, The First Affiliated Hospital of Sun Yat-sen University, Guangzhou, China, [9] Department of Liver Surgery, The First Affiliated Hospital of Sun Yat-sen University, Guangzhou, China

***Correspondence:**
Ming Kuang
kuangm@mail.sysu.edu.cn
Sui Peng
pengsui@vip.163.com

[†]These authors have contributed equally to this work

Background: Previous studies demonstrated a promising prognosis in advanced hepatocellular carcinoma (HCC) patients who underwent surgery, yet a consensus of which population would benefit most from surgery is still unreached.

Method: A total of 496 advanced HCC patients who initially underwent liver resection were consecutively collected. Least absolute shrinkage and selection operator (LASSO) regression was performed to select significant pre-operative factors for recurrence-free survival (RFS). A prognostic score constructed from these factors was used to divide patients into different risk groups. Survivals were compared between groups with log-rank test. The area under curves (AUC) of the time-dependent receiver operating characteristics was used to evaluate the predictive accuracy of prognostic score.

Result: For the entire cohort, the median overall survival (OS) was 23.0 months and the median RFS was 12.1 months. Patients were divided into two risk groups according to the prognostic score constructed with ALBI score, tumor size, tumor-invaded liver segments, gamma-glutamyl transpeptidase, alpha fetoprotein, and portal vein tumor thrombus stage. The median RFS of the low-risk group was significantly longer than that of the high-risk group in both the training (10.1 vs 2.9 months, $P<0.001$) and the validation groups (13.7 vs 4.6 months, $P=0.002$). The AUCs of the prognostic score in predicting survival were 0.70 to 0.71 in the training group and 0.71 to 0.72 in the validation group.

Conclusion: Surgery could provide promising survival for HCC patients at an advanced stage. Our developed pre-operative prognostic score is effective in identifying advanced-stage HCC patients with better survival benefit for surgery.

Keywords: hepatocellular carcinoma, tumor thrombosis, macrovascular invasion, surgery, prognostic score

INTRODUCTION

Yearly, about 365 thousand new cases of hepatocellular carcinoma (HCC) patients are diagnosed in China, and 319 thousand patients die of HCC (1, 2). The high morbidity and mortality make HCC a huge disease burden in China. Accordingly, over 50% of HCC patients are in an advanced stage at the first diagnosis (3). Patients at an advanced stage usually have a poor prognosis, especially those accompanied with macrovascular invasion.

No treatment was proven to be effective for advanced HCC patients until a large randomized clinical trial (RCT) claimed that sorafenib could prolong the overall survival (OS) of HCC patients at an advanced stage in 2008 (4). Later, lenvatinib was also introduced into the first-line treatment in 2018 (5). However, the median OS was only 8.1-9.8 months for patients with macrovascular invasion, which was far from satisfactory.

Over the past decade, lots of effort has been made to search for other approaches to improve the survival of advanced HCC patients. Resection is the most frequently applied curative treatment of HCC and is also generally performed among advanced-stage HCC patients in real clinical practice (3, 6). Patients were about three times more likely to receive resection than sorafenib (6). Evidence also showed that advanced HCC patients who underwent resection could have a significantly better survival than those in the non-resection group (7, 8). This was especially true for patients with macrovascular invasion, where the median survival could be prolonged by 1.77 years in the resection group if the patients had Child-pugh A stage liver function (9). Despite the reported survival benefits, the recommendation of surgery in advanced HCC is quite controversial. The guidelines of the American Association for the Study of Liver Diseases (AASLD) and the European Association for the Study of the Liver (EASL) took advanced HCC as a contradiction to surgery (10, 11). However, the guidelines of the Asian Pacific Association for the Study of the Liver (APASL) and the Japan Society of Hepatology (JHS) agreed that resection could be performed in some advanced HCC patients (12, 13). The differences between guidelines might be due to the huge heterogeneity within advanced HCC. Although some advanced HCC patients could reach a median survival of more than 4 years, others might have a similar survival with sorafenib treatment but still experience an invasive treatment procedure (9, 14–17). Therefore, finding out a super-selection of the population who might benefit most from surgery pre-operatively would help in proper treatment selection for advanced HCC patients.

Many factors influence the survival of advanced HCC patients, including tumor number, cancer cell differentiation, etc. (18). One of the most important prognostic factors is the stage of macrovascular invasion, especially the portal vein tumor thrombosis (PVTT). A study including 2093 advanced HCC patients showed that median survival could range from 0.91 to 4.13 years due to the different stages of PVTT (Vp4 to Vp1) (9). The stage of PVTT also influences the type and extent of surgery. Therefore, taking the stage of PVTT into consideration is necessary for the management of advanced-stage HCC patients. An EHBH-PVTT scoring system was established recently using four elements to predict survival in advanced HCC patients (19). However, the stage of PVTT was described in this study instead of being selected as a prognostic factor. To our knowledge, none of the published studies have evaluated the prognostic effect of the stage of PVTT.

Therefore, this article retrospectively analyzed HCC patients at an advanced stage who underwent resection, aiming to establish a prognostic score based on the stage of PVTT and other pre-operative clinical factors and to give some evidence on proper candidate selection for resection in advanced HCC.

METHOD

Patients Selection

This is a retrospective study based on a prospectively collected database from the First Affiliated Hospital of Sun Yat-sen University. From May 30th, 1995 to June 1st, 2017, 3 168 HCC patients who initially underwent liver resection were consecutively collected. HCC were diagnosed following the guidelines of the time (20–22). The inclusion criteria were as follows: a) primary HCC without previous treatment, b) Barcelona Clinic Liver Cancer (BCLC) stage C (23), c) Child-pugh stage A-B, and d) Eastern Cooperative Oncology Group (ECOG) grades 0-1. The exclusion criteria were: a) extrahepatic metastasis, b) patients who underwent palliative resection, or c) data of enhanced computed tomography (CT) or magnetic resonance (MR) not available. Eventually, 496 patients were included in this study.

Data Collection

At least 1 instance of enhanced CT or MR was performed within 1 month before resection for each patient. Tumor size, tumor number, and the stage of PVTT and hepatic vein tumor thrombus (HVTT) were evaluated on CT or MR, by two radiologists with over 5 years of experience. The stage of PVTT and HVTT were defined according to the stage system in Japan (18). PVTT were categorized as PVTT 4 (portal invasion at the main portal trunk), PVTT 3 (portal invasion at the first order branch), PVTT 2 (portal invasion at the second order branch), PVTT 1 (portal invasion at the third or more peripheral branch), and PVTT 0 (absence of portal invasion). HVTT were categorized as HVTT 3 (tumor thrombosis in the inferior vena cava), HVTT 2 (tumor thrombosis in a main hepatic vein), HVTT 1 (tumor thrombosis in a peripheral hepatic vein), and HVTT 0 (absence of HVTT). Patient characteristics including age, gender, and ECOG performance status at the time of surgery were collected. Latest results of laboratory tests, including levels of alpha fetoprotein (AFP), platelet (PLT), hemoglobin (HB), albumin (ALB), total bilirubin (TB), alanine transaminase (ALT), aspartate aminotransferase (AST), gamma-glutamyl transpeptidase (GGT), and prothrombin time (PT), were collected before surgery. Status of ascites, splenomegaly, and varicosity were also included in the analysis. Portal hypertension (PHT) was defined as esophageal varices or splenomegaly associated with a platelet count lower than 100×10^9/L (24).

The BCLC stage and Child-pugh grade were derived based on the radiology and laboratory findings.

Treatment and Follow-Up

Surgery was performed under general anesthesia by surgeons with 10–40 years of experience. The type of surgery was decided according to a routine discussion for each patient in the Department of Liver Surgery. Anatomic or non-anatomic resection was decided according to the tumor burden and liver function of the patients. The surgical approach was chosen based on the liver remnant, tumor location, and preference of the operator. Intraoperative ultrasound (US) was used to assist in operative evaluation.

Evaluation of recurrence was performed at the first month after initial resection and was repeated every 3 months for the first two years, and 3-6 months thereafter. Either US or CT was performed for evaluation during the follow-up. Once a focal in liver was detected by the US, the patient would receive CT or MR for further diagnosis. Recurrence was evaluated according to the criterion of HCC diagnosis in the EASL guideline. Treatment recommendations for recurrent HCC was made by the physician after evaluation of the tumor burden, liver function, and patient's common status. Curative treatments were recommended if possible, and the final decision was made by the patient.

Statistical Analysis

Patients were randomly divided into the training group (n=347) and the validation group (n=149) by a ratio of 7:3. Normal distribution test was performed for continuous variables. Continuous variables that obey normal distribution were presented as means ± SD and others as median and quartile. Categorical variables were presented as numbers and percentages. Differences between the training group and validation group were compared with the t-test for continuous variables and χ^2 test for categorical variables.

Recurrence-free survival (RFS) was defined as the time interval from the date of surgery to the date of first radiology confirmed recurrence according to the modified response criteria in solid tumors (25), the date of death from any cause, or to the date of the last follow-up visit. Overall survival (OS) was defined as the time interval from the date of surgery to the date of death from any cause or to the date of the last follow-up visit. The predicting model for RFS was constructed with the data of the training group. Least absolute shrinkage and selection operator (LASSO) regression followed by a stepwise analysis were performed to select factors to build the model. Time dependent Receiver Operating Characteristic (ROC) curve was used to calculate the area under the curve (AUC) for the evaluation of the model in both the training and the validation group. The cutoff was set to achieve the highest accuracy in the training group and was then applied to the validation group. Patients would be divided into the high-risk group and the low-risk group with this cutoff. Survival curves of RFS and OS in different risk groups were generated by the Kaplan–Meier method and compared by the log-rank test. Subgroup analyses were also performed according to whether the patients had the condition of ascites or PHT or thrombocytopenia or in Child-Pugh class B. Statistical significance was considered as a two-sided P value of less than 0.05. The above statistical analysis was performed with the STATA/MP 14.0.

RESULT

Patient Characteristics

Baseline characteristics of the training and validation groups were shown in **Table 1**. After excluding 85 patients with palliative resection, a total of 496 patients were enrolled. The majority of patients with HVTT were in HVTT 2 stage. As for the category of PVTT, only 17 patients had PVTT in the main trunk (3.4%). PVTT 2 and 3 stage accounted for 31.0% and 25.0% of all patients, respectively. Only 3.7% of the patients had a history of HCV affected, and 86.7% of the patients were HBsAg-positive. The majority of patients were in Child-Pugh stage A (90.1%). And most of the patients had tumors larger than 5cm (85.3%). The pre-treatment characteristics were similar between the training group and the validation group, except that the ratio of multiple lesions was higher in the training group (40.6% vs 29.5%, P=0.019).

Survival Outcomes

The median RFS of all patients in this study was 12.1 months, and the median OS was 23.0 months. One-year, 2-year, and 3-year RFS rates were 51.3%, 29.6%, and 23.4%, respectively. The corresponding rates of OS were 65.4%, 49.5%, and 42.4%, respectively. Survival rates were significantly different between PVTT 0-2 and PVTT 3-4. The median RFS was 6.3 months for patients with PVTT 0-2 and 3.5 months for patients with PVTT 3-4 (P<0.001). The corresponding median OS was 32.9 months and 12.1 months, respectively (P<0.001).

Survival Outcomes Development and Validation of a Prognostic Score

The score model was established based on the RFS data of the training group. Eventually, six factors were selected, which were the ALBI score (26), tumor size, the number of invaded liver segments, GGT, AFP, and the PVTT stage. The mark sheet was presented in **Table 2**. The score for each factor was determined by the coefficient in the stepwise Cox regression. Cutoff of the prognostic model was set to be 14, which could achieve the best AUC of the ROC curves. Patients in the training group were then divided into the low-risk group (score<14, n=148) and the high-risk group (score≥14, n=199). Median RFS of the low-risk group was significantly longer than that of the high-risk group (10.1 vs 2.9 months, P<0.001) (**Figure 1A**). The 6-month, 1-year, and 2-year RFS rates were 60.7%, 46.3%, and 38.0% for the low-risk group while the corresponding rates were only 27.4%, 19.4%, and 12.2% in the high-risk group, respectively. ROC curves for 6-month, 1-year, and 2-year RFS rates were presented in **Figure 2**. The corresponding AUCs were 0.71, 0.70, and 0.71 in the training group. Median OS was 44.3 months in the low-risk group, and only 13.1 months in the high-risk group (P<0.001) (**Figure 1B**).

TABLE 1 | Baseline characteristics of the training group and the validation group.

Variables		Total	Training	Validation	P value
Age (years)	≤65	434(87.5%)	305(87.9%)	129(86.6%)	0.684
	>65	62(12.5%)	42(12.1%)	20(13.4%)	
Tumor size (cm)	<=5	73(14.7%)	52(15.0%)	21(14.1%)	0.797
	>5	423(85.3%)	295(85.0%)	128(85.9%)	
	Median (IQR)	9.6 (6.5, 12.7)	9.6 (6.5, 12.9)	9.4 (6.4, 12.0)	0.552
Splenomegaly	No	275(55.4%)	187(53.9%)	88(59.1%)	0.288
	Yes	221(44.6%)	160(46.1%)	61(40.9%)	
Ascites	No	448(90.3%)	309(89.0%)	139(93.3%)	0.143
	Yes	48(9.7%)	38(11.0%)	10(6.7%)	
Child-Pugh stage	A	447(90.1%)	312(89.9%)	135(90.6%)	0.813
	B	49(9.9%)	35(10.1%)	14(9.4%)	
ALBI score	≤-2.6	203(40.9%)	140(40.3%)	63(42.3%)	0.688
	>-2.6	293(59.1%)	207(59.7%)	86(57.7%)	
Tumor number	Single	311(62.7%)	206(59.4%)	105(70.5%)	0.019
	Multiple	185(37.3%)	141(40.6%)	44(29.5%)	
	Median (IQR)	1.0 (1.0, 3.0)	1.0 (1.0, 4.0)	1.0 (1.0, 2.0)	0.003
PHT	No	424(85.5%)	296(85.3%)	128(85.9%)	0.861
	Yes	72(14.5%)	51(14.7%)	21(14.1%)	
AFP (ng/mL)	≤200	190(38.3%)	141(40.6%)	49(32.9%)	0.104
	>200	306(61.7%)	206(59.4%)	100(67.1%)	
PVTT class	0-2	355(71.6%)	252(72.6%)	103(69.1%)	0.429
	3-4	141(28.4%)	95(27.4%)	46(30.9%)	
HVTT class	0-1	359(72.4%)	251(72.3%)	108(72.5%)	0.973
	2-3	137(27.6%)	96(27.7%)	41(27.5%)	
NLR	≤2.2	206(41.5%)	143(41.2%)	63(42.3%)	0.824
	>2.2	290(58.5%)	204(58.8%)	86(57.7%)	
PLT (10^9/L)	≤100	29(5.8%)	18(5.2%)	11(7.4%)	0.339
	>100	467(94.2%)	329(94.8%)	138(92.6%)	
ALB (g/L)	>35	375(75.6%)	265(76.4%)	110(73.8%)	0.545
	≤35	121(24.4%)	82(23.6%)	39(26.2%)	
TB (umol/L)	≤34.2	464(93.5%)	324(93.4%)	140(94.0%)	0.807
	>34.2	32(6.5%)	23(6.6%)	9(6.0%)	
ALT (U/L)	≤40	241(48.6%)	166(47.8%)	75(50.3%)	0.610
	>40	255(51.4%)	181(52.2%)	74(49.7%)	
AST (U/L)	≤40	179(36.1%)	124(35.7%)	55(36.9%)	0.802
	>40	317(63.9%)	223(64.3%)	94(63.1%)	
GGT (U/L)	≤50	72(14.5%)	49(14.1%)	23(15.4%)	0.703
	>50	424(85.5%)	298(85.9%)	126(84.6%)	
HB (g/L)	≤120	107(21.6%)	81(23.3%)	26(17.4%)	0.144
	>120	389(78.4%)	266(76.7%)	123(82.6%)	
HBsAg	missing	3(0.6%)	1(0.3%)	2(1.3%)	0.258
	negative	63(12.7%)	42(12.1%)	21(14.1%)	
	positive	430(86.7%)	304(87.6%)	126(84.6%)	

IQR, interquartile range; PHT, portal hypertension; AFP, alpha fetoprotein; HVTT, hepatic vein tumor thrombosis; PVTT, portal vein tumor thrombosis; NLR, neutrophil to lymphocyte ratio; PLT, platelet; ALB, albumin; TB, total bilirubin; ALT, alanine transaminase; AST, aspartate aminotransferase; GGT, gamma-glutamyl transpeptidase; HB, hemoglobin.

TABLE 2 | The mark sheet of pre-operative score.

Variable	Score
ALBI score>-2.6	3
Tumor size >5cm	4
Tumor invaded liver segments ≥3	2
GGT >50U/L	4
AFP >200ng/mL	3
PVTT stage 3-4	3

Low-risk: sum of the score less than 14; High-risk: sum of the score no less than 14. GGT, gamma-glutamyl transpeptidase; AFP, alpha fetoprotein.

In the validation group, 53 patients were in the low-risk group while 96 were in the high-risk group. Median RFS was 13.7 months for the low-risk group and 4.6 months for the high-risk group (P=0.002) (**Figure 3A**). The 6-month, 1-year, and 2-year RFS rates were 75.1%, 51.8%, and 34.7% for the low-risk group. The corresponding rates were 40.2%, 26.8%, and 18.5% in the high-risk group, respectively. ROC curves for 6-month, 1-year, and 2-year RFS rates were presented in **Figure 4**. The corresponding AUCs were 0.72, 0.71, and 0.71 in the validation group. Median OS was not reached for the low-risk group but was 18.7 months for the high-risk group (P=0.001) (**Figure 3B**).

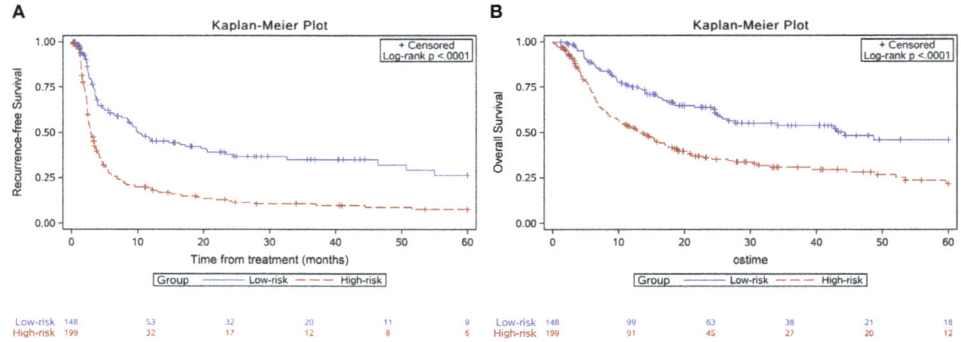

FIGURE 1 | Kaplan-Meier survival curves of the survival outcome in the training group. The recurrence free survival **(A)** and the overall survival **(B)** were both significantly longer in the low-risk group.

Subgroup analysis showed that, for patients with ascites, PHT, thrombocytopenia, or in Child-Pugh class B (128 out of 497), the RFS of the low-risk group was significantly higher than that of the high-risk group (10.0 vs. 3.3 months, $P<0.001$). Results were similar in patients without these conditions (RFS in low-risk group vs. high-risk group: 11.6 vs. 3.6 months, $P<0.001$).

DISCUSSION

In this study, we established a pre-operative prognostic score for advanced HCC patients to select an appropriate population at the advanced stage who could gain survival benefit from surgery. The score was easy to obtain with pre-operative clinical data and was well validated.

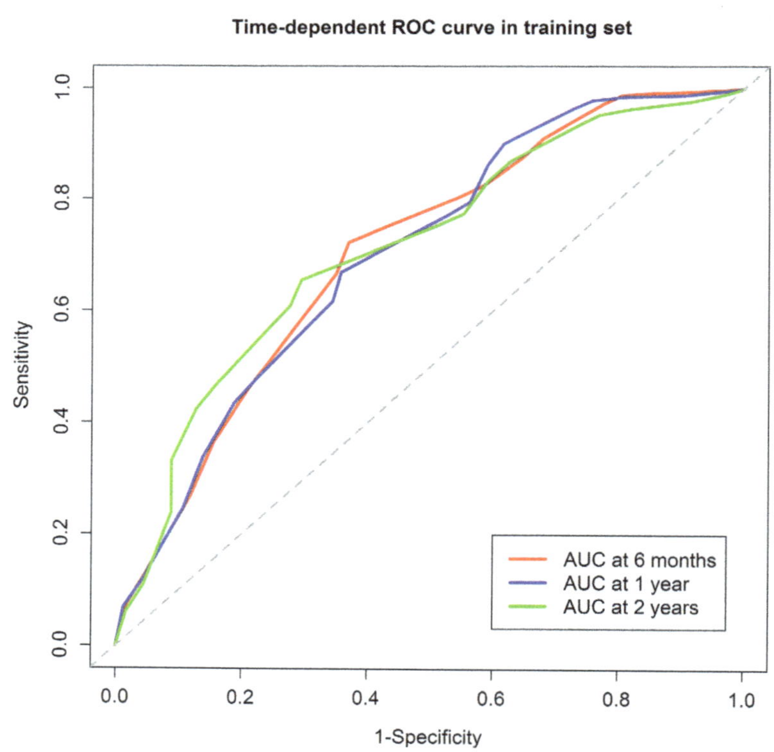

FIGURE 2 | The Receiver Operating Characteristic curves of the 6-month, 1-year, and 2-year recurrence free survival of the training group. The areas under curve were 0.71, 0.70, and 0.71, respectively.

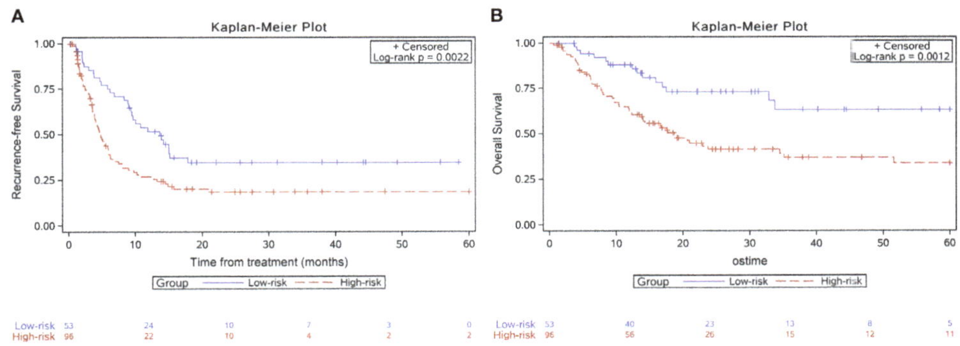

FIGURE 3 | Kaplan-Meier survival curves of the survival outcome in the validation group. The recurrence free survival **(A)** and the overall survival **(B)** were both significantly longer in the low-risk group.

Nowadays, systemic treatments are still the standard treatment for advanced stage HCC patients. Yet advanced HCC patients who undergo standard treatment are expected to have a median survival of only 8-13.6 months (4, 5, 27). In this article, advanced stage HCC patients who received resection could reach a median OS of 23.0 months, with 1-year and 3-year OS rates of 65.4% and 42.4%. These results are similar to a previous high-quality meta-analysis, with 1-year and 3-year OS rates of 62% and 42% for BCLC stage C patients (28). However, the survival result in our center is better than that reported in the EHBH-PVTT study (19), which was only 17.0 months even in the low-risk group. This might be due to the fact that the EHBH-PVTT study included more patients with PVTT 3 and mixed all PVTT stages together. However, survival outcomes could be distinct for patients with different PVTT stages (9). According to data in our center, patients with PVTT 2 had a median OS of 24.5 months,

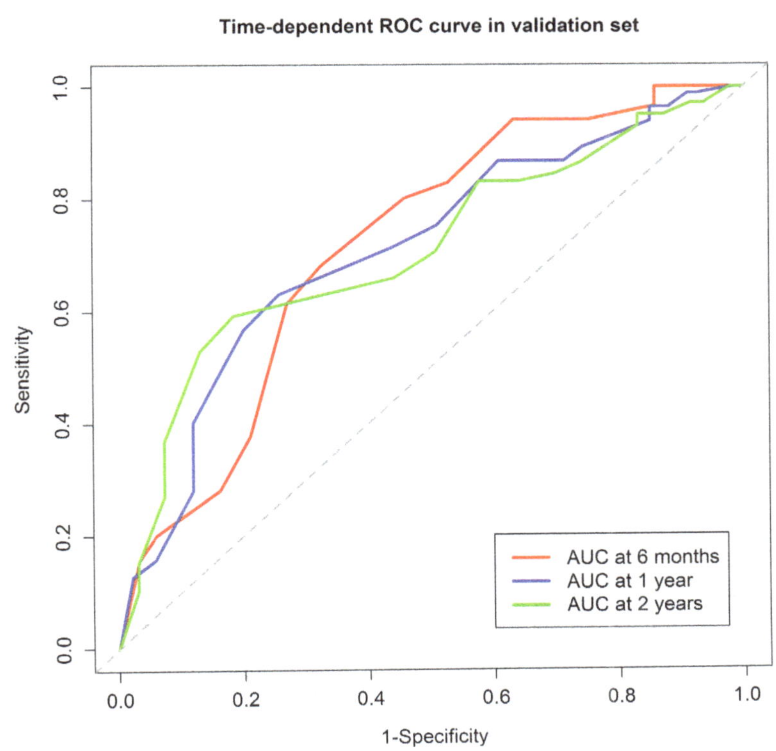

FIGURE 4 | The Receiver Operating Characteristic curves of the 6-month, 1-year, and 2-year recurrence free survival of the validation group. The areas under curve were 0.72, 0.71, and 0.71, respectively.

compared to only 10.6 months for patients with PVTT 3 (P=0.014). Neglection of the PVTT stages might lead to inadequate evaluation of survival benefit.

To our knowledge, this article is the first to establish a prognostic score on the basis of PVTT stage to help select a group of advanced HCC patients receiving surgery with a promising survival benefit. The score was based on pre-treatment clinical data so that patients could be divided into a high-risk group and a low-risk group before treatment selection. The median RFS of patients in the low-risk group was 10.9 months, and the median OS could reach 44.3 months, which was quite close to the OS of patients receiving resection in BCLC stage B in previous studies (29–31). The subgroup analysis of the phase III RCT of Sorafenib showed that no subgroup could achieve an OS longer than 15 months (32). Local therapy, such as transarterial chemoembolization (TACE), could achieve a median survival ranged from 13 to 35 months for non-TACE refractory patients (33). Survival for TACE-refractory patients was only 7 to 10.5 months. Despite the lack of direct comparison in this study, the survival advantage of resection in the low-risk group seemed to be superior to non-surgical treatments. The main cause of this promising result might be that resection has an obvious advantage in reducing tumor burden. Patients in the low-risk group tend to have better liver function, smaller tumors, and PVTT within the second order or more peripheral branch, which means anatomic resection (AR) is easier to achieve. AR is capable of eradicating potential micrometastases surrounding tumors (34), and was proven to be capable of providing better survival than non-AR (35). This might also contribute to the significant survival superiority of the low-risk group. Therefore, we recommend resection for advanced HCC patients who are estimated as low risk according to our score. On the other hand, the median OS for the high-risk group was 13.1 months, and the median RFS was only 2.9 months. One of the determining factors for the poor outcomes might be that more patients in the high-risk group had PVTT in the main trunk or the first-order branch. A previous study reported that the median survival was 0.91 years for patients with PVTT 4 and 1.58 years for patients with PVTT 3 (9). Radical removal of tumor thrombosis was difficult for these patients, which might cause an early recurrence. Therefore, resection should be carefully performed due to the limited survival and higher probability of severe complication in these patients. Prognosis of other treatments for these patients were incompetent as well. Jeong et al. investigated the efficacy of Sorafenib in patients with PVTT 3-4 and the median OS was only 3.1 months (36). TACE could achieve a median survival of 6.1 to 7.49 months, yet this is still unsatisfactory (37, 38). Further studies on other treatment strategies for this population are urgently needed. In our study, although the RFS were significantly different in the two groups, the median RFS was only 10.9 months even in the low-risk group. Although long-term survival could be achieved in selected advanced HCC patients, the recurrence rate was still quite high after resection. Evaluation of adjuvant and neoadjuvant therapies might be helpful to prolong survival for this population.

The composition of this score covers the three aspects of liver function, extent of the surgery, and tumor burden, which are also elements physician would consider clinically. The ALBI score and the level of GGT represent the liver function of the patient. The ALBI score involving bilirubin and albumin level was constructed in 2015 and was well validated in HCC patients (26, 39). The previous published EHBH-PVTT score selected bilirubin as the aspect of liver function. We considered our score might reflect liver function better. The number of tumor-invaded liver segments is the decisive factor of the planned extent of surgery and was only included in our score system. As for the tumor burden, most of the elements were similar in the two scores, except that we used the stage of PVTT as one of the prognostic factors. As mentioned above, survival differed a lot within different stages of PVTT. The EHBH cohort also concluded that stages of PVTT was associated with disease-free survival, yet this factor was not used for score construction. This might be due to the fact that the EHBH score used prognostic factors for OS while our score used factors for RFS. OS was largely affected by the status and treatment of recurrent tumors, which might cause bias in the retrospective analysis. Therefore, we considered that the construction of a prognostic score is better if based on RFS.

It is interesting that with a cutoff value of 14 in our score system, patients with poor liver function were all in the high-risk group even with smaller tumors, less invaded liver segments, lower AFP, and no PVTT in the main trunk or first-branches. Things were quite different in the prognostic system in early stages, where the tumor characteristics accounted for the majority of the prognostic model (40, 41). It seems that for patients in the advanced stage, liver function is the main limiting factor for long-term survival. Performance of surgery in patients with poor liver function should be considered with caution in the advanced stage.

There exist some limitations to this article. First, the approach of resection was not discussed in this article. Several studies showed that the approach of resection affected survival after surgery (42, 43). However, most patients in the advanced stage would receive open abdominal surgery for the complexity of the disease. Therefore, this might not affect the practicability of the prognostic score. Second, we did not make a comparison of resection to the standard treatment of advanced HCC in the two risk groups. This is because the proportion of patients receiving Sorafenib is quite low due to the limited cost-effectiveness. Further studies are needed for this comparison. Third, it should be noted that several conditions were not included during the development of the score, such as patients without preserved liver function (Child-Pugh score>8) and patients with extrahepatic metastasis. Clinically, curative resection on these patients were considered extremely difficult or might cause severe post-surgery complications. Evaluation on these patients was not practical. Therefore, this article only discussed long-term OS in patients who were evaluated as resectable clinically. Last, this study was conducted based on a single center cohort in China. Therefore, the generalizability of our results is limited in western populations and needs further validation.

In conclusion, we established an effective pre-operative score that could help to select a group of advanced HCC patients who might benefit from liver resection with promising long-term survival. We recommended resection for patients in the low-risk group.

AUTHOR CONTRIBUTIONS

Concept and design: MK, SP, HX, and S-LC. Data collection: HX, J-LL, M-MT, Z-WP, and S-TF. Acquisition, analysis, or interpretation of data: All authors. Drafting of the manuscript: HX, S-LC, SP, and MK. Critical revision of the manuscript for important intellectual content: SP, S-LC, and MK. Statistical analysis: QZ, T-FW, and XL. Supervision: MK and SP. All authors contributed to the article and approved the submitted version.

ACKNOWLEDGMENTS

The content of this manuscript has been presented in part at the international digestive disease forum, 2019 (44). We thank the Clinical Trials Unit, the First Affiliated Hospital of Sun Yat-sen University for providing statistical support for this study. No preregistration exists for the studies reported in this article.

REFERENCES

1. Siegel RL, Miller KD, Jemal A. Cancer statistics, 2018. *CA Cancer J Clin* (2018) 68:7–30. doi: 10.3322/caac.21442
2. Chen W, Sun K, Zheng R, Zeng H, Zhang S, Xia C, et al. Cancer incidence and mortality in China, 2014. *Chin J Cancer Res* (2018) 30:1–12. doi: 10.21147/j.issn.1000-9604.2018.01.01
3. Park J-W, Chen M, Colombo M, Roberts LR, Schwartz M, Chen P-J, et al. Global patterns of hepatocellular carcinoma management from diagnosis to death: the BRIDGE Study. *Liver Int* (2015) 35:2155–66. doi: 10.1111/liv.12818
4. Llovet JM, Ricci S, Mazzaferro V, Hilgard P, Gane E, Blanc J-F, et al. Sorafenib in advanced hepatocellular carcinoma. *N Engl J Med* (2008) 359:378–90. doi: 10.1056/NEJMoa0708857
5. Kudo M, Finn RS, Qin S, Han K-H, Ikeda K, Piscaglia F, et al. Lenvatinib versus sorafenib in first-line treatment of patients with unresectable hepatocellular carcinoma: a randomised phase 3 non-inferiority trial. *Lancet* (2018) 391:1163–73. doi: 10.1016/S0140-6736(18)30207-1
6. Roayaie S, Jibara G, Tabrizian P, Park J-W, Yang J, Yan L, et al. The role of hepatic resection in the treatment of hepatocellular cancer. *Hepatology* (2015) 62:440–51. doi: 10.1002/hep.27745
7. Zhong J-H, Ke Y, Gong W-F, Xiang B-D, Ma L, Ye X-P, et al. Hepatic resection associated with good survival for selected patients with intermediate and advanced-stage hepatocellular carcinoma. *Ann Surg* (2014) 260:329–40. doi: 10.1097/SLA.0000000000000236
8. Ruzzenente A, Capra F, Pachera S, Iacono C, Piccirillo G, Lunardi M, et al. Is liver resection justified in advanced hepatocellular carcinoma? Results of an observational study in 464 patients. *J Gastrointest Surg* (2009) 13:1313–20. doi: 10.1007/s11605-009-0903-x
9. Kokudo T, Hasegawa K, Matsuyama Y, Takayama T, Izumi N, Kadoya M, et al. Survival benefit of liver resection for hepatocellular carcinoma associated with portal vein invasion. *J Hepatol* (2016) 65:938–43. doi: 10.1016/j.jhep.2016.05.044
10. Heimbach JK, Kulik LM, Finn RS, Sirlin CB, Abecassis MM, Roberts LR, et al. AASLD guidelines for the treatment of hepatocellular carcinoma. *Hepatology* (2017) 67:358–80. doi: 10.1002/hep.29086
11. European Association for the Study of the Liver. Electronic address: easloffice@easloffice.eu, European Association For The Study Of The Liver. EASL Clinical Practice Guidelines: Management of hepatocellular carcinoma. *J Hepatol* (2018) 69:182–236. doi: 10.1016/j.jhep.2018.03.019
12. Omata M, Cheng A-L, Kokudo N, Kudo M, Lee JM, Jia J, et al. Asia-Pacific clinical practice guidelines on the management of hepatocellular carcinoma: a 2017 update. *Hepatol Int* (2017) 11:317–70. doi: 10.1007/s12072-017-9799-9
13. Kokudo N, Hasegawa K, Akahane M, Igaki H, Izumi N, Ichida T, et al. Evidence-based Clinical Practice Guidelines for Hepatocellular Carcinoma: The Japan Society of Hepatology 2013 update (3rd JSH-HCC Guidelines). *Hepatol Res* (2015) 45:123–7. doi: 10.1111/hepr.12464
14. Chok KSH, Cheung TT, Chan SC, Poon RTP, Fan ST, Lo CM. Surgical outcomes in hepatocellular carcinoma patients with portal vein tumor thrombosis. *World J Surg* (2014) 38:490–6. doi: 10.1007/s00268-013-2290-4
15. Xu J-F, Liu X-Y, Wang S, Wen H-X. Surgical treatment for hepatocellular carcinoma with portal vein tumor thrombus: a novel classification. *World J Surg Oncol* (2015) 13:86. doi: 10.1186/s12957-015-0493-x
16. Peng Z-W, Guo R-P, Zhang Y-J, Lin X-J, Chen M-S, Lau WY. Hepatic resection versus transcatheter arterial chemoembolization for the treatment of hepatocellular carcinoma with portal vein tumor thrombus. *Cancer* (2012) 118:4725–36. doi: 10.1002/cncr.26561
17. Matono R, Yoshiya S, Motomura T, Toshima T, Kayashima H, Masuda T, et al. Factors linked to longterm survival of patients with hepatocellular carcinoma accompanied by tumour thrombus in the major portal vein after surgical resection. *HPB (Oxford)* (2012) 14:247–53. doi: 10.1111/j.1477-2574.2011.00436.x
18. Kokudo T, Hasegawa K, Matsuyama Y, Takayama T, Izumi N, Kadoya M, et al. Liver resection for hepatocellular carcinoma associated with hepatic vein invasion: A Japanese nationwide survey. *Hepatology* (2017) 66:510–7. doi: 10.1002/hep.29225
19. Zhang X-P, Gao Y-Z, Chen Z-H, Chen M-S, Li L-Q, Wen T-F, et al. An Eastern Hepatobiliary Surgery Hospital/Portal Vein Tumor Thrombus scoring system as an aid to decision-making on hepatectomy for Hepatocellular Carcinoma patients with Portal Vein Tumor Thrombus: a multicenter study. *Hepatology* (2018) 69:2076–90. doi: 10.1002/hep.30490
20. European Association for Study of Liver, European Organisation for Research and Treatment of Cancer. EASL-EORTC clinical practice guidelines: management of hepatocellular carcinoma. *Eur J Cancer* (2012) 48:599–641. doi: 10.1016/j.ejca.2011.12.021
21. Bruix J, Sherman M, Llovet JM, Beaugrand M, Lencioni R, Burroughs AK, et al. Clinical management of hepatocellular carcinoma. In: *Conclusions of the barcelona-2000 EASL conference J Hepatol* 35:421–30. doi: 10.1016/S0168-8278(01)00130-1
22. Bruix J, Sherman M. Practice Guidelines Committee, American Association for the Study of Liver Diseases. Management of hepatocellular carcinoma. *Hepatology* (2005) 42:1208–36. doi: 10.1002/hep.20933
23. Bruix J, Reig M, Sherman M. Evidence-Based Diagnosis, Staging, and Treatment of Patients With Hepatocellular Carcinoma. *Gastroenterology* (2016) 150:835–53. doi: 10.1053/j.gastro.2015.12.041
24. Forner A, Llovet JM, Bruix J. Hepatocellular carcinoma. *Lancet* (2012) 379:1245–55. doi: 10.1016/S0140-6736(11)61347-0
25. Lencioni R, Llovet JM. Modified RECIST (mRECIST) assessment for hepatocellular carcinoma. *Semin Liver Dis* (2010) 30:52–60. doi: 10.1055/s-0030-1247132
26. Johnson PJ, Berhane S, Kagebayashi C, Satomura S, Teng M, Reeves HL, et al. Assessment of liver function in patients with hepatocellular carcinoma: a new evidence-based approach-the ALBI grade. *J Clin Oncol* (2015) 33:550–8. doi: 10.1200/JCO.2014.57.9151
27. Cheng A-L, Kang Y-K, Chen Z, Tsao C-J, Qin S, Kim JS, et al. Efficacy and safety of sorafenib in patients in the Asia-Pacific region with advanced hepatocellular carcinoma: a phase III randomised, double-blind, placebo-controlled trial. *Lancet Oncol* (2009) 10:25–34. doi: 10.1016/S1470-2045(08)70285-7

28. Hyun MH, Lee Y-S, Kim JH, Lee CU, Jung YK, Seo YS, et al. Hepatic resection compared to chemoembolization in intermediate- to advanced-stage hepatocellular carcinoma: A meta-analysis of high-quality studies. *Hepatology* (2018) 68:977–93. doi: 10.1002/hep.29883
29. Ng KK, Vauthey J-N, Pawlik TM, Lauwers GY, Regimbeau J-M, Belghiti J, et al. Is hepatic resection for large or multinodular hepatocellular carcinoma justified? Results from a multi-institutional database. *Ann Surg Oncol* (2005) 12:364–73. doi: 10.1245/ASO.2005.06.004
30. Kim H, Ahn SW, Hong SK, Yoon KC, Kim H-S, Choi YR, et al. Survival benefit of liver resection for Barcelona Clinic Liver Cancer stage B hepatocellular carcinoma. *Br J Surg* (2017) 104:1045–52. doi: 10.1002/bjs.10541
31. Wang B-W, Mok K-T, Liu S-I, Chou N-H, Tsai C-C, Chen I-S, et al. Is hepatectomy beneficial in the treatment of multinodular hepatocellular carcinoma? *J Formos Med Assoc* (2008) 107:616–26. doi: 10.1016/S0929-6646(08)60179-5
32. Bruix J, Raoul J-L, Sherman M, Mazzaferro V, Bolondi L, Craxì A, et al. Efficacy and safety of sorafenib in patients with advanced hepatocellular carcinoma: subanalyses of a phase III trial. *J Hepatol.* (2012) 57:821–9. doi: 10.1016/j.jhep.2012.06.014
33. Kodama K, Kawaoka T, Aikata H, Uchikawa S, Inagaki Y, Hatooka M, et al. Comparison of clinical outcome of hepatic arterial infusion chemotherapy and sorafenib for advanced hepatocellular carcinoma according to macrovascular invasion and transcatheter arterial chemoembolization refractory status. *J Gastroenterol Hepatol* (2018) 33:1780–6. doi: 10.1111/jgh.14152
34. Makuuchi M, Hasegawa H, Yamazaki S. Ultrasonically guided subsegmentectomy. *Surg Gynecol Obstet* (1985) 161:346–50. doi: 10.1055/s-2007-1022639
35. Shindoh J, Makuuchi M, Matsuyama Y, Mise Y, Arita J, Sakamoto Y, et al. Complete removal of the tumor-bearing portal territory decreases local tumor recurrence and improves disease-specific survival of patients with hepatocellular carcinoma. *J Hepatol* (2016) 64:594–600. doi: 10.1016/j.jhep.2015.10.015
36. Jeong SW, Jang JY, Shim KY, Lee SH, Kim SG, Cha S-W, et al. Practical Effect of Sorafenib Monotherapy on Advanced Hepatocellular Carcinoma and Portal Vein Tumor Thrombosis. *Gut Liver* (2013) 7:696–703. doi: 10.5009/gnl.2013.7.6.696
37. Zhao Y, Duran R, Chapiro J, Sohn JH, Sahu S, Fleckenstein F, et al. Transarterial Chemoembolization for the Treatment of Advanced-Stage Hepatocellular Carcinoma. *J Gastrointest Surg* (2016) 20:2002–9. doi: 10.1007/s11605-016-3285-x
38. Lv W-F, Liu K-C, Lu D, Zhou C-Z, Cheng D-L, Xiao J-K, et al. Transarterial chemoembolization for hepatocellular carcinoma combined with portal vein tumor thrombosis. *CMAR* (2018) 10:4719–26. doi: 10.2147/CMAR.S166527
39. Kao W-Y, Su C-W, Chiou Y-Y, Chiu N-C, Liu C-A, Fang K-C, et al. Hepatocellular Carcinoma: Nomograms Based on the Albumin-Bilirubin Grade to Assess the Outcomes of Radiofrequency Ablation. *Radiology* (2017) 285:162382–680. doi: 10.1148/radiol.2017162382
40. Zheng J, Chou JF, Gonen M, Vachharajani N, Chapman WC, Majella Doyle MB, et al. Prediction of Hepatocellular Carcinoma Recurrence Beyond Milan Criteria After Resection: Validation of a Clinical Risk Score in an International Cohort. *Ann Surg* (2017) 266:693–701. doi: 10.1097/SLA.0000000000002360
41. Cho CS, Gonen M, Shia J, Kattan MW, Klimstra DS, Jarnagin WR, et al. A novel prognostic nomogram is more accurate than conventional staging systems for predicting survival after resection of hepatocellular carcinoma. *J Am Coll Surgeons* (2008) 206:281–91. doi: 10.1016/j.jamcollsurg.2007.07.031
42. Lee JJ, Conneely JB, Smoot RL, Gallinger S, Greig PD, Moulton C-A, et al. Laparoscopic versus open liver resection for hepatocellular carcinoma at a North-American Centre: a 2-to-1 matched pair analysis. *HPB (Oxford)* (2015) 17:304–10. doi: 10.1111/hpb.12342
43. Yoon Y-S, Han H-S, Cho JY, Ahn KS. Total laparoscopic liver resection for hepatocellular carcinoma located in all segments of the liver. *Surg Endosc* (2010) 24:1630–7. doi: 10.1007/s00464-009-0823-6
44. Xiao H, Chen S-L, Tang M-M, Peng Z-W, Peng S, Kuang M. A pre-operative prognostic score for patients with advanced hepatocellular carcinoma (HCC) who underwent resection. *J Digest Dis* (2019) 20:S1 38–39. doi: 10.1111/1751-2980.12808

8

Diffuse Recurrence of Hepatocellular Carcinoma After Liver Resection: Transarterial Chemoembolization (TACE) Combined with Sorafenib Versus TACE Monotherapy

Wang Yao [1†], Miao Xue [1†], Mingjian Lu [2†], Yu Wang [1], Yue Zhao [1], Yanqin Wu [1], Wenzhe Fan [1] and Jiaping Li [1*]*

[1] Department of Interventional Oncology, the First Affiliated Hospital of Sun Yat-Sen University, Guangzhou, China,
[2] Department of Radiology, Affiliated Cancer Hospital & Institute of Guangzhou Medical University, Guangzhou, China

***Correspondence:**
Wenzhe Fan
fanwenzhe2007@126.com
Jiaping Li
yaowanggood@126.com

†These authors have contributed equally to this work and share first authorship

This study aims to compare the effectiveness and complications of transarterial chemoembolization (TACE) combined with sorafenib (S-TACE) and TACE monotherapy in HCC patients with diffuse recurrence (DR). This retrospective study was approved by our hospital ethics committee, and all patients provided informed consent. We retrospectively enrolled 356 DR patients from January 2005 to December 2014, who underwent either S-TACE or TACE monotherapy. Treatment complications, overall survival (OS) and progression-free survival (PFS) were evaluated. Survival curves were constructed using the Kaplan-Meier method and compared using a log-rank test. Our results found a significant difference between S-TACE and TACE monotherapy in the PFS and OS of HCC patients with early diffuse recurrence (EDR) (p=0.011 and 0.049, respectively). Patients with late diffuse recurrence (LDR) who underwent S-TACE had longer OS (median 24.0 vs. 16.0 months; p=0.044) compared with those in the TACE monotherapy group. Subgroup analysis revealed that S-TACE therapy resulted in higher OS of EDR patients with tumors > 5 cm and HBV-DNA >100 (p=0.036 and 0.035, respectively), compared with patients given TACE monotherapy. S-TACE therapy also resulted in better OS in LDR patients with AFP≥400 ng/ml, AFP<400 ng/ml, TB<28 g/L, TB>28 g/L, and a maximum tumor diameter < 5 cm (p=<0.001, 0.042, <0.001, <0.001, and <0.001, respectively). The rate of major complications in patients who underwent S-TACE was not significantly different to those who underwent TACE monotherapy (33.5% vs. 28.2%, p= 0.69). Overall, patients given S-TACE had better OS in both EDR and LDR patients, but only EDR patients had better PFS.

Keywords: transarterial chemoembolization, sorafenib, hepatocellular carcinoma, diffuse recurrence, liver resection

INTRODUCTION

Hepatocellular carcinoma (HCC) is the fifth most common type of tumor and the third largest cause of cancer-related deaths (1). Liver resection is a curative treatment method for HCC, however, only 9%–27% of HCC patients are eligible for surgical resection (2). Although radical hepatectomy can be therapeutically effective for small HCC, the recurrence rate remains high (3). Diffuse recurrence (DR) is defined as 10 or more new recurrent nodules with ill-defined tumor margins (4, 5). DR is divided into early diffuse recurrence (EDR) and late diffuse recurrence (LDR) based on the time to recurrence (6). According to the 2018 European Association for the Study of the Liver (EASL) HCC guidelines, DR is classified by multinodular recurrence, with transarterial chemoembolization (TACE) recommended as the optimal treatment. However, the efficacy of TACE is limited, and quick recurrence following this treatment can result in a worse prognosis according to the study of Choi et al. (7). So, new therapies are urgently needed.

In most circumstances, chemoembolization is the optimal treatment for multinodular recurrent HCC (8). TACE can prolong the survival of patients by preserving the liver function and treating multinodular asymptomatic tumors without macroscopic vascular invasion or extrahepatic spread (9, 10). Sorafenib, an oral multikinase inhibitor with antiproliferative and antiangiogenic activities, is recommended for patients with advanced-stage HCC (11, 12). Chao et al. combined TACE with sorafenib (S-TACE) in patients with multinodular, unresectable HCC. Of their patients, 81.5% did not have vascular invasion or extrahepatic spread. Their results found that S-TACE was well tolerated and efficacious in patients with multinodular HCC without vascular invasion and extrahepatic spread (13). However, the effects of S-TACE in patients with DR remains unknown.

Few reports have focused on studying or developing a treatment strategy for DR in patients with HCC who have undergone previous liver resection. The aim of this retrospective study was to compare the effectiveness and safety of S-TACE and TACE monotherapy in HCC patients with DR who have undergone a previous liver resection.

MATERIALS AND METHODS

Ethical Statement

Written informed consent was obtained from each patient prior to the treatment. The patients were sufficiently informed of the risks, benefits, and alternatives to both S-TACE and TACE monotherapy. The study protocol followed the ethical guidelines of the 1975 Declaration of Helsinki (as revised in Brazil in 2013). This retrospective study was approved by the institutional review board of our hospital.

Patient Selection

HCC was diagnosed according to the European Society of Digestive Oncology (14) and classified based on the Barcelona-Clinic Liver Cancer (BCLC) staging classification (15). The inclusion criteria were as follows: (a) patients with their first recurrence after liver resection; (b) aged 18–75 years; (c) with 10 or more new recurrent nodules; (d) with Eastern Cooperative Oncology Group performance status of 0 or 1; (e) with Child-Pugh classification of A or B. The exclusion criteria was: (a) patients with extrahepatic spread; (b) with serious medical comorbidities, such as dysfunction of the heart or kidneys, severe coagulation disorders, etc.; (c) with other current malignancies or a history of other malignancies besides HCC; (d) with vascular invasion; (e) patients who had undergone other treatments before this study (**Figure 1**).

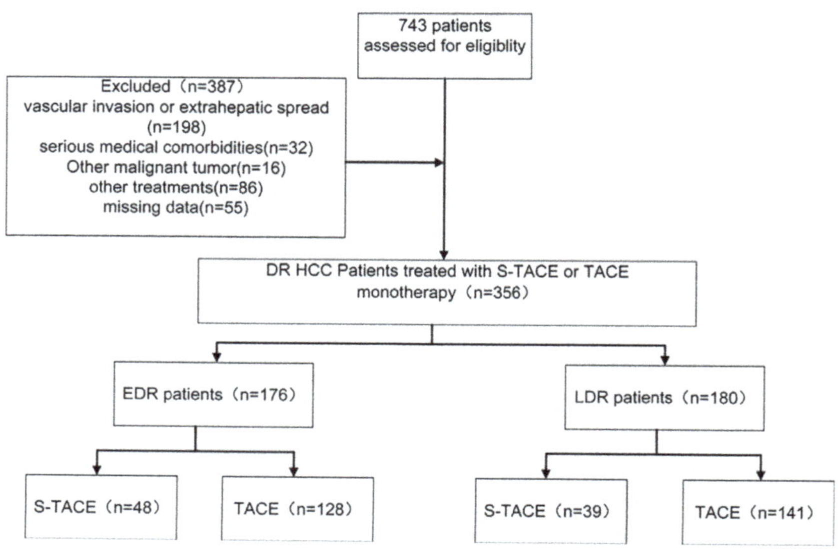

FIGURE 1 | Flowchart showed patient selection.

Transarterial Chemoembolization Procedure

All TACE procedures were performed by 1 of 3 interventional physicians. A 5F catheter (Terumo, Tokyo, Japan) or a 2.7F microcatheter (Renegade Hi-Flo Straight, Boston scientific, Natick, Mass; Progreat, Terumo, Tokyo, Japan) was employed for tumor-feeding artery superselective therapy. An emulsion of 5–20 ml lipiodol (Lipiodol; Guerbet, Aulnay-Sous-Bois, France) and 20–60 mg epirubicin (Pharmorubicin; Pfizer, New York, USA) were administered into the tumor-feeding vessels. The specific dose of lipiodol was determined based on the tumor number and volume. Then, 350–560 mm absorbable gelatin sponge particles (Gelfoam; Hangzhou Pharmaceutical, Linan, China) were administered into the tumor-feeding vessels. The embolization finishes when the radiocontrast agent stopped flowing for 5 cardiac cycles.

Sorafenib Management

Sorafenib therapy (daily dose, 400 mg BID) was initiated 2-5 days after the initial TACE and continued until the emergence of intolerance, refusal, and tumor progression. Sorafenib dose reduction was determined based on the presence of toxicity. If grade 3 or 4 adverse events (AEs)-defined by the National Cancer Institute Common Terminology Criteria for Adverse Events (16)-occurred, a dose adjustment (400 mg once daily) was performed until AEs were alleviated or eliminated. If grade 3 or 4 AEs continued after dose adjustment, sorafenib treatment would be halted until AEs were alleviated or eliminated.

Survival, Tumor Progression, and Safety

In this study, the primary endpoint evaluated was overall survival (OS), defined as the time HCC recurrence was diagnosed to the date the patient died for any reason. The secondary endpoint was progression-free survival (PFS), defined as the time HCC recurrence was diagnosed to the date on which the tumor progressed. HCC progression was defined as the appearance of local tumor progression, new HCC nodule, vascular invasion, or extrahepatic spread according to contrast-enhanced dynamic CT or MR imaging results. Treatment responses were divided according to the mRECIST standard into CR, PR, SD, and PD (17). Contrast-enhanced dynamic CT or MR results were discussed and confirmed by two radiologists.

We assessed the safety and toxicity of TACE and oral sorafenib administration in all patients, using the National Cancer Institute Common Terminology Criteria for Adverse Events. Grade 3–4 AE was defined as an event leading to substantial morbidity and disability (resulting in the unexpected loss of an organ), which resulted in increase in the level of care, hospital admission, length of hospital stay, or led to the adjustment or discontinuation of treatment protocols. Grade 3–4 AEs were considered major complications, other complications were regarded as minor.

Follow-Up

All patients were followed monthly for the first 3 months, then every 3 months until 2 years after TACE, and annually thereafter. Follow-up assessments included a detailed medical history, physical examination, laboratory tests, and chest and abdominal contrast-enhanced CT or MRI examination. When tumor progression occurred, the decision to perform repeated TACE was made by an MDT group.

Statistical Analyses

All statistical analyses were performed using SPSS software (version 24.0; SPSS, Chicago, IL, *USA*). Continuity correction and independent sample *t-tests* were used to analyze the quantitative data including age, ALB, TB, and maximal tumor diameter. Pearson x^2 and Fisher's exact tests were applied for qualitative data such as sex, cause of HCC, liver cirrhosis, AFP, HBV-DNA, ECOG, Child-Pugh class, and the incidence of complications. The cutoff value was calculated using R (TIBCO, Silicon Valley, CA). OS and PFS were calculated using the Kaplan-Meier method. The Kaplan-Meier survival estimates were compared using a x^2 statistic with a Log-Rank weighting scheme. Univariable and multivariable analyses were performed using the Cox proportional hazard regression model. All statistical tests were two-tailed, and a *p-value* <0.05 indicated a significant difference.

RESULTS

Optimal Cutoff Value for Distinguishing Early and Late Diffuse Recurrence

Recurrence was evaluated every 5 months to determine the optimal cutoff value for distinguishing between EDR and LDR. Eight months was found to be the optimal cutoff value, as shown in **Figure 2**. Clinicopathological data and outcomes after

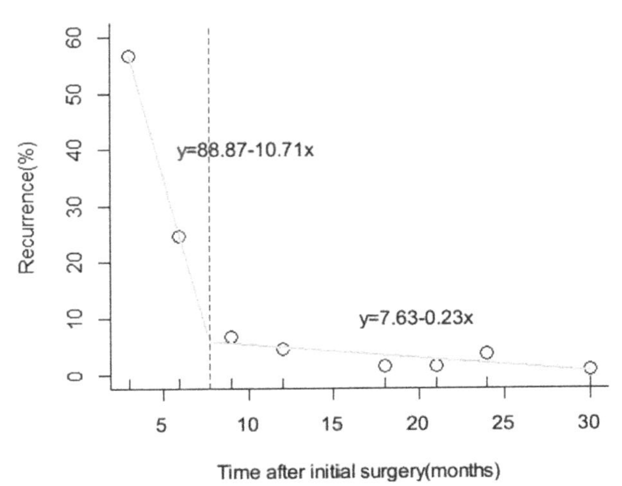

FIGURE 2 | Determination of the optimal cutoff value for early and late diffuse recurrence of hepatocellular carcinoma (HCC). The function of the two lines was y = 88.87 – 10.71x and y = 7.63 – 0 23x, respectively. The intercept value of the two lines was 8 months. 8 months was therefore defined as the optimal cutoff value to differentiate early and late diffuse recurrence of HCC.

recurrence were analyzed and compared between the EDR and LDR groups.

Patient Characteristics

Between January 2005 and December 2014, 356 patients at our hospital developed DR after initial liver resection. Follow-up data were collected until December 30, 2017. Patients were divided into 2 groups (the EDR group and LDR group) according to recurrence type. In the EDR group, 48 cases (27%) were in the S-TACE group and 128 cases (73%) were in the TACE monotherapy group. In the LDR group, 39 cases (22%) were in the S-TACE group and 141 cases (77%) were in the TACE monotherapy group. Median age of the EDR patients was 55.0±11.7 and 56.0±11.9 years in S-TACE and TACE monotherapy groups, respectively. The median age of the LDR patients was 52.0±12.8, 57.0±12.3 years in S-TACE and TACE monotherapy groups, respectively. There was no significant difference in the baseline characteristics of the EDR and LDR groups (**Table 1**, **Table 2**). All baseline characteristics were collected before TACE. The median follow-up time was 52 months (range, 2–62 months) in the EDR group and 63 months (range, 3–86 months) in the LDR group. There were 123 cases (70%) in the EDR group and 96 cases (53%) in the LDR group where the patient died during the follow-up period. The mean duration of sorafenib treatment was 11 months (range, 1–23 months).

TABLE 1 | Baseline patient characteristics of early diffuse recurrence (EDR) patients.

Characteristic	S-TACE (n=48)	TACE (n=128)	P value
Sex			0.789
Male	42(87.5)	110(85.9)	
Female	6(12.5)	18(14.1)	
Age(y)			0.565
Median±SD	55.0±11.7	56.0±11.9	
Range	26–77	22–78	
Cause of HCC			0.514
HBV	39(81.3)	109(85.2)	
HCV	4(8.3)	9(7.1)	
Alcohol	1(2.1)	3(2.3)	
Other	4(8.3)	7(5.4)	
Liver cirrhosis	33(68.8)	101(78.9)	0.160
ALB(g/L)			0.124
Median±SD	36.0±6.7	37.0±6.3	
Range	27-73	24-66	
TB (umol/L)			0.618
Median± SD	25.5±6.3	27.0±13.4	
Range	11–44	5–90	
AFP(ng/ml)			0.053
≥400	21(43.8)	78(60.9)	
<400	27(56.3)	50(39.1)	
HBV-DNA			0.051
≥100	31(64.6)	53(41.4)	
<100	17(35.4)	75(58.6)	
ECOG			0.891
0	42(87.5)	111(86.7)	
1	6(12.5)	17(13.3)	
Child-Pugh			0.508
A	41(85.4)	114(89.1)	
B	7(14.6)	14(10.9)	
Maximal tumor diameter(cm)			0.181
Median ± SD	5.0±2.6	4.0±2.9	
Range	2.0-13.0	1.0-13.0	

Except where indicated, data are numbers of patients. Data in parentheses are percentages and were calculated by using the total number of patients in each group as the denominator.

TABLE 2 | Baseline patient characteristics of late diffuse recurrence (LDR) patients.

Characteristic	S-TACE (n=39)	TACE (n=141)	P value
Sex			0.247
Male	36(92.3)	127(90.1)	
Female	3(7.7)	14(9.9)	
Age(y)			0.428
Mean±SD	52.0±12.8	57.0±12.3	
Range	22–76	22-78	
Cause of HCC			0.613
HBV	33(84.6)	124(87.9)	
HCV	3(7.7)	6(4.3)	
Alcohol	1(2.6)	4(2.8)	
Other	2(5.1)	7(5.0)	
Liver cirrhosis	31(79.5)	110(78.0)	0.844
ALB(g/L)			0.262
Mean±SD	36.0±4.4	35.0±6.3	
Range	27–47	24–66	
TB (umol/L)			0.088
Mean ± SD	21.0±10.1	14.9±9.8	
Range	7.9-39.0	7.6-41.0	
AFP(ng/ml)			0.833
≥400	19(48.7)	66(46.8)	
<400	20(51.3)	75(53.2)	
HBV-DNA(U/ml)			0.062
≥100	10(25.6)	59(41.8)	
<100	29(74.4)	82(58.2)	
ECOG			0.247
0	33(84.6)	107(75.9)	
1	6(15.4)	34(24.1)	
Child-Pugh			0.276
A	32(82.1)	125(88.7)	
B	7(17.9)	16(11.3)	
Maximal tumor diameter(cm)			0.279
Mean ± SD	6.0±3.3	5.0±3.2	
Range	1.0–15.0	1.0–16.0	

Except where indicated, data are numbers of patients. Data in parentheses are percentages and were calculated by using the total number of patients in each group as the denominator.

Recurrence-Free Survival and Overall Survival

In the EDR group, median OS was 17.5 months (95% CI: 14.3, 19.7 months) and 11.0 months (95% CI: 9.9, 12.1 months) in the S-TACE and TACE monotherapy groups, respectively. The median PFS was 5.0 months (95%CI: 3.9, 6.1 months) and 4.0 months (95% CI: 3.4, 4.6 months) in the S-TACE and TACE monotherapy groups, respectively. There was a significant difference in OS and PFS (log-rank test, p=0.011 and p=0.049, respectively) between the two groups (**Figure 3**).

In LDR group, median OS was 24.0 months (95% CI: 19.1, 28.9 months) and 16.0 months (95% CI: 14.6, 17.4 months) in S-TACE and TACE monotherapy groups, respectively. The median PFS was 8.0 months (95% CI: 6.9, 9.1 months) and 5.0 months (95% CI: 4.3, 5.7 months) in the S-TACE and TACE monotherapy groups, respectively. There was a significant difference in OS (log-rank test, p=0.044) between the two groups, but not for PFS (log-rank test, p= 0.176) (**Figure 3**).

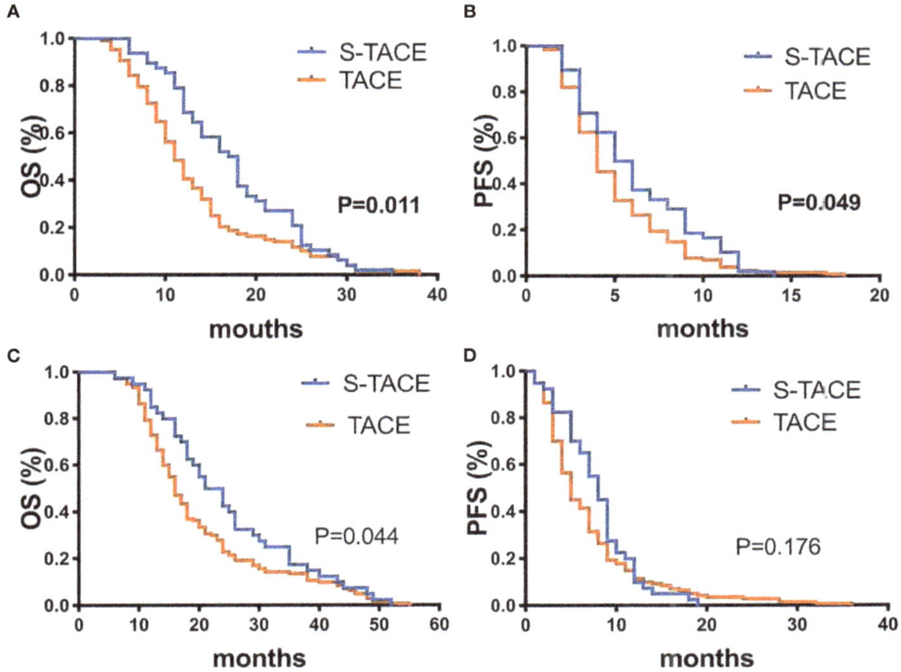

FIGURE 3 | Kaplan-Meier curves showed overall survival **(A)** and Progression-free survival **(B)** in the S-TACE and complications of transarterial chemoembolization (TACE) groups in patients with early diffuse recurrence (EDR). Kaplan-Meier curves showed overall survival **(C)** and Progression-free survival **(D)** in the S-TACE and complications of transarterial chemoembolization (TACE) groups for patients with late diffuse recurrence (LDR).

Overall, the LDR group had better OS and PFS (p< 0.001) than the EDR group. In subgroup analysis, the LDR group had better OS (p<0.001) and PFS (p=0.031) than the EDR group when S-TACE was performed. When TACE was performed, the LDR group had better OS (p<0.001) and PFS (p<0.001) than the EDR group (**Figure 4**).

Univariate and Multivariate Analysis

Univariate analysis of EDR patients found that the factors related to OS were HBV-DNA and maximum tumor size (p = 0.023 and 0.008, respectively) (**Table 3**). Multivariate analysis found that HBV-DNA and maximum tumor size were found to be independent predictors of poor OS in EDR patients (p= and 0.030 and 0.010, respectively) (**Table 3**).

Univariate analysis found that in the LDR group, AFP, TB, HBV-DNA, and maximum tumor size were associated with OS (p=0.002, 0.041, 0.038, and 0.003, respectively) (**Table 4**). In multivariate regression analysis, AFP, TB, and maximum tumor size were found to be independent predictors of poor OS in LDR patients (p=0.008, 0.043, 0.045) (**Table 4**).

Subgroup Analysis

In EDR patients, S-TACE therapy resulted in higher OS than TACE monotherapy in tumors with a maximum diameter of >5 cm and HBV-DNA>100 group (p= 0.036 and 0.035, respectively). There was no significant difference between S-TACE and TACE monotherapy in tumors with a maximum diameter of < 5 cm and HBV<100 group (p=0.105 and 0.099, respectively) (**Figure 5**). In LDR patients, patients given S-TACE therapy had better OS than those given TACE monotherapy in patients with AFP≥400 ng/ml, AFP<400 ng/ml, TB<28 g/L, TB>28 g/L, and maximum diameter of tumor < 5 cm group (p<0.001,<0.001, <0.001, <0.001, and <0.001, respectively). There was no significant difference between patients given S-TACE and TACE monotherapy with tumors > 5 cm (p=0.113) (**Figure 6**).

Complications

There were no deaths in either the EDR or LDR group within 30 days after treatment. Major and minor complications are reported in **Tables 5** and **6**. There was no significant difference in major complications between the EDR and LDR groups (33.5% vs. 28.2%, p = 0.69). By the end of the follow-up period, 47 patients (53%) had discontinued sorafenib administration, including 24 (50%) patients in the EDR group and 23 (59%) patients in the LDR group because of serious AEs. Most patients (97.9%) experienced at least one AE (see **Table 5** and **Table 6**).

In the EDR group, the major AEs that were experienced by at least 10% of patients were abdominal pain (11.3%) and hand-foot skin reaction (33.3%). Others major AEs included diarrhea (8.0%), hypertension (8.3%), gastrointestinal hemorrhage (6.3%), and fever (6.3%). There was no significant difference in occurrence of AEs between the S-TACE and TACE monotherapy groups

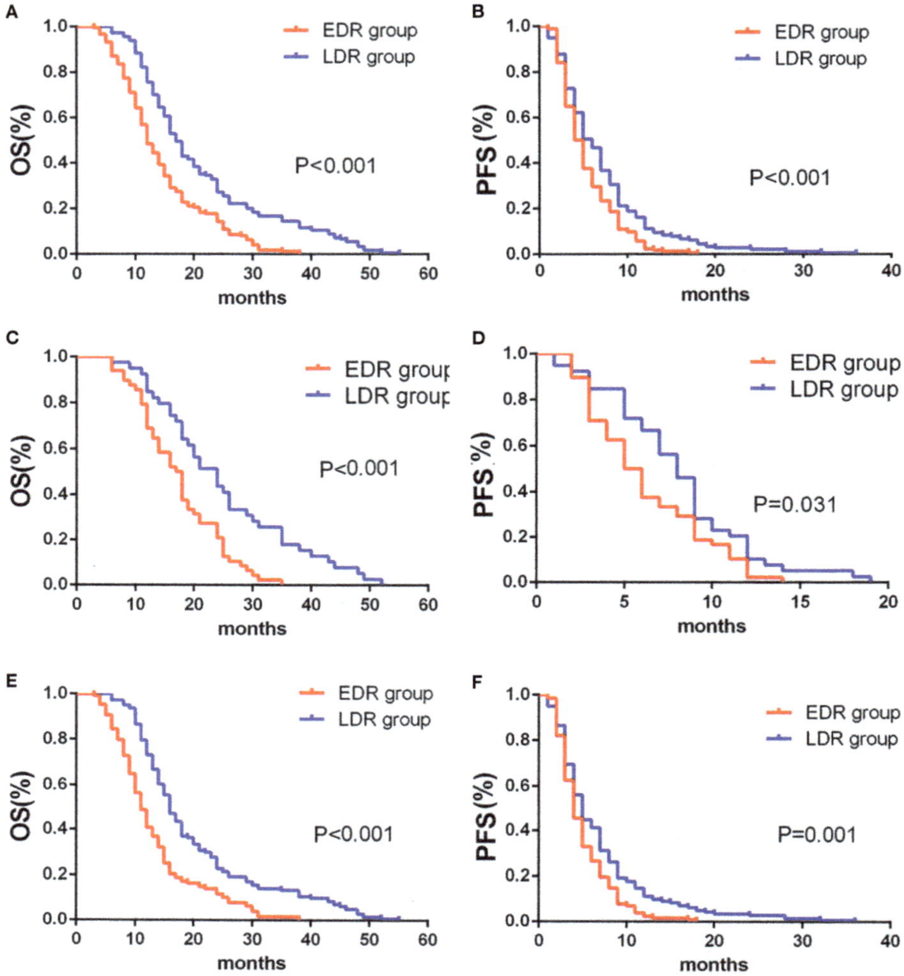

FIGURE 4 | Kaplan-Meier curves showed overall survival **(A)** and Progression-free survival **(B)** in the early diffuse recurrence (EDR) and late diffuse recurrence (LDR) groups. Kaplan-Meier curves showed overall survival **(C)** and Progression-free survival **(D)** in the EDR and LDR groups for patients with S-TACE. Kaplan-Meier curves showed overall survival **(E)** and Progression-free survival **(F)** in the EDR and LDR groups for patients with complications of transarterial chemoembolization (TACE) alone.

TABLE 3 | Univariable and multivariable analysis of prognostic factors for OS in early diffuse recurrence (EDR) patients.

Factor	Univariate analysis			Multivariate analysis		
	P Value	Hazard ratio	95%CI	P Value	Hazard ratio	95%CI
Sex	0.912	0.972	(0.583, 1.620)	NA	–	–
Age	0.991	0.998	(0.730, 1.364)	NA	–	–
Cause of HCC	0.949	1.007	(0.822, 1.233)	NA	–	–
Liver cirrhosis	0.752	0.946	(0.668, 1.338)	NA	–	–
AFP	0.143	1.257	(0.926, 1.707)	NA	–	–
ALB	0.380	0.989	(0.964, 1.014)	NA	–	–
TB	0.460	1.004	(0.993, 1.016)	NA	–	–
HBV-DNA	0.023	1.424	(1.049, 1.933)	0.030	1.403	(1.032,1.906)
ECOG	0.196	1.338	(0.861, 2.080)	NA	–	–
Child-Pugh	0.462	0.823	(0.490, 1.383)	NA	–	–
Maximum tumor size	0.008	1.500	(1.112, 2.025)	0.010	1.482	(1.097,2.002)

–, no data; CI, confidence interval; NA, not applicable.

TABLE 4 | Univariable and multivariable analysis of prognostic factors for OS in late diffuse recurrence (LDR) patients.

Factor	Univariate analysis			Multivariate analysis		
	P Value	Hazard ratio	95%CI	P Value	Hazard ratio	95%CI
Sex	0.998	1.001	(0.605, 1.654)	NA	–	–
Age	0.242	0.992	(0.979, 1.005)	NA	–	–
Cause of HCC	0.709	0.917	(0.581, 1.447)	NA	–	–
Liver cirrhosis	0.719	0.937	(0.656, 1.338)	NA	–	–
AFP	0.002	1.621	(1.189, 2.208)	0.008	1.545	(1.122, 2.126)
ALB	0.066	1.330	(0.981, 1.803)	NA	–	–
TB	0.041	0.698	(0.495, 0.985)	0.043	0.698	(0.494, 0.988)
HBV-DNA	0.038	1.384	(1.018, 1.879)	0.091	1.310	(0.957, 1.793)
ECOG	0.627	0.900	(0.589, 1.377)	NA	–	–
Child-Pugh	0.535	0.870	(0.561, 1.350)	NA	–	–
Maximum tumor size	0.003	1.584	(1.166, 2.154)	0.045	1.389	(1.007, 1.915)

–, no data; CI, confidence interval; NA, not applicable.

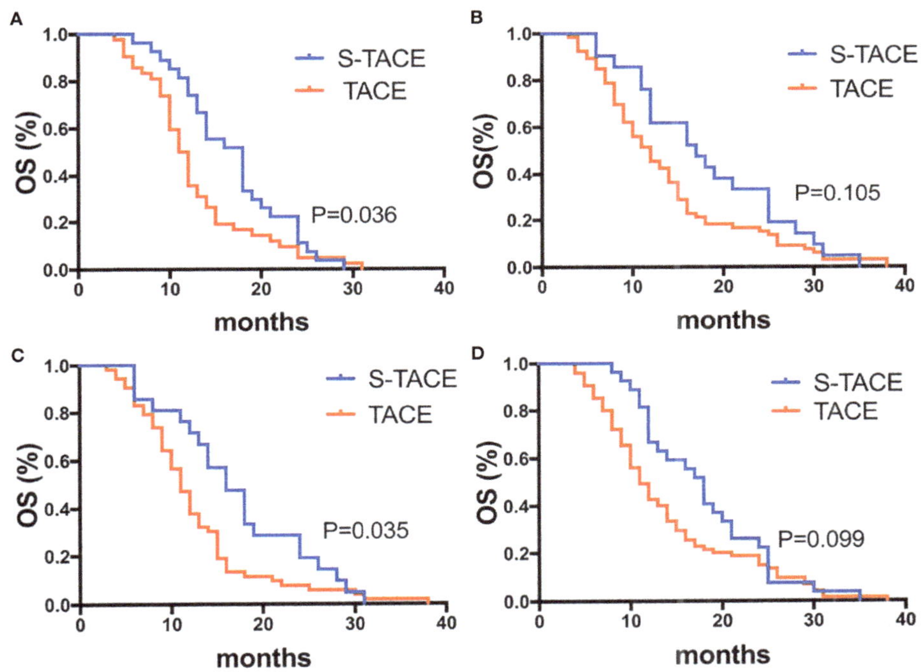

FIGURE 5 | Kaplan-Meier curves showed overall survival in the S-TACE and complications of transarterial chemoembolization (TACE) groups in patients with early diffuse recurrence (EDR) [**(A)** maximum diameter of tumor size > 5cm, **(B)** maximum diameter of tumor size < 5cm, **(C)** HBV-DNA>100, **(D)** HBV-DNA<100].

(**Table 5**). In the LDR group, the major AEs that were experienced by at least 10% of patients were abdominal pain (18.9%), hand-foot skin reaction (23.1%), and hypertension (10.4%). Others major AEs included vomiting (5.0%), fever (7.2%), fatigue (7.2%), diarrhea (6.1%), ascites (3.9%), and gastrointestinal hemorrhage (5.1%). There was no significant difference in occurrence of AEs between the S-TACE and TACE monotherapy groups (**Table 6**). Most abdominal pain was caused by the TACE therapy, and could be relieved by morphine or flurbiprofen axetil. Hand-foot skin reactions and hypertension were caused by sorafenib. About half of the hand-foot skin reactions were relieved by using lubricant or regressed within several months. Angiotensin receptor blockers were used to effectively relieve hypertension caused by sorafenib. All major AEs were treated without AE-related death and patients recovered with in two weeks.

DISCUSSION

Recurrence rate after liver resection is high in HCC patients (5–7, 18). A short interval from resection of HCC to recurrence leads to worse outcomes. Most patients with recurrence were not eligible for repeated hepatectomy due to being DR patients. TACE is the optimal treatment method for these patients (18, 19). In addition, sorafenib is recommended for unresectable HCC. Recently, various reports have shown that the combination of TACE and

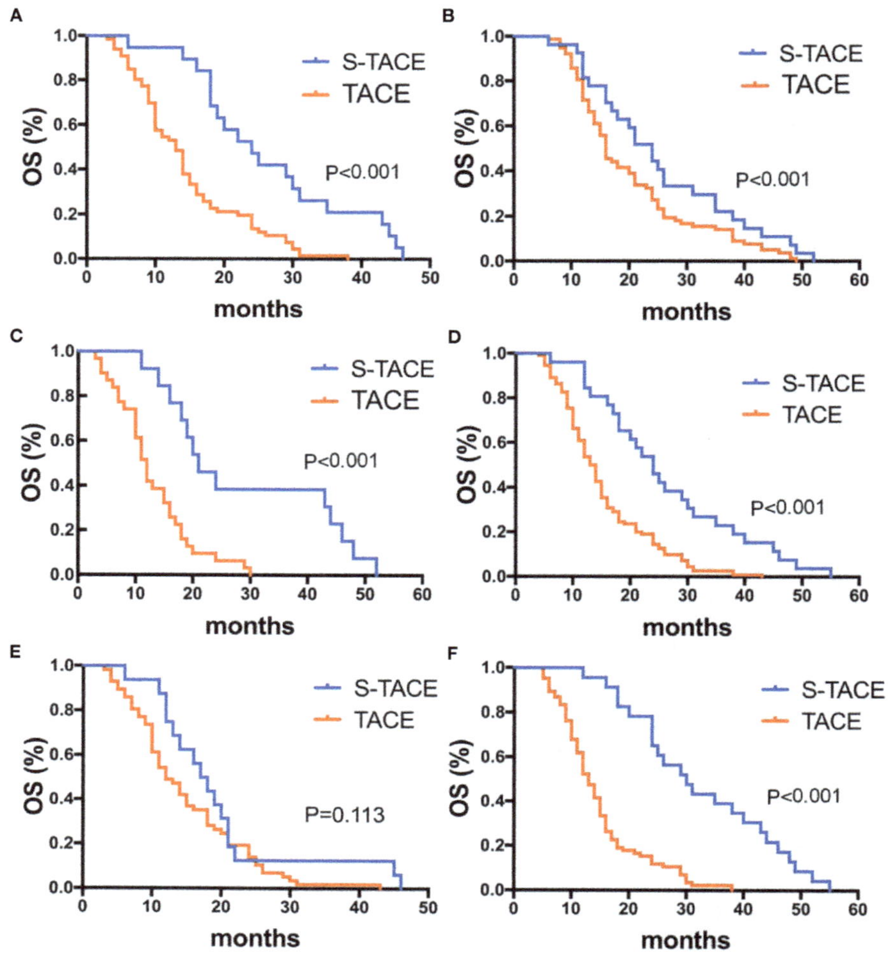

FIGURE 6 | Kaplan-Meier curves showed overall survival in the S-TACE and complications of transarterial chemoembolization (TACE) groups in patients with late diffuse recurrence (LDR) [**(A)** AFP≥400 ng/ml, **(B)** AFP<400 ng/ml, **(C)** TB>28 g/L, **(D)** TB < 28 g/L, **(E)** maximum diameter of tumor size> 5 cm, **(F)** maximum diameter of tumor size< 5 cm].

sorafenib resulted in better clinical outcomes than TACE monotherapy in multinodular HCC without vascular invasion or extra hepatic spread (9, 10, 13). Our study revealed that compared with TACE monotherapy, S-TACE could effectively prolong OS in EDR and LDR patients, which was consistent with the results of abovementioned previous studies.

Our data indicated that S-TACE could significantly improve OS in patients with EDR and LDR. Jung Ho Park reported that postoperative early multinodular recurrence was associated with the presence of portal vein tumor thrombi and intrahepatic metastases, and this form of recurrence was found to have a grave prognosis compared with that in late multinodular recurrence (20). Our findings supported these results and suggested that multiple comprehensive treatments should be applied in these patients. In addition, TACE induced ischemic or hypoxic changes which led to increased VEGF activity in surviving cancer tissue (21). Therefore, the use of a potent multikinase inhibitor, such as sorafenib, could limit the proliferative, proangiogenic, and/or antiapoptopic effects of VEGF expression, which could restrict tumor growth after TACE (12). This result corroborated the findings of a previous study reporting that S-TACE was suitable for metachronous, multicentric HCC nodules (22). Our study also demonstrated that S-TACE could improve the efficacy of multinodular recurrence.

In our study, the S-TACE combination showed little advantage over TACE monotherapy in LDR patients. This may be related to the fact that late recurrence is usually associated with underlying liver conditions, such as cirrhosis or active hepatitis (23). Patients with late recurrence might die due to poor liver functions; thus, the advantages of S-TACE would not be present in these patients. Thus, anti-viral therapy and liver protection should be recommended for these patients. In addition, multiple tumors, satellite nodules, and tumors greater than 5 cm were independent risk factors for late recurrence according to Xu et al. (24). Thus, S-TACE should be employed early for patients when the tumor load is high.

TABLE 5 | Number (percentage) of patients reporting AEs in early diffuse recurrence (EDR) patients by CTCAE grading[1].

Adverse Event	S-TACE (n=48)		TACE Monotherapy (n=128)		P Value
	Grade 1–2	Grade 3–4	Grade 1–2	Grade 3–4	
Diarrhea	23(47.9)	4(8.3)	67(52.3)	10(7.8)	0.605
Abdominal pain	29(60.4)	7(14.6)	77 (60.2)	13 (10.2)	0.810
Ascites	5(10.4)	1(2.1)	13(10.2)	3(2.4)	0.995
Vomiting	30(62.5)	1(2.1)	93 (72.7)	4(3.2)	0.169
Fatigue	34(70.8)	2(4.2)	77(60.2)	4(3.2)	0.167
Fever	34(70.8)	3(6.3)	102 (79.7)	8 (6.3)	0.189
Headache	7(14.6)	1(2.1)	13 (10.2)	3 (2.4)	0.461
Upper respiratory infection	5 (10.5)	0(0)	10 (7.8)	1(0.8)	0.696
PLT decreased	9(18.8)	2(4.2)	16(12.5)	6(4.5)	0.360
WBC decreased	8(16.7)	3 (6.3)	19(14.8)	4(3.2)	0.500
Anaemia	4 (8.3)	1(2.1)	13(10.2)	3 (2.4)	0.703
Hand-foot skin reaction	31 (64.6)	16 (33.3)	–	–	NA
Hypertension	13(27.1)	4 (8.3)	–	–	NA
Hair loss	7 (14.6)	0 (0)	–	–	NA
Gastrointestinal hemorrhage	6(12.6)	3(6.3)	–	–	NA
Epistaxis	7 (14.6)	0 (0)	–	–	NA

CTCAE grading[1]: National Cancer Institute (NCI) Common Terminology Criteria for Adverse Events (CTCAE) version 4.0; –, no data; NA, not applicable; PLT, Platelets; WBC, White blood cell.

TABLE 6 | Number (percentage) of patients reporting AEs in late diffuse recurrence (LDR) patients by CTCAE grading[1].

Adverse Event	S-TACE (n=39)		TACE Monotherapy (n=141)		P Value
	Grade 1–2	Grade 3–4	Grade 1–2	Grade 3–4	
Diarrhea	21(53.8)	2(5.2)	63(44.7)	9(6.4)	0.332
Abdominal pain	25(64.1)	6(15.4)	95(67.4)	28(19.9)	0.537
Ascites	4(10.2)	2(5.1)	18(12.8)	5(3.5)	0.855
Vomiting	11(28.2)	3(7.7)	31(21.9)	6(4.3)	0.266
Fatigue	19(48.7)	3(7.7)	69(48.9)	10(7.1)	0.994
Fever	16(41.0)	4(10.4)	59(41.8)	9(6.4)	0.882
Headache	7(17.9)	0(0)	21(14.9)	3(2.1)	0.849
Upper respiratory infection	4(10.4)	0(0)	8(5.7)	2(1.4)	0.496
PLT decreased	6(15.4)	1(2.6)	18(12.8)	6(4.3)	0.855
WBC decreased	5(12.8)	0(0)	13(9.2)	3(2.1)	0.765
Anaemia	3(7.7)	0(0)	16(11.3)	5(3.5)	0.262
Hand-foot skin reaction	28(71.8)	9(23.1)	–	–	NA
Hypertension	11(28.2)	4(10.4)	–	–	NA
Hair loss	3(7.7)	0(0)	–	–	NA
Gastrointestinal hemorrhage	4(10.4)	2(5.1)	–	–	NA
Epistaxis	3(7.7)	0(0)	–	–	NA

CTCAE grading[1]: National Cancer Institute (NCI) Common Terminology Criteria for Adverse Events (CTCAE) version 4.0; –, no data; NA, not applicable; PLT, Platelets; WBC, White blood cell.

In terms of risk factors for EDR and LDR, we found that tumor size and HBV-DNA were associated with EDR, while AFP, TB, and tumor size were related to LDR. This could be related to the larger maximum tumor size and higher AFP level, which indicated a higher tumor load leading to poor prognosis (25, 26). Therefore, combined therapies should be applied to higher tumor loads, which would help to improve OS. Additionally, our study indicated that the OS of LDR patients was much longer than that of EDR patients, regardless of the treatment. This may be due to EDR recurrence being accompanied by more malignant biological behaviors.

In our study, most AEs in the LDR or EDR group through S-TACE or TACE monotherapy were grade 1 or 2 and could be easily controlled. These results were consistent with those of the previous studies (13, 27, 28). Importantly, no lethal AEs were reported in patients with S-TACE, and all major serious AEs were in remission after treatment. Our observations were consistent with those of previous studies reporting that S-TACE was not associated with a significantly greater incidence/severity of adverse events than TACE monotherapy (29). Most patients in both the LDR and EDR groups discontinued sorafenib because of serious AEs. Serious hand-foot skin reaction and abdominal pain were common reasons for discontinuation of sorafenib. Since the mechanism of hand-skin reaction and abdominal pain was unknown, they were difficult to treat.

Our study had several limitations. First, this study was retrospective, which may reduce the reliability of data leading to selection bias. Second, EDR and LDR were not determined histologically or genetically. So, it was difficult to explain why there were different prognoses and risk factors in LDR and EDR patients, and we could not provide individualized treatment. We suggest that genome sequencing of HCC would be a key next step for this research. Third, the limited number of patients were insufficient for subgroup analysis. Consequently, a multi-center prospective randomized controlled trial is needed to confirm our findings. Fourth, the administration of sorafenib could be improved in this study; we should closely follow-up with patients and take positive measures when serious AEs occur. Finally, a higher rate of patients discontinuing sorafenib could influence the effect of S-TACE.

In conclusion, S-TACE resulted in improved outcomes in EDR patients including OS and PFS, especially in patients with a maximum tumor diameter > 5 cm and HBV-DNA>100, in comparison with TACE monotherapy. In LDR patients, there was significantly better OS in the S-TACE group, especially for patients with AFP>400 mg/L, AFP<400 mg/L, TB>28 g/L, TB<28 g/L, and a maximum tumor diameter > 5 cm.

AUTHOR CONTRIBUTIONS

WY, JL, and WF conceptualized the study and contributed to the investigation. WY, MX, and ML performed the formal analysis, were in charge of the projection administration, and wrote the original draft. YQW and YZ were in charge of the data curation and methodology. YW was in charge of the software. All authors contributed to the article and approved the submitted version.

ACKNOWLEDGMENTS

The authors thank Hui Zhu, MD, for her editorial assistance. We also thank Hongyu Wang, PhD, Jialiang Wei, PhD, and Jian Guo, PhD, for they help in collecting the clinical data.

REFERENCES

1. El-Serag HB, Rudolph KL. Hepatocellular carcinoma: epidemiology and molecular carcinogenesis. *Gastroenterology* (2007) 132:2557–76. doi: 10.1053/j.gastro.2007.04.061
2. Cherqui D, Laurent A, Mocellin N, Tayar C, Luciani A, Van Nhieu JT, et al. Liver resection for transplantable hepatocellular carcinoma: long-term survival and role of secondary liver transplantation. *Ann Surg* (2009) 250:738–46. doi: 10.1097/sla.0b013e3181bd582b
3. Prashant B, Marc A, Eric V, Daniel C, Gilles P, Antonio S, et al. Salvage versus primary liver transplantation for early hepatocellular carcinoma: do both strategies yield similar outcomes? *Ann Surg* (2016) 264:155–63. doi: 10.1097/sla.0000000000001442
4. Kim JM, Yi NJ, Kwon CHD, Lee KW, Suh KS, Joh JW. Early disseminated recurrence after liver resection in solitary hepatocellular carcinoma. *Ann Surg Treat Res* (2018) 94:129–34. doi: 10.4174/astr.2018.94.3.129
5. Kotoh K, Enjoji M, Arimura E, Morizono S, Kohjima M, Sakai H, et al. Scattered and rapid intrahepatic recurrences after radio frequency ablation for hepatocellular carcinoma. *World J Gastroenterol* (2005) 11:6828–32. doi: 10.3748/wjg.v11.i43.6828
6. Poon RT, Fan ST, Ng IO, Lo CM, Liu CL, Wong J. Different risk factors and prognosis for early and late intrahepatic recurrence after resection of hepatocellular carcinoma. *Cancer* (2000) 89:500–7. doi: 10.1002/1097-0142(20000801)89:3<500::AID-CNCR4>3.0.CO;2-O
7. Choi GH, Kim DH, Kang CM, Kim KS, Choi JS, Lee WJ, et al. Prognostic factors and optimal treatment strategy for intrahepatic nodular recurrence after curative resection of hepatocellular carcinoma. *Ann Surg Oncol* (2008) 15:618–29. doi: 10.1245/s10434-007-9671-6
8. Del Pozo AC, Lopez P. Management of hepatocellular carcinoma. *Clin Liver Dis* (2007) 11:305–21. doi: 10.1016/j.cld.2007.04.007
9. Lo CM, Ngan H, Tso WK, Liu CL, Lam CM, Poon RT, et al. Randomized controlled trial of transarterial lipiodol chemoembolization for unresectable hepatocellular carcinoma. *Hepatology* (2002) 35:1164–71. doi: 10.1053/jhep.2002.33156
10. Llovet JM, Real MI, Montana X, Planas R, Coll S, Aponte J, et al. Arterial embolisation or chemoembolisation versus symptomatic treatment in patients with unresectable hepatocellular carcinoma: a randomised controlled trial. *Lancet* (2002) 359:1734–9. doi: 10.1016/s0140-6736(02)08649-x
11. Abou-Alfa GK, Schwartz L, Ricci S, Amadori D, Santoro A, Figer A, et al. Phase II study of sorafenib in patients with advanced hepatocellular carcinoma. *J Clin Oncol* (2006) 24:4293–300. doi: 10.1200/JCO.2005.01.3441
12. Liu L, Cao Y, Chen C, Zhang X, McNabola A, Wilkie D, et al. Sorafenib blocks the RAF/MEK/ERK pathway, inhibits tumor angiogenesis, and induces tumor cell apoptosis in hepatocellular carcinoma model PLC/PRF/5. *Cancer Res* (2006) 66:11851–8. doi: 10.1158/0008-5472.CAN-06-1377
13. Chao Y, Chung YH, Han G, Yoon JH, Yang J, Wang J, et al. The combination of transcatheter arterial chemoembolization and sorafenib is well tolerated and effective in Asian patients with hepatocellular carcinoma: final results of the START trial. *Int J Cancer* (2015) 136:1458–67. doi: 10.1002/ijc.29126
14. Verslype C, Rosmorduc O, Rougier P. Hepatocellular carcinoma: ESMO-ESDO Clinical Practice Guidelines for diagnosis, treatment and follow-up. *Ann Oncol* (2012) 23:vii41–8. doi: 10.1093/annonc/mds225
15. Llovet JM, Bru C, Bruix J. Prognosis of hepatocellular carcinoma: the BCLC staging classification. *Semin Liver Dis* (1999) 19:329–38. doi: 10.1055/s-2007-1007122
16. Trotti A, Colevas AD, Setser A, Rusch V, Jaques D, Budach V, et al. CTCAE v3.0: development of a comprehensive grading system for the adverse effects of cancer treatment. *Semin Radiat Oncol* (2003) 13:176–81. doi: 10.1016/s1053-4296(03)00031-6
17. Lencioni R, Llovet JM. Modified RECIST (mRECIST) assessment for hepatocellular carcinoma. *Semin Liver Dis* (2010) 30:52–60. doi: 10.1055/s-0030-1247132
18. Poon RT, Fan ST, Lo CM, Liu CL, Wong J. Intrahepatic recurrence after curative resection of hepatocellular carcinoma: long-term results of treatment and prognostic factors. *Ann Surg* (1999) 229:216–22. doi: 10.1097/00000658-199902000-00009
19. Minagawa M, Makuuchi M, Takayama T, Kokudo N. Selection criteria for repeat hepatectomy in patients with recurrent hepatocellular carcinoma. *Ann Surg* (2003) 238:703–10. doi: 10.1097/01.sla.0000094549.11754.e6
20. Park JH, Koh KC, Choi MS, Lee JH, Yoo BC, Paik SW, et al. Analysis of risk factors associated with early multinodular recurrences after hepatic resection for hepatocellular carcinoma. *Am J Surg* (2006) 192:29–33. doi: 10.1016/j.amjsurg.2005.11.010
21. Li X, Feng GS, Zheng CS, Zhuo CK, Liu X. Expression of plasma vascular endothelial growth factor in patients with hepatocellular carcinoma and effect of transcatheter arterial chemoembolization therapy on plasma vascular endothelial growth factor level. *World J Gastroenterol* (2004) 10:2878–82. doi: 10.3748/wjg.v10.i19.2878
22. Sansonno D, Lauletta G, Russi S, Conteduca V, Sansonno L, Dammacco F. Transarterial chemoembolization plus sorafenib: a sequential therapeutic scheme for HCV-related intermediate-stage hepatocellular carcinoma: a randomized clinical trial. *Oncologist* (2012) 17:359–66. doi: 10.1634/theoncologist.2011-0313
23. Yamamoto Y, Ikoma H, Morimura R, Konishi H, Murayama Y, Komatsu S, et al. Optimal duration of the early and late recurrence of hepatocellular carcinoma after hepatectomy. *World J Gastroenterol* (2015) 21:1207–15. doi: 10.3748/wjg.v21.i4.1207
24. Xu XF, Xing H, Han J, Li ZL, Lau WY, Zhou YH, et al. Risk Factors, Patterns, and Outcomes of Late Recurrence After Liver Resection for Hepatocellular

Carcinoma: A Multicenter Study From China. *JAMA Surg* (2019) 154:209–17. doi: 10.1001/jamasurg.2018.4334

25. Vitale A, Lai Q, Farinati F, Bucci L, Giannini EG, Napoli L, et al. Utility of Tumor Burden Score to Stratify Prognosis of Patients with Hepatocellular Cancer: Results of 4759 Cases from ITA.LI.CA Study Group. *J Gastrointest Surg* (2018) 22:859–71. doi: 10.1007/s11605-018-3688-y
26. Kobayashi A, Miyagawa S, Miwa S, Nakata T. Prognostic impact of anatomical resection on early and late intrahepatic recurrence in patients with hepatocellular carcinoma. *J Hepatobiliary Pancreat Surg* (2008) 15:515–21. doi: 10.1007/s00534-007-1293-7
27. Abdel-Rahman O, Elsayed ZA. Combination trans arterial chemoembolization (TACE) plus sorafenib for the management of unresectable hepatocellular carcinoma: a systematic review of the literature. *Dig Dis Sci* (2013) 58:3389–96. doi: 10.1007/s10620-013-2872-x
28. Cabrera R, Pannu DS, Caridi J, Firpi JR, Soldevila-Pico C, Morelli G, et al. The combination of sorafenib with transarterial chemoembolisation for hepatocellular carcinoma. *Aliment Pharmacol Ther* (2011) 34:205–13. doi: 10.1016/s2468-1253(17)30156-5
29. Geschwind JF, Gholam PM, Goldenberg A, Mantry P, Martin RC, Piperdi B, et al. Use of Transarterial Chemoembolization (TACE) and Sorafenib in Patients with Unresectable Hepatocellular Carcinoma: US Regional Analysis of the GIDEON Registry. *Liver Cancer* (2016) 5:37–46. doi: 10.1159/000367757

Efficacy of Laparoscopic Hepatectomy *versus* Open Surgery for Hepatocellular Carcinoma with Cirrhosis

Yu Pan [1,2†], Shunjie Xia [1,2†], Jiaqin Cai [3], Ke Chen [1,2] and Xiujun Cai [1,2*]*

[1] Department of General Surgery, Sir Run Run Shaw Hospital, School of Medicine, Zhejiang University, Zhejiang, China, [2] Key Laboratory of Endoscopic Technique Research of Zhejiang Province, Hangzhou, China, [3] Department of Plastic Surgery, Sir Run Run Shaw Hospital, School of Medicine, Zhejiang University, Zhejiang, China

***Correspondence:**
Xiujun Cai
srrsh_cxj@zju.edu.cn
Ke Chen
chenke68@zju.edu.cn

†These authors have contributed equally to this work

Background: The role of laparoscopic hepatectomy (LH) in hepatocellular carcinoma (HCC) with cirrhosis remains controversial and needs to be further assessed. The present meta-analysis aimed to compare the surgical and oncological outcomes of LH with those of open hepatectomy (OH) for HCC with cirrhosis.

Methods: The PubMed, Embase, and Cochrane Library databases were searched for studies comparing LH and OH until Mar 2021. Weighted mean differences (WMDs), odds ratios (ORs), and hazard ratios (HRs) were calculated for continuous, dichotomous, and long-term variables, respectively, with 95% confidence intervals (CIs). Subgroup analysis was performed according to different resection types: major resection and minor resection. The meta-analysis was performed using the STATA 12.0.

Results: A total of 16 case-matched studies (784 patients in the LH group and 1,191 patients in the OH group.) were included in this meta-analysis. In terms of primary outcomes, LH was associated with decreased overall complication rate (OR 0.57; 95% CI 0.46 to 0.71; P <0.01), major complication rate (OR 0.52; 95% CI 0.33 to 0.82; P < 0.01), postoperative mortality (OR 0.27; 95% CI 0.11 to 0.66; P <0.01), 1-y overall survival (OS) rate (HR 0.48; 95% CI 0.31 to 0.73; P <0.01), 2-y OS (HR 0.61; 95% CI 0.45 to 0.83; P < 0.01), and 5-y OS (0.67; 95% CI 0.53 to 0.85; P < 0.01). With respect to secondary outcomes, blood loss (WMD −69.16; 95% CI −101.72 to −36.61; P < 0.01), length of hospitalization (LOH) (WMD −2.65; 95% CI −3.41 to −1.89; P < 0.01), minor complication rate (OR 0.70; 95% CI 0.53 to 0.94; P = 0.02), postoperative liver failure (OR 0.60; 95% CI 0.38 to 0.95; P = 0.03), and postoperative ascites (OR 0.44; 95% CI 0.28 to 0.72; P < 0.01) was lower in LH than in OH. No significant differences in operation time (P = 0.07), transfusion rate (P = 0.05), 1-, 2-, and 5-year DFS rate (1-year, P = 0.08; 2-year, P = 0.08; 5-year, P = 0.23) were noted between LH and OH. Subgroup analysis based on minor resection revealed that LH had similar favored outcomes in comparison with those in the overall pooled analysis. However, LH had a longer operation time than OH in the setting of major resection (P < 0.01).

Conclusion: LH is technically feasible and safe for selected HCC patients with cirrhosis. LH can achieve favored short-term and long-term oncological outcomes in minor liver resection. Laparoscopic major hepatectomy (LMH) seems to offer some advantages over the open approach; however concerns about surgical and oncological safety remain. More evidence on LMH is warranted before expanding its indication to patients with cirrhosis.

Keywords: laparoscopic hepatectomy, hepatocellular carcinoma, cirrhosis, prognosis, meta-analysis

INTRODUCTION

Hepatocellular carcinoma (HCC) is the most common primary cancer of the liver and one of the leading causes of cancer-related deaths worldwide (1, 2). Hepatectomy is the commonly used curative treatment strategy for very early- and early-stage HCC patients with preserved liver function. In the early 1990s, with the inception of laparoscopic techniques, initial reports on laparoscopic hepatectomy (LH) were published (3, 4). Since then, the laparoscopic approach has been increasingly accepted in the field of liver surgery. Laparoscopic techniques have been shown to expedite recovery, improve postoperative pain, and result in better cosmesis than the open approach. In the statement of the First International Consensus Conference for Laparoscopic Liver Resection, laparoscopic left lateral segmentectomy was identified as the gold standard approach (5). In 2014, the Second International Consensus Conference for Laparoscopic Liver Resection recommended laparoscopic minor hepatectomy as the standard surgical practice (6).

Most patients with HCC commonly have chronic hepatitis and cirrhosis making liver resection technically demanding. Liver resection is a challenging procedure in the setting of cirrhosis owing to elevated portal pressure and impaired coagulation function in patients with this condition. A retrospective study by Neeff et al. reported that the severity of cirrhosis was correlated with perioperative mortality after hepatectomy (7). The development of devices and techniques for hemostasis has allowed bleeding control in LH. Several efforts have been made to promote the adoption of LH in the treatment of HCC with cirrhosis (8–11). Given the advantages of laparoscopic surgery in terms of minimal invasiveness, LH is expected to be more beneficial for HCC patients with cirrhosis. Several meta-analyses have reported that patients with cirrhosis undergoing LH experienced less blood loss, fewer postoperative complications, and shorter hospital stays than those undergoing open resection (12, 13). Most studies included in these meta-analyses were retrospective and limited to laparoscopic minor resection. Since then, one randomized clinical trial (RCT) and several case-matched studies focusing on HCC with cirrhosis have reported the favored surgical outcomes of LH (14–16). Furthermore, major liver resection is an important curative modality for HCC. Recently, laparoscopic major hepatectomy (LMH) for selected patients with cirrhosis has been reported by several experienced surgeons in a few medical centers (17, 18). Hence, in this study, we aimed to compare the surgical and oncological outcomes of LH with those of open hepatectomy (OH) for HCC with cirrhosis by collecting high-quality case-matched studies.

METHODS

Search Strategy

This systematic review was conducted in accordance with the Preferred Reporting Items for Systematic Reviews and Meta-Analyses (PRISMA) guidelines (19). Electronic databases including PubMed, Embase, and Cochrane Library were searched. The search strategy for Pubmed was as follows: (((("Minimally Invasive Surgical Procedures"[Mesh]) OR "Laparoscopy"[Mesh])) AND "Liver Cirrhosis"[Mesh]) AND "Liver Neoplasms"[Mesh]) and similar strategy was performed in other databases. The references of the retrieved results were also manually reviewed to obtain more related articles as possible. The final search was conducted in Mar 2021. No institutional review board approval or patient written consent was necessary because only published data were used.

Study Selection

Case-matched studies written in English and comparing the outcomes of OH *vs* LH for HCC in patients with cirrhosis were considered for inclusion. The exclusion criteria were as follows: (i). reviews, editorials, case reports, abstracts, or letters; (ii). studies including patients without cirrhosis or those with unproven cirrhosis; (iii). studies including patients who underwent robotic or hybrid procedures; (iv). overlapped studies; (v). studies that did not report at least three of the primary outcomes.

Data Extraction

After the initial screening, full-text versions of the selected articles were obtained. Two reviewers (SX and KC), as well as an independent third reviewer (YP) in cases in which consensus could not be reached, individually assessed each article and rejected those that failed to meet the inclusion criteria. The following items were extracted: year of publication, study design, sample size, country of study, patient characteristics, and outcome measures. The primary outcomes were overall complication rate, major complication rate, postoperative mortality, overall survival (OS) rate, and disease-free survival (DFS) rate. The secondary outcomes were operation time, blood loss, transfusion rate, length of hospitalization (LOH), minor complication rate, postoperative ascites, and postoperative liver failure (POLF). The Newcastle-Ottawa scale (NOS) was used to evaluate the quality of observational studies (http://www.ohri.ca/programs/clinical_epidemiology/oxford.asp). The NOS scores were ≥7, were considered of high quality. According to previous studies, minor resection was defined as hepatectomy of fewer than three sections and major resection was defined as hepatectomy of more than three sections (20–22). Clavien–Dindo classification was used to grade postoperative complications and a major complication was defined as Clavien–Dindo ≥3; otherwise, the complication was defined as minor (23).

Statistical Analysis

Dichotomous variables were evaluated using odds ratios (ORs) with 95% confidence intervals (95% CIs), and continuous variables were analyzed using the weighted mean differences (WMDs) with 95% CIs. The hazard ratio (HR) was used as a summary statistic for long-term outcomes (survival analysis), as described by Tierney et al. (24). Medians were converted to means using the formula described by Hozo et al. (25). According to the Higgins I^2 statistic, heterogeneities <25, 25 to 50, and >50% were defined as low, moderate, and high, respectively (26). A fixed-effects model was used for studies with low or moderate statistical heterogeneity (27), whereas a random-effects model was used for studies with high statistical heterogeneity (28). Subgroup analysis was performed according to different resection types: major resection and minor resection. Funnel plots were used to estimate the potential publication bias. $P<0.05$ was considered statistically significant. The meta-analysis was performed using the STATA 12.0.

RESULTS

Study Characteristics

This meta-analysis was registered to PROSPERO (https://www.crd.york.ac.uk/prospero/) with an ID of CRD42020161775. The search strategy initially retrieved 501 records. After the exclusion of irrelevant studies by screening the abstracts, the full texts of 28 potentially relevant articles were obtained for assessment. Twelve studies were excluded due to overlapping data, inclusion of patients without cirrhosis, unavailable statistical data, non-comparative studies, non-case matched studies (8, 9, 29–38). Sixteen studies were eventually included (15–18, 39–50). The PRISMA flowchart of the literature review is presented in **Figure 1**.

The characteristics of the included studies are summarized in **Table 1**. A total of 1,975 patients from both Eastern and Western countries were pooled in this meta-analysis: 784 patients in the LH group and 1,191 patients in the OH group. To balance the basic characteristics, the propensity score matching method was used in 12 out of 16 retrospective studies, whereas the case-matched method was used in the others. Detail of matched characteristics was summarized in **Supplementary Table 1**. Nine studies focused on minor liver resection, and five studies reported outcomes limited to patients who underwent major liver resection. Ten studies reported the conversion rate of LH,

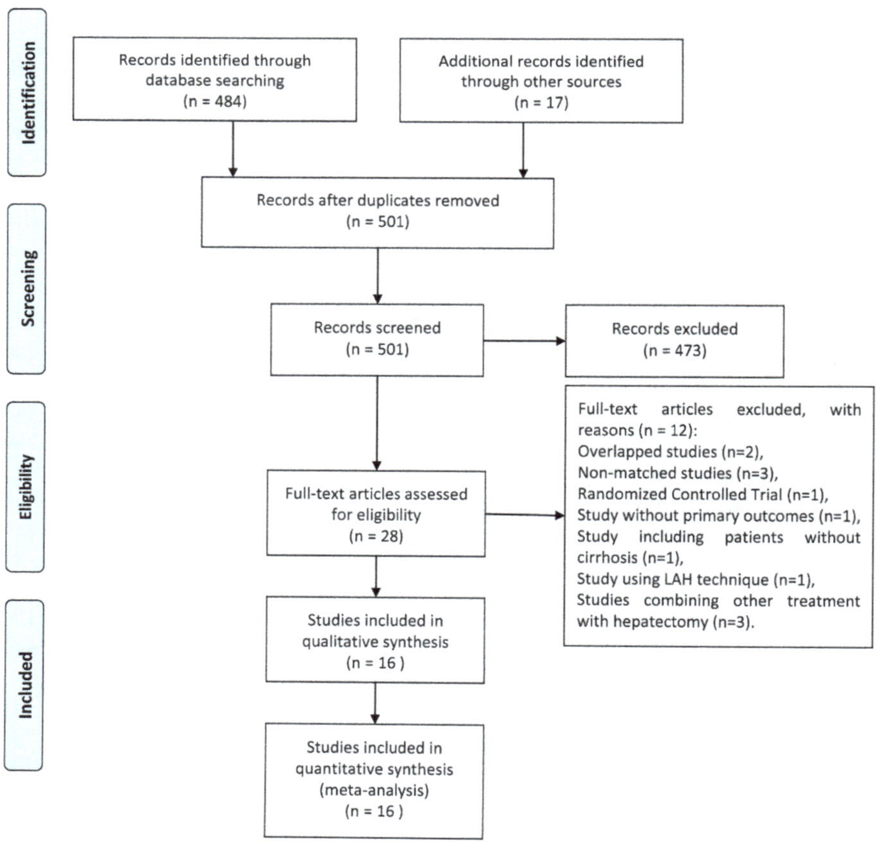

FIGURE 1 | Flow chart of the studies included in the meta-analysis.

TABLE 1 | The basic characteristics of included studies.

study	year	Country	Study design	sample size (LH/OH)	Mean age (LH/OH)	Gender (M/F) (LH/OH)	Childs-Pugh A:B ratio (LH/OH)	tumor size (LH/OH)	tumor pattern (LH/OH)	conversion rate	resection type	Matched method
Belli et al.	2007	Italy	R	23 vs 23	59.5 vs 62.4	13/10 vs 14/9	23/0 vs 23/0	3.1 vs 3.2	NA	0	minor	M
Truant et al.	2011	France	R	36 vs 53	60.6 vs 63.3	31/5 vs 47/6	36/0 vs 53/0	2.9 vs 3.1	34/2 vs 44/9	NA	minor	M
Memeo et al.	2014	France	R	45 vs 45	62 vs 60	35/10 vs 37/8	44/1 vs 43/2	3.2 vs 3.7	NA	0	minor	M
Komatsu et al.	2016	Japan	R	38 vs 38	61.5 vs 61.7	34/4 vs 33/5	38/0 vs 38/0	4.75 vs 8.5	19/19 vs 22/16	34.21%	major	M
Cheung et al.	2016	China	R	110 vs 330	60 vs 61	80/30 vs 258/72	110/0 vs 330/0	2.6 vs 2.85	100/10 vs 292/38	5.5%	minor	PSM
Jiang et al.	2016	China	R	59 vs 59	51 vs 50	42/17 vs 38/21	59/0 vs 59/0	3 vs 3	59/0 vs 59/0	5.1%	minor	PSM
Yoon et al.	2017	Korea	R	33 vs 33	56.03 vs 57.33	23/10 vs 26/7	33/0 vs 33/0	3.31 vs 2.96	NA	NA	major	PSM
Xu et al.	2018	China	R	32 vs 32	53.5 vs 52	28/4 vs 28/4	32/0 vs 32/0	4 vs 6.2	29/3 vs 29/3	NA	major	PSM
Kim et al.	2018	Korea	R	18 vs 36	55.7 vs 54.6	13/5 vs 22/14	18/0 vs 36/0	2.9 vs 3.66	18/0 vs 36/0	0	minor	PSM
Sandro et al.	2018	Italy	R	75 vs 75	68.6 vs 67.1	33/42 vs 24/51	65/10 vs 63/12	2.5 vs 2.5	66/9 vs 65/10	7.6%	minor	PSM
Delvecchio et al.	2020		RM	38 vs 84	75 vs 74.3	29/9 vs 61/23	37/1 vs 82/2	4 vs 7	33/5 vs 68/18	NA	major	PSM
Cheung et al.	2020	China	R	24 vs 96	63 vs 62	20/4 vs 81/15	24/0 vs 96/0	4.5 vs 4.8	18/6 vs 75/21	NA	major	PSM
Hobeika et al.	2020	France	R	124 vs 124	63 vs 63	98/26 vs 101/13	NA	NA	NA	16.8%	minor	PSM
Yamamoto et al.	2020	Japan	R	58 vs 58	71 vs 72	39/19 vs 30/28	45/13 vs 45/13	1.7 vs 1.6	NA	NA	minor	PSM
Inoue et al.	2020	Japan	R	28 vs 28	73 vs 72	19/9 vs 18/10	28/0 vs 27/1	2.4 vs 2.4	NA	12.70%	NA	PSM
Fu et al.	2021	China	R	43 vs 77	52 vs 56	33/10 vs 59/18	43/0 vs 70/0	2.5 vs 2.5	NA	2.0%	NA	PSM

LH laparoscopic hepatectomy, OH open hepatectomy, M male, F female, NA not available, R retrospective, RM retrospective multicenter, PSM propensity score-matched.

TABLE 2 | The qualities of included studies evaluated using the Newcastle-Ottawa Quality Assessment Scale.

Study	Selection	Comparability	Outcomes	Total
	1. Representativeness of exposed cohort 2. Selection of nonexposed cohort 3. Ascertainment of exposure 4. Outcome not present at the start of the study		1. Assessment of outcomes 2. Length of follow-up 3. Adequacy of follow-up	
Belli et al.	****	**	**	********
Truant et al.	****	**	***	*********
Memeo et al.	****	**	***	*********
Cheung et al.	****	**	***	*********
Jiang et al.	****	**	*	*******
Komatsu et al.	****	**	**	********
Yoon et al.	****	**	**	********
Sandro et al.	****	**	**	********
Xu et al.	****	**	**	********
Kim et al.	****	**	**	********
Delvecchio et al.	****	**	***	*********
Cheung et al.	****	**	***	*********
Hobeika et al.	****	**	*	*******
Yamamoto et al.	****	**	***	*********
Inoue et al.	****	**	*	*******
Fu et al.	****	**	*	*******

**1 score.*

which ranged from 0 to 34.21%. Surgical techniques including inflow occlusion method, parenchymal transection technique, and hemostasis method, were summarized in **Supplementary Table 2**. All studies were considered to be of adequate quality for the meta-analysis, as presented in **Table 2**.

Intraoperative Outcomes

All 16 pooled studies reported the operation time. Compared with the OH group, the LH group achieved a comparable operation time (WMD 19.33, 95% CI −1.67 to 40.34; P = 0.07; **Figure 2A**). According to 15 studies reporting intraoperative blood loss, our meta-analysis found blood loss was less in the LH than that in the OH groups (WMD −69.16; 95% CI −101.72 to −36.61; P < 0.01; **Figure 2B**). Similarly the occurrence of transfusion in LH was less than that in OH (OR 0.63; 95% CI 0.40 to 1.00; P = 0.05; **Figure 2C**).

Postoperative Outcomes

A shorter LOH was observed in LH (WMD −2.65; 95% CI −3.41 to −1.89; P < 0.01; **Figure 3A**). Postoperative complications were recorded in fifteen studies. The LH group had a decreased risk of overall postoperative complications (OR 0.57; 95% CI 0.46 to 0.71; P < 0.01; **Figure 3B**). Moreover, 15 studies reported postoperative mortalities. On the basis of these data, LH had a lower mortality rate (OR 0.27; 95% CI 0.11 to 0.66; P < 0.01; **Figure 3C**). To clarify the influence of LH on postoperative complications, we classified postoperative complications into minor complications and major complications.

With respect to the overall postoperative complications, the LH group had more favorable minor complication rate (OR 0.70; 95% CI 0.53 to 0.94; P = 0.02; **Figure 4A**) and major complication rate (OR 0.52; 95% CI 0.33 to 0.82; P < 0.01; **Figure 4B**) than OH. We also evaluated some detailed complications specifically associated with liver resection in patients with cirrhosis, including POLF and ascites. The LH group had less POLF (OR 0.60; 95% CI 0.38 to 0.95; P = 0.03; **Figure 4C**) and ascites (OR 0.44; 95% CI 0.28 to 0.72; P < 0.01; **Figure 4D**) than the OH group.

Long-Term Outcomes

Twelve studies reported the long-term outcomes including OS and DFS rates. The data showed that LH had more favorable 1-, 2-, and 5-year OS rate (1-year: HR 0.48; 95% CI 0.31 to 0.73; P < 0.01; **Figure 5A**; 2-year: HR 0.61; 95% CI 0.45 to 0.83; P < 0.01; **Figure 5C**; 5-year: HR 0.67; 95% CI 0.53 to 0.85; P < 0.01; **Figure 5E**) than OH. As for the DFS rate, LH had comparable outcomes to OH in terms of 1-, 2-, and 5-year DFS rates (1-year: HR 0.73; 95% CI 0.52 to 1.04; P = 0.08; **Figure 5B**; 2-year: HR 0.86; 95% CI 0.73 to 1.02; P =0.08; **Figure 5D**; 5-year: HR 0.90; 95% CI 0.75 to 1.07; P = 0.23; **Figure 5F**).

Subgroup Analysis

Given that the included studies enrolled patients who underwent different extents of liver resection, subgroup analysis was conducted according to the resection extent (minor or major resection), as shown in **Table 3**. In accordance with the overall analysis, LH was associated with less blood loss, shorter LOH, fewer postoperative complications and mortalities, better 1-year, 2-year, and 5-year OS rate in minor resection subgroup analysis. Notably, in the major resection subgroup analysis, the LH group had a longer operation time, shorter LOH, and fewer postoperative complications than the OH group. Moreover, there was no difference in the OS and DFS rates between the LH and OH groups in the major resection subgroup analysis.

Sensitivity Analysis and Publication Bias

Sensitivity analyses were conducted by excluding the highest-weighted study in each pooled analysis. These exclusions did not alter the results of cumulative analyses. A funnel plot based on overall postoperative complications was performed to assess

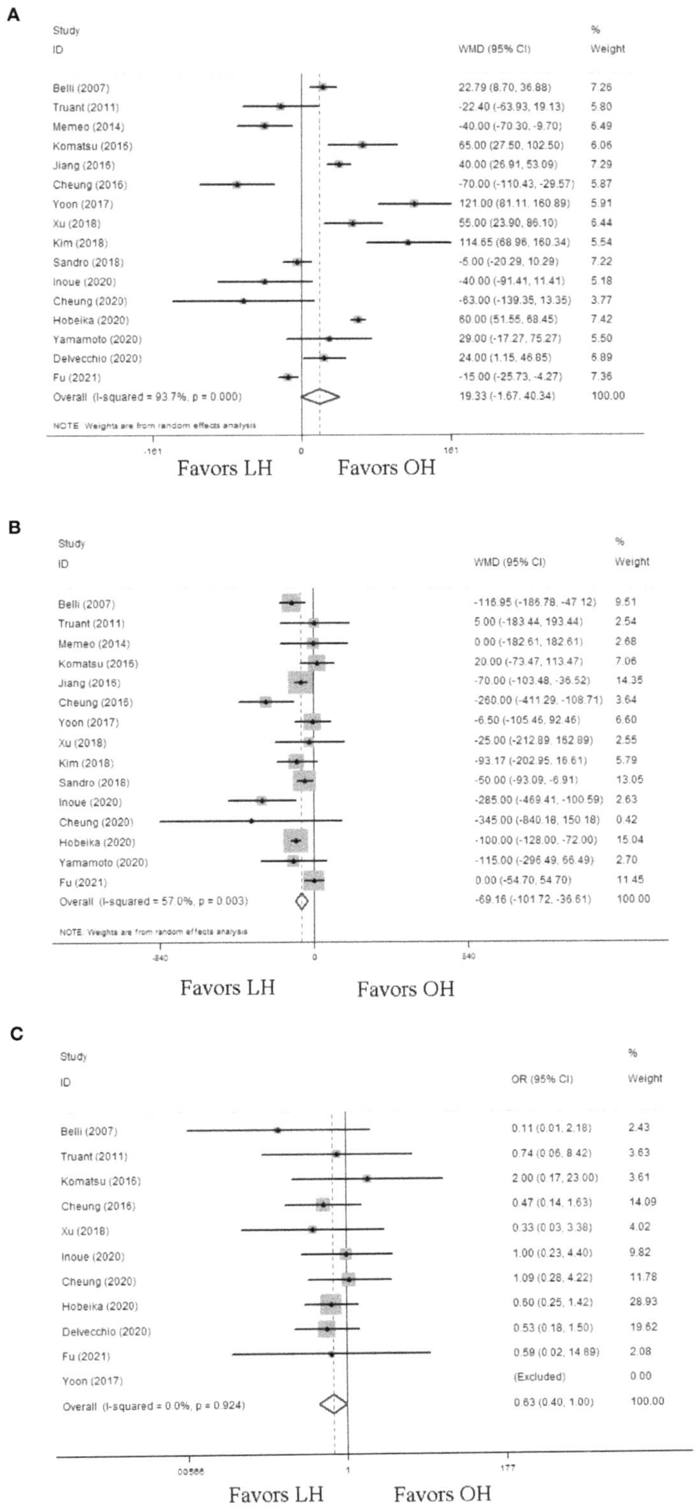

FIGURE 2 | Forest plots of intraoperative outcomes, **(A)** operation time, **(B)** blood loss, **(C)** transfusion rate.

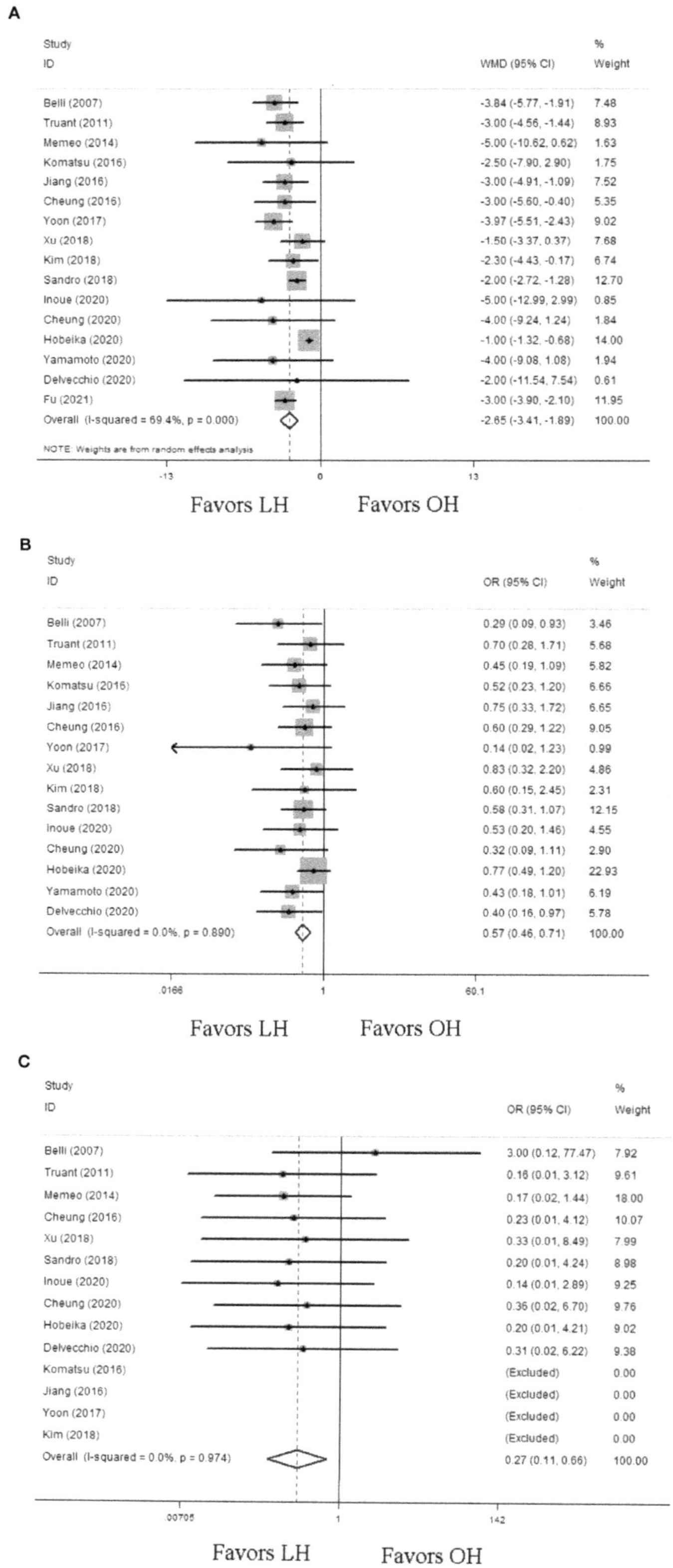

FIGURE 3 | Forest plots of postoperative outcomes, **(A)** length of postoperative hospitalization, **(B)** overall postoperative complication, **(C)** postoperative mortality.

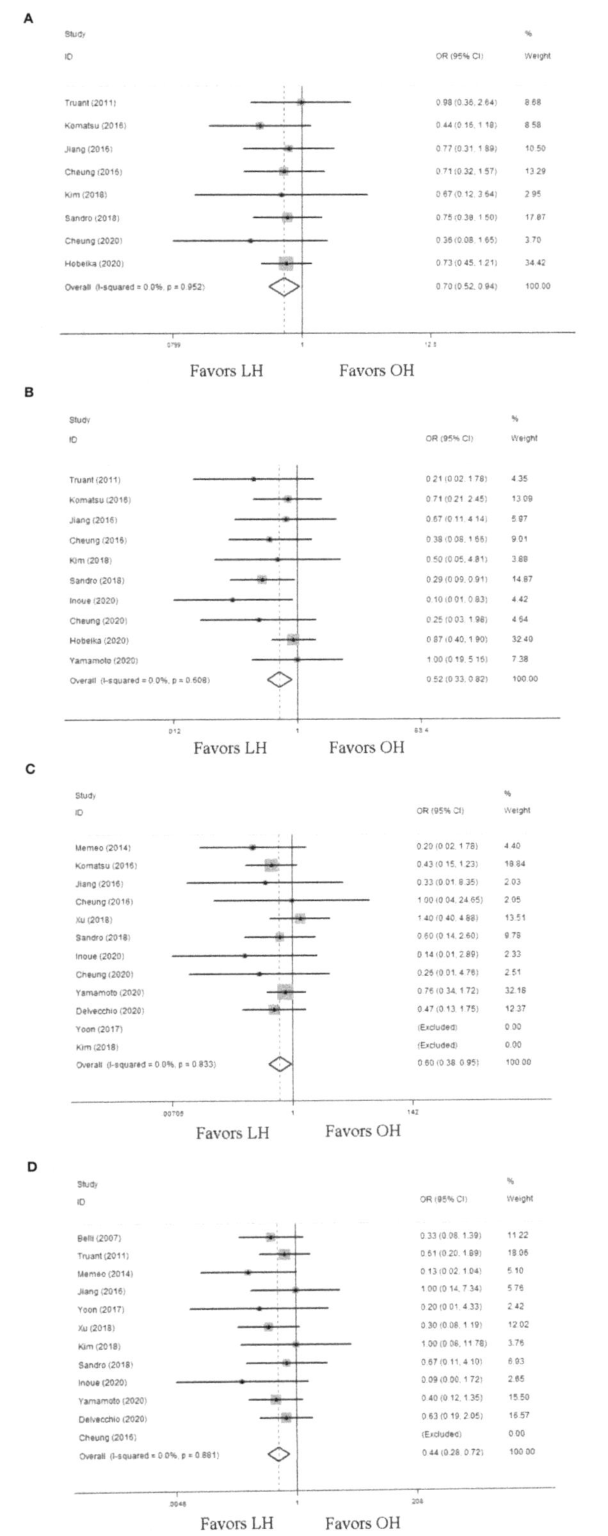

FIGURE 4 | Forest plots of postoperative complication in detail, **(A)** minor complication, **(B)** major complication, **(C)** postoperative liver failure, **(D)** ascites.

publication bias. No significant publication bias was detected by visual inspection of the funnel plot, in which the pooled studies were almost symmetrical and none of them were outside the 95% CI (**Figure 6**).

DISCUSSION

OH is a well-established curative treatment for HCC. However, patients with poor liver functional reserve, such as those with cirrhosis, are at higher risk of undergoing OH with a large surgical incision, wide extent of resection, and relatively large amount of blood loss. LH is emerging as a promising alternative approach for HCC patients with cirrhosis. Several previous meta-analyses have evaluated the advantages and disadvantages of LH (**Table 4**). Studies by Twaij et al. and Chen et al. identified significantly decreased overall postoperative complications, mortality, blood loss, and LOH in the LH group (12, 13). Goh et al. reported that LH was associated with better oncological outcomes (51). However, most studies included in those meta-analyses were retrospective studies with small sample sizes, which are prone to biases. Recently, several high-quality articles comparing LH and OH for HCC with cirrhosis have been published (14–18). To minimize the selection bias, this systematic review and meta-analysis pooled 16 case-matched retrospective studies. Comparisons were made between LH and OH for HCC in patients with cirrhosis, along with subgroup analysis according to different surgical extents.

Consistent with previous studies, the main findings obtained from our meta-analysis showed that patients who underwent LH presented notable oncological advantages in terms of 1-, 2-, and 5-year OS and 1-year DFS. In addition, our meta-analysis showed that LH was associated with lower postoperative morbidity, lower mortality, less blood loss, and shorter LOH than OH.

The primary concern with LH was bleeding control during transection in the setting of cirrhosis. The impact of cirrhosis on portal vein pressure and coagulation, and the movement restriction in laparoscopic surgery, make bleeding control challenging and increase the conversion risk. Truant et al. reported that uncontrolled bleeding accounted for 57.1% (4/7) of total conversion (42). Similarly, Sandro et al. also reported that one-third (2/7) of patients underwent conversion because of bleeding (15). With the accumulation of surgical experience, bleeding control during transection has been established by using the Pringle maneuver, compression with or without hemostatic material, clipping, suturing, temporary clamp for vessels, and various energy devices. Simultaneously, decreased intraoperative blood loss has been achieved with the application of appropriate pneumoperitoneum pressure, which reduces venous bleeding, and a magnified operating view, which allows meticulous manipulation. In this meta-analysis, the blood loss in the LH group was less than that in the OH group, as reported in previous studies. The considerable decrease in blood loss with the LH procedure means a decreased risk of transfusion. Accordingly, a lower transfusion rate in the LH group was observed in the present study.

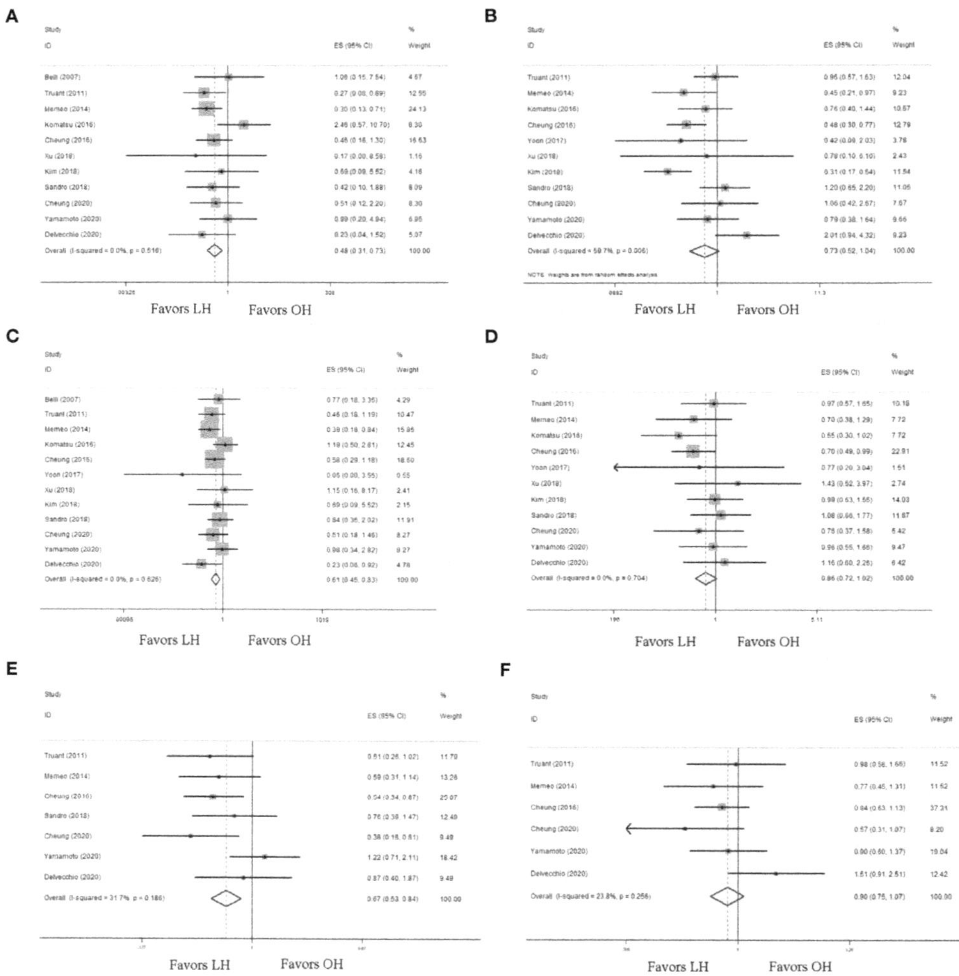

FIGURE 5 | Forest plots of long-term outcomes, **(A)** 1-y overall survival rate, **(B)** 1-y disease-free survival rate, **(C)** 2-y overall survival rate, **(D)** 2-y disease-free survival rate, **(E)** 5-y overall survival rate, **(F)** 5-y disease-free survival rate.

Decreased blood loss, avoidance of large incisions and meticulous manipulation alleviate the surgical trauma. The minimally invasive approach reduces the risk of acute or delayed systematic adverse events and subsequent postoperative morbidity and mortality. The overall complication rate of LH was approximately 22.8% (169/741), which was significantly lower than that of OH (34.9%, 389/1,114). Recently, Goh et al. examined 400 cases of LH and reported a postoperative morbidity of 18.8%, which is equivalent to the present study (52). A similar result was observed in that OH had a nearly four-fold risk of postoperative death in comparison with LH (OR = 0.28).

Hepatectomy can lead to refractory ascites in patients with cirrhosis, which can be fatal. By preserving the integrity of the abdominal wall and reducing surgery-induced injury to the area surrounding the liver, disruption of collateral blood and lymphatic flow is minimized in the laparoscopic approach. Further analysis of postoperative complications revealed that the LH group had less postoperative ascites. The LH group had fewer major and minor complications as than the OH group. Furthermore, in the setting of LH, minor complications were predominant, accounting for 75.8% (91/120) of the overall complications, which was significantly higher than that in OH (68.2%, 176/258). Therefore, it can be deduced that LH is technically safe and tends to have fewer and milder complications.

Reduced surgical trauma, fewer postoperative events, and enhanced recovery resulted in shorter LOH and lower medical costs. More importantly, the present study demonstrated that patients undergoing LH had better oncological outcomes, including 1-, 2-, 5-year OS and 1-year DFS. Although no statistical difference was found in 2- and 5-year DFS owing to the inclusion of limited studies, a trend of favoring LH was observed. We speculated that the better prognosis of LH patients might lie in the less compression during laparoscopic manipulation, which prevented tumor cell metastasis. In addition, the minimally invasive approach resulted in faster recovery of the immune and nutritional status, which may also contribute to better prognosis.

TABLE 3 | Subgroup analysis of outcomes based on the surgical extents.

Outcomes	Included studies	Sample size	I2	Pooled mode	Pooled effect	P value
Operation time						
All	16	1975	93.7%	Random	WMD:19.33(-1.67,40.34)	0.07
Minor resection	9	1351	93.9%	Random	WMD:14.80(-11.24,40.85)	0.27
Major resection	5	448	84.7%	Random	WMD:47.24(5.52,89.00)	0.03
Blood loss						
All	15	1853	57.0%	Random	WMD:-69.16(-101.72,-36.61)	<0.01
Minor resection	9	1351	34.3%	Fixed	WMD:-84.75(-112.22,-57.29)	<0.01
Major resection	4	326	0.0%	Fixed	WMD:-1.97(-65.34,61.40)	0.95
Transfusion						
All	10	1381	7.3%	Fixed	OR:0.63(0.40,1.00)	0.05
Minor resection	4	823	0.0%	Fixed	OR:0.52(0.27.1.02)	0.06
Major resection	4	382	0.0%	Fixed	OR:0.71(0.34,1.49)	0.36
LOH						
All	16	1975	69.4%	Random	WMD:-2.65(-3.41,-1.89)	<0.01
Minor resection	9	1351	70.8%	Random	WMD:-2.45(-3.33,-1.57)	<0.01
Major resection	5	448	4.6%	Random	WMD:-2.99(-4.11,-1.86)	<0.01
Overall complication						
All	15	1859	0.0%	Fixed	OR:0.57(0.46,0.71)	<0.01
Minor resection	9	1351	0.0%	Fixed	OR:0.61(0.48,0.78)	<0.01
Major resection	5	448	0.0%	Fixed	OR:0.47(0.30,0.75)	<0.01
Minor complication						
All	8	1295	0.0%	Fixed	OR:0.70(0.53,0.94)	0.02
Minor resection	6	1099	0.0%	Fixed	OR:0.76(0.55,1.03)	0.08
Major resection	2	196	0.0%	Fixed	OR:0.41(0.18,0.95)	0.04
Major complication						
All	10	1467	0.0%	Fixed	OR:0.52(0.33,0.82)	<0.01
Minor resection	7	1215	0.0%	Fixed	OR:0.57(0.34,0.94)	0.03
Major resection	2	196	0.0%	Fixed	OR:0.54(0.19,1.56)	0.26
Mortality						
All	10	1425	0.0%	Fixed	OR:0.27(0.11,0.66)	<0.01
Minor resection	6	1063	0.0%	Fixed	OR:0.26(0.08,0.83)	0.02
Major resection	3	306	0.0%	Fixed	OR:0.34(0.06,1.94)	0.22
POLF						
All	10	1352	0.0%	Fixed	OR:0.60(0.38,0.95)	0.03
Minor resection	5	914	0.0%	Fixed	OR:0.63(0.33,1.21)	0.17
Major resection	4	382	0.0%	Fixed	OR:0.60(0.31,1.17)	0.14
Ascites						
All	11	971	0.00%	Fixed	OR:0.44(0.28,0.72)	<0.01
Minor resection	7	663	0.00%	Fixed	OR:0.48(0.27,0.86)	0.01
Major resection	3	252	0.00%	Fixed	OR:0.43(0.18,1.02)	0.05
1-year OS						
All	11	1367	32.90%	Fixed	HR:0.48(0.31,0.73)	<0.01
Minor resection	7	985	0%	Fixed	HR:0.42(0.26,0.68)	<0.01
Major resection	4	382	36.4%	Fixed	HR:0.72(0.30,1.74)	0.46
2-year OS						
All	12	1433	0.00%	Fixed	HR:0.61(0.45,0.83)	<0.01
Minor resection	7	985	0%	Fixed	HR:0.59(0.42,0.85)	<0.01
Major resection	5	448	31.7%	Fixed	HR:0.66(0.37,1.17)	0.16
5-year OS						
All	7	1127	31.70%	Fixed	HR:0.67(0.53,0.85)	<0.01
Minor resection	5	885	35%	Fixed	HR:0.69(0.53,0.90)	<0.01
Major resection	2	242	55.8%	Random	HR:0.57(0.26,1.30)	0.18
1-year DFS						
All	11	1387	59.70%	Random	HR:0.73(0.52,1.04)	0.08
Minor resection	6	939	67.10%	Random	HR:0.63(0.41,0.96)	0.03
Major resection	5	448	22.3%	Fixed	HR:1.03(0.69,1.56)	0.88
2-year DFS						
All	11	1387	0%	Fixed	HR:0.86(0.73,1.02)	0.08
Minor resection	6	939	0%	Fixed	HR:0.87(0.72,1.05)	0.15
Major resection	5	448	0%	Fixed	HR:0.83(0.59,1.17)	0.29
5-year DFS						
All	6	781	23.80%	Fixed	HR:0.90(0.75,1.07)	0.23

(Continued)

TABLE 3 | Continued

Outcomes	Included studies	Sample size	I2	Pooled mode	Pooled effect	P value
Minor resection	4	735	0%	Fixed	HR:0.87(0.71,1.06)	0.16
Major resection	2	242	81.9%	Random	HR:0.95(0.37,2.44)	0.91

LOH length of hospitalization, CI confidence interval, WMD weighted mean difference, OR odds ratio, POLF postoperative liver failure, HR hazard ratio, OS overall survival, DFS disease-free survival disease-free survival.

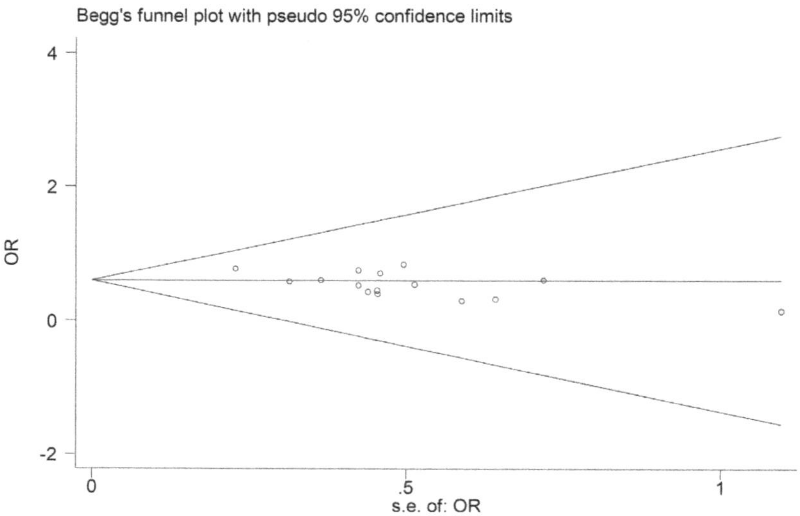

FIGURE 6 | Funnel plots of postoperative complication.

TABLE 4 | Summary of outcomes reported by previous meta-analysis and present meta-analysis.

Study	Latest literature search	Included studies	Study characteristics	Operation time	Blood loss	Blood transfusion	postoperative morbidity	postoperative mortality	LOH	1-year OS	5-year OS	1-year DFS	5-year DFS
Twaij et al.	2013.8	4	R&RM	E	FLH	FLH	FLH	NA	FLH	NA	NA	NA	NA
Chen et al.	2015.3	7	R&RM	E	FLH	FLH	FLH	E	FLH	E	FLH	E	E
Goh et al.	2016.11	5	R&RM	NA	NA	NA	NA	NA	NA	FLH	FLH	FLH	E
Present study	2021.3	16	RM	E	FLH	FLH	FLH	FLH	FLH	FLH	FLH	E	E

LOH length of hospitalization, OS overall survival, DFS disease-free survival, R retrospective study, RM retrospective matched study, RCT randomized clinical trial, E equivalent, FLH favors laparoscopic hepatectomy, NA not available.

Unlike previous meta-analyses on this issue, the present study performed subgroup analysis based on the surgical extent, which was necessary to eliminate such heterogeneity among the studies. The present study found that the results of subgroup analysis based on minor resection were in line with the results of the overall analysis, however, the results of subgroup analysis based on major resection should be cautiously interpreted, although only three studies were included. As expected, LMH was a potential alternative to its open counterpart, and it maintained the advantage of shorter LOH and fewer postoperative complications as in laparoscopic minor hepatectomy. However, LMH had a longer operation time than the open approach, suggesting that this procedure is technically demanding. Notably, Komatsu et al. reported a conversion rate of 34.21% in the LMH group, reflecting the steep learning curve of LMH in the setting of HCC with cirrhosis. Comprehensive liver function assessment and a good understanding of the liver anatomy, as well as ample surgical expertise, are the most important factors for successful LMH. Emerging evidence proving the value of LMH may lead to the expansion of the indication of LH to HCC patients with cirrhosis.

Our review has notable strengths as follows: (i) all included studies were case-matched studies, which balanced the baseline characteristics and reduced the selection bias, (ii) more detailed data than in other meta-analyses were extracted and analyzed, and (iii) "HR" instead of "OR" was applied in analyzing time-to-event data, such OS and DFS. Nevertheless, the present meta-analysis also had several limitations. First, most of the included studies were retrospective studies which adversely affected the overall quality of the evidence. Although the baseline characteristics of confounding factors were balanced in all included retrospective studies, the allocation of patients was rarely described in the included studies, which inevitably resulted in selection bias. Second, none of the included studies prospectively has calculated the sufficient sample size to identify differences between OH and LH. Several studies with small sample sizes presented the initial experience of surgeons in performing LH, although those surgeons might have a high level of expertise in OH. The lack of sufficient sample size and quality control of the surgical techniques might also bring bias. Third, LH is considered as an emerging and potentially better alternative to OH. It can't be guaranteed that all results, including LH with poor outcomes, were reported, and no mandatory registration is required in observational studies, which can be a source of publication bias.

CONCLUSION

In summary, this systematic review and meta-analysis comparing LH and OH demonstrated that LH can be safely performed in selected HCC patients with cirrhosis. LH offers favorable short-term outcomes and long-term oncological outcomes in minor liver resections. Although LMH seems to offer some advantages over the open approach, concerns about surgical and oncological safety remain. More evidence on LMH is warranted before expanding its indication to patients with cirrhosis.

AUTHOR CONTRIBUTIONS

Conception and design: X-JC and YP. Administrative support: X-JC. Provision of study material or patients: YP, KC, and S-JX. Collection and assembly of data: KC, S-JX, and J-QC. Data analysis and interpretation: YP. Manuscript writing: all authors. All authors contributed to the article and approved the submitted version.

REFERENCES

1. Njei B, Rotman Y, Ditah I, Lim JK. Emerging trends in hepatocellular carcinoma incidence and mortality. *Hepatol (Baltimore Md)* (2015) 61 (1):191–9. doi: 10.1002/hep.27388
2. El-Serag HB. Hepatocellular carcinoma. *New Engl J Med* (2011) 365 (12):1118–27. doi: 10.1056/NEJMra1001683
3. Reich H, McGlynn F, DeCaprio J, Budin R. Laparoscopic excision of benign liver lesions. *Obstetrics Gynecol* (1991) 78(5 Pt 2):956–8.
4. Katkhouda N, Fabiani P, Benizri E, Mouiel J. Laser resection of a liver hydatid cyst under videolaparoscopy. *Br J Surg* (1992) 79(6):560–1. doi: 10.1002/bjs.1800790628
5. Buell JF, Cherqui D, Geller DA, O'Rourke N, Iannitti D, Dagher I, et al. The international position on laparoscopic liver surgery: The Louisville Statement, 2008. *Ann Surg* (2009) 250(5):825–30. doi: 10.1097/sla.0b013e3181b3b2d8
6. Takahara T, Wakabayashi G, Beppu T, Aihara A, Hasegawa K, Gotohda N, et al. Long-term and perioperative outcomes of laparoscopic versus open liver resection for hepatocellular carcinoma with propensity score matching: a multi-institutional Japanese study. *J Hepato-biliary-pancreatic Sci* (2015) 22 (10):721–7. doi: 10.1002/jhbp.276
7. Neeff H, Mariaskin D, Spangenberg HC, Hopt UT, Makowiec F. Perioperative mortality after non-hepatic general surgery in patients with liver cirrhosis: an analysis of 138 operations in the 2000s using Child and MELD scores. *J Gastrointestinal Surg: Off J Soc Surg Alimentary Tract* (2011) 15(1):1–11. doi: 10.1007/s11605-010-1366-9
8. Tarantino G, Magistri P, Serra V, Berardi G, Assirati G, Ballarin R, et al. Laparoscopic Liver Resection of Right Posterior Segments for Hepatocellular Carcinoma on Cirrhosis. *J Laparoendoscopic Adv Surg Techniq Part A* (2017) 27(6):559–63. doi: 10.1089/lap.2016.0506
9. Siniscalchi A, Ercolani G, Tarozzi G, Gamberini L, Cipolat L, Pinna AD, et al. Laparoscopic versus Open Liver Resection: Differences in Intraoperative and Early Postoperative Outcome among Cirrhotic Patients with Hepatocellular Carcinoma-A Retrospective Observational Study. *HPB Surg: World J Hepatic Pancreatic Biliary Surg* (2014) 2014:871251. doi: 10.1155/2014/871251
10. Worhunsky DJ, Dua MM, Tran TB, Siu B, Poultsides GA, Norton JA, et al. Laparoscopic hepatectomy in cirrhotics: safe if you adjust technique. *Surg Endoscopy* (2016) 30(10):4307–14. doi: 10.1007/s00464-016-4748-6
11. Cannon RM, Saggi B, Buell JF. Evaluation of a laparoscopic liver resection in the setting of cirrhosis. *HPB: Off J Int Hepato Pancreato Biliary Assoc* (2014) 16(2):164–9. doi: 10.1111/hpb.12098
12. Twaij A, Pucher PH, Sodergren MH, Gall T, Darzi A, Jiao LR. Laparoscopic vs open approach to resection of hepatocellular carcinoma in patients with known cirrhosis: systematic review and meta-analysis. *World J Gastroenterol* (2014) 20(25):8274–81. doi: 10.3748/wjg.v20.i25.8274
13. Chen J, Bai T, Zhang Y, Xie ZB, Wang XB, Wu FX, et al. The safety and efficacy of laparoscopic and open hepatectomy in hepatocellular carcinoma patients with liver cirrhosis: a systematic review. *Int J Clin Exp Med* (2015) 8 (11):20679–89.
14. El-Gendi A, El-Shafei M, El-Gendi S, Shawky A. Laparoscopic Versus Open Hepatic Resection for Solitary Hepatocellular Carcinoma Less Than 5 cm in Cirrhotic Patients: A Randomized Controlled Study. *J Laparoendoscopic Adv Surg Techniq Part A* (2018) 28(3):302–10. doi: 10.1089/lap.2017.0518
15. Di Sandro S, Bagnardi V, Najjar M, Buscemi V, Lauterio A, De Carlis R, et al. Minor laparoscopic liver resection for Hepatocellular Carcinoma is safer than minor open resection, especially for less compensated cirrhotic patients: Propensity score analysis. *Surg Oncol* (2018) 27(4):722–9. doi: 10.1016/j.suronc.2018.10.001
16. Kim WJ, Kim KH, Kim SH, Kang WH, Lee SG. Laparoscopic Versus Open Liver Resection for Centrally Located Hepatocellular Carcinoma in Patients With Cirrhosis: A Propensity Score-matching Analysis. *Surg Laparoscopy Endoscopy Percutaneous Techniq* (2018) 28(6):394–400. doi: 10.1097/sle.0000000000000569
17. Yoon YI, Kim KH, Kang SH, Kim WJ, Shin MH, Lee SK, et al. Pure Laparoscopic Versus Open Right Hepatectomy for Hepatocellular Carcinoma in Patients With Cirrhosis: A Propensity Score Matched Analysis. *Ann Surg* (2017) 265(5):856–63. doi: 10.1097/sla.0000000000002072
18. Xu HW, Liu F, Li HY, Wei YG, Li B. Outcomes following laparoscopic versus open major hepatectomy for hepatocellular carcinoma in patients with cirrhosis: a propensity score-matched analysis. *Surg Endoscopy* (2018) 32 (2):712–9. doi: 10.1007/s00464-017-5727-2
19. Moher D, Liberati A, Tetzlaff J, Altman DG. Preferred reporting items for systematic reviews and meta-analyses: the PRISMA statement. *J Clin Epidemiol* (2009) 62(10):1006–12. doi: 10.1016/j.jclinepi.2009.06.005
20. Strasberg SM. Nomenclature of hepatic anatomy and resections: a review of the Brisbane 2000 system. *J Hepato-biliary-pancreatic Surg* (2005) 12(5):351–5. doi: 10.1007/s00534-005-0999-7

21. Hasegawa Y, Nitta H, Takahara T, Katagiri H, Baba S, Takeda D, et al. Safely extending the indications of laparoscopic liver resection: When should we start laparoscopic major hepatectomy? *Surg Endoscopy* (2017) 31(1):309–16. doi: 10.1007/s00464-016-4973-z
22. Goh BKP, Teo JY, Lee SY, Kam JH, Cheow PC, Jeyaraj P, et al. Critical appraisal of the impact of individual surgeon experience on the outcomes of laparoscopic liver resection in the modern era: collective experience of multiple surgeons at a single institution with 324 consecutive cases. *Surg Endoscopy* (2018) 32(4):1802–11. doi: 10.1007/s00464-017-5864-7
23. Dindo D, Demartines N, Clavien PA. Classification of surgical complications: a new proposal with evaluation in a cohort of 6336 patients and results of a survey. *Ann Surg* (2004) 240(2):205–13. doi: 10.1097/01.sla.0000133083.54934.ae
24. Tierney JF, Stewart LA, Ghersi D, Burdett S, Sydes MR. Practical methods for incorporating summary time-to-event data into meta-analysis. *Trials* (2007) 8:16. doi: 10.1186/1745-6215-8-16
25. Hozo SP, Djulbegovic B, Hozo I. Estimating the mean and variance from the median, range, and the size of a sample. *BMC Med Res Method* (2005) 5:13. doi: 10.1186/1471-2288-5-13
26. Higgins JP, Thompson SG, Deeks JJ, Altman DG. Measuring inconsistency in meta-analyses. *BMJ (Clin Res ed)* (7414) (2003) 327:557–60. doi: 10.1136/bmj.327.7414.557
27. Mantel N, Haenszel W. Statistical aspects of the analysis of data from retrospective studies of disease. *J Natl Cancer Institute* (1959) 22(4):719–48.
28. DerSimonian R, Laird N. Meta-analysis in clinical trials. *Controlled Clin Trials* (1986) 7(3):177–88. doi: 10.1016/0197-2456(86)90046-2
29. Yamashita Y, Ikeda T, Kurihara T, Yoshida Y, Takeishi K, Itoh S, et al. Long-term favorable surgical results of laparoscopic hepatic resection for hepatocellular carcinoma in patients with cirrhosis: a single-center experience over a 10-year period. *J Am Coll Surgeons* (2014) 219(6):1117–23. doi: 10.1016/j.jamcollsurg.2014.09.003
30. Cheung TT, Ma KW, She WH, Dai WC, Tsang SHY, Chan ACY, et al. Pure laparoscopic hepatectomy with augmented reality-assisted indocyanine green fluorescence versus open hepatectomy for hepatocellular carcinoma with liver cirrhosis: A propensity analysis at a single center. *Asian J Endoscopic Surg* (2018) 11(2):104–11. doi: 10.1111/ases.12492
31. Cheung TT, Poon RT, Yuen WK, Chok KS, Jenkins CR, Chan SC, et al. Long-term survival analysis of pure laparoscopic versus open hepatectomy for hepatocellular carcinoma in patients with cirrhosis: a single-center experience. *Ann Surg* (2013) 257(3):506–11. doi: 10.1097/SLA.0b013e31827b947a
32. Vega EA, Kutlu OC, Joechle K, De La Cruz N, Ko D, Conrad C. Preoperative Prognosticators of Safe Laparoscopic Hepatocellular Carcinoma Resection in Advanced Cirrhosis: a Propensity Score Matching Population-Based Analysis of 1799 Western Patients. *J Gastrointestinal Surg: Off J Soc Surg Alimentary Tract* (2019) 23(6):1157–65. doi: 10.1007/s11605-019-04139-7
33. Jin H, Yin Z, Zhou Y, Ma T, Jian Z. Safety and Feasibility of a Laparoscopy-Assisted Non-Anatomic Resection Technique for Hepatocellular Carcinoma Located at Right Posterior Segments in Cirrhotic Patients: A Case-Controlled Study with Propensity Score Matching. *Digestive Surg* (2018) 35(5):411–8. doi: 10.1159/000480359
34. Lee KF, Chong CN, Wong J, Cheung YS, Wong J, Lai P. Long-term results of laparoscopic hepatectomy versus open hepatectomy for hepatocellular carcinoma: a case-matched analysis. *World J Surg* (2011) 35(10):2268–74. doi: 10.1007/s00268-011-1212-6
35. Sposito C, Battiston C, Facciorusso A, Mazzola M, Muscarà C, Scotti M, et al. Propensity score analysis of outcomes following laparoscopic or open liver resection for hepatocellular carcinoma. *Br J Surg* (2016) 103(7):871–80. doi: 10.1002/bjs.10137
36. Tanaka S, Takemura S, Shinkawa H, Nishioka T, Hamano G, Kinoshita M, et al. Outcomes of Pure Laparoscopic versus Open Hepatic Resection for Hepatocellular Carcinoma in Cirrhotic Patients: A Case-Control Study with Propensity Score Matching. *Eur Surg Res Europaische Chirurgische Forschung Recherches Chirurgicales Europeennes* (2015) 55(4):291–301. doi: 10.1159/000439274
37. Wu X, Huang Z, Lau WY, Li W, Lin P, Zhang L, et al. Perioperative and long-term outcomes of laparoscopic versus open liver resection for hepatocellular carcinoma with well-preserved liver function and cirrhotic background: a propensity score matching study. *Surg Endoscopy* (2019) 33(1):206–15. doi: 10.1007/s00464-018-6296-8
38. Kanazawa A, Tsukamoto T, Shimizu S, Kodai S, Yamazoe S, Yamamoto S, et al. Impact of laparoscopic liver resection for hepatocellular carcinoma with F4-liver cirrhosis. *Surg Endoscopy* (2013) 27(7):2592–7. doi: 10.1007/s00464-013-2795-9
39. Belli G, Fantini C, D'Agostino A, Cioffi L, Langella S, Russolillo N, et al. Laparoscopic versus open liver resection for hepatocellular carcinoma in patients with histologically proven cirrhosis: short- and middle-term results. *Surg Endoscopy* (2007) 21(11):2004–11. doi: 10.1007/s00464-007-9503-6
40. Komatsu S, Brustia R, Goumard C, Perdigao F, Soubrane O, Scatton O. Laparoscopic versus open major hepatectomy for hepatocellular carcinoma: a matched pair analysis. *Surg Endoscopy* (2016) 30(5):1965–74. doi: 10.1007/s00464-015-4422-4
41. Memeo R, de'Angelis N, Compagnon P, Salloum C, Cherqui D, Laurent A, et al. Laparoscopic vs. open liver resection for hepatocellular carcinoma of cirrhotic liver: a case-control study. *World J Surg* (2014) 38(11):2919–26. doi: 10.1007/s00268-014-2659-z
42. Truant S, Bouras AF, Hebbar M, Boleslawski E, Fromont G, Dharancy S, et al. Laparoscopic resection vs. open liver resection for peripheral hepatocellular carcinoma in patients with chronic liver disease: a case-matched study. *Surg Endoscopy* (2011) 25(11):3668–77. doi: 10.1007/s00464-011-1775-1
43. Cheung TT, Dai WC, Tsang SH, Chan AC, Chok KS, Chan SC, et al. Pure Laparoscopic Hepatectomy Versus Open Hepatectomy for Hepatocellular Carcinoma in 110 Patients With Liver Cirrhosis: A Propensity Analysis at a Single Center. *Ann Surg* (2016) 264(4):612–20. doi: 10.1097/sla.0000000000001848
44. Jiang X, Liu L, Zhang Q, Jiang Y, Huang J, Zhou H, et al. Laparoscopic versus open hepatectomy for hepatocellular carcinoma: long-term outcomes. *J BUON: Off J Balkan Union Oncol* (2016) 21(1):135–41.
45. Delvecchio A, Conticchio M, Ratti F, Gelli M, Anelli FM, Laurent A, et al. Laparoscopic major hepatectomy for hepatocellular carcinoma in elderly patients: a multicentric propensity score–based analysis. *Surg Endoscopy* (2020). doi: 10.1007/s00464-020-07843-7
46. Fu XT, Tang Z, Chen JF, Shi YH, Liu WR, Gao Q, et al. Laparoscopic hepatectomy enhances recovery for small hepatocellular carcinoma with liver cirrhosis by postoperative inflammatory response attenuation: a propensity score matching analysis with a conventional open approach. *Surg Endoscopy* (2021) 35(2):910–20. doi: 10.1007/s00464-020-07710-5
47. Inoue Y, Yokohama K, Ohama H, Tsuchimoto Y, Terazawa T, Asai A, et al. Efficacy and safety of laparoscopic hepatectomy for hepatocellular carcinoma comorbid with cirrhosis. *Przeglad Gastroenterol* (2020) 15(3):225–33. doi: 10.5114/pg.2020.99039
48. Cheung TT, Ma KW, She WH, Dai WC, Tsang SHY, Chan ACY, et al. Pure laparoscopic versus open major hepatectomy for hepatocellular carcinoma with liver F4 cirrhosis without routine Pringle maneuver - A propensity analysis in a single center. *Surg Oncol* (2020) 35:315–20. doi: 10.1016/j.suronc.2020.09.012
49. Hobeika C, Nault JC, Barbier L, Schwarz L, Lim C, Laurent A, et al. Influence of surgical approach and quality of resection on the probability of cure for early-stage HCC occurring in cirrhosis. *JHEP Rep: Innovation Hepatol* (2020) 2(6):100153. doi: 10.1016/j.jhepr.2020.100153
50. Yamamoto M, Kobayashi T, Oshita A, Abe T, Kohashi T, Onoe T, et al. Laparoscopic versus open limited liver resection for hepatocellular carcinoma with liver cirrhosis: a propensity score matching study with the Hiroshima Surgical study group of Clinical Oncology (HiSCO). *Surg Endoscopy* (2020) 34 (11):5055–61. doi: 10.1007/s00464-019-07302-y
51. Goh EL, Chidambaram S, Ma S. Laparoscopic vs open hepatectomy for hepatocellular carcinoma in patients with cirrhosis: A meta-analysis of the long-term survival outcomes. *Int J Surg (London England)* (2018) 50:35–42. doi: 10.1016/j.ijsu.2017.12.021
52. Goh BKP, Lee SY, Teo JY, Kam JH, Jeyaraj PR, Cheow PC, et al. Changing trends and outcomes associated with the adoption of minimally invasive hepatectomy: a contemporary single-institution experience with 400 consecutive resections. *Surg Endoscopy* (2018) 32(11):4658–65. doi: 10.1007/s00464-018-6310-1

10

Unresectable Hepatocellular Carcinoma: Transcatheter Arterial Chemoembolization Combined with Microwave Ablation vs. Combined with Cryoablation

Jialiang Wei[1†], *Wei Cui*[2†], *Wenzhe Fan*[1], *Yu Wang*[1] *and Jiaping Li*[1*]

[1] Department of Interventional Oncology, The First Affiliated Hospital, Sun Yat-sen University, Guangzhou, China,
[2] Department of Interventional Therapy, Cancer Center, Guangdong Provincial People's Hospital, Guangdong Academy of Medical Sciences, School of Medicine, South China University of Technology, Guangzhou, China

***Correspondence:**
Jiaping Li
jiapingli3s@126.com

† These authors have contributed equally to this work

Background: Transcatheter arterial chemoembolization (TACE) combined with ablation has been widely used for treating unresectable hepatocellular carcinoma (HCC). However, the technique with which TACE should be combined for it to be more effective remains unknown.

Purpose: To retrospectively evaluate the efficacy and safety of TACE combined with microwave ablation (MWA) vs. TACE combined with cryoablation (CRA) in treating unresectable HCC.

Materials and Methods: From January 2011 to December 2018, 108 patients diagnosed with unresectable HCC were divided into either the TACE-MWA group (n = 48) or TACE-CRA group (n = 60). Overall survival (OS) and time to progression (TTP) were compared between the two groups. To reduce potential bias, a propensity score matching (PSM) was performed. Complications were observed. Kaplan-Meier survival curves were constructed and compared using the log-rank test.

Results : The baseline characteristics of the two groups were balanced. The median OS was 20.9 months (95% CI 14.3–27.6 months) in the TACE-MWA group and 13.0 months (95% CI 8.8–17.1 months) in the TACE-CRA group (P = 0.096). The median TTP was 8.8 months (95% CI 4.3–13.4 months) in the TACE-MWA group and 9.3 months (95% CI 7.1–11.5 months) in the TACE-CRA group (P = 0.675). After PSM, 48 patients remained in each group. The median OS in the TACE-MWA and TACE-CRA groups was 20.9 months (95% CI 14.3–27.6 months), and 13.5 months (95% CI 8.4–18.6 months, P = 0.100), respectively. The median TTP in the TACE-MWA and TACE-CRA groups was 8.8 months (95% CI 4.3–13.4 months), and 8.6 months (95% CI 3.1–14.2 months, P = 0.909), respectively. The overall incidence rate of ablation-related complications was lower in the TACE-MWA group than in the TACE-CRA group (66.7 vs. 88.3%, P = 0.006). Multivariate analysis showed that the presence of portal vein tumor thrombus (PVTT) and the maximum diameter of intrahepatic tumor were significant prognostic factors for OS and TTP.

Conclusion: The efficacy of TACE-MWA and TACE-CRA in the treatment of unresectable HCC was comparable. TACE-MWA was more promising because of a lower complication rate, especially with regard to thrombocytopenia. Further prospective randomized controlled trials are required to validate our findings.

Keywords: hepatocellular carcinoma, transcatheter arterial chemoembolization, microwave ablation, cryoablation, combination therapy

INTRODUCTION

Hepatocellular carcinoma (HCC) has moved upward to become the fourth most common cause of cancer-related death in the world (1, 2). Transcatheter arterial chemoembolization (TACE) is the first-line treatment for patients with unresectable, intermediate-stage HCC, and also effective in patients with advanced-stage HCC (2, 3). However, tumor recurrence and metastasis often occur due to incomplete embolization, tumor neovascularization, the lack of vascular access to the tumor, and difficulties associated with super selective embolization. The long-term efficacy of TACE alone is thus not satisfactory (4–7), and combining other therapies with TACE has become a strategy. TACE combined with ablation therapy, targeted molecular therapy, and radioactive seed implantation have been effective to varying degrees (8–10).

Percutaneous local ablation therapies, such as radiofrequency ablation (RFA), microwave ablation (MWA), and cryoablation (CRA) are recommended in HCC patients with Barcelona Clinic Liver Cancer (BCLC) stage 0 or A who are not candidates for surgery. The main methods employed now are RFA and MWA (2). Previous studies have found that MWA was comparable in efficacy and safety to RFA in treating small and medium-size intrahepatic tumors (11). Relative to RFA and MWA, CRA has an advantage in treating unresectable HCC due to its specific mechanism of action, such as the formation of a visual ice-ball, less damage to the adjacent great blood vessels or organs, less severe pain, and the activation of cyroimmunlogy in tumor (12). A previous study found no significant difference between RFA and CRA in the treatment of stage I and II HCC (13). There are relatively few comparative studies on the treatment of HCC by MWA vs. CRA, especially for large HCC. However, for large unresectable HCC, ablation monotherapy is rarely reported. Combination therapy has become a common treatment strategy to improve local control and decrease distant recurrence, (9).

TACE combined with ablation therapy has been shown to be safe and effective (10). Compared with TACE alone or ablation alone, TACE combined with ablation can significantly improve the efficacy for two specific reasons: (1) after TACE, the blood supply to tumor can be reduced, thereby making ablation more effective; (2) the iodide oil deposited by the TACE procedure can allow guidance during ablation under unenhanced CT scan (14, 15). Previous studies have found that TACE combined with MWA or RFA can prolong the overall survival of patients than TACE alone (6, 8, 16). In large unresectable HCC cases, although there was no significant difference between MWA and RFA in terms of the efficacy and safety, MWA has some advantages, including consistently higher intratumor temperature, faster ablation time, multiple applicators, less heat sink effect and a wider range (17, 18). Our previous study confirmed that TACE combined with CRA can improve overall survival in patients with HCC when compared with TACE alone (12). However, it is not clear whether TACE combined with MWA or TACE combined with CRA is more effective (9, 19–21). In this study, we aim to evaluate comparative differences in the efficacy and safety of TACE combined with MWA and TACE combined with CRA for the treatment of patients with unresectable HCC.

MATERIALS AND METHODS

Study Design

This is a retrospective study from our center. The study was approved by the ethics committee of our hospital and conducted in accordance with the guidelines of the Helsinki declaration. Written informed consent was waived because the study was retrospective.

The study inclusion criteria were as follows: (a) 18–75 years old; (b) newly diagnosed with HCC, according to EASL or AASLD guidelines (3, 22); (c) BCLC stage B or C, without candidacy for surgical resection or transplantation; (d) Child-Pugh class A or B; (e) laboratory tests values (platelet count $>60 \times 10^9$/L, hemoglobin concentration >85 g/L, prothrombin time elevated >6 s); (f) normal renal function (serum creatinine concentration 1.5 times or lower than the upper limit of the normal range), and (g) a performance status score of 0–2 in the eastern cooperative tumor group (ECOG). We excluded patients exhibiting any of the following: the obstruction of the main portal vein, previous liver resection, as well as a history of liver transplantation, treatments such as radioactive seed implantation, targeted therapy or systemic chemotherapy.

From January 2010 to December 2018, 218 patients received either TACE-MWA or TACE-CRA. A total of 110 patients were excluded (**Figure 1**). Finally, a total of 108 patients were enrolled, and TACE was the first-line treatment. All patients either had no indication for surgery or refused surgery after multidisciplinary discussion with the same team. All patients were informed of the advantages and disadvantages of MWA and CRA, including expected treatment outcome, treatment-related morbidity, and cost. The choice of ablation modalities was ultimately made by patients and their authorized representatives. Patients were divided into the TACE-MWA group and TACE-CRA group based on the treatment they received.

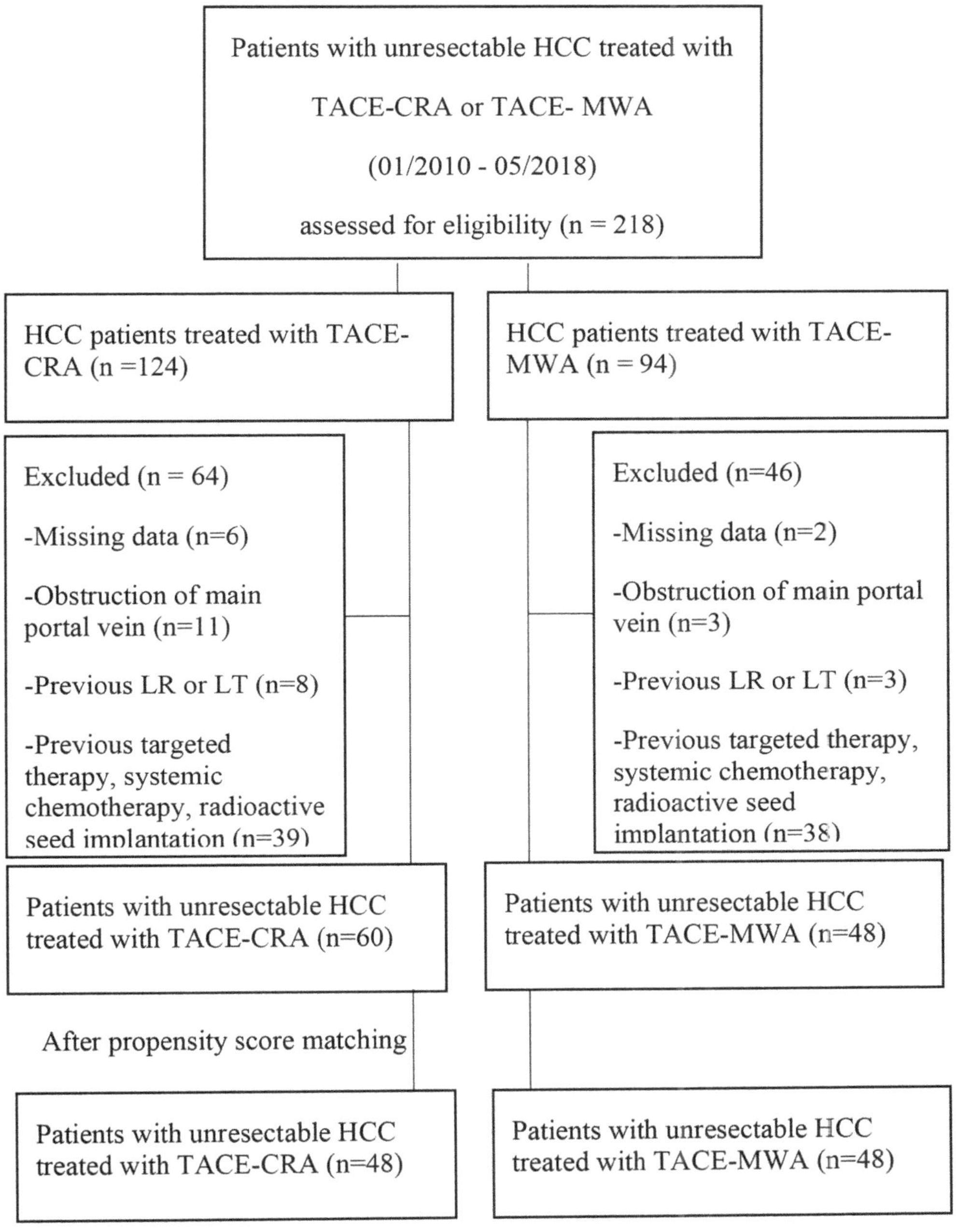

FIGURE 1 | Flowchart shows patients selection. HCC, hepatocellular carcinoma; CRA, cryoablation; MWA, microwave ablation; TACE, transcatheter arterial chemoembolization; LR, liver resection; LT, liver transplantation.

TACE Protocol

TACE was performed by three radiologists (JL, YW, and WF), with over 10–20 years of interventional experience. TACE was performed as previously described (23, 24). A selective 5-Fr YASHIRO or RH catheter was briefly introduced, and a visceral angiogram was performed to evaluate hepatic artery supply. Patients received the super selective catheterization of the hepatic artery supplied by the distal tumor with 2.7-F micro-catheter (Progreat; Terumo), and 5–20 ml lipiodol (Lipiodol; Guerbet, Roissy, France) mixed with 20–40 mg epirubicin (Pfizer, Wuxi, China) were slowly injected until the blood flow slowed. Finally, 350–560 μm of polyvinyl alcohol particles (Alicon Pharmaceutical, Hangzhou, China) were injected to reduce tumor blood flow if necessary. All patients received contrast-enhanced dynamic CT or MR imaging within 2 weeks before the first TACE. After the first TACE, ablation was performed within 2 weeks. Tumor response was evaluated with enhanced CT at 4–6 weeks after treatment according to the mRECIST guidelines. Based on the evaluation of results, TACE was given on-demand treatment.

Percutaneous Microwave Ablation Procedure

If CT or MRI reexamination showed that the intrahepatic lesion was still not regressing after the first TACE, MWA was offered to patients who were not expected to have complete tumor necrosis after a second TACE session. In the TACE-MWA group, percutaneous MWA was generally performed by the same team of doctors in 2 weeks after the first TACE procedure. Most of the patients were under conscious sedation. General anesthesia was reserved for cases in which intra-procedural pain became problematic. MWA was performed using the MTC-3C microwave therapy instruments (Vison-China Medical Devices R&D Institute, Nanjing, China) set to a frequency of 2,450 MHz±10% and an output power of 5–120 W. The microwave antenna was a 15-gauge cooling unipolar needle, either 150 or 180 mm long. MWA output power was 50–80 W applied for 5–10 min per ablation depending on the specific situation. Ablations can lead to coagulation necrosis using microwave less than four antenna to achieve a suitable ablation volume.

Percutaneous Cryoablation Procedure

Similarly, the efficacy of the first TACE was evaluated, and if the intrahepatic lesion was still not regressing, CRA was offered to patients who were not expected to have complete tumor necrosis after a second TACE session. All percutaneous CRA procedures in the TACE-CRA group were performed by the same team of doctors who performed the first TACE procedure. The CRA procedure was performed using techniques previously described (12). Most of the patients tolerated to the procedure under conscious sedation, although a general anesthetic was used for cases where intra-procedural pain was problematic. CRA is a process that uses extreme cold to destroy or damage tissue (25). Procedures were guided by computed tomography. The CRA procedures were performed using an argon-based cryoablation system (Cryo-Hit, Galil Medical, Yokneam, Israel) and 17-gauge cryoablation applicators. One to five applicators were used to achieve an ice ball that completely encompassed the tumor with a 5 mm or greater margin of uninvolved liver beyond the tumor. The CRA procedure took more than one session in such situations.

Assessment of Response and Follow-Up Protocol

The primary end point was overall survival (OS), which was defined as the time from the beginning of the first TACE treatment to death or the last follow-up. The secondary endpoints included tumor response and time to tumor progression (TTP), which was defined as the time from the beginning of the first TACE treatment to radiologic tumor progression, death, or the last follow-up. Tumor evaluation indicators included objective response rate (ORR) and disease control rate (DCR), as described in the modified Response Evaluation Criteria in Solid Tumors (mRECIST) (26). ORR refers to the proportion of patients whose tumors shrank to a certain amount and remained unchanged for a certain period of time, including complete response (CR) and partial response (PR) cases. DCR refers to the proportion of patients whose tumors shrank or stabilized for a certain period of time, including CR, PR, and stable disease (SD) cases. Complications were observed clinically during admission and assessed by telephone interview after discharge. They were graded according to the Common Terminology Criteria for Adverse Events (CTCAE, version 3.0) (27).

Statistical Analysis

All statistical analyses were performed using SPSS software version 23.0 software (IBM SPSS, Chicago, IL). Continuous variables between the two groups were expressed as median ± SD, and compared using the Student's t-test. Categorical variables were expressed as percentage and frequency, and compared using the χ^2 test. Survival curves were constructed using the Kaplan-Meier method and were compared using the log-rank test. Univariate and multivariate analyses with various parameters were performed using Cox's regression model with proportional hazards. The relative prognostic significance of the variables in predicting the overall survival rate and the time to tumor progression rate or metastasis was assessed using multivariate Cox proportional hazards regression analysis and logistic regression analysis, respectively. To minimize the selection bias, a 1:1 propensity score matching (PSM) was performed using the nearest-neighbor matching method with a caliper distance of 0.1 without replacement. All independent variables were entered into the propensity model. All statistical tests were two-tailed, and $P < 0.05$ were considered statistically significant.

RESULTS

Patients

The baseline characteristics are presented in **Table 1**. No significant differences were observed between the TACE-MWA group and the TACE-CRA group before and after PSM (**Table 1**). In both TACE-MWA and TACE-CRA groups, the median number of the TACE procedure performed was 2 (range 1–7). In TACE-MWA and TACE-CRA groups, the median number of the ablation procedure performed was 2.0 (range 1–3) and 1.0 (range 1–5), respectively.

Tumor Response

Six patients (12.5%) in the TACE-MWA group vs. 4 patients (6.7%) in the TACE-CRA group had a CR, while 29 patients (60.8%) in the TACE-MWA group vs. 16 patients (26.7%) in the TACE-CRA group had a PR. 35 patients (60.4%) in the TACE-MWA group vs. 20 patients (33.3%) in the TACE-CRA group achieved an objective response ($P = 0.161$). 44 patients (91.7%) in the TACE-MWA group vs. 45 patients (75%) in the TACE-CRA group achieved disease control ($P < 0.001$). Additionally, 15 patients (25%) in the TACE-CRA group and 4 patients (8.3%) in the TACE-MWA group had a PD.

Complications

No unexpected treatment-related deaths were observed. Complications after ablation therapy and TACE are shown in

TABLE 1 | Patients characteristics.

Parameter	Overall series			Propensity score-matched pairs		
	TACE + CRA N = 60 (%)	TACE + MWA N = 48 (%)	P-value	TACE + CRA N = 48 (%)	TACE + MWA N = 48 (%)	P-value
Sex			>0.999			0.726
Female	6 (10.0)	5 (10.4)		4 (8.3)	5 (10.4)	
Male	54 (90.0)	43 (89.6)		44 (91.7)	43 (89.6)	
Age (y), mean ± SD	52.9 ± 11.4	54.7 ± 10.3	0.415	51.9 ± 11.2	54.7 ± 10.3	0.207
≤ 60	38 (63.3)	31 (64.6)	0.893	33 (68.8)	31 (64.6)	0.665
> 60	22 (36.7)	17 (35.4)		15 (31.2)	17 (35.4)	
ECOG PS			0.490			0.305
0	26 (43.3)	24 (50.0)		19 (39.6)	24 (50.0)	
1	34 (56.7)	24 (50.0)		29 (60.4)	24 (50.0)	
HBsAg			>0.999			0.726
Positive	54 (90.0)	44 (91.7)		43 (89.6)	44 (91.7)	
Negative	6 (10.0)	4 (8.3)		5 (10.4)	4 (8.3)	
HCV			>0.999			0.557
Positive	2 (3.3)	1 (2.1)		2 (4.2)	1 (2.1)	
Negative	58 (96.7)	47 (97.9)		46 (95.8)	47 (97.9)	
Cirrhosis			0.314			0.529
Yes	33 (55.0)	31 (64.6)		28 (58.3)	31 (64.6)	
No	27 (45.0)	17 (35.4)		20 (41.7)	17 (35.4)	
Ascites			0.915			0.805
Yes	12 (20.0)	10 (20.8)		11 (22.9)	10 (20.8)	
No	48 (80.0)	38 (79.2)		37 (77.1)	38 (79.2)	
Tumor diameter (cm)	11.8 ± 5.3	11.5 ± 4.9	0.748	12.4 ± 5.5	11.5 ± 4.9	0.403
> 10	39 (65.0)	26 (54.2)	0.253	33 (68.8)	26 (54.2)	0.142
≤ 10	21 (35.0)	22 (45.8)		15 (31.2)	22 (45.8)	
No. of tumors			0.341			0.660
Solitary	15 (25)	16 (33.3)		14 (29.2)	16 (33.3)	
Multiple	45 (75)	32 (66.7)		34 (70.8)	32 (66.7)	
Tumor growth pattern			0.139			0.138
With capsule	18 (30)	21 (43.7)		14 (29.2)	21 (43.7)	
Infiltrative	42 (70)	27 (56.3)		34 (70.8)	27 (56.3)	
AFP level (ng/ml)			0.762			0.539
≤ 400	32 (53.3)	27 (56.3)		24 (50.0)	27 (56.3)	
> 400	28 (46.7)	21 (43.7)		24 (50.0)	21 (43.7)	
PVTT statue			0.861			0.681
Yes	24 (40.0)	20 (41.7)		22 (45.8)	20 (41.7)	
No	36 (60.0)	28 (58.3)		26 (54.2)	28 (58.3)	

ECOG PS, eastern cooperative oncology group performance status; HBsAg, hepatitis B surface antigen; HCV, hepatitis C virus; PVTT, portal vein tumor thrombosis; AFP, α-Fetoprotein; HCC, hepatocellular carcinoma.

Tables 2, 3. The most common complications after ablation were fever, abdominal pain, local skin frostbite, hemorrhage, and thrombocytopenia. The most common grade 1–2 complications were abdominal pain and thrombocytopenia in the TACE-CRA group. Three patients suffered from local skin frostbite in the TACE-CRA group. Four patients in the TACE-CRA group who suffered from grade 3–4 thrombocytopenia were treated with recombinant human interleukin-11 to assist with recovery. One patient developed a liver abscess after CRA. New ascites appeared in another patient after CRA. No cryoshock, liver failure, pneumonia, acute myocardial infarction, hepatorenal syndrome, or other severe complication happened in either group after ablation therapy.

Survival

The median follow-up duration was 77.7 months (95% CI: 22.7, 132.6 months). At the last follow-up, 16 patients in TACE-MWA group and 9 patients in TACE-CRA group were still alive. The median OS was 20.9 months (95% CI 14.3–27.6 months) in TACE-MWA group, and 13.0 months (95% CI 8.8–17.1 months)

TABLE 2 | Complications related to CRA/MWA in the two group.

Complications	TACE-CRA (*N* = 60)		TACE-MWA (*N* = 48)		*P*-Value	
	Any grade (%)	Grade 3–4 (%)	Any grade (%)	Grade 3–4 (%)	Any grade (%)	Grade 3–4 (%)
Overall incidence	53 (88.3)	7 (11.7)	32 (66.7)	2 (4.2)	0.006	0.293
Fever	7 (11.7)	0	5 (10.4)	0	0.837	...
Abdominal pain	38 (70.0)	4 (6.7)	25 (52.1)	2 (4.2)	0.057	0.888
Frostbite/burns	3 (5.0)	0	0	0	0.326	...
Pleural effusion	4 (6.7)	0	0	0	0.190	...
Hemorrhage	1 (1.7)	0	0	0	...	...
Thrombocytopenia	25 (41.7)	4 (6.7)	4 (8.3)	0	0.000	0.190
New ascites	1 (1.7)	0	0	0	...	...
Liver abscess	1 (1.7)	0	0	0	...	...

TABLE 3 | Complications related to TACE in the two group.

Complications	TACE-CRA (*N* = 60, %)	TACE-MWA (*N* = 48, %)	*P*-Value
Overall incidence	45 (75%)	38 (79.2)	0.610
Fever,	35 (58.3)	22 (45.8)	0.259
Abdominal pain, grade 1–2	39 (65%)	19 (39.6)	0.348
Nausea/vomiting, grade 1–2	6 (10)	9 (18.6)	0.010
New ascites	5 (8.3)	0	...
Liver dysfunction, grade 1–2	0	1 (2.1)	...
Pleural effusion	0	1 (2.1)	...

in TACE-CRA group ($P = 0.096$). The median TTP was 8.8 months (95% CI 4.3–13.4 months) in the TACE-MWA group, and 9.3 months (95% CI 7.1–11.5 months) in the TACE-CRA group ($P = 0.675$). There was no statistically significant difference in OS or TTP between the two groups (**Figures 2A,B**). After 1:1 PSM, 48 patients remained in each group. All variables were matched between the two groups (**Table 1**). The median OS in the TACE-MWA and TACE-CRA groups was 20.9 months (95% CI 14.3–27.6 months), and 13.5 months (95% CI 8.4–18.6 months, $P = 0.100$), respectively. The median TTP in the TACE-MWA and TACE-CRA groups was 8.8 months (95% CI 4.3–13.4 months), and 8.6 months (95% CI 3.1–14.2 months, $P = 0.909$), respectively (**Figures 2C,D**). Univariate analysis showed that the presence of ascites, presence of portal vein tumor thrombus (PVTT), maximum diameter of intrahepatic tumor, tumor growth pattern, and α-fetoprotein level were associated with OS and TTP ($P < 0.05$) (**Tables 4, 5**). Multivariate analysis showed that the presence of PVTT and the maximum diameter of intrahepatic tumor were statistically significant prognostic factors for OS and TTP ($P < 0.05$) (**Tables 4, 5; Figures 3A,B**).

DISCUSSION

In this study, we first evaluated the safety and efficacy of treating unresectable HCC with TACE-MWA vs. TACE-CRA. There were no statistically significant differences in the median OS (20.9 vs. 13.0 months, $P = 0.096$) and median TTP (8.8 vs. 9.3 months, $P = 0.675$) between the TACE-MWA and TACE-CRA groups, respectively; however, our results showed that MWA has fewer complications than CRA in treating unresectable HCC.

Many previous studies have demonstrated that combination therapy is significantly more effective in patients with unresectable HCC (8, 9, 12, 20, 28–30). Ginsburg et al. (31) found that a median OS of TACE plus MWA of about 42.6 months, and complete local tumor response rate was 76.6% (49 of 64 tumors). Ginsburg et al. (31) also inferred that the BCLC stage was associated with OS. Zheng et al. (8) showed that the median TTP and OS of TACE-MWA were 12.5 and 26.6 months, respectively, and that tumor size and number were associated with TTP and OS. Ni et al. (32) obtained a median OS for TACE plus MWA was 21.5 months. In our study, we found that the median TTP and OS of patients in the TACE-MWA group were 8.8 and 18.4 months, respectively, and the local tumor response rate was significantly lower than that in Ginsburg et al. (31). We think the main reason is the huge difference in tumor size between the two studies. In Zheng et al. (8) the average tumor size in the TACE-MWA group was similar to that observed in our study, and the TTP and OS were slightly longer; however, there was no description of tumor capsule and the ECOG score. In our study, the OS of patients in the TACE-MWA group was similar to that observed in Ni et al. (32) however, 67 (77.9%) patients in that study had no portal vein invasion.

Xu et al. (33) divided patients into the TACE-CRA group and CRA alone group, and found that the size and number of tumors in the TACE-CRA group were larger than those in the CRA alone group before treatment. Nevertheless, the 4- and 5-year survival rates of patients in the TACE-CRA group were higher than those in the CRA alone group. Huang Chen et al. (34) designed a prospective study to evaluate the effectiveness of TACE combined with cryoablation vs. TACE alone, and discovered that the complete remission rate and total effective rate of the combination group were significantly higher than those of the TACE group. The aforementioned studies showed that TACE combined with CRA could bring added benefits to patients with unresectable HCC. The effect of combined

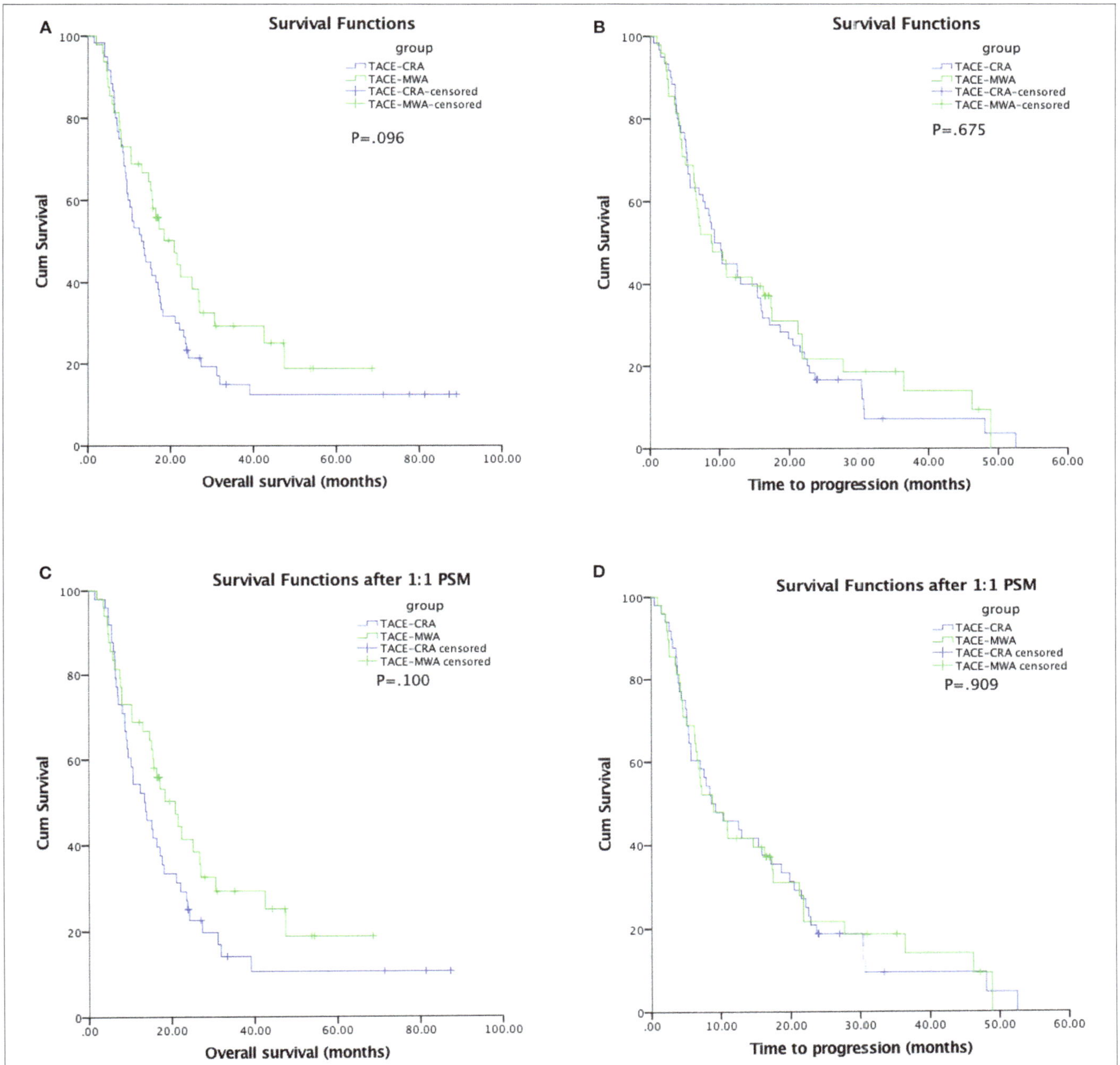

FIGURE 2 | (A) Kaplan-Meier curves of overall survival (OS) in patients with hepatocellular carcinoma treated with TACE-MWA (n = 48; median OS, 20.9 months) and TACE-CRA (n = 60; median OS, 13.0 months; P = 0.096). **(B)** Kaplan-Meier curves of time to progression (TTP) in patients with hepatocellular carcinoma treated with TACE-MWA (n = 48; median TTP, 8.8 months) and TACE-CRA (n = 60; median TTP, 9.3 months; P = 0.675). **(C)** Kaplan-Meier curves of overall survival (OS) in patients with hepatocellular carcinoma treated with TACE-MWA (n = 48; median OS, 20.9 months) and TACE-CRA (n = 48; median OS, 13.5 months; P = 0.100). **(D)** Kaplan-Meier curves of time to progression (TTP) in patients with hepatocellular carcinoma treated with TACE-MWA (n = 48; median TTP, 8.8 months) and TACE-CRA (n = 48; median TTP, 8.6 months; P = 0.909).

treatment was significantly better than that of TACE or CRA alone, and no major complications occurred.

In previous studies, some scholars believed that CRA reduced local tumor progression (35) and was suitable for patients with large intrahepatic tumor diameter (29, 33). The maximum diameter of intrahepatic tumors in the TACE-CRA group was larger than that in the TACE-MWA group. Although there was no significant difference, the diameter of tumor was still closely related to survival time (12). Additionally, there was no statistically significant difference in ORR between the two groups;

TABLE 4 | Univariate and multivariate analysis of predictors of OS.

Factor	Univariate analysis		Multivariate analysis	
	HR	*P*-value	HR	*P*-value
Group (TACE-CRA vs. TACE-MWA)	0.688 (0.442, 1.072)	0.099	...	...
Sex (male vs. female)	1.356 (0.625, 2.944)	0.441	...	...
Age (>60 vs. ≤60 y)	0.631 (0.400, 0.997)	0.049	0.928 (0.521, 1.653)	0.801
ECOG (1 vs. 0)	1.018 (0.661, 1.567)	0.937	...	...
HBsAg (positivity vs. negativity)	0.937 (0.451, 1.944)	0.861	...	...
Cirrhosis (Presence vs. absence)	1.458 (0.928, 2.291)	0.102	...	...
Ascites (Presence vs. absence)	2.132 (1.277, 3.559)	0.004	1.414 (0.751, 2.662)	0.283
PVTT (Presence vs. absence)	2.449 (1.584, 3.785)	0.000	1.928 (1.113, 3.282)	0.016
Maximum diameter of intrahepatic tumor (>10 vs. ≤10 cm)	2.414 (1.513, 3.851)	0.000	2.020 (1.225, 3.331)	0.006
Tumor growth pattern (infiltrative vs. with capsule)	1.634 (1.026, 2.602)	0.039	11.259 (0.748, 2.120)	0.386
No. classification of intrahepatic tumor (multiple vs. solitary)	0.638 (0.389, 1.048)	0.076	...	...
α-Fetoprotein (> 400 vs. ≤ 400 ng/ml)	1.994 (1.291, 3.081)	0.002	1.602 (0.988, 2.599)	0.056

TABLE 5 | Univariate and multivariate analysis of predictors of TTP.

Factor	Univariate analysis		Multivariate analysis	
	HR	*P*-value	HR	*P*-value
Group (TACE-CRA vs. TACE-MWA)	0.916 (0.606, 1.383)	0.676	0.948 (0.606, 1.483)	0.815
Sex (male vs. female)	1.228 (0.615, 2.456)	0.560	...	...
Age (> 60 vs. ≤ 60 y)	0.733 (0.477, 1.126)	0.156	...	...
ECOG (1 vs. 0)	1.306 (0.864, 1.974)	0.205	...	...
HBsAg (positivity vs. negativity)	0.660 (0.341, 1.280)	0.219	...	...
Cirrhosis (Presence vs. absence)	1.454 (0.948, 2.228)	0.086	...	...
Ascites (Presence vs. absence)	2.287 (1.388, 3.769)	0.001	1.431 (0.759, 2.698)	0.268
PVTT (Presence vs. absence)	2.219 (1.465, 3.360)	0.000	1.650 (1.007, 2.704)	0.047
Maximum diameter of intrahepatic tumor (>10 vs. ≤10 cm)	2.551 (1.646, 3.953)	0.000	2.111 (1.308, 3.407)	0.002
Tumor growth pattern (infiltrative vs. with capsule)	1.737 (1.115, 2.706)	0.015	1.418 (0.871, 2.310)	0.160
No. classification of intrahepatic tumor (multiple vs. solitary)	0.727 (0.458, 1.153)	0.176	...	...
α-Fetoprotein (> 400 vs. ≤ 400 ng/ml)	1.717 (1.139, 2.587)	0.010	1.379 (0.851, 2.237)	0.192

however, DCR in the TACE-MWA group was significantly higher than in the TACE-CRA group. Thus, we believe that TACE-MWA can produce a relatively good outcome in selected patients.

We recorded no mortality in either group, similar to a multicenter Italian study showing that microwave ablation is associated with a low rate of major complications (36). The most common complication after ablation in both groups was abdominal pain, which is considered a common symptom of post-ablation syndrome. In the TACE-CRA group, 3 patients (5%) suffered local skin frostbite, which gradually recovered after rewarming. This underscores the importance of protecting adjacent skin during cryoablation. In our center, we used 1–2 sterile rubber gloves filled with warm water to wrap around the ablation needle puncture site to avoid frostbite. One patient who developed an abscess was treated successfully with ultrasound-guided catheterization and drainage of the hepatic abscess, repeated drainage tube flushing, and anti-infection treatment 2 weeks after CRA. After CRA, one patient suffered from hypoproteinemia and a small amount of ascites, which resolved after intensive nutritional support treatment and the infusion of human blood albumin injection. The ascites was attributed to liver dysfunction secondary to the ablation procedure. In the TACE-CRA group, four patients developed serious thrombocytopenia. This is significantly higher than the TACE-MWA group, and in concordance with the results of a previous study (21). However, platelets returned to normal range after platelet-raising therapy, including platelet infusion and recombinant human interleukin-11.

Our study has some limitations. First, it was a single-center, retrospective study, and there was a selection bias. Some patients refused surgery even after discussion with multidisciplinary team, which could have influenced the results of this study. Although we had applied PSM, selection bias was still unavoidable. Second, the number of patients in the two groups was relatively small. Other disadvantages exist in the study design as well. Although there was no significant difference in baseline data between the two groups, some degree of selection bias was unavoidable. Well-designed, multicenter

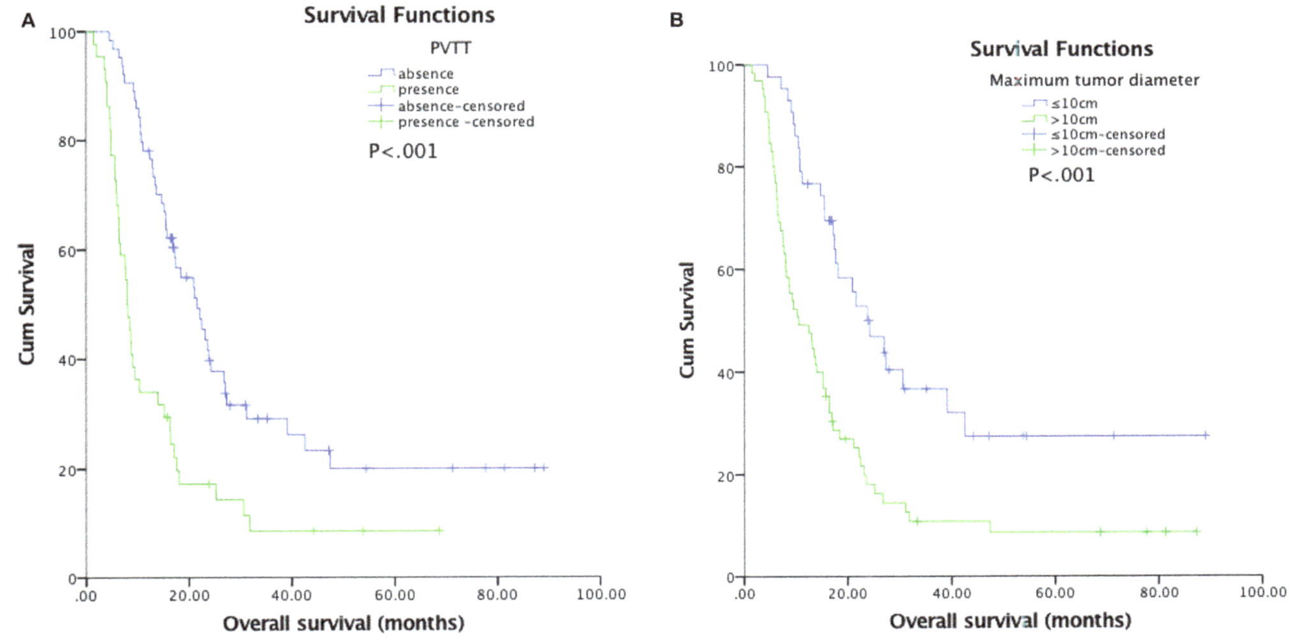

FIGURE 3 | (A) Kaplan-Meier curves of overall survival (OS) in patients with hepatocellular carcinoma with presence of PVTT ($n = 44$; median OS, 8.0 months) and absence of PVTT ($n = 64$; median OS, 21.6 months; $P < 0.001$). However, multivariable analysis showed that the difference had significant between the two groups ($P = 0.016$). **(B)** Kaplan-Meier curves of overall survival (OS) in patients with hepatocellular carcinoma with a maximum tumor diameter ≤10 cm ($n = 43$; median OS, 24.3 months) or >10 cm ($n = 65$; median OS, 10.6 months; $P < 0.001$). However, multivariable analysis showed that the difference had significant between the two groups ($P = 0.006$).

randomized controlled trials are needed to determine the long-term safety and effects of TACE-MWA and TACE-CRA in treating HCC patients that are deemed unresectable at the time of initial diagnosis.

In conclusion, TACE-MWA and TACE-CRA appear to have equal efficacy in the treatment of unresectable HCC, with TACE-MWA having the added benefit of causing fewer complications in selected patients.

AUTHOR CONTRIBUTIONS

JL and WC: study conception and design. JW, WC, and WF: data collection and data analysis and interpretation. JW, WC, YW, and WF: manuscript writing and manuscript revise. All authors: manuscript review and final approval of manuscript.

REFERENCES

1. Villanueva A, Longo DL. Hepatocellular carcinoma. *N Engl J Med.* (2019) 380:1450–62. doi: 10.1056/NEJMra1713263
2. Yang JD, Hainaut P, Gores GJ, Amadou A, Plymoth A, Roberts LR. A global view of hepatocellular carcinoma: trends, risk, prevention and management. *Nat Rev Gastroenterol Hepatol.* (2019) 16:589–604. doi: 10.1038/s41575-019-0186-y
3. European Association for the Study of the Liver. Electronic address eee, European Association for the Study of the L. EASL clinical practice guidelines: management of hepatocellular carcinoma. *J Hepatol.* (2018) 69:182–236. doi: 10.1016/j.jhep.2018.03.019
4. Zhou B, Yan Z, Liu R, Shi P, Qian S, Qu X, et al. Prospective study of transcatheter arterial chemoembolization (Tace) with ginsenoside rg3 versus Tace alone for the treatment of patients with advanced hepatocellular carcinoma. *Radiology.* (2016) 280:630–9. doi: 10.1148/radiol.2016150719
5. Sciarra A, Ronot M, Di Tommaso L, Raschioni C, Castera L, Belghiti J, et al. TRIP: a pathological score for transarterial chemoembolization resistance individualized prediction in hepatocellular carcinoma. *Liver Int.* (2015) 35:2466–73. doi: 10.1111/liv.12844
6. Shimose S, Tanaka M, Iwamoto H, Niizeki T, Shirono T, Aino H, et al. Prognostic impact of transcatheter arterial chemoembolization (TACE) combined with radiofrequency ablation in patients with unresectable hepatocellular carcinoma: comparison with TACE alone using decision-tree analysis after propensity score matching. *Hepatol Res.* (2019) 49:919–28. doi: 10.1111/hepr.13348
7. Ren B, Wang W, Shen J, Li W, Ni C, Zhu X. Transarterial chemoembolization (TACE) combined with sorafenib versus TACE alone for unresectable hepatocellular carcinoma: a propensity score matching study. *J Cancer.* (2019) 10:1189–96. doi: 10.7150/jca.28994
8. Zheng L, Li HL, Guo CY, Luo SX. Comparison of the efficacy and prognostic factors of transarterial chemoembolization plus microwave ablation versus transarterial chemoembolization alone in patients with a large solitary or multinodular hepatocellular carcinomas. *Korean J Radiol.* (2018) 19:237–46. doi: 10.3348/kjr.2018.19.2.237

9. Li W, Ni CF. Current status of the combination therapy of transarterial chemoembolization and local ablation for hepatocellular carcinoma. *Abdom Radiol.* (2019) 44:2268–75. doi: 10.1007/s00261-019-01943-2
10. Zhang L, Hu P, Chen X, Bie P. Transarterial chemoembolization (TACE) plus sorafenib versus TACE for intermediate or advanced stage hepatocellular carcinoma: a meta-analysis. *PLoS ONE.* (2014) 9:e100305. doi: 10.1371/journal.pone.0100305
11. Lei Zhang NW, Shen Q, Cheng W, Qian G-J. Therapeutic efficacy of percutaneous radiofrequency ablation versus microwave ablation for hepatocellular carcinoma. *PLoS ONE.* (2013) 8:e76119. doi: 10.1371/journal.pone.0076119
12. Cui W, Fan W, Huang K, Wang Y, Lu M, Yao W, et al. Large hepatocellular carcinomas: treatment with transarterial chemoembolization alone or in combination with percutaneous cryoablation. *Int J Hyperthermia.* (2018) 35:239–45. doi: 10.1080/02656736.2018.1493235
13. Xu J, Noda C, Erickson A, Mokkarala M, Charalel R, Ramaswamy R, et al. Radiofrequency ablation vs. cryoablation for localized hepatocellular carcinoma: a propensity-matched population study. *Anticancer Res.* (2018) 38:6381–6. doi: 10.21873/anticanres.12997
14. Hyun D, Cho SK, Shin SW, Park KB, Park HS, Choo SW, et al. Early stage hepatocellular carcinomas not feasible for ultrasound-guided radiofrequency ablation: comparison of transarterial chemoembolization alone and combined therapy with transarterial chemoembolization and radiofrequency ablation. *Cardiovasc Intervent Radiol.* (2016) 39:417–25. doi: 10.1007/s00270-015-1194-0
15. Tanaka M, Ando E, Simose S, Hori M, Kuraoka K, Ohno M, et al. Radiofrequency ablation combined with transarterial chemoembolization for intermediate hepatocellular carcinoma. *Hepatol Res.* (2014) 44:194–200. doi: 10.1111/hepr.12100
16. Yuan W, Yang MJ, Xu J, Yan ZP, Liu R, Qu XD, et al. Radiofrequency ablation combined with transarterial chemoembolization for specially located small hepatocellular carcinoma. *Technol Cancer Res Treat.* (2018) 17:1533033818788529. doi: 10.1177/1533033818788529
17. Caroline J. Simon DED, William W. Mayo-Smith. microwave ablation: principles and applications. *RadioGraphics.* (2005) 25:S69–83. doi: 10.1148/rg.25si055501
18. Poulou LS, Botsa E, Thanou I, Ziakas PD, Thanos L. Percutaneous microwave ablation vs. radiofrequency ablation in the treatment of hepatocellular carcinoma. *World J Hepatol.* (2015) 7:1054–63. doi: 10.4254/wjh.v7.i8.1054
19. Abdelaziz A, Elbaz T, Shousha HI, Mahmoud S, Ibrahim M, Abdelmaksoud A, et al. Efficacy and survival analysis of percutaneous radiofrequency versus microwave ablation for hepatocellular carcinoma: an egyptian multidisciplinary clinic experience. *Surg Endosc.* (2014) 28:3429–34. doi: 10.1007/s00464-014-3617-4
20. Nault JC, Sutter O, Nahon P, Ganne-Carrie N, Seror O. Percutaneous treatment of hepatocellular carcinoma: state of the art and innovations. *J Hepatol.* (2018) 68:783–97. doi: 10.1016/j.jhep.2017.10.004
21. Wu S, Hou J, Ding Y, Wu F, Hu Y, Jiang Q, et al. Cryoablation versus radiofrequency ablation for hepatic malignancies: a systematic review and literature-based analysis. *Medicine.* (2015) 94:e2252. doi: 10.1097/MD.0000000000002252
22. Heimbach JK, Kulik LM, Finn RS, Sirlin CB, Abecassis MM, Roberts LR, et al. AASLD guidelines for the treatment of hepatocellular carcinoma. *Hepatology.* (2018) 67:358–80. doi: 10.1002/hep.29086
23. Zhang Y, Huang G, Wang Y, Liang L, Peng B, Fan W, et al. Is salvage liver resection necessary for initially unresectable hepatocellular carcinoma patients downstaged by transarterial chemoembolization? Ten years of experience. *Oncologist.* (2016) 21:1–8. doi: 10.1634/theoncologist.2016-0094
24. Zhang Y, Fan W, Wang Y, Lu L, Fu S, Yang J, et al. Sorafenib with and without transarterial chemoembolization for advanced hepatocellular carcinoma with main portal vein tumor thrombosis: a retrospective analysis. *Oncologist.* (2015) 20:1417–24. doi: 10.1634/theoncologist.2015-0196
25. Song KD. Percutaneous cryoablation for hepatocellular carcinoma. *Clin Mol Hepatol.* (2016) 22:509–15. doi: 10.3350/cmh.2016.0079
26. Lencioni R, Llovet J. Modified RECIST (mRECIST) assessment for hepatocellular carcinoma. *Semin Liver Dis.* (2010) 30:52–60. doi: 10.1055/s-0030-1247132
27. Sacks D, McClenny TE, Cardella JF, Lewis CA. Society of interventional radiology clinical practice guidelines. *J Vasc Interv Radiol.* (2003) 14(9 Pt 2):S199–202. doi: 10.1097/01.RVI.0000094584.83406.3e
28. Takuma Y, Takabatake H, Morimoto Y, Toshikuni N, Kayahara T, Makino Y, et al. comparison of combined Transcatheter arterial chemoembolization and radiofrequency ablation with surgical resection by using propensity score matching in patients with hepatocellular carcinoma within Milan criteria. *Radiology.* (2013) 269:927–37. doi: 10.1148/radiol.13130387
29. Wang C, Wang H, Yang W, Hu K, Xie H, Hu KQ, et al. Multicenter randomized controlled trial of percutaneous cryoablation versus radiofrequency ablation in hepatocellular carcinoma. *Hepatology.* (2015) 61:1579–90. doi: 10.1002/hep.27548
30. Shibata T, Shibata T, Maetani Y, Isoda H, Hiraoka M. Radiofrequency ablation for small hepatocellular carcinoma: prospective comparison of internally cooled electrode and expandable electrode. *Radiology.* (2006) 238:346–53. doi: 10.1148/radiol.2381041848
31. Ginsburg M, Zivin SP, Wroblewski K, Doshi T, Vasnani RJ, Van Ha TG. Comparison of combination therapies in the management of hepatocellular carcinoma: transarterial chemoembolization with radiofrequency ablation versus microwave ablation. *J Vasc Interv Radiol.* (2015) 26:330–41. doi: 10.1016/j.jvir.2014.10.047
32. Ni JY, Sun HL, Chen YT, Luo JH, Chen D, Jiang XY, et al. Prognostic factors for survival after transarterial chemoembolization combined with microwave ablation for hepatocellular carcinoma. *World J Gastroenterol.* (2016) 20:17483–90. doi: 10.3748/wjg.v20.i46.17483
33. Xu KC, Niu LZ, Zhou Q, Hu YZ, Guo DH, Liu ZP, et al. Sequential use of transarterial chemoembolization and percutaneous cryosurgery for hepatocellular carcinoma. *World J Gastroenterol.* (2009) 15:3664–9. doi: 10.3748/wjg.15.3664
34. Huang C, Zhuang W, Feng H, Guo H, Tang Y, Chen H, et al. Analysis of therapeutic effectiveness and prognostic factor on argon-helium cryoablation combined with transcatheter arterial chemoembolization for treatment of advanced of advanced hepatocellular carcinoma. *J Cancer Res Ther.* (2016) 12:148–52. doi: 10.4103/0973-1482.200605
35. Rong G, Bai W, Dong Z, Wang C, Lu Y, Zeng Z, et al. Long-term outcomes of percutaneous cryoablation for patients with hepatocellular carcinoma within Milan criteria. *PLoS ONE.* (2015) 10:e0123065. doi: 10.1371/journal.pone.0123065
36. Livraghi T, Meloni F, Solbiati L, Zanus G. Complications of microwave ablation for liver tumors: results of a multicenter study. *Cardiovasc Intervent Radiol.* (2011) 35:868–74. doi: 10.1007/s00270-011-0241-8

11

Importance of Microvascular Invasion Risk and Tumor Size on Recurrence and Survival of Hepatocellular Carcinoma After Anatomical Resection and Non-Anatomical Resection

Haoyu Hu[1], Shuo Qi[1], Silue Zeng[1], Peng Zhang[1], Linyun He[1], Sai Wen[1], Ning Zeng[1,2], Jian Yang[1,2], Weiqi Zhang[1], Wen Zhu[1,2], Nan Xiang[1,2] and Chihua Fang[1,2]*

[1] Department of Hepatobiliary Surgery, Zhujiang Hospital, Southern Medical University, Guangzhou, China, [2] Guangdong Provincial Clinical and Engineering Center of Digital Medicine, Guangzhou, China

***Correspondence:**
Chihua Fang
fangch_dr@163.com

Purpose: To establish a valid prediction model to prognose the occurrence of microvascular invasion (MVI), and to compare the efficacy of anatomic resection (AR) or non-anatomic resection (NAR) for hepatocellular carcinoma (HCC).

Methods: Two hundred twenty-eight patients with HCC who underwent surgical treatment were enrolled. Their hematological indicators, MRI imaging features, and outcome data were acquired.

Result: In the multivariable analysis, alpha-fetoprotein >15 ng/mL, neutrophil to lymphocyte ratio >3.8, corona enhancement, and pertumoral hypointensity on hepatobiliary phase were associated with MVI. According on these factors, the AUROC of the predictive model in the primary and validation cohorts was 0.884 (95% CI: 0.829, 0.938) and 0.899 (95% CI: 0.821, 0.967), respectively. Patients with high risk of MVI or those with low risk of MVI but tumor size >5 cm in the AR group were associated with a lower rate of recurrence and death than patients in the NAR group; however, when patients are in the state of low-risk MVI with tumor size >5 cm, there is no difference in the rate of recurrence and death between AR and NAR.

Conclusion: Our predictive model for HCC with MVI is convenient and accurate. Patients with high-risk of MVI or low-risk of MVI but tumor size >5 cm executing AR is of great necessity.

Keywords: hepatocellular carcinoma, microvascular invasion, prediction model, tumor size, hepatectomy

KEY POINTS

- We have developed a convenient and accurate predictive-model by combining hematological indicators with imaging features.
- It can assist surgeons choose the optimized surgical approach.
- Then it would eventually help to improve the recurrence-free and long-term survival rate of patients.

INTRODUCTION

Vascular invasion of hepatocellular carcinoma (HCC) include macrovascular invasion and microvascular invasion in pathology, both of which are predictors of poor prognosis after surgical resection or liver transplantation (1, 2). The 5-year recurrence rate of HCC patients with microvascular invasion after radical hepatic resection is reportedly as high as 70%, and tumor recurrence rate exceeds 35% even after liver transplantation (3, 4).

Though preoperative radiological techniques such as CT and MRI are feasible to detect macrovascular invasion (5), recording the presence of microvascular invasion (MVI) is still challenging since it requires histopathological examination of surgically resected specimen (6). Early prediction of MVI in hepatocellular carcinoma remains elusive. Studies have shown that microvascular violation of state can be reflected by specific clinical hematological indicators, such as des-gamma-carboxyprothrombin (PIVKA-II), alpha-fetoprotein (AFP), and peripheral neutrophil to lymphocyte ratio (NLR) (7, 8); also, it can be predicted by tumor size, multiple tumor nodules, tumor rough edges, incomplete capsule, and nuclear magnetic resonance arterial peritumoral enhancement imaging characteristics and changes in peritumoral hepatobiliary specific density of microvessels (9–12). Currently, Radiomics is the most popular method for microvascular invasion assessment and prediction (13). Despite the potential of Radiomics to guide clinical decision making, there is a lack of standardized evaluation toward numerous published Radiomics studies; moreover, Radiomics necessitates interdisciplinary cooperation. These two factors are the reason why Radiomics is difficult to be implemented in many hospitals. Therefore, a simple and effective method capable of predicting the incidence of MVI prior to surgery is urgently needed to improve prognosis after radical resection in patients with HCC.

Additionally, it has been reported that anatomical resection (AR) of the liver can be useful in isolating microvascular metastases while removing lesions (14, 15). However, multicenter retrospective studies revealed no significant difference between AR and non-anatomical resection (NAR) in terms of tumor-free survival and long-term survival post-operatively (16). In the current study, we aim to establish a valid prediction model to prognose the occurrence of microvascular invasion, and apply this model to compare the efficacy of AR or NAR in the treatment of patients retrospectively.

PATIENTS AND METHODS

In this study, 228 patients with HCC who underwent surgical treatment at Zhujiang Hospital, Southern Medical University, from January 2012 to June 2018 were enrolled by the following criteria. Inclusion criteria: (1) pathological diagnosis of HCC; (2) hematological indicators processed within 15 days before surgery, including complete blood count, alpha-fetoprotein (AFP) and imaging examinations; (3) Child-Pugh classification of liver function as A; (4) surgery performed under the guidance of 3D reconstructed images; exclusion criteria: (1) palliative tumor resection; (2) primary angiographic diagnosis of cancerous thrombosis; (3) patients who received preoperative radiotherapy, chemotherapy, TACE, or targeted therapy as the initial treatment such as sorafenib, anti-PD-1/PDL-1; (4) follow-up time <12 months. Finally, a total of 228 patients were included in the study. The patients were divided into two independent cohorts at a ratio of 7:3 using a random number table. One hundred sixty patients constituted the training cohort and the remaining 68 formed the validation cohort. Ethics committee approval was approved by the Institutional Ethics Review Board of Zhujiang Hospital, Southern Medical University (ethics number:2018-GDYK-001), and clinical data of the above patients were collected and analyzed retrospectively.

Data Acquisition

1) Hematological indicators: complete blood count, liver function, AFP, HBV, and HCV antigen/antibody, and HBV deoxyribonucleic acid (HBV-DNA).
2) Imaging examination: MRI was performed with the patient relaxed in a supine position. The positioning image adopts breath-hold fast spoiled gradient echo sequences and fast imaging employing steady-state acquisition (FIESTA) on the coronal plane. The magnetic resonance spectrum (MRS) scan uses a single-element spot-resolved spectrum sequence, and the scanning time is about 1 min. For gadoxetic acid (Primovist or Eovist; Bayer Schering Pharma, Berlin, Germany)-enhanced MRI, the following images were obtained using a fat-suppressed 3-dimensional gradient-echo T1-weighted sequence (volumetric interpolated breath-hold examination, Siemens or T1 high-resolution isotropic volume examination, Philips): arterial phase (20–35 s), portal phase (60 s), delayed phase (3 min), and hepatobiliary phase (HBP) (20 min). The scanning delay time for arterial phase imaging was determined using MR fluoroscopic monitoring.

Analysis of Hematological Indicators

NLR is the ratio of neutrophil count to lymphocyte count. The obtained hematological index is established with the ROC curve of pathological MVI information. If the area under the curve (AUC) $\geqq$0.6, the cutoff value corresponding to the Youden index is obtained, and the variables are classified into two categories; if the AUC <0.6, the classification criteria for each hematological index are determined through the literature report.

Analysis of Imaging Data

Preoperative MR images were retrospectively evaluated using a Picture Archiving and Communication System (PACS; Pathspeed, GE Medical Systems Integrated Imaging Solutions, Mt. Prospect, IL, USA). Image analysis was performed by two abdominal radiologists (Li Xinming and Lin Huan, with 7 and 6 years of experience in hepatic MRI, respectively) who were unaware of information on clinical, laboratory, pathologic, and follow-up results. The two reviewers evaluated

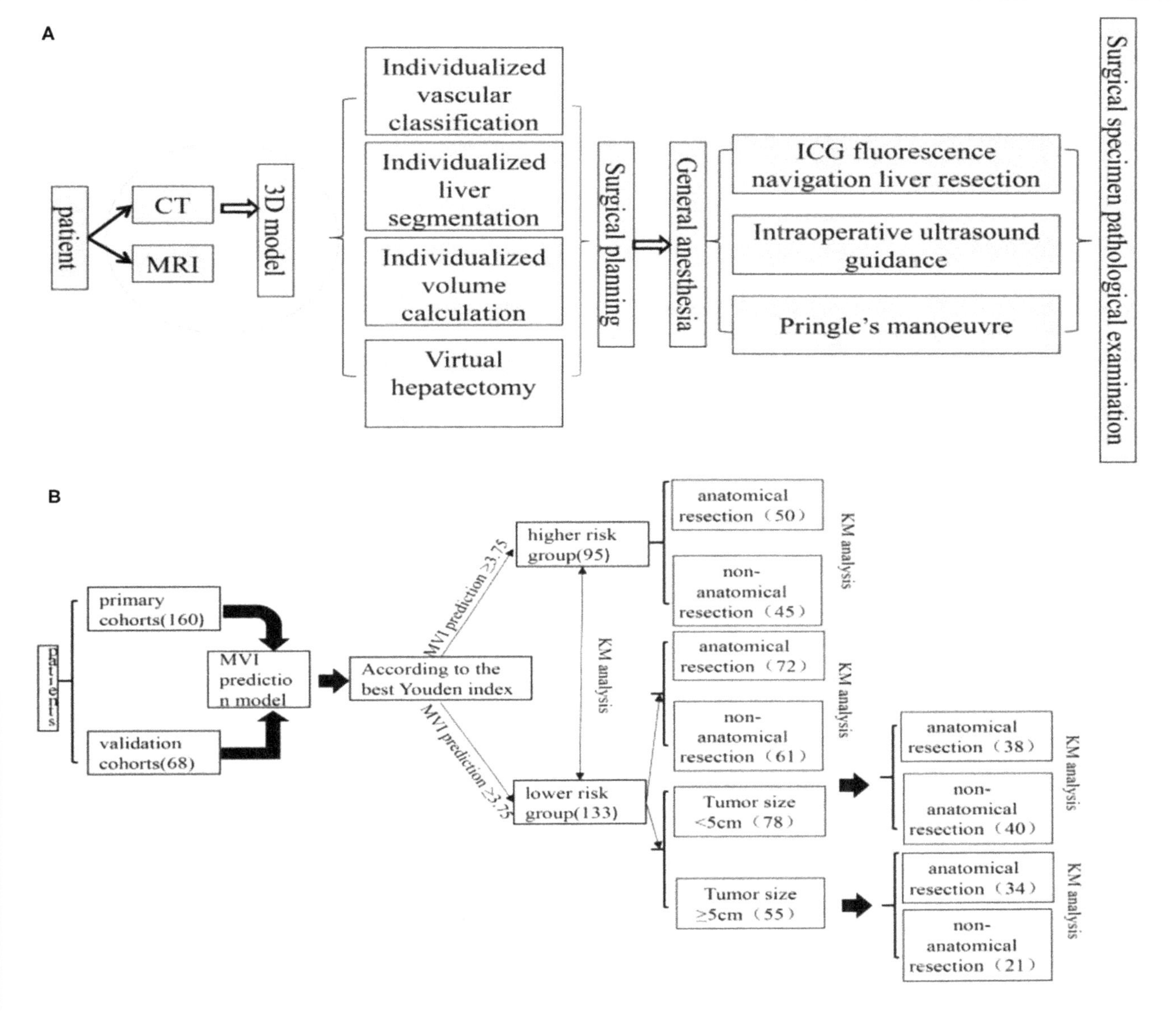

FIGURE 1 | Surgical planning and procedure **(A)** and flow chart of manuscript design **(B)**. KM, Kaplan-Meier.

the following imaging features for each HCC independently: (a) arterial rim enhancement (17), means in the arterial phase existing irregularity like enhancement with relatively hypovascular central areas; (b) corona enhancement (C E) (18), known as the transient enhancement of the perilesional parenchyma. The enhancement of the perilesional parenchyma fades in the portal venous phase and is resolved by the 3-min delayed phase; (c) radiological capsule (18), defined as a peripheral rim of smooth hyperenhancement in the portal venous or delayed phase; (d) tumor margin (19), categorized as non-smooth margin, showing as non-nodular tumors with an out-of-shape margin that had the edge-peaked distribution, or smooth margin, showing as nodular tumors with smooth outline in the HBP images; (e) tumor hypointensity on HBP (20), means comparing with the surrounding liver, the tumor shows lower signal intensity on HBP; (f) peritumoral hypointensity on HBP(HY-HBP) (21), defined as wedge-shaped or flame-like hypointense area of hepatic parenchyma located outside of the tumor margin on HBP.

Surgical Planning and Procedure

All patients completed a three-dimensional visualization analysis before surgery (22). The procedure of surgical planning is shown in **Figure 1A**. Most resections were intended to be anatomic according to the vascular topological relationship. However, in a few patients with peripheral lesions and portal hypertension or suboptimal liver function, partial resection including the tumor and an intended 1–2 cm margin were performed.

Pathological Analysis

All surgical specimens were examined by two pathologists to detect the presence of MVI. The histologic parameters ordinarily included pathological grade, size, number, surgical margin, and MVI status of the resected tumor were based on the practice guidelines for the pathological diagnosis of primary liver cancer: 2015 update (23). MVI was defined as the presence of a tumor in a microportal vein, microhepatic vein, or a capsular vessel of the surrounding liver tissue lined by the endothelium that was visible only on microscopy.

Follow-Up

Follow-up examinations were conducted 1 month after surgery and then every 2–3 months using laboratory findings (complete blood count, serum AFP, and liver function). Abdominal ultrasonography and contrast-enhanced CT or MR were performed every 3 months. The patients were followed-up once every 3–4 months post-operatively until death or dropout from the follow-up program. A diagnosis of recurrence of HCC was based on CT and/or MRI and elevated serum a-fetoprotein (AFP) levels. Most of the patients were observed according to the recommendation guidelines for diagnosis and management of liver diseases by the Chinese "Guidelines for the Diagnosis and Treatment of Primary Hepatocellular Carcinoma (2017 edition)."

Statistical Analysis

Univariate logistic regression analyses were performed to determine factors with MVI risk; multivariate analyses with an adjusted odds-ratio (OR) regression model were conducted to construct the MVI risk model from multi-scale hematological indicators and Radiomic signatures. The candidate clinical variables were sex, age, history of hepatic virus infection (0, negative; 1, history of HBV, HBV + HCVB), history of cirrhosis (0, absent; 1, present), AST (0, ≦34 U/L; 1, >34 U/L), ALT (0, ≦40 U/L; 1, >40 U/L), PT (0, ≦13 s, 1, >13 s), TBil (0, ≥35 g/L, 1 <35 g/L), AFP (0, ≦15 ng/mL; 1, >15 ng/mL), NLR (0, ≦3.8; 1, >3.8), Tumor size (0, ≤5 cm; 1 >5 cm). Radiologic features included arterial rim enhancement, arterial peritumoral enhancement, tumor margin, radiological capsule, tumor hypointensity on HBP, and peritumoral hypointensity on HBP. In order to partition the patients into high- and low-risk MVI groups, the optimal cutoff value for the risk scores was determined via area under the ROC curve (AUROC) analysis using the Youden index.

The rate of HCC recurrence and survival between the AR and NAR groups based on MVI risk in the prediction model was subsequently compared. In subgroup analysis, this rate in the two groups was assessed based on high risk of MVI based on the prediction model. Also, In the MVI low-risk group, the tumor diameter of 5 cm was used as the cut-off point to compare the survival difference between AR and NAR flow of manuscript design showed in **Figure 1B**. All statistical analyses were performed using SPSS version 25.0 (SPSS Inc., Chicago, IL, USA). The level of statistical significance was set at $P < 0.05$.

TABLE 1 | Baseline characteristics of study patients.

Variable	Primary cohort	Validation cohort	*P*-value
Age(Mean ± SD, years)	50.74 ± 11.58	51.25 ± 12.08	0.766
M/F ratio	129/31	51/17	0.341
History of hepatic virus infection			0.148
Yes/No	128/32	41/17	
Liver cirrhosis			0.549
Presence/Absence	76/84	35/33	
AFP level (median, Q, ng/mL)	24.50 (4.15, 332.00)	4.710 (2.388, 54.69)	0.059
NLR level (median, Q)	2.46 (1.64, 5.74)	2.92 (1.93, 4.98)	0.259
ALT (Mean ± SD, U/L)	43.42 ± 37.88	39.43 ± 38.79	0.471
AST (median, Q, U/L)	35 (24, 45)	27 (21, 47)	0.122
TBil (median, Q, μmol/L)	13.77 ± 3.53	16.87 ± 1.98	0.911
ALB (Mean ± SD, g/L)	39.50 ± 5.59	38.44 ± 1.91	0.141
PT (Mean ± SD,*10^9)	13.65 ± 1.51	13.78 ± 1.04	0.533
Intraoperative blood loss, (median, Q, mL)	400 (200, 600)	300 (200, 575)	0.255
Anatomical resection			>0.999
Yes/Not	86/74	36/32	
Anatomical lobectomy			0.812
Segment	10	6	
1 lobe	30	12	
2 lobe	45	18	
≥3 lobe	1	0	
Tumor size (Mean ± SD, cm)	5.44 ± 3.17	4.14 ± 2.26	0.076
Satellite nodules	20	11	0.6836
Tumor number			0.603
1/2/3	140/18/2	57/9/2	
Capsule formation			0.149
Presence/Absence	70/90	37/31	
Pathological grade			0.611
Well differentiated	26	8	
Moderately differentiated	111	48	
Poorly differentiated	23	12	
MVI			0.446
Presence/Absence	56/104	20/48	
Arterial rim enhancement			0.197
Presence/Absence	76/84	37/31	
corona enhancement			0.317
Presence/Absence	81/79	37/31	
Tumor margin(rough)			0.229
Presence/Absence	95/65	31/37	
Radiological capsule			0.883
Presence/Absence	90/70	40/28	
Tumor hypointensity on HBP			>0.999
Presence/Absence	141/19	60/8	
Peritumoral hypointensity on HBP			0.148
Presence/Absence	84/76	28/40	

AFP, alpha fetoprotein; NLR, neutrophil to lymphocyte ratio; ALT, alanine aminotransferase; AST, aspartate aminotransferase; PT, prothrombin time; TBil, total bilirubin; ALB, albumin; MVI, microvascular invasion.

TABLE 2 | Univariable and multivariable analysis of preoperative data for presence of microvascular invasion in the primary cohort.

Variable	Univariable analysis		Multivariable analysis	
	OR (95% CI)	*P*-value	OR (95% CI)	*P*-value
History of hepatic virus infection	0.83 (0.39, 1.75)	0.625		
Liver cirrhosis	0.85 (0.54, 1.35)	0.494		
AFP >15 ng/mL	5.15 (2.40, 11.08)	< 0.001	4.30 (1.61, 11.48)	0.002
NLR >3.8	7.44 (3.60, 15.39)	< 0.001	4.21 (1.70, 10.39)	0.002
Platelet count >100 (10^9/L)	1.86 (0.58, 5.99)	0.300		
ALT	1.09 (0.55, 2.13)	0.809		
AST	2.10 (1.07, 4.13)	0.031	1.31 (0.52, 3.32)	0.567
TBil	0.75 (0.25, 2.25)	0.610		
ALB	0.90 (0.47, 1.73)	0.753		
PT	0.87 (0.44, 1.73)	0.70		
Tumor size	1.30 (0.68, 2.50)	0.426		
Arterial rim enhancement	0.46 (0.24, 0.90)	0.02	0.62 (0.25, 1.59)	0.321
Corona enhancement	6.64 (3.12, 14.11)	0.001	5.40 (2 04, 14.30)	< 0.001
Tumor margin	1.37 (0.70, 2.69)	0.354		
Radiological capsule	1.06 (0.55, 2.04)	0.870		
Tumor hypointensity on HBP	1.40 (0.51, 3.85)	0.509		
Peritumoral hypointensity on HBP	7.99 (3.62, 17.64)	< 0.001	8.06 (2 96, 21.93)	< 0.001

HBP, hepatobiliary phase.

TABLE 3 | Multivariable analysis of risk factors of MVI and measurement of the MVI risk score.

Variable	Multivariable analysis		B coefficient	Points
	OR (95% CI)	*P*-value		
AFP >15 ng/mL	4.71 (1.79, 12.39)	0.002	1.55	1.5
NLR >3.8	4.05 (1.68, 9.75)	0.002	1.40	1
corona enhancement	5.96 (2.34, 15.19)	< 0.001	1.78	2
Peritumoral hypointensity on HBP	8.37 (3.12, 22.41)	< 0.001	2.12	2

Multivariable logistic regression model was carried out by using stepwise backward variable selection. The scaled coefficients were simplified by rounding them to nearest half. The MVI risk score is obtained by adding the total number of points scored in each of the 4 variables.

RESULTS

Patient Characteristics

The baseline data of the patients are shown in **Table 1** as the primary cohort and validation cohort. Among the two cohorts, male patients predominate over females. There were no differences between the two cohorts. Also, the size of the tumor in the primary cohort is 5.44 ± 3.17 cm and 4.14 ± 2.26 cm in the validation cohort, which shows no significant difference ($P = 0.076$). Histopathology shows that the number of MVI cases in the two groups is 56 and 20, respectively, with no significant difference.

The six risk factors related to MVI were screened by single factor logistic regression analysis using laboratory hematology examination indicators and typical imaging characteristics, respectively: AFP >15 ng/mL (OR: 5.647, $P < 0.001$), NLR >3.8 (OR: 7.970, $P < 0.001$), AST >34 U/L (OR: 2.724, $P = 0.003$), Arterial rim enhancement (OR: 0.492, $P = 0.03$), corona enhancement (C E, OR: 6.319; $P < 0.001$), peritumoral hypointensity on HBP (PH-HBP, OR: 7.510; $P < 0.001$), as shown in **Table 2**; and AFP >15 ng/mL (OR: 5.411; 95% CI: 2.093, 13.990; $P < 0.001$), NLR >3.8 (OR: 3.977; 95% CI: 1.689, 9.368; $P = 0.002$), C E (OR: 6.183; 95% CI: 2.478, 15.429; $P < 0.001$), PH-HBP (OR: 8.754; 95% CI: 3.355, 22.843; $P < 0.001$; **Table 3**); the MVI prediction model is: MVI risk = 1.5 × AFP + 1 × NLR + 2 × C E + 2 × PH-HBP, obtained by adding the total number of points scored in each of the four independent risk factors. The highest score is 6.5, and the lowest score is 0. Through the multi-factor logistic regression analysis in **Table 3**. A forest plot of independent predictors of MVI with odds-ratio and a nomogram plot for predicting MVI risk (**Figure 2A**) and the above four factors was constructed (**Figure 2B**). In the primary cohort, the AUROC (**Figure 2C**) of the nomogram was 0.887 (95% CI: 0.835, 0.939). In order to distinguish the MVI high-risk group and the low-risk group from the whole sample, we obtained an optimal cutoff value of 3.75.

Model Validation

A calibration analysis of the MVI prediction model showed high coherence between the observed risk and the predicted risk ($P = 0.200$) in the primary cohort (**Figure 3A**) and validation cohort (**Figure 3B**); meanwhile, the AUROC of the model in the

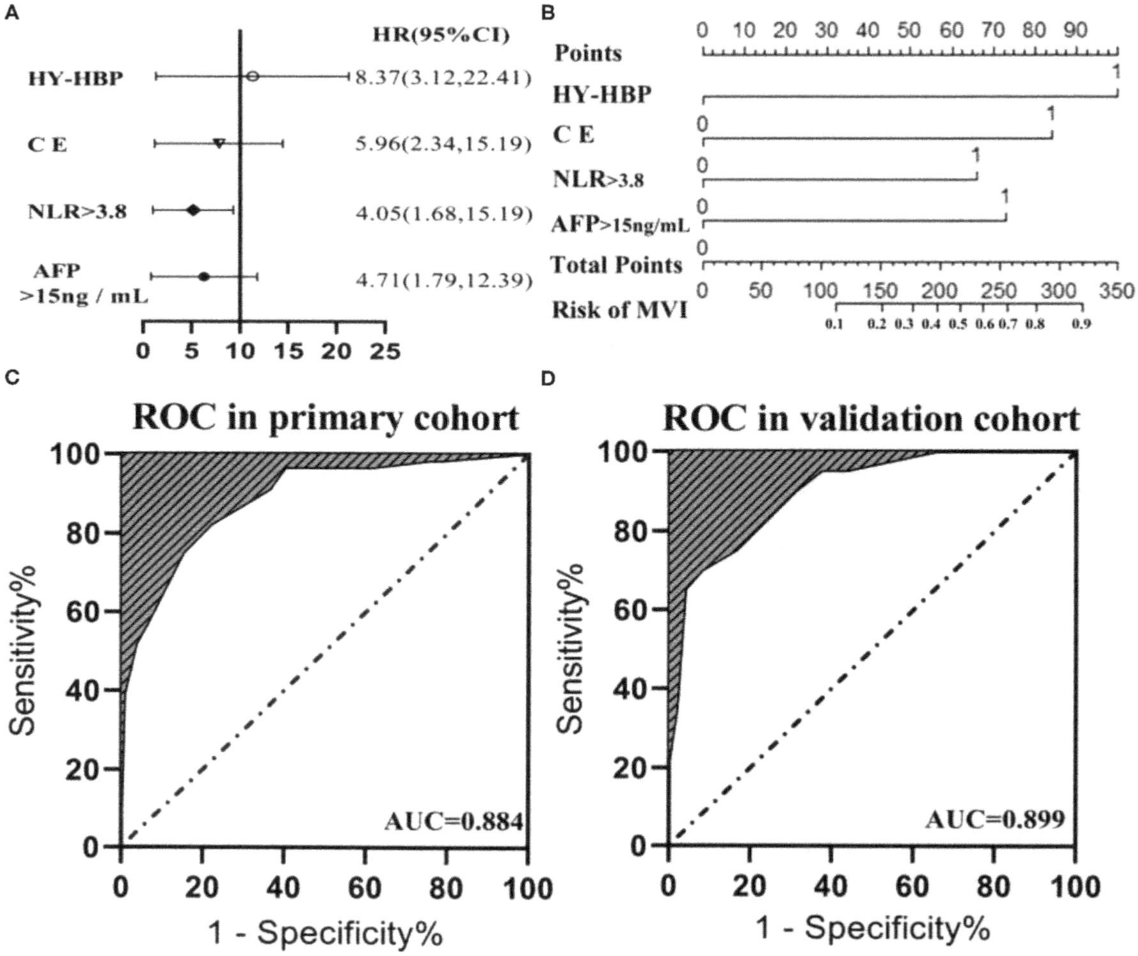

FIGURE 2 | (A) Forest plot of independent predictors of MVI with odds-ratio (OR) multivariate regression model. **(B)** The model presented with a nomogram scaled by the proportional regression coefficient of each risk variables. The area under the receiver operating characteristic curve (AUROC) for the MVI prediction model: **(C)** AUROC was 0.884 in the primary cohorts; **(D)** AUROC was 0.899 in the validation cohorts.

validation cohort (**Figure 2D**) was 0.899 (95% CI: 0.821, 0.967), with the sensitivity of 0.750, the specificity of 0.833, and accuracy of 0.794.while in the primary cohort the average AUROC was 0 884 (95% CI: 0.829, 0.938) and its sensitivity, specificity, and accuracy were 0.824, 0.779, and 0.795, respectively.

Figure 3C presents the decision curve. It shows that if the threshold probability is within a range from 0.01 to 0.92, the use of nomogram model can bring more net benefit than the patient of complete intervention or no intervention at all.

Recurrence and Survival

The primary cohort and the validation cohort were organized into one cohort, and then divided into a MVI high-risk group and a MVI low-risk group by the MVI prediction model. The median recurrence time in the high-risk group was 18 months, and 28 months in the low-risk group. The difference was statistically significant ($P = 0.003$; **Figure 4A**). The 3- and 5-year survival rates of the higher-risk group were 56.09 and 71.59%, respectively, which were significantly lower than the 32.01% and 54.47% of the lower risk group ($p = 0.001$; **Figure 4B**). The 5-year overall recurrence rate of the AR in the high-risk group was 58.00% lower than the 5-year recurrence rate (81.20%) of the NAR (**Figure 4C**). The 3- and 5-year survival rates were significantly better in the group than in the NAR group. Similarly, in the MVI low-risk group, AR was higher than NAR in terms of 3- and 5-year recurrence rate, and survival rate (**Figures 4D–F**). Meanwhile, we obtained similar results of recurrence and survival to those obtained for real MVI treated with AR or NAR (**Supplementary Figure 1**).

In the high-risk group, tumor size was further considered as a risk factor affecting tumor recurrence and long-term survival in patients undergoing anatomical resection (AR)/non-anatomical resection (NAR). When the tumor size was ≦5 cm, the recurrence ($P = 0.039$) rate of the AR group was significantly lower than that of the NAR group (**Supplementary Figure 2A**), while the survival ($P = 0.011$) rate

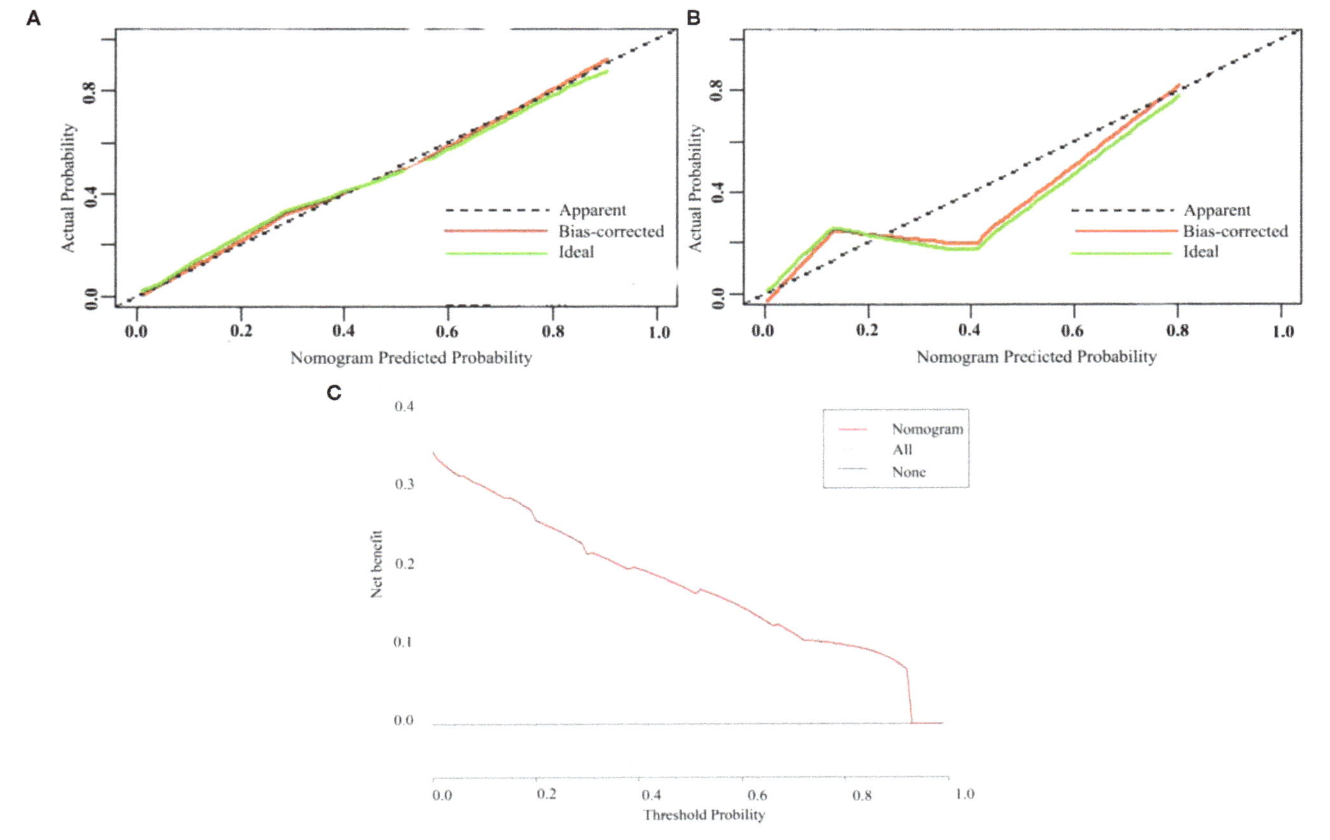

FIGURE 3 | Calibration curve of MVI prediction model in primary cohort **(A)** and validation cohort **(B)**. **(C)** Presents the decision curve for all patients.

of the AR group was significantly higher than that of the NAR group (**Supplementary Figure 2B**). Similarly, when the tumor size reached >5 cm, the recurrence rate and survival rate of the AR group and NAR group were the same as when the tumor size was ≤5 cm (**Supplementary Figures 2D,E**).

However, in the low-risk group, we found that the median recurrence time of patients undergoing AR was 34 months for tumor size ≦5 cm, and 17 months in NAR liver resection. But, there was no significant difference between the two ($P = 0.182$; **Figure 5A**). The median survival time of patients with anatomical hepatectomy and non-anatomical hepatectomy was 36 and 24 months, respectively. Also, there was no significant difference from each other ($P = 0.909$; **Figure 5B**). For patients with tumors size >5 cm, the 5-year recurrence rate of patients undergoing anatomical liver resection was 48.0%, which was significantly lower than 82.8% of patients in NAR ($P < 0.001$; **Figure 5C**). Similarly, the 5-year survival rate of the AR group was also higher than that of the NAR group (73.0 vs. 14.2%; $P < 0.001$; **Figure 5D**).

DISCUSSION

In this work, a predictive model for HCC MVI is established by combining hematological indicators with imaging characteristics. The model includes alpha-fetoprotein, neutrophil-lymphocyte ratio, corona enhancement, and peritumoral hypointensity on HBP images, which is convenient and accurate. Anatomical liver resection is beneficial to the long-term survival of patients with high-risk of MVI. While in the lower risk group, anatomical liver resection for patients with tumors >5 cm in size will be more conducive to long-term survival. For those with a size ≦5 cm, both methods are acceptable.

MVI and AFP have been proved as independent risk factors of early recurrence and poor overall survival after liver cancer liver resection; the correlation between them has been dramatically focused. Furthermore, it also has attracted much scholars' attention to the epidemiological and molecular biological relationship between tumors and inflammation (24–26). The NLR reflects the antagonism of the body against tumors by refiecting the relative changes in neutrophil and lymphocyte counts. A recent study found that NLR >3.0–3.2 is an independent risk factor for MVI (8). Analogously, there was meta-analysis finding that NLR does have a significant correlation with vascular invasion. The analysis of 17 research also found that their NLR cutoff value range is from 1.51 to 5.0 (27). In our study, the cutoff value of NLR is 3.8, which is consistent with those researches.

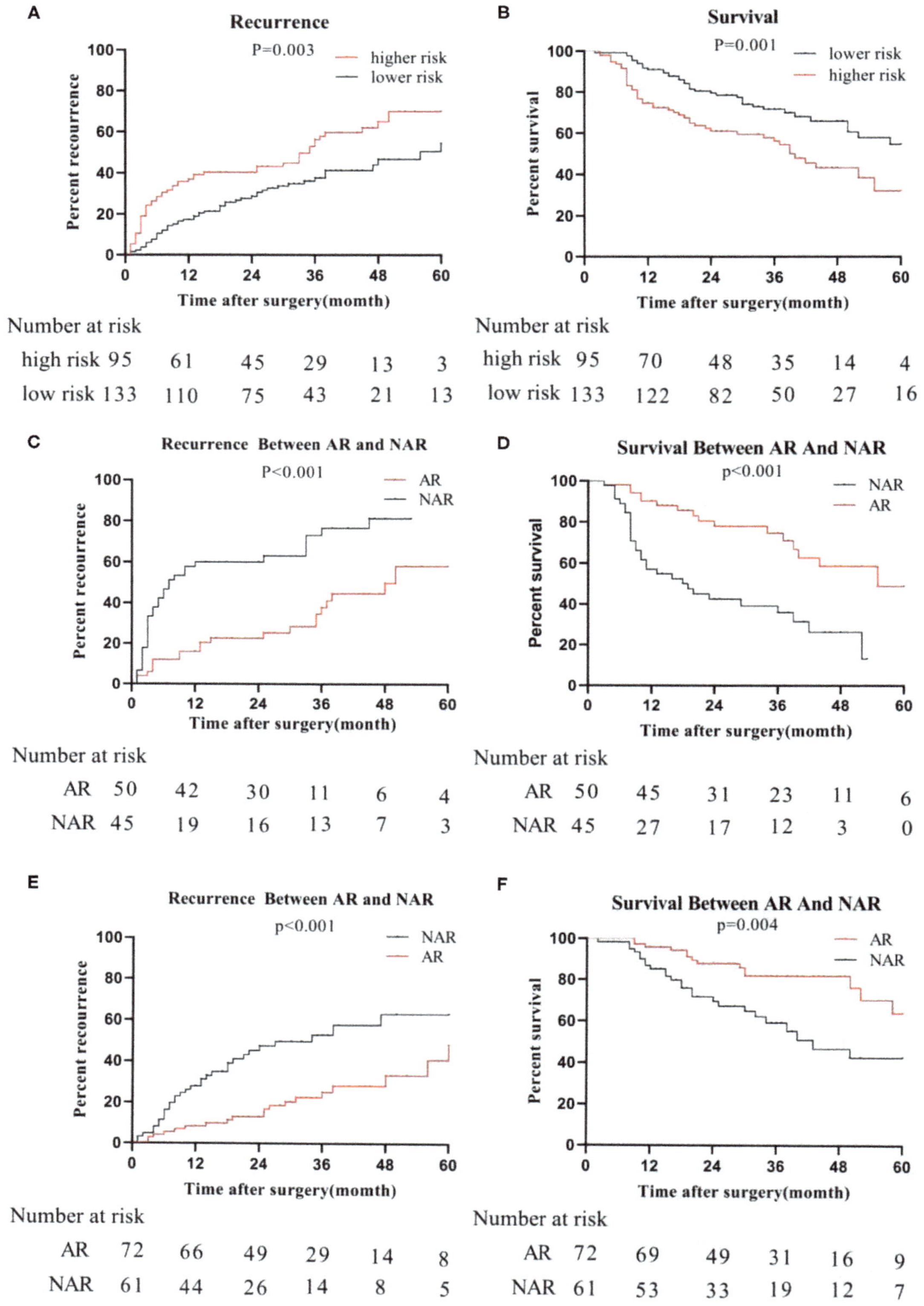

FIGURE 4 | Recurrence and survival of the whole cohort; we organize the primary cohort and the validation cohort into one cohort, recurrence-rate **(A)** and survival-rate **(B)** comparison between higher risk group and lower risk group; in higher risk group, recurrence-rate **(C)** survival -rate **(D)** comparison between AR and NAR; in lower risk group, recurrence-rate **(E)** and survival -rate **(F)** comparison between AR and NAR.

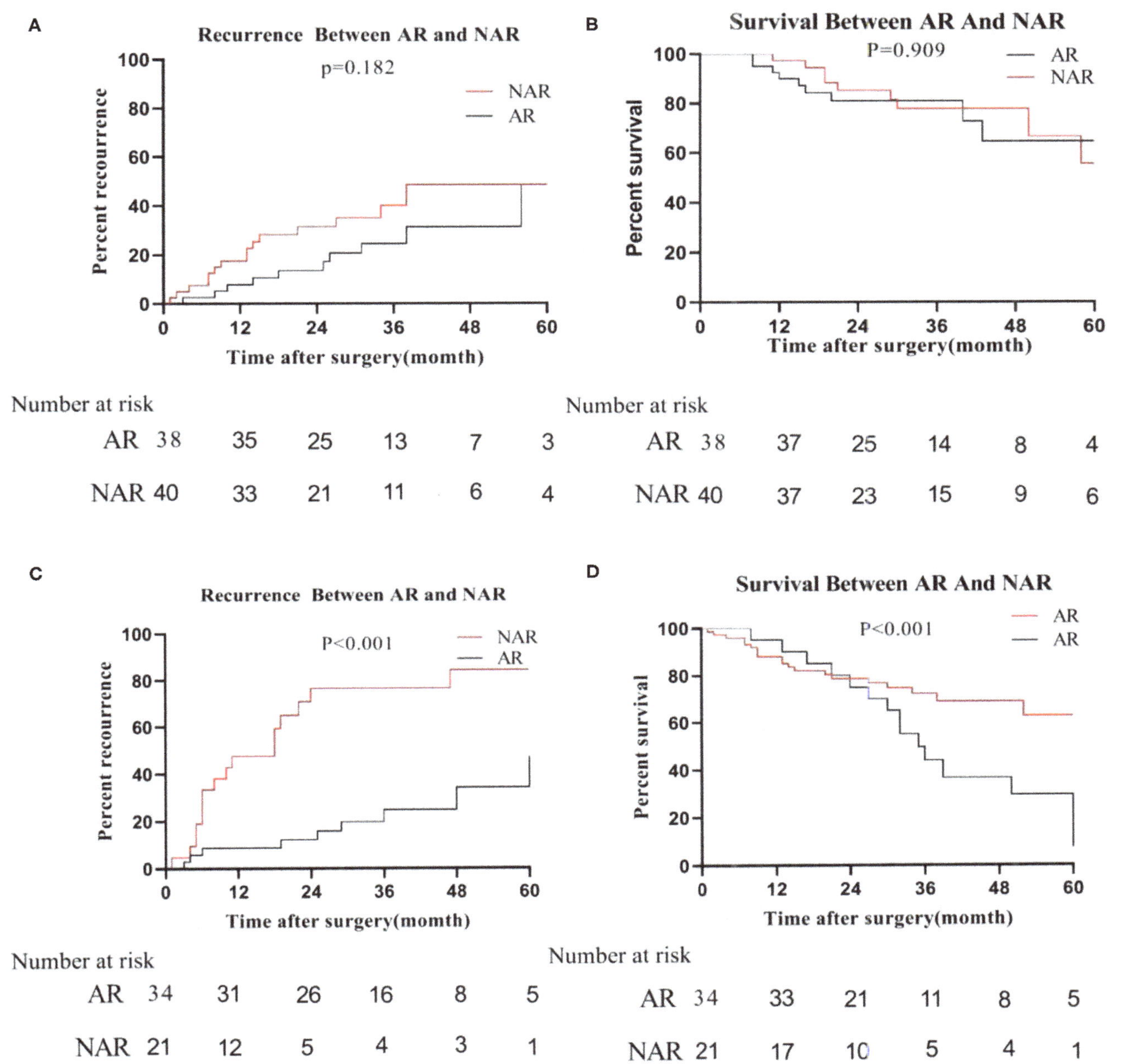

FIGURE 5 | In the low-risk group, recurrence **(A)** and survival **(B)** between AR and NAR when tumor size ≦5 cm; recurrence **(C)** and survival **(D)** between AR and NAR when tumor size >5 cm.

Gadoxetic acid-enhanced MRI scanning could increase the detection rate of micro hepatocellular carcinoma significantly; besides, some studies have discovered that specific characteristics of MRI could be used as typical features of imaging diagnostic MVI, such as incomplete imaging capsule, coronal enhancement in arterial phase, peritumoral hypointensity on HBP images. Lee et al. (28) found that arterial peritumoral enhancement, non-smooth tumor margin, peritumoral hypointensity on HBP were characteristic risk factors that are indicating microvascular invasion of HCC. In this study, significant correlations were found between peritumoral hypointensity on HBP, corona enhancement, and MVI, and this model was included for this purpose.

Early prediction of MVI risk can benefit preoperative individualized treatment plans, which is a consensus among scholars. Xu et al. (13) constructed a predictive MVI model extracted from CT images using Radiomics technology, which obtained satisfactory prediction results (AUC = 0.909). However, the process is complicated since the feature extraction of Radiomics requires algorithms to be developed by science and engineering technicians. It is currently hard to be acknowledged and being put into clinical practice owing to the over-fitting or under-fitting of many algorithms to imaging. Many studies are focusing on the prediction of MVI based on preoperative hematological indicators, but the prediction effect is poor (0.744–0.774) (29). Our prediction model, which integrates hematological indicators with radiology imaging features is concise and operable. Furthermore, it has a higher prediction accuracy than Radiomics and single hematology index prediction models. The AUROC in the test cohort is 0.887, and the AUROC in the verification cohort is 0.938.

The presence of MVI will result in increased early recurrence rates and reduced long-term survival. In this study, all patients were divided into a higher-risk group and a lower-risk group by the Yoden index. The 3- and 5-year survival of the higher-risk group were lower than those of the lower-risk group (56.09 vs. 71.59%, 32.01 vs. 54.47%; $p = 0.019$). Our study finds that performing anatomical liver resection in high-risk groups of MVI is beneficial to patients' long-term survival. When Professor Makuuchi determined the definition of anatomical hepatectomy, he believed that a gross resection of the tumor-bearing liver removes not only the tumor visible to the naked eye but also microvascular invasion that is difficult to detect (30), which has been affirmed by many studies and is also consistent with the findings of our study. Also, some researchers revealed that AR or NAR for HCC with MVI did not influence the recurrence-free survival or OS rates after hepatectomy in the modern era (16).

However, our study discovered that even in the MVI low-risk group, patients with HCC could obtain long-time survival when performing AR. In order to eliminate the effect of different tumor diameters on recurrence and survival after liver resection, we performed a further analysis using the tumor diameter of 5 cm as the cutoff value according to the literature. In the low-risk group, whether patients undergoing anatomical liver resection did not affect their tumor-free survival rate and survival rate. However, performing anatomical liver resection for patients with tumor diameters >5 cm is beneficial to long-term survival. The probable reason is that larger tumor size is associated with capsular invasion, satellite nodules, tumor thrombi, and non-invasive growth patterns (31). Moreover, larger HCC tumor size stimulates invasive behavior.

Also, several shortcomings existed in this study. A single-center retrospective study and the number of data enrolled is insufficient, which might lead to some bias of the data. Dates were not further divided by tumor sizes during the enrollment process, which would also have an impact on the patient's prognosis. Some studies found that different tumor sizes (31, 32) and the shortest distance from the edge of the tumor to the plane of surgical margin (33–35) would significantly affect post-operative outcomes, yet no further discussion was done in the survival analysis in this study. The issues mentioned above need to be analyzed by further multi-center and extensive sample data. This work is ongoing in our center.

In summary, we have developed and validated a novel score for predicting MVI risk in patients with HCC. Due to a high risk of early tumor recurrence, our findings suggest that patients with high MVI risk should undergo AR rather than NAR at the time of initial treatment allocation. Furthermore, in patients with lower MVI risk when tumor size >5 cm executing AR is of great necessity, also.

AUTHOR CONTRIBUTIONS

CF contributed to the conception of the study. HH performed the study. HH, SQ, SZ, and PZ contributed significantly to analysis and manuscript preparation. HH, SQ, LH, and SW performed the data analyses and wrote the manuscript. HH, NZ, JY, WZhang, WZhu, and NX helped perform the analysis with constructive discussions. All authors contributed to the article and approved the submitted version.

ACKNOWLEDGMENTS

Thanks to Li Xinmin and Lin Huan from the Department of Radiology of Zhujiang Hospital Affiliated to Southern Medical University for the imaging analysis.

REFERENCES

1. Lim KC, Chow PK, Allen JC, Chia GS, Lim M, Cheow PC, et al. Microvascular invasion is a better predictor of tumor recurrence and overall survival following surgical resection for hepatocellular carcinoma compared to the Milan criteria. *Ann Surg.* (2011) 254:108–13. doi: 10.1097/SLA.0b013e31821ad884
2. Shetty K, Timmins K, Brensinger C, Furth EE, Rattan S, Sun W, et al. Liver transplantation for hepatocellular carcinoma validation of present selection criteria in predicting outcome. *Liver Transpl.* (2004) 10:911–8. doi: 10.1002/lt.20140
3. Zimmerman MA, Ghobrial RM, Tong MJ, Hiatt JR, Cameron AM, Hong J, et al. Recurrence of hepatocellular carcinoma following liver transplantation: a review of preoperative and postoperative prognostic indicators. *Arch Surg.* (2008) 143:182–8. doi: 10.1001/archsurg.2007.39
4. Banerjee S, Wang DS, Kim HJ, Sirlin CB, Chan MG, Korn RL, et al. A computed tomography radiogenomic biomarker predicts microvascular invasion and clinical outcomes in hepatocellular carcinoma. *Hepatology.* (2015) 62:792–800. doi: 10.1002/hep.27877
5. European Association for the Study of the Liver. EASL clinical practice guidelines: management of hepatocellular carcinoma. *J Hepatol.* (2018) 69:182–236. doi: 10.1016/j.jhep.2018.03.019
6. Rodriguez-Peralvarez M, Luong TV, Andreana L, Meyer T, Dhillon AP, Burroughs AK. A systematic review of microvascular invasion in hepatocellular carcinoma: diagnostic and prognostic variability. *Ann Surg Oncol.* (2013) 20:325–39. doi: 10.1245/s10434-012-2513-1
7. Lee S, Kang TW, Song KD, Lee MW, Rhim H, Lim HK, et al. Effect of microvascular invasion risk on early recurrence of hepatocellular carcinoma after surgery and radiofrequency ablation. *Ann Surg.* (2019) 273:564–71. doi: 10.1097/SLA.0000000000003268

8. Nitta H, Allard M, Sebagh M, Karam V, Ciacio O, Pittau G, et al. Predictive model for microvascular invasion of hepatocellular carcinoma among candidates for either hepatic resection or liver transplantation. *Surgery.* (2019) 165:1168–75. doi: 10.1016/j.surg.2019.01.012
9. Pan Y, Chen J, Fang A, Wang X, Chen J, Wang J, et al. A nomogram predicting the recurrence of hepatocellular carcinoma in patients after laparoscopic hepatectomy. *Cancer Commun.* (2019) 39:55. doi: 10.1186/s40880-019-0404-6
10. Lei Z, Li J, Wu D, Xia Y, Wang Q, Si A, et al. Nomogram for preoperative estimation of microvascular invasion risk in hepatitis B virus-related hepatocellular carcinoma within the Milan criteria. *JAMA Surg.* (2016) 151:356–63. doi: 10.1001/jamasurg.2015.4257
11. Renzulli M, Brocchi S, Cucchetti A, Mazzotti F, Mosconi C, Sportoletti C, et al. Can current preoperative imaging be used to detect microvascular invasion of hepatocellular carcinoma? *Radiology.* (2016) 279:432–42. doi: 10.1148/radiol.2015150998
12. Chandarana H, Robinson E, Hajdu CH, Drozhinin L, Babb JS, Taouli B. Microvascular invasion in hepatocellular carcinoma: is it predictable with pretransplant MRI? *AJR Am J Roentgenol.* (2011) 196:1083–9. doi: 10.2214/AJR.10.4720
13. Xu X, Zhang H, Liu Q, Sun S, Zhang J, Zhu F, et al. Radiomic analysis of contrast-enhanced CT predicts microvascular invasion and outcome in hepatocellular carcinoma. *J Hepatol.* (2019) 70:1133–44. doi: 10.1016/j.jhep.2019.02.023
14. Zhao H, Chen C, Gu S, Yan X, Jia W, Mao L, et al. Anatomical versus non-anatomical resection for solitary hepatocellular carcinoma without macroscopic vascular invasion: a propensity score matching analysis. *J Gastroenterol Hepatol.* (2017) 32:870–8. doi: 10.1111/jgh.13603
15. Hasegawa K, Kokudo N, Imamura H, Matsuyama Y, Aoki T, Minagawa M, et al. Prognostic impact of anatomic resection for hepatocellular carcinoma. *Ann Surg.* (2005) 242:252–9. doi: 10.1097/01.sla.0000171307.37401.db
16. Hidaka M, Eguchi S, Okuda K, Beppu T, Shirabe K, Kondo K, et al. Impact of anatomical resection for hepatocellular carcinoma with microportal invasion (vp1): a multi-institutional study by the Kyushu Study Group of Liver Surgery. *Ann Surg.* (2020) 271:339–46. doi: 10.1097/SLA.0000000000002981
17. Kawamura Y, Ikeda K, Hirakawa M, Yatsuji H, Sezaki H, Hosaka T, et al. New classification of dynamic computed tomography images predictive of malignant characteristics of hepatocellular carcinoma. *Hepatol Res.* (2010) 40:1006–14. doi: 10.1111/j.1872-034X.2010.00703.x
18. Choi JY, Lee J, Sirlin CB. CT and MR imaging diagnosis and staging of hepatocellular carcinoma: Part II. Extracellular agents, hepatobiliary agents, and ancillary imaging features. *Radiology.* (2014) 273:30–50. doi: 10.1148/radiol.14132362
19. Ariizumi S, Kitagawa K, Kotera Y, Takahashi Y, Katagiri S, Kuwatsuru R, et al. A non-smooth tumor margin in the hepatobiliary phase of gadoxetic acid disodium (Gd-EOB-DTPA)-enhanced magnetic resonance imaging predicts microscopic portal vein invasion, intrahepatic metastasis, and early recurrence after hepatectomy in patients with hepatocellular carcinoma. *J Hepatobiliary Pancreat Sci.* (2011) 18:575–85. doi: 10.1007/s00534-010-0369-y
20. Kitao A, Matsui O, Yoneda N, Kozaka K, Kobayashi S, Koda W, et al. Hypervascular hepatocellular carcinoma: correlation between biologic features and signal intensity on gadoxetic acid-enhanced MR images. *Radiology.* (2012) 265:780–9. doi: 10.1148/radiol.12120226
21. Kim KA, Kim MJ, Jeon HM, Kim KS, Choi JS, Ahn SH, et al. Prediction of microvascular invasion of hepatocellular carcinoma: usefulness of peritumoral hypointensity seen on gadoxetate disodium-enhanced hepatobiliary phase images. *J Magn Reson Imaging.* (2012) 35:629–34. doi: 10.1002/jmri.22876
22. Fang C, Zhang P, Qi X. Digital and intelligent liver surgery in the new era: prospects and dilemmas. *EBioMedicine.* (2019) 41:693–701. doi: 10.1016/j.ebiom.2019.02.017
23. Cong WM, Bu H, Chen J, Dong H, Zhu YY, Feng LH, et al. Practice guidelines for the pathological diagnosis of primary liver cancer: 2015 update. *World J Gastroenterol.* (2016) 22:9279–87. doi: 10.3748/wjg.v22.i42.9279
24. Ishizuka M, Nagata H, Takagi K, Iwasaki Y, Shibuya N, Kubota K. Clinical significance of the C-reactive protein to albumin ratio for survival after surgery for colorectal cancer. *Ann Surg Oncol.* (2016) 23:900–7. doi: 10.1245/s10434-015-4948-7
25. Cescon M, Bertuzzo VR, Ercolani G, Ravaioli M, Odaldi F, Pinna AD. Liver transplantation for hepatocellular carcinoma: role of inflammatory and immunological state on recurrence and prognosis. *World J Gastroenterol.* (2013) 19:9174–82. doi: 10.3748/wjg.v19.i48.9174
26. Chan AW, Chan SL, Wong GL, Wong VW, Chong CC, Lai PB, et al. Prognostic Nutritional Index (PNI) predicts tumor recurrence of very early/early stage hepatocellular carcinoma after surgical resection. *Ann Surg Oncol.* (2015) 22:4138–48. doi: 10.1245/s10434-015-4516-1
27. Wang Y, Peng C, Cheng Z, Wang X, Wu L, Li J, et al. The prognostic significance of preoperative neutrophil-lymphocyte ratio in patients with hepatocellular carcinoma receiving hepatectomy: a systematic review and meta-analysis. *Int J Surg.* (2018) 55:73–80. doi: 10.1016/j.ijsu.2018.05.022
28. Lee S, Kim SH, Lee JE, Sinn DH Park CK. Preoperative gadoxetic acid–enhanced MRI for predicting microvascular invasion in patients with single hepatocellular carcinoma. *J Hepatol.* (2017) 67:526–34. doi: 10.1016/j.jhep.2017.04.024
29. Nitta H, Allard M, Sebagh M, Ciacio O, Pittau G, Vibert E, et al. Prognostic value and prediction of extratumoral microvascular invasion for hepatocellular carcinoma. *Ann Surg Oncol.* (2019) 26:2568–76. doi: 10.1245/s10434-019-07365-0
30. Makuuchi M, Hasegawa H, Yamazaki S. Ultrasonically guided subsegmentectomy. *Surg Gynecol Obstet.* (1985) 161:346–50.
31. Wu G, Wu J, Wang B, Zhu X, Shi X, Ding Y. Importance of tumor size at diagnosis as a prognostic factor for hepatocellular carcinoma survival: a population-based study. *Cancer Manag Res.* (2018) 10:4401–10. doi: 10.2147/CMAR.S177663
32. Kluger MD, Salceda JA, Laurent A, Tayar C, Duvoux C, Decaens T, et al. Liver resection for hepatocellular carcinoma in 313 western patients: tumor biology and underlying liver rather than tumor size drive prognosis. *J Hepatol.* (2015) 62:1131–40. doi: 10.1016/j.jhep.2014.12.018
33. Wang H, Yu H, Qian YW, Cao ZY, Wu MC, Cong WM. Impact of surgical margin on the prognosis of early hepatocellular carcinoma (</=5 cm): a propensity score matching analysis. *Front Med.* (2020) 7:139. doi: 10.3389/fmed.2020.00139
34. Aoki T, Kubota K, Hasegawa K, Kubo S, Izumi N, Kokudo N, et al. Significance of the surgical hepatic resection margin in patients with a single hepatocellular carcinoma. *Br J Surg.* (2020) 107:113–20. doi: 10.1002/bjs.11329
35. Yang P, Si A, Yang J, Cheng Z, Wang K, Li J, et al. A wide-margin liver resection improves long-term outcomes for patients with HBV-related hepatocellular carcinoma with microvascular invasion. *Surgery.* (2019) 165:721–30. doi: 10.1016/j.surg.2018.09.016

12

Comprehensive Analysis to Identify the Epithelial–Mesenchymal Transition-Related Immune Signatures as a Prognostic and Therapeutic Biomarkers in Hepatocellular Carcinoma

Guozhi Wu[1,2,3†], Yuan Yang[1,2,3†], Yu Zhu[1,4†], Yemao Li[1,2,3], Zipeng Zhai[1,2,3], Lina An[1,2,3], Min Liu[2,3], Ya Zheng[2,3], Yuping Wang[2,3], Yongning Zhou[2,3*] and Qinghong Guo[2,3*]

[1] The First Clinical Medical College, Lanzhou University, Lanzhou, China, [2] Department of Gastroenterology, The First Hospital of Lanzhou University, Lanzhou, China, [3] Gansu Key Laboratory of Gastroenterology, Lanzhou University, Lanzhou, China, [4] Department of Hematology, the First Hospital of Lanzhou University, Lanzhou, China

***Correspondence:**
Qinghong Guo
guoza@sohu.com
Yongning Zhou
zhouyn@lzu.edu.cn

†These authors have contributed equally to this work

Background: Hepatocellular carcinoma (HCC) is a highly heterogeneous disease with the high rates of the morbidity and mortality due to the lack of the effective prognostic model for prediction.

Aim: To construct a risk model composed of the epithelial–mesenchymal transition (EMT)-related immune genes for the assessment of the prognosis, immune infiltration status, and chemosensitivity.

Methods: We obtained the transcriptome and clinical data of the HCC samples from The Cancer Genome Atlas (TCGA) and The International Cancer Genome Consortium (ICGC) databases. The Pearson correlation analysis was applied to identify the differentially expressed EMT-related immune genes (DE-EMTri-genes). Subsequently, the univariate Cox regression was introduced to screen out the prognostic gene sets and a risk model was constructed based on the least absolute shrinkage and selection operator-penalized Cox regression. Additionally, the receiver operating characteristic (ROC) curves were plotted to compare the prognostic value of the newly established model compared with the previous model. Furthermore, the correlation between the risk model and survival probability, immune characteristic, and efficacy of the chemotherapeutics were analyzed by the bioinformatics methods.

Results: Six DE-EMTri-genes were ultimately selected to construct the prognostic model. The area under the curve (AUC) values for 1-, 2-, and 3- year were 0.773, 0.721, and 0.673, respectively. Stratified survival analysis suggested that the prognosis of the low-score group was superior to the high-score group. Moreover, the univariate and multivariate analysis indicated that risk score [hazard ratio (HR) 5.071, 95% CI 3.050, 8.432; HR 4.396, 95% CI 2.624, 7.366; $p < 0.001$] and stage (HR 2.500, 95% CI 1.721, 3.632; HR 2.111, 95% CI 1.443, 3.089; $p < 0.001$) served as an independent predictive factors in HCC. In addition, the macrophages, natural killer (NK) cells, and regulatory T

(Treg) cells were significantly enriched in the high-risk group. Finally, the patients with the high-risk score might be more sensitive to cisplatin, doxorubicin, etoposide, gemcitabine, and mitomycin C.

Conclusion: We established a reliable EMTri-genes-based prognostic signature, which may hold promise for the clinical prediction.

Keywords: hepatocellular carcinoma (HCC), epithelial-mesenchymal-transition (EMT), overall survival (OS), immune infiltration, chemosensitivity

INTRODUCTION

Hepatocellular carcinoma (HCC) has become the sixth most common carcinomas with a high mortality rate worldwide (1, 2). Asians and Pacific Islanders have the highest morbidity (4.7 per 100,000 people) and mortality (2.8 per 100,000 people) rates among the young adults, whereas Blacks have the highest morbidity (26.9 per 100,000 people) and mortality (18.6 per 100,000 people) rates among the middle-aged persons during the years 2000–2010 (3). The chronic inflammation, induced by infection of hepatitis C virus (HCV) or hepatitis B virus (HBV), alcohol, non-alcoholic fatty liver disease (NAFLD), and so on, is the main mechanism driving the occurrence and development of liver cancer (4–8). However, many patients with HCC with high-risk factors are often diagnosed with advanced status, resulting in a 5-year survival of only about 10% (9).

Epithelial–mesenchymal transition (EMT) is a process in which the epithelial cells lose the connection and polarity during the embryogenesis, leading to a migrating mesenchymal phenotype (10). It is widely accepted that EMT plays crucial roles in the different biological and pathological processes of HCC including tumor progression, metastasis after chemotherapy treatments, and anticancer drugs resistance (11–13). Among them, EMT tumor drug resistance gradually arouses the attention of the researchers. Increasing studies have reported that EMT is involved in the drugs resistance in the plenty of cancers such as HCC (14), breast cancer (15, 16), pancreatic cancer (17), and bladder cancer (18). With respect to the mechanism of EMT-mediated chemotherapy resistance, several studies have found that transforming growth factor-β (TGF-β) (19, 20), Wnt (21, 22), Hedgehog (21, 23), p53 (24), and phosphatidylinositol 3-kinase (PI3K)/Akt (22, 25) signaling pathways involved in drugs resistance are closely related to EMT. In addition, the development of cell resistance to drug-induced apoptosis and the local effect of tumor microenvironment (TME) are also two factors driving EMT-mediated drug resistance (26). Through modulating the course of EMT and the immune response, the TME-related exosomes may also mediate the drug resistance process (27).

Some genes have been found to be involved in EMT. For example, the activation of TGF-β downstream signals is a key molecular event in the induction of EMT (19, 20, 28). Besides, the stimulation of fibroblast-derived CXCL14/ACKR2 pathway proceeds the EMT process, as demonstrated by a reduction of the expression level of the epithelial marker E-cadherin and increased the expression of the mesenchymal biomarkers (N-cadherin and vimentin) (29, 30). Mounting data have already found that the EMT-related genes are associated with the onset and progression of the tumors. In lung cancer, midkine (MDK) enhances the EMT capability of the cancer cells by TGF-β, Wnt, and Notch2 signaling pathways (31–33). An experiment has demonstrated that the suppression of ficolins (FCNs) can upregulate TGF-β, which, in turn, activates the downstream pathways to inhibit EMT in HCC (34). Additionally, it is found in colorectal cancer that secreted phosphoprotein 1 (SPP1) can promote the metastasis of the cancer cells by activating EMT (35).

Various novel signatures have been established recently to uncover the potential mechanisms of cancer and the application prospects of the biomarkers associated with the onset of tumor progression (36–38). In this study, we established a prognostic model based on differentially expressed EMT-related immune genes (EMTri-genes) to perform the prognosis prediction in the patients with HCC. Next, the functional enrichment analyses were utilized to explore the underlying regulatory mechanisms of the signature. Moreover, the correlations between the signature and immune infiltration status and chemosensitivity were assessed by the single-sample gene set enrichment analysis (ssGSEA) and the R package pRRophetic, respectively.

METHODS

Retrieval and Download of the Data From the TCGA-LIHC and the ICGC Liver Cancer - RIKEN, Japan (LIRI-JP) Datasets

The RNA sequencing and clinical data for the patients with HCC were retrieved and downloaded from The Cancer Genome Atlas-Liver Hepatocellular Carcinoma (TCGA-LIHC) dataset (https://tcga-data.nci.nih.gov/tcga/) and the International Cancer Genome Consortium (ICGC) portal (https://dcc.icgc.org/projects/LIRI-JP), respectively. The former dataset was regarded as a training cohort with 365 cases, while another considered as a validation cohort of 231 patients. Next, the EMT-related genes were obtained from the Molecular Signatures Database (MSigDB) (http://software.broadinstitute.org/gsea/msigdb). Meanwhile, immune-related genes list was downloaded from the ImmPort website (http://www.immport.org). Thereafter, 576 of EMT-related genes and 1,626 of immune-related genes were identified in this study (**Appendices 1, 2**).

Screening out EMT-Related Immune Genes

To screen for the EMTri-genes, the Pearson correlation coefficient was set to be larger than 0.4 and $p < 0.001$. Subsequently, R package limma was utilized to perform the identification of the differentially expressed EMTri-genes (DE-EMTri-genes) by setting up a threshold of log2 fold change (FC) ≥ 2 along with a false discovery rate (FDR) < 0.05 in the training cohort.

Establishment of a Risk Model for the Direct Evaluation of the Risk Scores

First, the univariate Cox analysis was used to screen for the overall survival (OS)-related genes. In addition, the protein–protein interaction (PPI) and gene–gene interaction (GGI) network based on these OS-related genes were constructed by the Search Tool for the Retrieval of Interacting Genes/Proteins (STRING) database (http://string-db.org/) in order to explore the potential regulatory relationships of these genes. Subsequently, we performed the Lasso regression, with 10-fold cross-validation and *p*-value of 0.05, for variable selection based on the significant results of the univariate analysis. The Lasso regression run for a total of 1,000 cycles and the random stimulus for each cycle was set to 1,000. Genes with frequency more than 100 were chosen to perform the Cox proportional hazards regression so as to construct the prognostic model. We calculated the area under the curve (AUC) value of each model and connected each AUC value into a curve. The calculation would not be suspended until the curve reached its maximum value, at which point the model would be listed as optimal. Additionally, we plotted the 1-, 2-, and 3-year receiver operating characteristic (ROC) curves to reflect the prognostic accuracy. Next, the risk scores [formula: $\sum_{i=1}^{n}$ $(expression\ level\ ofgene^{*}regression\ coefficient)$] were calculated for each patient to distinguish between the high- and low-risk groups in accordance with the median of the risk scores. Besides, the principal component analysis (PCA) and t-statistic stochastic neighborhood embedding (t-SNE) were utilized for the visualization of the samples distribution in the two groups by using R package Stats and Rtsne, respectively. The Kaplan–Meier method was conducted to verify the survival duration differences between the two groups. Accordingly, the survival curves and forest plot were drawn. A logistic regression model was established by using the rms package in R software and the nomogram was used for visualization. The variables included in the model construction were age, gender, grade, stage, T, N, and M, respectively. Subsequently, the calibration curve was drawn to make a comparison of the predicted and real results.

Stratified Analysis

The stratified survival analyses were conducted based on the several clinicopathological characteristics including the age; sex; tumor, node, and metastasis (TNM) stages; and clinical stages. The HCC samples were classified into T1/T2 (the diameter of isolated tumor >2 cm, with vascular invasion; or multiple tumors, the diameter <5 cm) and T3/T4 (single or multiple tumors, involving the main branches of the portal vein or hepatic vein) according to the TNM system of the American Joint Committee on Cancer (AJCC), eighth edition. Moreover, the patients with HCC were categorized as N0 (node negative) and N1 (regional lymph node metastasis) according to the lymph node metastasis. Based on the distant metastasis, the patients with HCC were divided into M0 (no distant metastasis) and M1 (with distant metastasis). In addition, the patients with HCC were also categorized as stage I/II (early stage) and stage III/IV (advanced stage).

Enrichment Analysis

Differentially expressed genes (DEGs) were entered into the Gene Ontology (GO) (http://www.geneontology.org/) and the Kyoto Encyclopedia of Genes and Genomes (KEGG) (http://www.genome.jp/kegg/) websites to obtain the enriched GO terms and significant KEGG pathways. These analyses were performed by the clusterProfiler package implemented in the R package (log2FC > 1.5 and $p < 0.05$ were the critical values).

Tumor Immune Infiltration Status Assessment

The ssGSEA based on the R package gene set variation analysis (GSVA) was used to investigate the enrichment levels of the immune cells and corresponding immune-related functions between the two risk groups. The HCC samples used for analysis were extracted from the TCGA-LIHC and the LIRI-JP dataset, respectively.

Evaluation of Constructed Model in Clinical Practice

The half-maximal inhibitory concentration (IC50) was calculated by using the R package pRRophetic for administrating the chemotherapeutic drugs, such as cisplatin, doxorubicin, gemcitabine, mitomycin C, vinblastine, and sorafenib, to predict the chemosensitivity in the different risk score groups. Subsequently, the Wilcoxon signed-rank test was adopted to compare the IC50 between the two groups.

RESULTS

Screening for EMT-Related Immune Genes and Construction of the Risk Models for the Evaluation of Prognosis

The flow diagram of this study is presented in **Figure 1**. The Pearson correlation coefficient analysis was utilized to identify the EMTri-genes. As a result, 456 of EMTri-genes were obtained from the TCGA-LIHC cohort and then 55 of the DE-EMTri-genes were identified (**Figures 2A,B**). Next, the OS-related genes with significant difference were identified via the univariate Cox regression analysis and included in the Lasso regression analysis to establish the prognostic models based on the *RBP2*, *MAPT*, *BIRC5*, *PLXNA1*, *CHGA*, and *SPP1* genes (**Figures 2C,D**). The risk score formula is as follows: risk score $= 0.013023617745279 \times$ messenger RNA (mRNA) expression level of *RBP2*+ $0.262079957422771 \times$ mRNA expression level of *MAPT*+ $0.141033589913412 \times$ mRNA expression level of *BIRC5*+ $0.0443117549486775 \times$ mRNA expression level of *PLXNA1*+ $0.0236121577329352 \times$ mRNA expression level of *CHGA*+ $0.0594398057536237 \times$ mRNA expression level of *SPP1*. Network of the PPI and GGI was shown in **Figures 2E,F**. The risk scores for the patients with HCC in the training

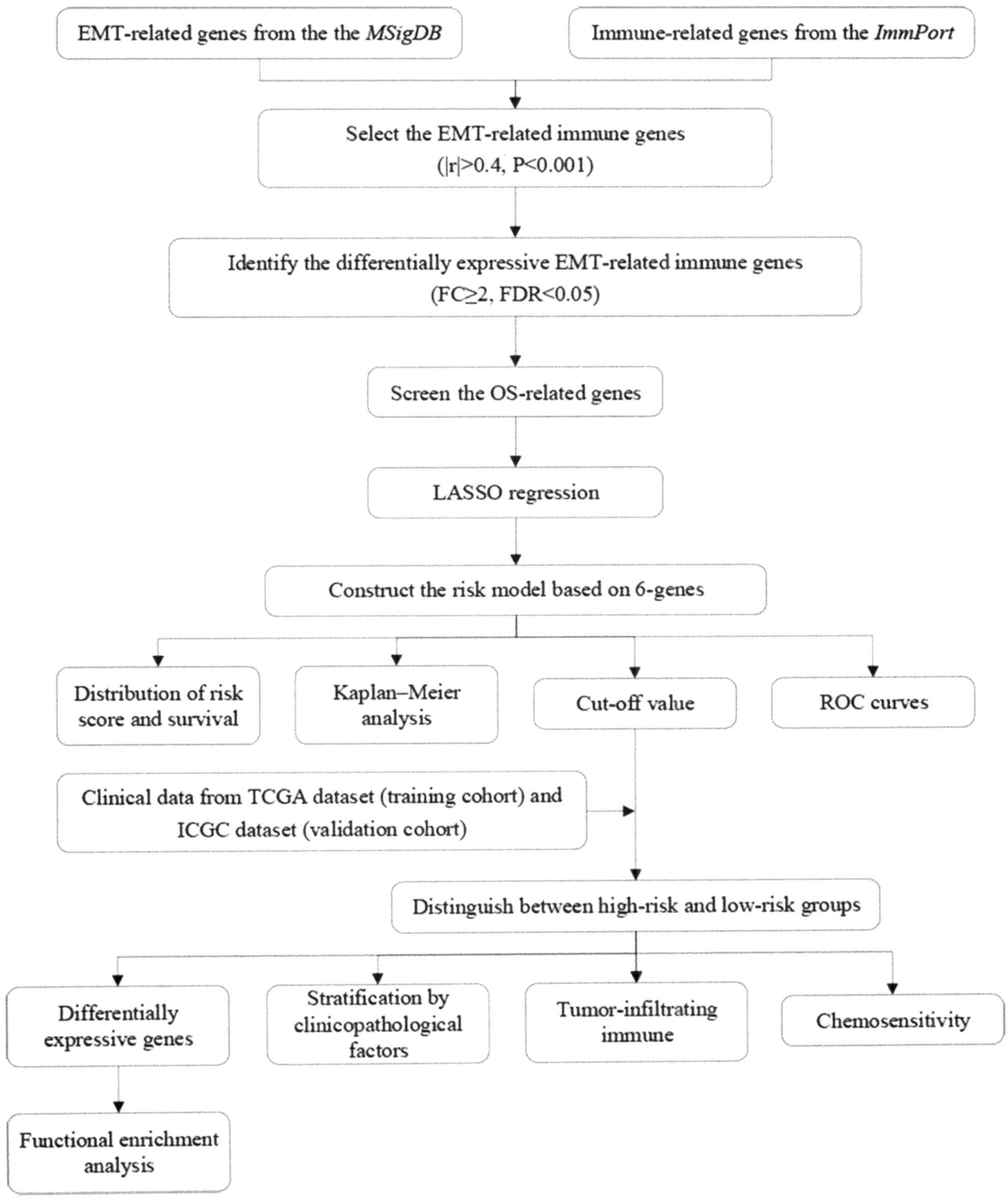

FIGURE 1 | Flow diagram of the study.

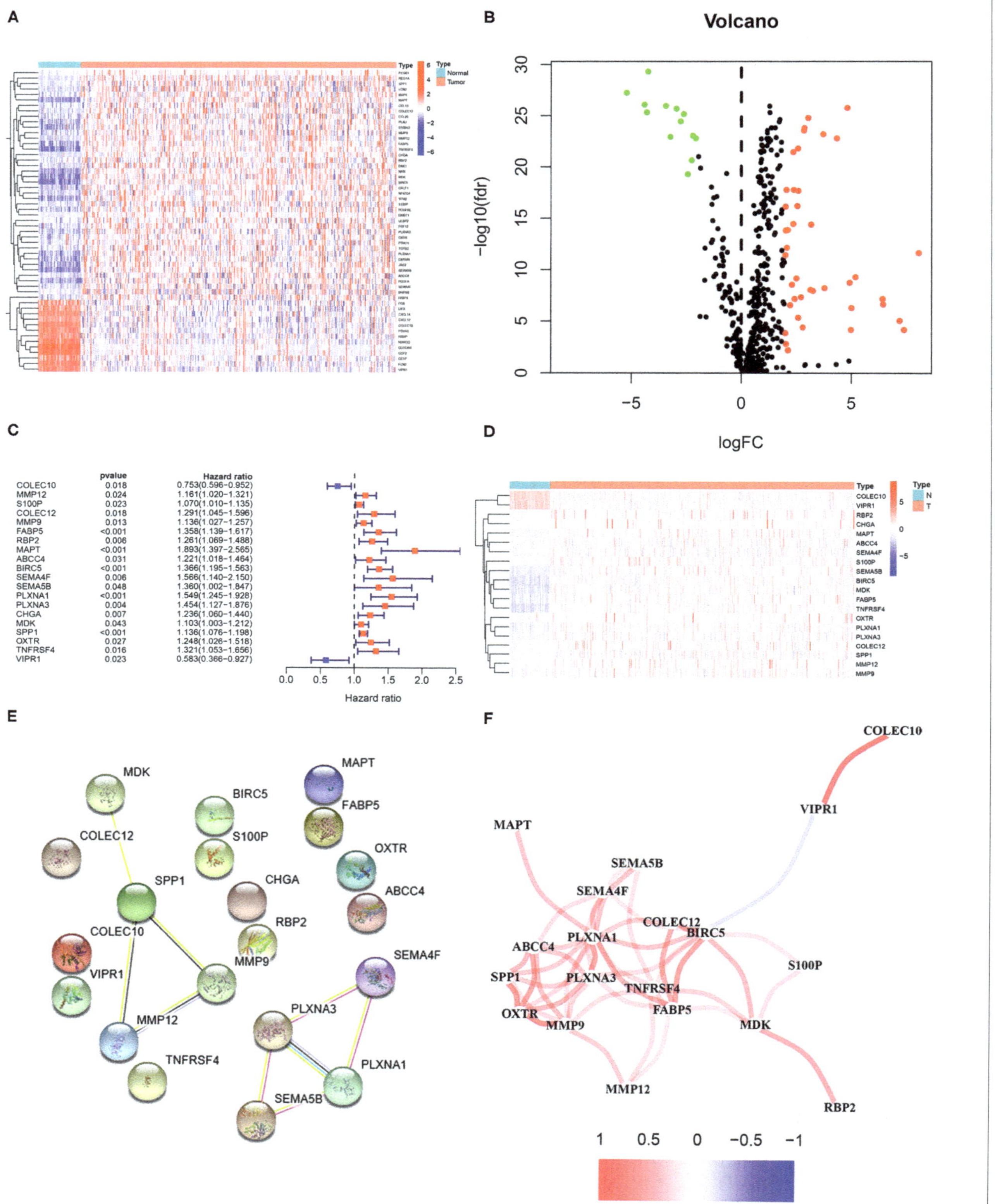

FIGURE 2 | Identification of the epithelial–mesenchymal transition (EMT)-related immune genes with the differential expression and overall survival (OS)-related genes as well as plotting of the protein–protein interaction (PPI) and gene–gene interaction (GGI). **(A)** The heatmap and **(B)** volcano plots of the differentially expressed (DE)-EMT-related immune genes in hepatocellular carcinoma (HCC). **(C)** The forest and **(D)** heatmap plots of the OS-related genes based on the univariate Cox regression analysis. Network plot of **(E)** the PPI and **(F)** GGI.

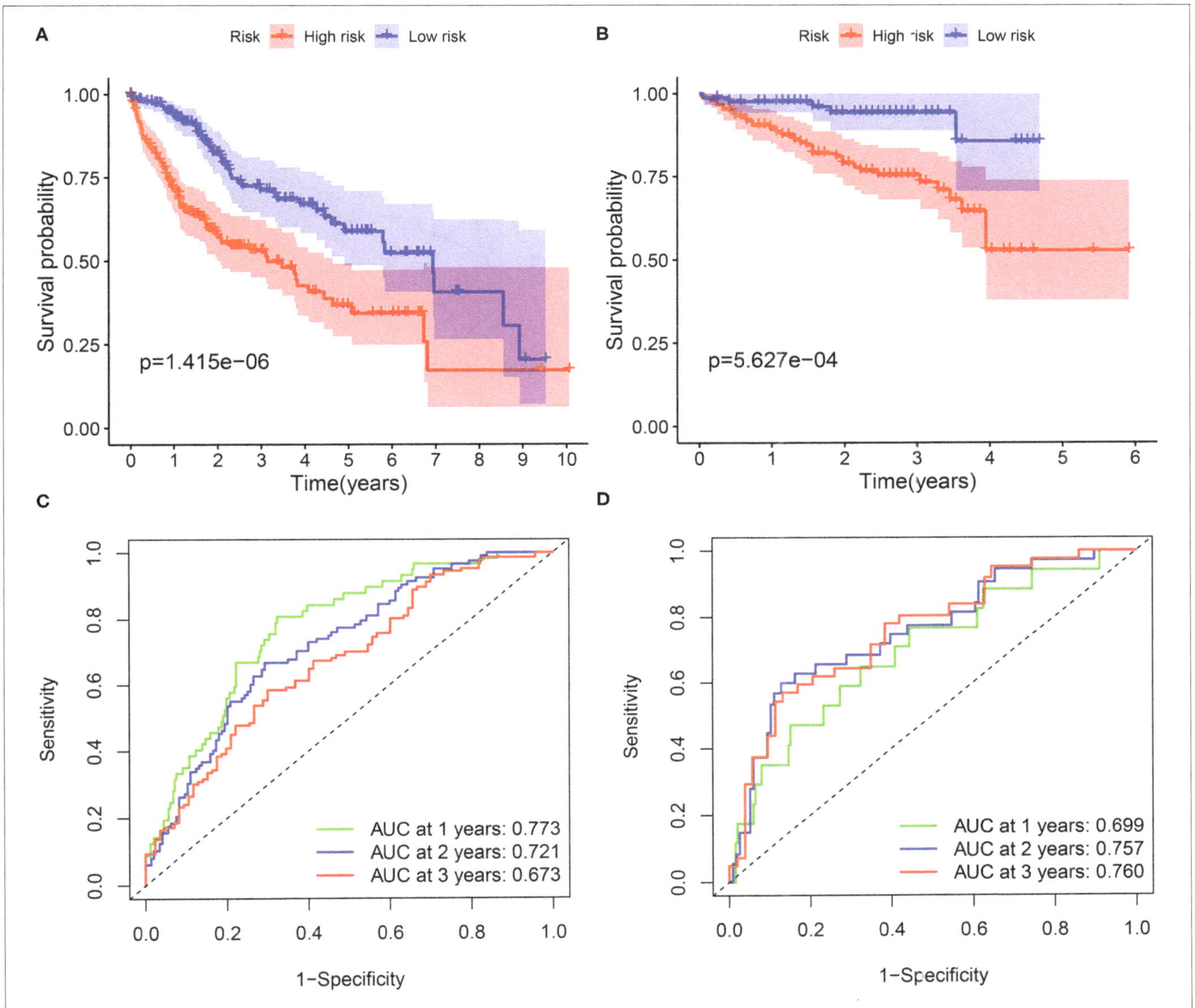

FIGURE 3 | The Kaplan–Meier analysis and the construction of prognostic model based on *FABP5*, *MAPT*, *BIRC5*, *PLXNA1*, and *SPP1* genes. The survival curves in the **(A)** training cohort and **(B)** validation cohort. The 1-, 2-, and 3-year receiver operating characteristic (ROC) curves for assessing the prognostic performance of the gene signature in **(C)** The Cancer Genome Atlas (TCGA) dataset and **(D)** the International Cancer Genome Consortium (ICGC) dataset.

cohort were calculated and the patients were then separated into the different risk groups according to the median score. Subsequently, the Kaplan–Meier survival analysis suggested that, compared to the high-risk group, the low-risk group associated with longer OS (**Figure 3A**). The ROC curves for 1-, 2-, and 3- year were drawn and the corresponding AUC values were 0.773, 0.721, and 0.673, respectively (**Figure 3C**). The risk score and survival time distribution of each patient were illustrated in **Figures 4A,C**. For the enhanced visualization property, the PCA and t-SNE methods were adopted to provide the good separation display effects (**Figures 4E,G**). The logistic regression model constructed by the age, gender, grade, stage, T, N, and M was visualized by the nomogram (**Figure 5A**). The calibration curves showed sufficient consistency between the predicted and real findings (**Figures 5B–D**).

Verifying Prognostic DE-EMT-Related Immune Gene Signature Based on the International Cancer Genome Consortium Dataset

The ICGC dataset that serves as a validation cohort was utilized to confirm the prognostic value, demonstrated by the TCGA database, of DE-EMTri-genes-based signature. Meanwhile, the risk scores were also calculated for all the patients in the validation dataset to distinguish between the different risk

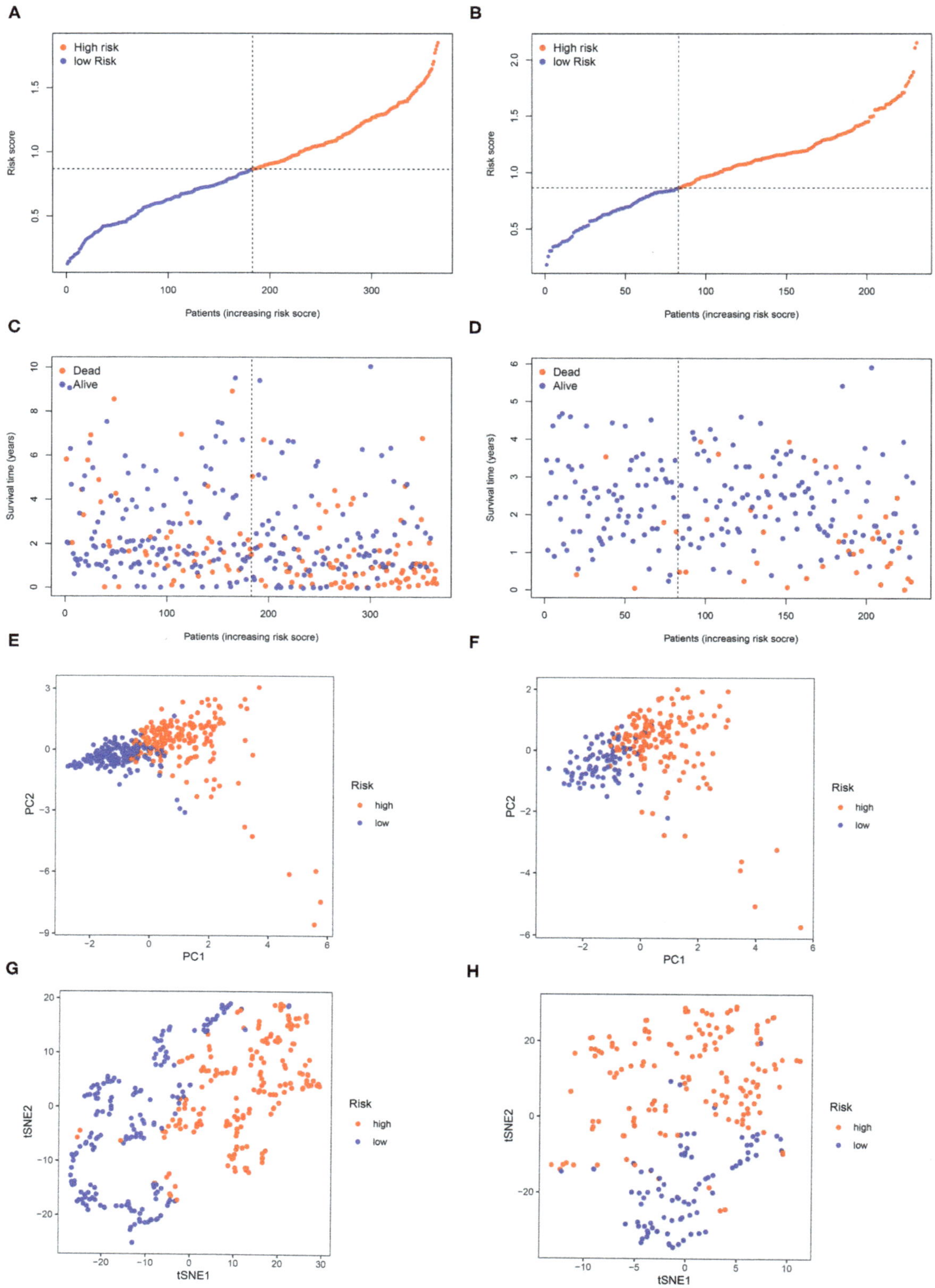

FIGURE 4 | The risk score and survival time distribution of each patient. Risk score distribution in **(A)** the TCGA dataset and **(B)** the ICGC dataset. Survival time distribution in **(C)** the TCGA dataset and **(D)** principal component analysis (PCA) in **(E)** the TCGA dataset and **(F)** the ICGC dataset. t-statistic stochastic neighborhood embedding (t-SNE) in **(G)** the TCGA dataset and **(H)** the ICGC dataset.

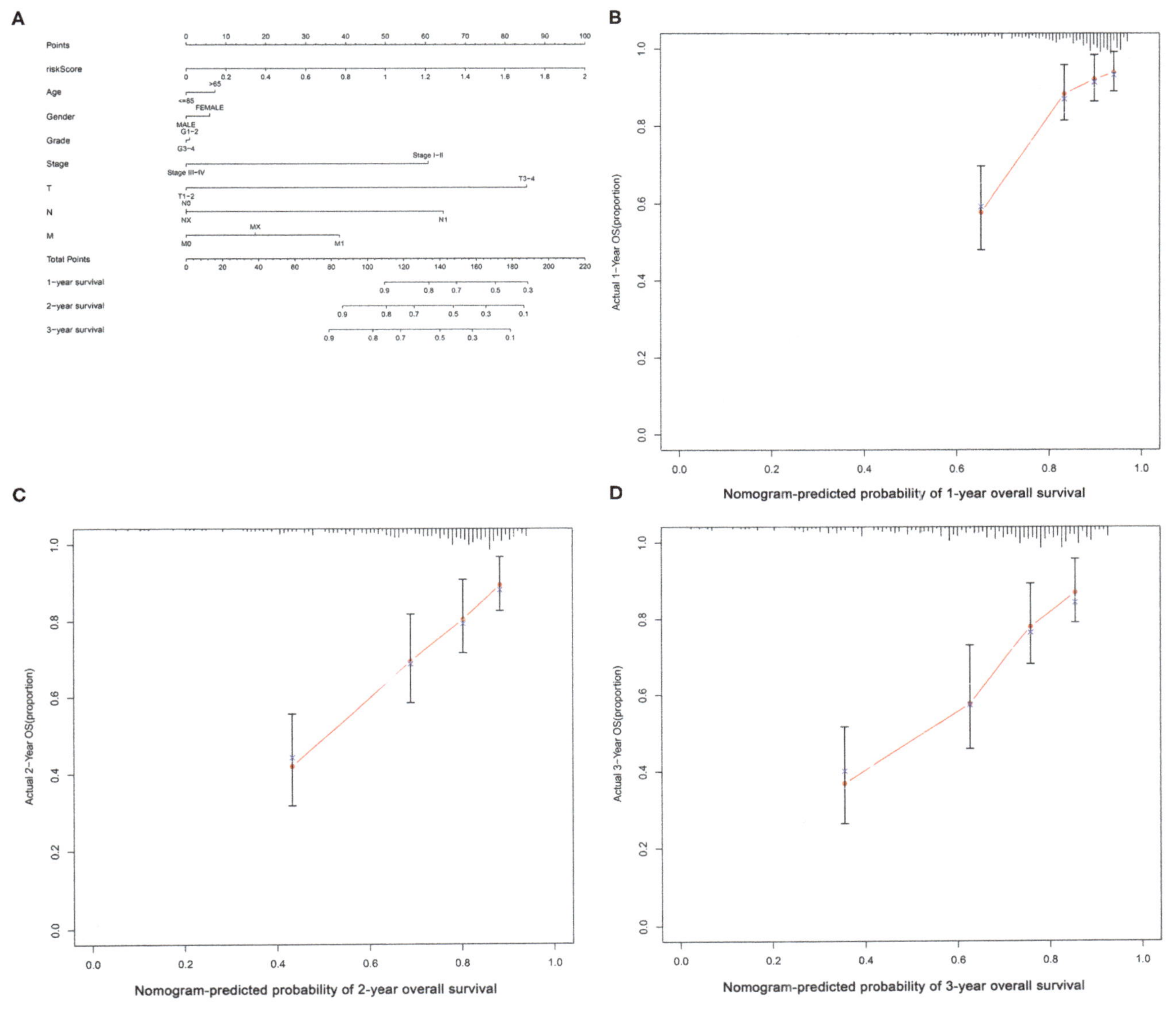

FIGURE 5 | Nomogram of the logistic regression model and calibration curves. **(A)** Nomogram; nomogram-predicted probability of **(B)** 1-year, **(C)** 2-year and **(D)** 3-year OS.

groups. The survival curves showed an increased survival time in low-risk group, which was in line with the training cohort (**Figure 3B**). Lastly, it was concluded that 1-, 2-, and 3-year AUC of the EMTri-genes graded as 0.699, 0.757, and 0.760 in the validation results (**Figure 3D**), indicating a powerful predictive capacity of the signature. Similarly, the risk score and survival status distribution of the patients with HCC were plotted as well as the PCA and t-SNE methods were performed and the results were consistent with that of the TCGA dataset (**Figures 4B,D,F,H**).

Clinicopathological Characteristics Analysis

As illustrated in **Figure 6**, significant survival differences between the two groups, stratified by the various clinicopathological characteristics, including age $\geq$ 65 years ($p < 0.003$), age < 65 years ($p < 0.001$), male ($p < 0.001$), G1–G2 ($p = 0.002$), stage I–II ($p < 0.001$), and stage III–IV ($p = 0.022$), were observed. The corresponding validation results were displayed in **Supplementary Figure S3**.

Assessment of the Independent Prognostic Value of These Six Genes Status for Overall Survival

Risk score was identified as an independent predictive parameter between the different risk groups according to the univariate and multivariate Cox regression analysis. The univariate analysis illustrated a significant correlation between the risk score and OS in the training and validation cohorts (HR 5.071, 95%

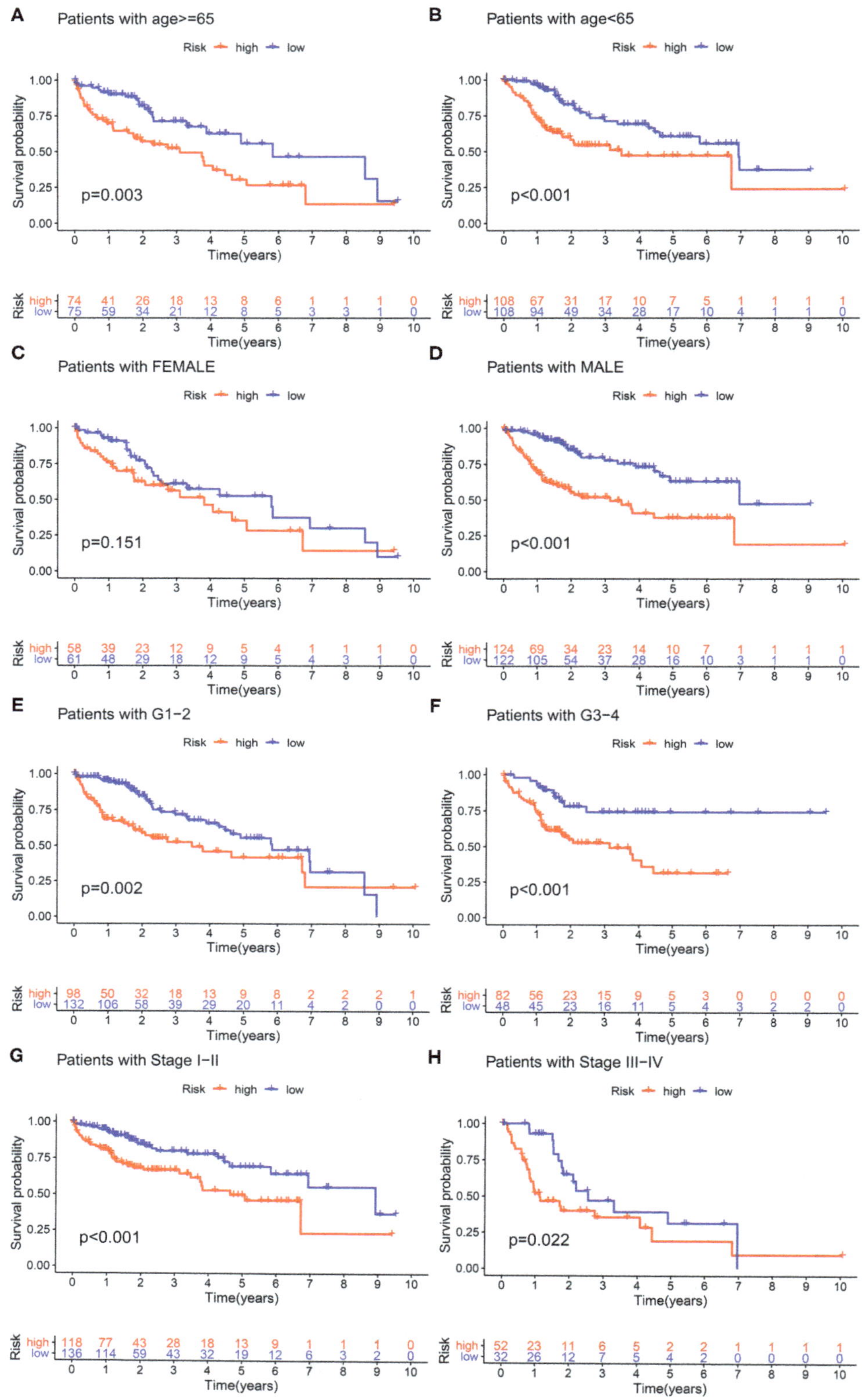

FIGURE 6 | Clinicopathological characteristics analysis. Survival probability stratified by age **(A,B)**, gender **(C,D)**, grade **(E,F)**, and stage **(G,H)**.

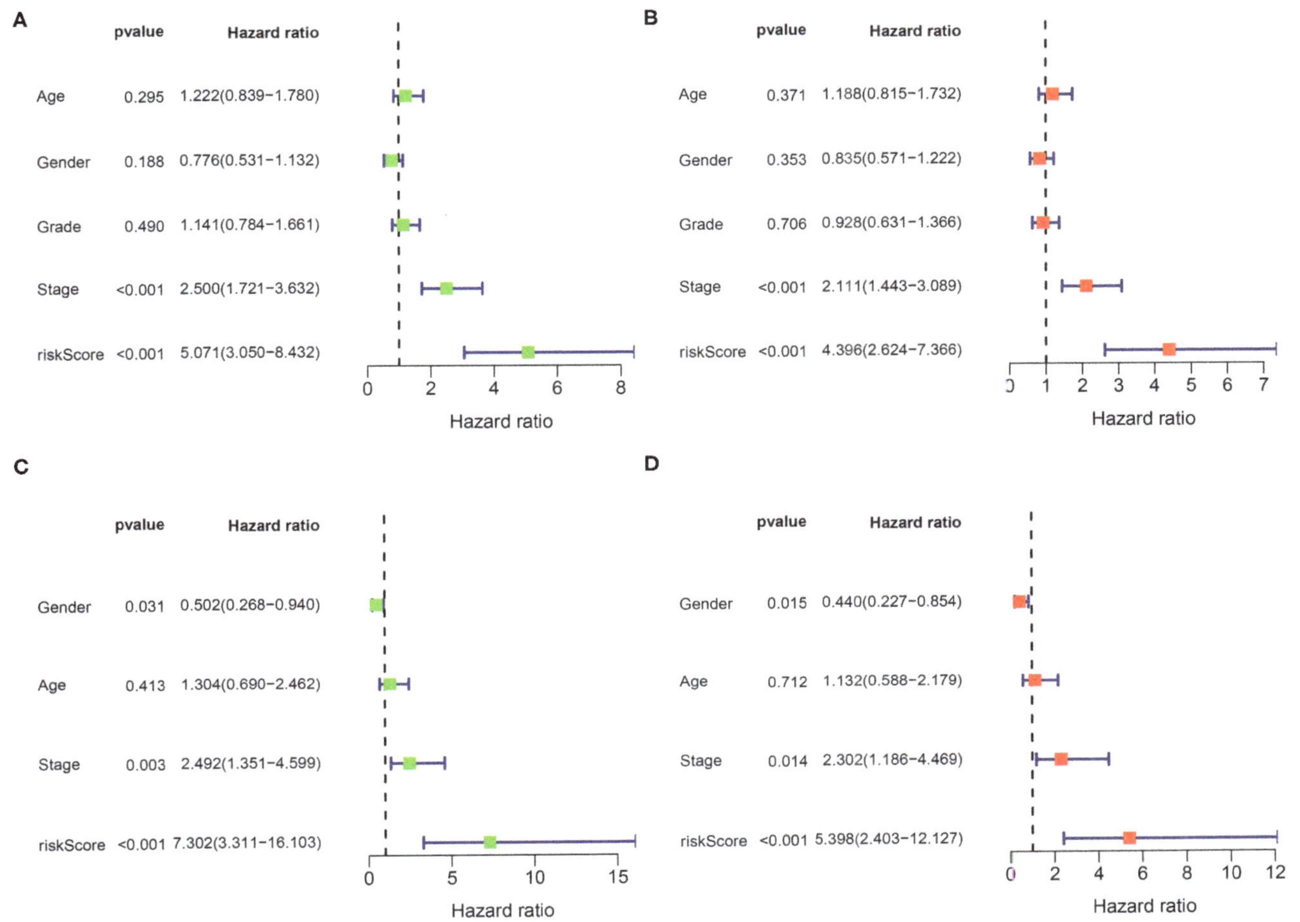

FIGURE 7 | Univariate and multivariate analysis for the identification of the predictive factors. The forest plots of **(A)** the univariate and **(B)** multivariate results show that the risk score [hazard ratio (HR) 5.071, 95% CI 3.050, 8.432; HR 4.396, 95% CI 2.624, 7.366; $p < 0.001$] and stage (HR 2.500, 95% CI 1.721, 3.632; HR 2.111, 95% CI 1.443, 3.089; $p < 0.001$) are associated with poor prognosis in the TCGA dataset. The forest plots of **(C)** the univariate and **(D)** multivariate analysis in the ICGC dataset.

CI 3.050, 8.432, $p < 0.001$; HR 7.302, 95% CI 3.311, 16.103, $p < 0.001$; **Figures 7A,C**). In the multivariate analysis that excluded the confounding factors, a significant association between the risk score and OS was still observed (HR 4.396, 95% CI 2.624, 7.366, $p < 0.001$; HR 5.398, 95% CI 2.403, 12.127, $p < 0.001$; **Figures 7B,D**).

Enrichment Analysis to Identify the DE-EMT-Related Immune Function Signatures

The GO and KEGG enrichment analyses were conducted to explore the biological process and signaling pathway of the DEGs between the different risk groups. As a result, the GO analysis revealed that the DEGs significantly enriched in extracellular matrix (ECM) structural constituent and calcium-dependent protein binding according to the TCGA (**Supplementary Figure S1**) and the ICGC datasets (**Supplementary Figure S2**). In addition, the ECM–receptor interaction and interleukin-17 (IL-17) signaling pathway were found to be with marked significance through the KEGG pathway enrichment analysis based on the two cohorts (**Figures 8A,B**).

Immune Infiltration Status Analysis

To assess the relationship between the signature and TME, the infiltrating levels of the immune cells and specified immune-related functions were analyzed via the ssGSEA based on the R package GSVA. Combined with the training and validation cohorts, the macrophages, natural killer (NK) cells, and regulatory T (Treg) cells occurred significantly more often in the tissues of the high-risk group, suggesting that these immune cells might be involved in the onset of the cancer progression (**Figure 9A**). Meanwhile, the results of immune function enrichment analysis demonstrated that the type I interferon (IFN-I) response and type II IFN (IFN-II) response were correlated with the high risk scores (**Figure 9C**), indicating that the immune cells probably exert their roles through

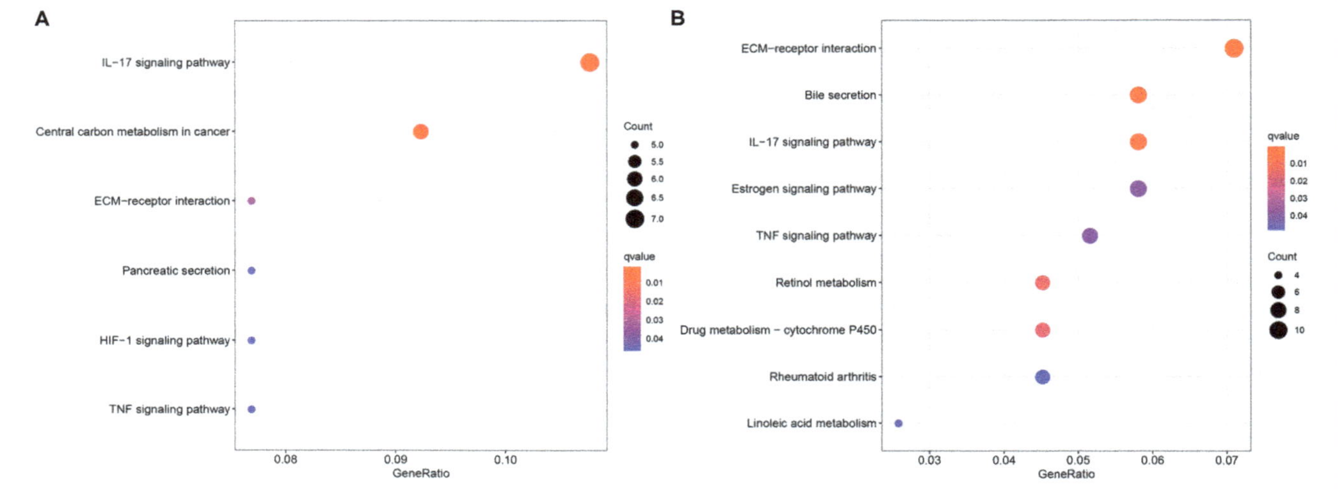

FIGURE 8 | Enrichment of the Kyoto Encyclopedia of Genes and Genomes (KEGG) analysis. Bubble plot of the KEGG analysis based on **(A)** the TCGA dataset and **(B)** the ICGC dataset.

these two pathways. The validation results were presented in **Figures 9B,D**.

Evaluation of Chemosensitivity Based on the Constructed Risk Assessment Model

To evaluate the chemosensitivity differences between the two groups, the R package pRRophetic was utilized to calculate the IC50 value. In the high-risk group, cisplatin, doxorubicin, gemcitabine, and mitomycin C have lower IC50 values (i.e., higher chemosensitivity) (**Supplementary Figures S4A–D**). However, the IC50 of vinblastine was higher, suggesting that the high-risk population was less sensitive to chemotherapy with this drug (**Supplementary Figure S4E**). Additionally, no significant difference of chemosensitivity for sorafenib between the two risk groups was observed (**Supplementary Figure S4F**).

DISCUSSION

Hepatocellular carcinoma refers to the malignancies in the liver and the multiple factors play vital roles in the process of pathogenesis. The new diagnosed cases and mortality of HCC are gradually increasing worldwide (39). Moreover, due to the late detection, the survival time of the patients with HCC is significantly shortened. Therefore, there is an urgent need to find out the biomarkers related to the clinicopathological signatures and prognosis of HCC to help in the early diagnosis of HCC. In this study, we constructed a risk model based on the signatures of the EMTri-genes and provided a favorable performance to evaluate the corresponding prognostic value, immune infiltration status, and chemosensitivity to HCC.

Previous studies have established the prognostic models grounded on the different immune-related genes (40, 41), but the signatures are not convenient for the clinical application because of too many genes involved in the establishment of the model. In this study, *RBP2*, *MAPT*, *BIRC5*, *PLXNA1*, *CHGA*, and *SPP1* were identified as the OS-related genes and used for modeling. An *in vitro* test revealed that the high expression of *RBP2*was correlated with the poor disease-free survival (DFS) and OS (42), suggesting its prognostic value in HCC. Besides, the previous studies based on the bioinformatics analysis reported that *MAPT* (43), *BIRC5* (44), *PLXNA1* (45), *CHGA* (46), and *SPP1* (37) were used for the construction of the prognostic model and probably influenced the OS time of the patients with HCC. Since the results have not yet been validated externally, our analyses add further credibility to these findings.

The constructed risk model was then utilized to distinguish the high- and low-risk group among the patients with HCC. Subsequently, the univariate and multivariate regressions were employed to analyze the differences in OS between the two groups and the results demonstrated that the survival time of the two risk groups differed significantly indicating the effective prognostic value of the signature.

It is noteworthy to mention that the DEGs selected in accordance with the different risk groups are involved in the tumor-related pathways such as ECM–receptor interaction and IL-17 signaling pathway. Studies have found that not only ECM has been proved to be essentially responsible for the promotion of the invasion, metastasis, and EMT process of the cancer cells (47–49), but changes in its composition promote the cancer formation and progression as well as mediate drug resistance by blocking effective drug delivery (50–52). For example, the elevated levels of the matrix metalloproteinases (MMPs) are usually associated with an undesirable prognosis and a higher risk of recurrence in the breast cancer (53). Tumor-associated macrophages (TAMs) have been found to directly result in the degradation of ECM and promote the invasion of the tumor cells by secreting the proteolytic enzymes (MMP-2 and MMP-9) and stromal-associated proteins (51, 54). Moreover, the infiltrated macrophages secrete the enzymes and cytokines to promote ECM stiffness (55), which, in turn, lead to the tumor proliferation,

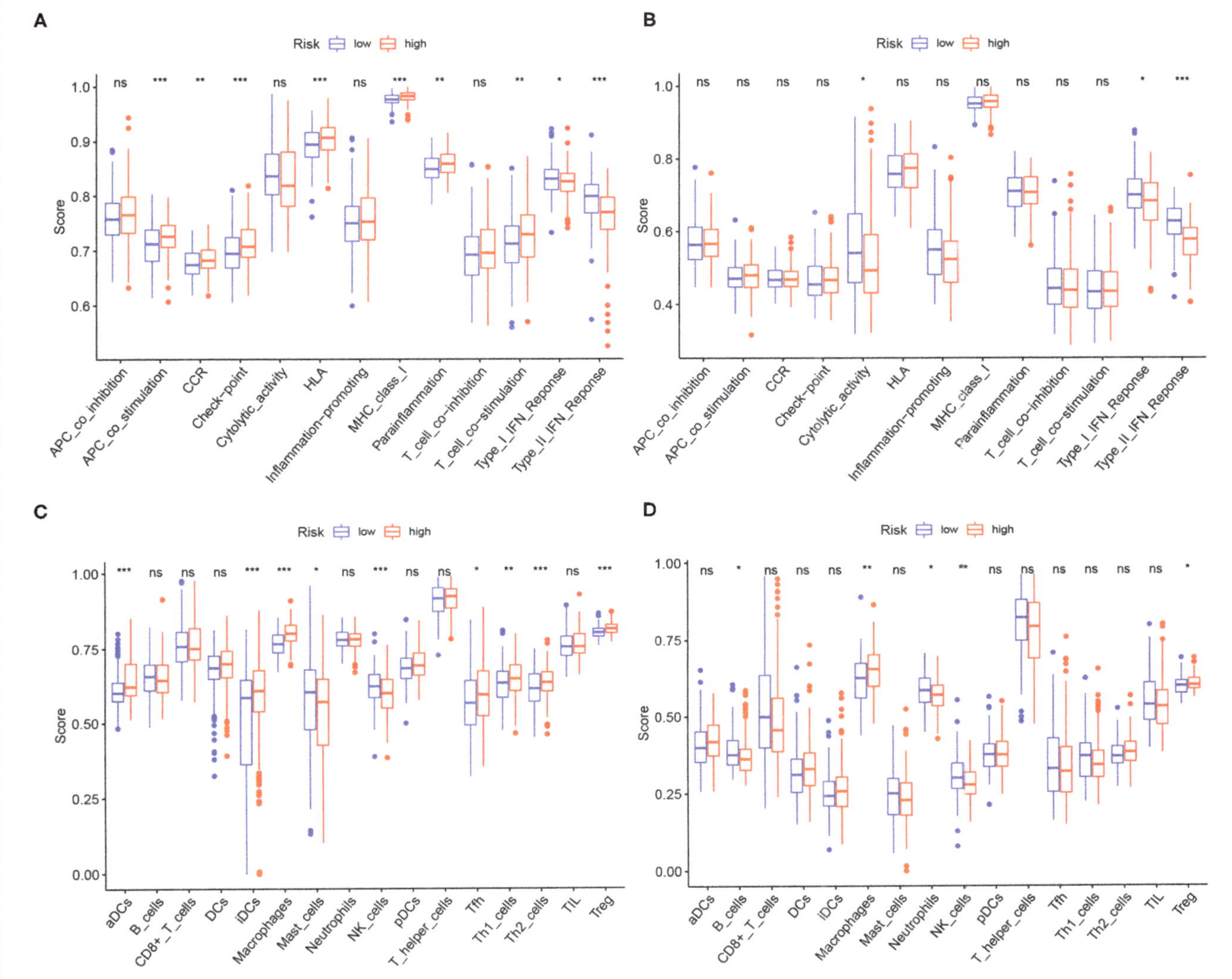

FIGURE 9 | Relationships between the risk score, immune infiltration cells, and immune functions. The high-risk scores were positively correlated with infiltration of the macrophages, natural killer (NK) cells, and regulatory T (Treg) cells both in **(A)** the TCGA dataset and **(B)** the ICGC dataset. The high-risk scores were positively correlated with type I IFN response and type II IFN response both in **(C)** the TCGA dataset and **(D)** the ICGC dataset.

migration, invasion, and drug resistance (51). With respect to the role of the inflammatory cytokines IL-17 signaling pathway, the mounting data showed that IL-17 positively correlated with the tumor proliferation, progression, and metastasis in various malignancies such as prostate cancer (56), colorectal cancer (57), lung cancer (58), and HCC (59).

To investigate the relationship between the risk scores and immune cells infiltration, we analyzed the tumor immune infiltration signatures in the tissues of HCC, concluding that infiltrating the NK cells, Treg cells, and macrophages may be involved in the development of cancer. Recent attentions have been paid to the role of the tumor-infiltrating immune in cancer. Current chemotherapy and radiotherapy regimens can promote the antigen exposure on the tumor surface, thereby stimulating the accumulation of the Treg cells (60). However, the abundance of the Treg cells in the tumor tissues is generally associated with the poor clinical prognosis. In contrast, depletion of the Treg cells can effectively improve to activate the anticancer immunity and NK cell proliferation. For example, the anti-CTLA4 (61) and anti-CCR4 (62) antibodies have been shown to reduce the Treg cells infiltration and enhance antitumor immune responses. Similarly, chemotherapy also increases the infiltration of the TAMs in the tumor tissues and the activated TAMs also make promotion on the tumor progression by secreting proinflammatory cytokine such as interleukin-6 (IL-6) (63). Depletion of the TAMs and inhibition of differentiation to M2 phenotype significantly enhance the antitumor effects of chemotherapy by activating the antitumor T-cell responses (64, 65). Different from the Treg cells and macrophages, NK cell infiltration is associated with longer survival time and is expected to enhance the antitumor responses (66). Interestingly, many novel targeted drugs are designed to exert their antitumor activity by the NK cell-mediated antibody-dependent cell-mediated cytotoxicity (ADCC) (67). The interaction between the immune cells and the corresponding enrichment pathway is expected to be a potential anticancer therapeutic target.

Previous studies only evaluated the infiltration status of the immune cells in the TME. However, they did not explore the specific functions in which these cells are involved. IFN-I and IFN-II responses are known to be involved in antitumor immune response by activating the NK cells, suppressing the activity of the Treg cells, and the differentiation to M2 of TAMs (68). In this study, the immune cells (such as the NK cells, Treg cells, and macrophages) might be involved in the cancer immunity through modulating IFN-I. IFN-I is generally thought to promote the cytotoxic T lymphocytes (CTLs) antitumor responses and suppress the proliferation of the cancer cells (69, 70). On one hand, IFN-I can increase the cytotoxicity of the NK cells and the CD8+ T cells against the tumor cells (71). On the other hand, IFN-I is capable of prolonging the survival time of the CD8+ T cells and protect them from attacking the natural cytotoxicity receptor 1 (NCR1)-mediated NK cells (72, 73). In addition, IFN-I can decrease the immunosuppression of the Treg cells by upregulating phosphodiesterase 4 (PD4) and downregulating cyclic AMP (cAMP) (74). Moreover, IFN-I signaling is able to enhance the inflammation responses by the macrophages through regulating the secretion of the IL-1β and IL-18, promoting antitumor immune response (75). Nevertheless, there have been evidences that IFN-I also exerts the immunosuppressive effects. IFN-I can upregulate the abundance of the Treg cells and promote indoleamine 2,3-dioxygenase (IDO) expression (an immunosuppressive enzyme produced by the macrophages) and PD-L1 (an IFN-I-responsive gene that suppresses CTL activity) as well as the level of the checkpoint antagonists that suppress the antitumor immune responses (76–80). IFN-I signals may have opposite endings under the different conditions; therefore, the mechanism of IFN-I in antitumor immune response needs further external verification.

Lastly, based on the constructed model, IC50 values were calculated to assess the chemosensitivity of drugs authorized by the AJCC. As a result, cisplatin, doxorubicin, etoposide, gemcitabine, and mitomycin C seem to be more suitable for the treatment of the patients with HCC with the high-risk scores. However, sorafenib, approved as the first-line treatment option for HCC nowadays, did not show any significant superiority in the high- or low-risk groups. These results could provide a direction for the clinical trials that evaluate the applicability of these therapies.

In comparison with the recently published studies (81), this study selected the six EMT-related genes that are different from Bian et al. study and tried a novel and similar algorithm (Lasso regression) to construct the risk assessment model. We divided the patients with HCC into the two risk populations and further revealed the correlations between the immune infiltration status and risk scores as well as assessed the chemosensitivity of the approved drugs for HCC. Nevertheless, there are a few shortcomings in this study. First and foremost, our model was established and verified based on the public datasets (the TCGA and the ICGC) but lacked experimental data to validate. Furthermore, the raw data for all of the analyses were relatively insufficient; hence, it is necessary to increase the sample size in the future studies. Moreover, the potential mechanisms of IFN-I and IFN-II in the antitumor immunity need to be further explored. Last but not least, this study is presently based on the signal-dimensional analyzing frame. Transcriptome level data mining methods have been improved but the development of multi-omics approach has shown potential in the future. The application of single-cell multi-omics technique helps to provide a more complete map of the gene regulatory networks in the complex tissues. Through the effective multi-omics analysis relations among the public datasets, the optimal models will be able to be constructed in order to improve the predictive performance (82–85).

CONCLUSIONS

In conclusion, this study constructed the six-genes-based signature that has a great predictive value for the prognosis of HCC. Based on this signature, we found that infiltration of the NK cells, Treg cells, and macrophages was significantly associated with the high-risk scores and IFN might be involved in the progression of HCC. In addition, we also provided a reference for the clinical selection of the authorized chemotherapy drugs in the different populations. The underlying mechanisms of the immune infiltration deserve further exploration.

AUTHOR CONTRIBUTIONS

GW, YY, and YZhu contributed to the conception and design. YZho and QG contributed to the administrative support. YY, YL, ZZ, and LA contributed to the provision of the study materials or patients. GW, ML, YZhe, and YW contributed to the collection and assembly of the data. GW, YY, and YZhu contributed to the data analysis and interpretation. All the authors contributed to the writing and final approval of the manuscript.

ACKNOWLEDGMENTS

Thanks to the Gansu Key Laboratory of Gastroenterology and Department of Gastroenterology and the First Hospital of Lanzhou University for their support.

REFERENCES

1. Ferenci P, Fried M, Labrecque D, Bruix J, Sherman M, Omata M, et al. Hepatocellular carcinoma (HCC): a global perspective. *J Clin Gastroenterol.* (2010) 44:239–45. doi: 10.1097/MCG.0b013e3181d46ef2
2. Ferlay J, Soerjomataram I, Dikshit R, Eser S, Mathers C, Rebelo M, et al. Cancer incidence and mortality worldwide: sources, methods and major patterns in GLOBOCAN 2012. *Int J Cancer.* (2015) 136:E359–86. doi: 10.1002/ijc.29210
3. Altekruse S, Henley S, Cucinelli J, McGlynn K. Changing hepatocellular carcinoma incidence and liver cancer mortality rates in the United States. *Am J Gastroenterol.* (2014) 109:542–53. doi: 10.1038/ajg.2014.11
4. Davila JA, Morgan RO, Shaib Y, McGlynn KA, El-Serag HB. Hepatitis C infection and the increasing incidence of hepatocellular carcinoma: a population-based study. *Gastroenterology.* (2004) 127:1372–80. doi: 10.1053/j.gastro.2004.07.020
5. Fattovich G, Stroffolini T, Zagni I, Donato F. Hepatocellular carcinoma in cirrhosis: incidence and risk factors. *Gastroenterology.* (2004) 127(5 Suppl. 1):S35–50. doi: 10.1053/j.gastro.2004.09.014
6. El-Serag HB, Kanwal F. Epidemiology of hepatocellular carcinoma in the United States: where are we? Where do we go? *Hepatology.* (2014) 60:1767–75. doi: 10.1002/hep.27222
7. Kim H, El-Serag H. The Epidemiology of Hepatocellular Carcinoma in the USA. *Curr Gastroenterol Rep.* (2019) 21:17. doi: 10.1007/s11894-019-0681-x
8. Seeff LB. Introduction: the burden of hepatocellular carcinoma. *Gastroenterology.* (2004) 127(5 Suppl. 1):S1–4. doi: 10.1053/j.gastro.2004.09.010
9. Altekruse SF, McGlynn KA, Reichman ME. Hepatocellular carcinoma incidence, mortality, and survival trends in the United States from 1975 to 2005. *J Clin Oncol.* (2009) 27:1485–91. doi: 10.1200/JCO.2008.20.7753
10. Nieto MA, Huang RY, Jackson RA, Thiery JP. EMT: 2016. *Cell.* (2016) 166:21–45. doi: 10.1016/j.cell.2016.06.028
11. Hay ED. An overview of epithelio-mesenchymal transformation. *Acta Anat.* (1995) 154:8–20. doi: 10.1159/000147748
12. Kalluri R, Weinberg RA. The basics of epithelial-mesenchymal transition. *J Clin Invest.* (2009) 119:1420–8. doi: 10.1172/JCI39104
13. Song R, Song H, Liang Y, Yin D, Zhang H, Zheng T, et al. Reciprocal activation between ATPase inhibitory factor 1 and NF-κB drives hepatocellular carcinoma angiogenesis and metastasis. *Hepatology.* (2014) 60:1659–73. doi: 10.1002/hep.27312
14. Xiao S, Chang RM, Yang MY, Lei X, Liu X, Gao WB, et al. Actin-like 6A predicts poor prognosis of hepatocellular carcinoma and promotes metastasis and epithelial-mesenchymal transition. *Hepatology.* (2016) 63:1256–71. doi: 10.1002/hep.28417
15. Huang J, Li H, Ren G. Epithelial-mesenchymal transition and drug resistance in breast cancer (Review). *Int J Oncol.* (2015) 47:840–8. doi: 10.3892/ijo.2015.3084
16. Yamashita N, Tokunaga E, Iimori M, Inoue Y, Tanaka K, Kitao H, et al. Epithelial paradox: clinical significance of coexpression of E-cadherin and vimentin with regard to invasion and metastasis of breast cancer. *Clin Breast Cancer.* (2018) 18:e1003–9. doi: 10.1016/j.clbc.2018.02.002
17. Arumugam T, Ramachandran V, Fournier KF, Wang H, Marquis L, Abbruzzese JL, et al. Epithelial to mesenchymal transition contributes to drug resistance in pancreatic cancer. *Cancer Res.* (2009) 69:5820–8. doi: 10.1158/0008-5472.CAN-08-2819
18. McConkey DJ, Choi W, Marquis L, Martin F, Williams MB, Shah J, et al. Role of epithelial-to-mesenchymal transition (EMT) in drug sensitivity and metastasis in bladder cancer. *Cancer Metastasis Rev.* (2009) 28:335–44. doi: 10.1007/s10555-009-9194-7
19. Teicher BA, Holden SA, Ara G, Chen G. Transforming growth factor-beta in *in vivo* resistance. *Cancer Chemother Pharmacol.* (1996) 37:601–9. doi: 10.1007/s002800050435
20. Li J, Liu H, Yu J, Yu H. Chemoresistance to doxorubicin induces epithelial-mesenchymal transition via upregulation of transforming growth factor β signaling in HCT116 colon cancer cells. *Mol Med Rep.* (2015) 12:192–8. doi: 10.3892/mmr.2015.3356
21. Wu Y, Ginther C, Kim J, Mosher N, Chung S, Slamon D, et al. Expression of Wnt3 activates Wnt/β-catenin pathway and promotes EMT-like phenotype in trastuzumab-resistant HER2-overexpressing breast cancer cells. *Mol Cancer Res.* (2012) 10:1597–606. doi: 10.1158/1541-7786.MCR-12-0155-T
22. Wang H, Deng G, Ai M, Xu Z, Mou T, Yu J, et al. Hsp90ab1 stabilizes LRP5 to promote epithelial-mesenchymal transition via activating of AKT and Wnt/β-catenin signaling pathways in gastric cancer progression. *Oncogene.* (2019) 38:1489–507. doi: 10.1038/s41388-018-0532-5
23. Della Corte CM, Bellevicine C, Vicidomini G, Vitagliano D, Malapelle U, Accardo M, et al. *SMO* gene amplification and activation of the hedgehog pathway as novel mechanisms of resistance to anti-epidermal growth factor receptor drugs in human lung cancer. *Clin Cancer Res.* (2015) 21:4686–97. doi: 10.1158/1078-0432.CCR-14-3319
24. Zheng T, Yin D, Lu Z, Wang J, Li Y, Chen X, et al. Nutlin-3 overcomes arsenic trioxide resistance and tumor metastasis mediated by mutant p53 in Hepatocellular Carcinoma. *Mol Cancer.* (2014) 13:133. doi: 10.1186/1476-4598-13-133
25. Lin YH, Wu MH, Liao CJ, Huang YH, Chi HC, Wu SM, et al. Repression of microRNA-130b by thyroid hormone enhances cell motility. *J Hepatol.* (2015) 62:1328–40. doi: 10.1016/j.jhep.2014.12.035
26. Du B, and Shim JS. Targeting Epithelial-Mesenchymal Transition (EMT) to overcome drug resistance in cancer. *Molecules.* (2016) 21:965. doi: 10.3390/molecules21070965
27. Zhang J, Song Q, Wu M, Zheng W. The emerging roles of exosomes in the chemoresistance of hepatocellular carcinoma. *Curr Med Chem.* (2021) 28:93–109. doi: 10.2174/0929867327666200130103206
28. Xia L, Huang W, Tian D, Zhang L, Qi X, Chen Z, et al. Forkhead box Q1 promotes hepatocellular carcinoma metastasis by transactivating ZEB2 and VersicanV1 expression. *Hepatology.* (2014) 59:958–73. doi: 10.1002/hep.26735
29. Lin Y, Ma Q, Li L, Wang H. The CXCL12-CXCR4 axis promotes migration, invasiveness, and EMT in human papillary thyroid carcinoma B-CPAP cells via NF-κBsignaling. *Biochem Cell Biol.* (2018) 96:619–26. doi: 10.1139/bcb-2017-0074
30. Sjöberg E, Meyrath M, Milde L, Herrera M, Lövrot J, Hägerstrand D, et al. A novel ACKR2-dependent role of fibroblast-Derived CXCL14 in epithelial-to-mesenchymal transition and metastasis of breast cancer. *Clin Cancer Res.* (2019) 25:3702–17. doi: 10.1158/1078-0432.CCR-18-1294
31. Katsuno Y, Lamouille S, Derynck R. TGF-β signaling and epithelial-mesenchymal transition in cancer progression. *CurrOpin Oncol.* (2013) 25:76–84. doi: 10.1097/CCO.0b013e32835b6371
32. Grupp K, Melling N, Bogoevska V, Reeh M, Uzunoglu F, El Gammal A, et al. Expression of ICAM-1, E-cadherin, periostin and midkine in metastases of pancreatic ductal adenocarcinomas. *Exp Mol Pathol.* (2018) 104:109–13. doi: 10.1016/j.yexmp.2018.01.005
33. Shin D, Jo J, Kim S, Choi M, Han C, Choi B, et al. Midkine is a potential therapeutic target of tumorigenesis, angiogenesis, and metastasis in non-small cell lung cancer. *Cancers.* (2020) 12:2402. doi: 10.3390/cancers120 92402
34. Yang G, Liang Y, Zheng T, Song R, Wang J, Shi H, et al. FCN2 inhibits epithelial-mesenchymal transition-induced metastasis of hepatocellular carcinoma via TGF-β/Smadsignaling. *Cancer Lett.* (2016) 378:80–6. doi: 10.1016/j.canlet.2016.05 007
35. Xu C, Sun L, Jiang C, Zhou H, Gu L, Liu Y, et al. SPP1, analyzed by bioinformatics methods, promotes the metastasis in colorectal cancer by activating EMT pathway. *Biomed Pharmacother.* (2017) 91:1167–77. doi: 10.1016/j.biopha.2017.05.056
36. Song Q, Wang H, Bao J, Pullikuth AK, Li KC, Miller LD, et al. Systems biology approach to studying proliferation-dependent prognostic subnetworks in breast cancer. *Sci Rep.* (2015) 5:12981. doi: 10.1038/srep12981
37. Liu T, Wu H, Qi J, Qin C, Zhu Q. Seven immune-related genes prognostic power and correlation with tumor-infiltrating immune cells in hepatocellular carcinoma. *Cancer Med.* (2020) 9:7440–52. doi: 10.1002/cam4.3406
38. Yang Y, Wu G, Li Q, Zheng Y, Liu M, Zhou L, et al. Angiogenesis-related immune signatures correlate with prognosis, tumor microenvironment, and therapeutic sensitivity in hepatocellular carcinoma. *Front Mol Biosci.* (2021) 8:690206. doi: 10.3389/fmolb.2021.690206
39. Bray F, Ferlay J, Soerjomataram I, Siegel RL, Torre LA, Jemal A. Global cancer statistics 2018: GLOBOCAN estimates of incidence and mortality worldwide for 36 cancers in 185 countries. *CA Cancer J Clin.* (2018) 68:394–424. doi: 10.3322/caac.21492

40. Ouyang G, Yi B, Pan G, Chen X. A robust twelve-gene signature for prognosis prediction of hepatocellular carcinoma. *Cancer Cell Int.* (2020) 20:207. doi: 10.1186/s12935-020-01294-9
41. Zhang J, Chen G, Zhang J, Zhang P, Ye Y. Construction of a prognostic model based on nine immune-related genes and identification of small molecule drugs for hepatocellular carcinoma (HCC). *Am J Transl Res.* (2020) 12:5108–30.
42. Wang ZY, Yang J, Liu CK, Shen SQ. High expression of retinoblastoma-binding protein 2 (RBP2) in patients with hepatocellular carcinoma and its prognostic significance. *Med Sci Monit.* (2017) 23:2736–44. doi: 10.12659/MSM.905262
43. Qi L, Wang L, Huang J, Jiang M, Diao H, Zhou H, et al. Activated amelogenin Y-linked (AMELY) regulation and angiogenesis in human hepatocellular carcinoma by biocomputation. *Oncol Lett.* (2013) 5:1075–9. doi: 10.3892/ol.2013.1122
44. Chaudhary K, Poirion OB, Lu L, Garmire LX. Deep learning-based multi-omics integration robustly predicts survival in liver cancer. *Clin Cancer Res.* (2018) 24:1248–59. doi: 10.1158/1078-0432.CCR-17-0853
45. Hu B, Yang XB, Sang XT. Molecular subtypes based on immune-related genes predict the prognosis for hepatocellular carcinoma patients. *Int Immunopharmacol.* (2021) 90:107164. doi: 10.1016/j.intimp.2020.107164
46. Zhang X, Zhang H, Shen B, Sun XF. Chromogranin-A expression as a novel biomarker for early diagnosis of colon cancer patients. *Int J Mol Sci.* (2019) 20:2919. doi: 10.3390/ijms20122919
47. Rahbari NN, Kedrin D, Incio J, Liu H, Ho WW, Nia HT, et al. Anti-VEGF therapy induces ECM remodeling and mechanical barriers to therapy in colorectal cancer liver metastases. *Sci Transl Med.* (2016) 8:360ra135. doi: 10.1126/scitranslmed.aaf5219
48. Yan P, He Y, Xie K, Kong S, Zhao W. *In silico* analyses for potential key genes associated with gastric cancer. *PeerJ.* (2018) 6:e6092. doi: 10.7717/peerj.6092
49. Bao Y, Wang L, Shi L, Yun F, Liu X, Chen Y, et al. Transcriptome profiling revealed multiple genes and ECM-receptor interaction pathways that may be associated with breast cancer. *Cell Mol Biol Lett.* (2019) 24:38. doi: 10.1186/s11658-019-0162-0
50. Biancur DE, Kimmelman AC. The plasticity of pancreatic cancer metabolism in tumor progression and therapeutic resistance. *BiochimBiophys Acta Rev Cancer.* (2018) 1870:67–75. doi: 10.1016/j.bbcan.2018.04.011
51. Najafi M, Farhood B, Mortezaee K. Extracellular matrix (ECM) stiffness and degradation as cancer drivers. *J Cell Biochem.* (2019) 120:2782–90. doi: 10.1002/jcb.27681
52. Mohan V, Das A, Sagi I. Emerging roles of ECM remodeling processes in cancer. *Semin Cancer Biol.* (2020) 62:192–200. doi: 10.1016/j.semcancer.2019.09.004
53. Radisky ES, Radisky DC. Matrix metalloproteinases as breast cancer drivers and therapeutic targets. *Front Biosci.* (2015) 20:1144–63. doi: 10.2741/4364
54. Afik R, Zigmond E, Vugman M, Klepfish M, Shimshoni E, Pasmanik-Chor M, et al. Tumor macrophages are pivotal constructors of tumor collagenous matrix. *J Exp Med.* (2016) 213:2315–31. doi: 10.1084/jem.20151193
55. Lech M, Anders HJ. Macrophages and fibrosis: how resident and infiltrating mononuclear phagocytes orchestrate all phases of tissue injury and repair. *BiochimBiophys Acta.* (2013) 1832:989–97. doi: 10.1016/j.bbadis.2012.12.001
56. Wang X, Yang L, Huang F, Zhang Q, Liu S, Ma L, et al. Inflammatory cytokines IL-17 and TNF-α up-regulate PD-L1 expression in human prostate and colon cancer cells. *Immunol Lett.* (2017) 184:7–14. doi: 10.1016/j.imlet.2017.02.006
57. Razi S, BaradaranNoveiry B, Keshavarz-Fathi M, Rezaei N. IL-17 and colorectal cancer: from carcinogenesis to treatment. *Cytokine.* (2019) 116:7–12. doi: 10.1016/j.cyto.2018.12.021
58. Wu F, Xu J, Huang Q, Han J, Duan L, Fan J, et al. The role of interleukin-17 in lung cancer. *Mediators Inflamm.* (2016) 2016:8494079. doi: 10.1155/2016/8494079
59. Hu Z, Luo D, Wang D, Ma L, Zhao Y, Li L. IL-17 activates the IL-6/STAT3 signal pathway in the proliferation of hepatitis B virus-related hepatocellular carcinoma. *Cell PhysiolBiochem.* (2017) 43:2379–90. doi: 10.1159/000484390
60. Tanaka A, Sakaguchi S. Regulatory T cells in cancer immunotherapy. *Cell Res.* (2017) 27:109–18. doi: 10.1038/cr.2016.151
61. Liakou CI, Kamat A, Tang DN, Chen H, Sun J, Troncoso P, et al. CTLA-4 blockade increases IFNgamma-producing CD4+ICOShi cells to shift the ratio of effector to regulatory T cells in cancer patients. *Proc Natl Acad Sci USA.* (2008) 105:14987–92. doi: 10.1073/pnas.0806075105
62. Sugiyama D, Nishikawa H, Maeda Y, Nishioka M, Tanemura A, Katayama I, et al. Anti-CCR4 mAb selectively depletes effector-type FoxP3+CD4+ regulatory T cells, evoking antitumor immune responses in humans. *Proc Natl Acad Sci USA.* (2013) 110:17945–50. doi: 10.1073/pnas.1316796110
63. Chanmee T, Ontong P, Konno K, Itano N. Tumor-associated macrophages as major players in the tumor microenvironment. *Cancers.* (2014) 6:1670–90. doi: 10.3390/cancers6031670
64. DeNardo D, Brennan D, Rexhepaj E, Ruffell B, Shiao S, Madden S, et al. Leukocyte complexity predicts breast cancer survival and functionally regulates response to chemotherapy. *Cancer Discov.* (2011) 1:54–67. doi: 10.1158/2159-8274.CD-10-0028
65. Komohara Y, Fujiwara Y, Ohnishi K, Takeya M. Tumor-associated macrophages: potential therapeutic targets for anti-cancer therapy. *Adv Drug Deliv Rev.* (2016) 99(Pt B):180–5. doi: 10.1016/j.addr.2015.11.009
66. Coca S, Perez-Piqueras J, Martinez D, Colmenarejo A, Saez MA, Vallejo C, et al. The prognostic significance of intratumoral natural killer cells in patients with colorectal carcinoma. *Cancer.* (1997.79: 2320–8.3.
67. Zhang C, Hu Y, Shi C. Targeting natural killer cells for tumor immunotherapy. *Front Immunol.* (2020) 11:60. doi: 10.3389/fimmu.2020.00060
68. Parker B, Rautela J, Hertzog P. Antitumour actions of interferons: implications for cancer therapy. *Nat Rev Cancer.* (2016) 16:131–44. doi: 10.1038/nrc.2016.14
69. Moschos S, Varanasi S, Kirkwood JM. Interferons in the treatment of solid tumors. *Cancer Treat Res.* (2005) 126:207–41. doi: 10.1007/0-387-24361-5_9
70. Budhwani M, Mazzieri R, Dolcetti R. Plasticity of type I interferon-mediated responses in cancer therapy: from anti-tumor immunity to resistance. *Front Oncol.* (2018) 8:322. doi: 10.3389/fonc.2018.00322
71. Zitvogel L, Galluzzi L, Kepp O, Smyth M, Kroemer G. Type I interferons in anticancer immunity. *Nat Rev Immunol.* (2015) 15:405–14. doi: 10.1038/nri3845
72. Crouse J, Bedenikovic G, Wiesel M, Ibberson M, Xenarios I, Von Laer D, et al. Type I interferons protect T cells against NK cell attack mediated by the activating receptor NCR1. *Immunity.* (2014) 40:961–73. doi: 10.1016/j.immuni.2014.05.003
73. Xu HC, Grusdat M, Pandyra AA, Polz R, Huang J, Sharma P, et al. Type I interferon protects antiviral CD8+ T cells from NK cell cytotoxicity. *Immunity.* (2014) 40:949–60. doi: 10.1016/j.immuni.2014.05.004
74. Bacher N, Raker V, Hofmann C, Graulich E, Schwenk M, Baumgrass R, et al. Interferon-α suppresses cAMP to disarm human regulatory T cells. *Cancer Res.* (2013) 73:5647–56. doi: 10.1158/0008-5472.CAN-12-3788
75. Novikov A, Cardone M, Thompson R, Shenderov K, Kirschman KD, Mayer-Barber KD, et al. *Mycobacterium tuberculosis* triggers host type I IFN signaling to regulate IL-1β production in human macrophages. *J Immunol.* (2011) 187:2540–7. doi: 10.4049/jimmunol.1100926
76. Mansfield AS, Heikkila PS, Vaara AT, von Smitten KA, Vakkila JM, Leidenius MH. Simultaneous Foxp3 and IDO expression is associated with sentinel lymph node metastases in breast cancer. *BMC Cancer.* (2009) 9:231. doi: 10.1186/1471-2407-9-231
77. Terawaki S, Chikuma S, Shibayama S, Hayashi T, Yoshida T, Okazaki T, et al. IFN-α directly promotes programmed cell death-1 transcription and limits the duration of T cell-mediated immunity. *J Immunol.* (2011) 186:2772–9. doi: 10.4049/jimmunol.1003208
78. Yang X, Zhang X, Fu ML, Weichselbaum RR, Gajewski TF, Guo Y, et al. Targeting the tumor microenvironment with interferon-β bridges innate and adaptive immune responses. *Cancer Cell.* (2014) 25:37–48. doi: 10.1016/j.ccr.2013.12.004
79. Benci JL, Xu B, Qiu Y, Wu TJ, Dada H, Twyman-Saint Victor C, et al. Tumor interferon signaling regulates a multigenic resistance program to immune checkpoint blockade. *Cell.* (2016) 167:1540–54.e12. doi: 10.1016/j.cell.2016.11.022
80. Snell LM, McGaha TL, Brooks DG. Type I interferon in chronic virus infection and cancer. *Trends Immunol.* (2017) 38:542–57. doi: 10.1016/j.it.2017.05.005

81. Bian S, Ni W, Zhu M, Song Q, Zhang J, Ni R, et al. Identification and validation of the N6-methyladenosine RNA methylation regulator YTHDF1 as a novel prognostic marker and potential target for hepatocellular carcinoma. *Front Mol Biosci.* (2020) 7:604766. doi: 10.3389/fmolb.2020.604766
82. Song Q, Su J, Miller L, Zhang W. scLM: automatic detection of consensus gene clusters across multiple single-cell datasets. *Genomics Proteomics Bioinformatics.* (2020). doi: 10.1016/j.gpb.2020.09.002. [Epub ahead of print].
83. Su J, Song Q, Qasem S, O'Neill S, Lee J, Furdui C, et al. Multi-omics analysis of brain metastasis outcomes following craniotomy. *Front Oncol.* (2020) 10:615472. doi: 10.3389/fonc.2020.615472
84. Song Q, Su J. DSTG: deconvoluting spatial transcriptomics data through graph-based artificial intelligence. *Briefings Bioinformatics.* (2021) 22:bbaa414. doi: 10.1093/bib/bbaa414
85. Song Q, Su J, Zhang W. scGCN is a graph convolutional networks algorithm for knowledge transfer in single cell omics. *Nat Commun.* (2021) 12:3826. doi: 10.1038/s41467-021-24172-y

13

The N6-Methyladenosine Modification and its Role in mRNA Metabolism and Gastrointestinal Tract Disease

Teng Cai [1,2], Lawrence Lawer Atteh [1], Xianzhuo Zhang [1], Chongfei Huang [1], Mingzhen Bai [1], Haidong Ma [1], Chao Zhang [1], Wenkang Fu [1], Long Gao [1], Yanyan Lin [3,4] and Wenbo Meng [1,3,4*]*

[1] The First Clinical Medical College, Lanzhou University, Lanzhou, China, [2] Gansu Province Key Laboratory Biotherapy and Regenerative Medicine, Lanzhou, China, [3] The Department of General Surgery, The First Hospital of Lanzhou University, Lanzhou, China, [4] Gansu Province Institute of Hepatopancreatobiliary Surgery, Lanzhou, China

***Correspondence:**
Wenbo Meng
mengwb@lzu.edu.cn
Yanyan Lin
ldyy_linyy@lzu.edu.cn

The N6-methyladenosine (m6A) modification is the most abundant internal modification of messenger RNA (mRNA) in higher eukaryotes. Under the actions of methyltransferase, demethylase and methyl-binding protein, m6A resulting from RNA methylation becomes dynamic and reversible, similar to that from DNA methylation, and this effect allows the generated mRNA to participate in metabolism processes, such as splicing, transport, translation, and degradation. The most common tumors are those found in the gastrointestinal tract, and research on these tumors has flourished since the discovery of m6A. Overall, further analysis of the mechanism of m6A and its role in tumors may contribute to new ideas for the treatment of tumors. m6A also plays an important role in non-tumor diseases of the gastrointestinal tract. This manuscript reviews the current knowledge of m6A-related proteins, mRNA metabolism and their application in gastrointestinal tract disease.

Keywords: N6-methyladenosine, mRNA metabolism, gastrointestinal tract, tumor, non-tumor diseases

INTRODUCTION

Epigenetics refers to heritable changes in gene expression or cell phenotypes that usually occur without alteration of the DNA sequence but rather result in slight or substantial modifications to DNA or RNA. To date, more than 100 types of RNA modifications, including mRNA, tRNA, rRNA, and lncRNA modifications, have been discovered (1). The most common modification of RNA is methylation, and the N6-methyladenosine (m6A) modification is the most common modification of mammalian mRNA (2).

m6A is a posttranscriptional modification through which a methyltransferase methylates the 6th nitrogen atom of adenine (A). m6A was first detected on mRNA in hepatocellular carcinoma cells (3) and later on non-coding RNAs such as miRNA (4), circRNA (5), lncRNA (6), and snRNA (7). Similar to the results observed with DNA methylation, the m6A modification of mRNA is a reversible and dynamic modification process catalyzed by the actions of methylases and demethylases. The rapid development of immune coprecipitation and RNA sequencing technology in recent years has led to great progress in research on the m6A modification of mRNA, which have led to a deeper understanding of the mechanism of m6A and its role, particularly in tumors. In this paper, the relationship between m6A-related proteins, mRNA metabolism and digestive system tumors is described in detail.

DISCOVERY AND DISTRIBUTION OF m6A

The m6A modification of mRNA is a posttranscriptional modification in which the 6th nitrogen atom of adenine is methylated by a methyltransferase (8). This modification can affect the stability, splicing, transport, nucleation and translation of mRNA (9–12). m6A was first discovered in bacteria by Dunn and Smith (13). In 1974, Desrosiers et al. (3) observed the methylation of mRNA in liver cancer cells and found that m6A accounted for ~80% of modifications and could be regarded as the most important mode of methylation. In general, m6A can be found on many eukaryotic (14–18) and viral (19–21) mRNAs. Although m6A was discovered early and is widely distributed, the related research progress has been slow due to technical limitations. However, the presence of m6A has gained recognition, and two studies in 2012 (8, 9) detected more than 12,000 m6A sites in human and mouse cells, including more than 7,000 types of mRNAs and more than 300 types of lncRNAs. m6A mainly clusters around stop codons, 3′ untranslated regions (3′ UTRs) and internal long exons of mRNA, and the sites are highly conserved. In other words, m6A modification mainly occurs in the highly conserved sequence RRACH (R = G or A; H = A, C, or U). This modification also occurs on other RNAs, such as tRNA and rRNA, but the related conserved sequence is different from that found for mRNA (9). In addition to the type of RNA, the distribution of m6A is specific in human tissues. For example, the content of m6A in the liver, kidney and brain is significantly higher than that in other tissues (8), which indicates that m6A may also play a vital role in the differentiation and development of tissues and organs. Furthermore, m6A expression varies among cancer cell lines and is closely related to the self-renewal of tumor stem cells in tumorigenesis (22).

m6A-RELATED ENZYMES

The discovery of fat mass and obesity-associated protein (FTO), a type of m6A demethylase (23), revealed that the m6A modification of mRNA is a dynamic and reversible process influenced by three enzymes: methyltransferases ("writers"), demethylases ("erasers") and methyl binding proteins ("readers") (**Figure 1**).

m6A Writers

The m6A methyltransferase complex comprises methyltransferase-like 3 (METTL3), methyltransferase-like 14 (METTL14) and Wilms tumor 1-associated protein (WTAP). The complex utilizes S-adenosylmethionine (SAM) as the methyl group donor to methylate the 6th nitrogen atom of adenine to form m6A. METTL3, which is also called MT-A70, was the earliest discovered m6A methyltransferase and was originally isolated and purified from HeLa cells (24). METTL3 has SAM-binding activity and is highly conserved (25, 26). Because almost all m6A methylation modifications are lost after METTL3 knockdown (27), METTL3 is a key component of the m6A methyltransferase complex and the only methyltransferase that is currently known to bind to SAM. METTL14, another member of the methyltransferase complex, showed high (43%) homology to METTL3 (28). As observed in previous studies, the knockdown of METTL14 in HeLa cells decreases the m6A methylation level; thus, METTL14 is another important component of the m6A methyltransferase complex (28). Although METTL14 exhibits high homology with METTL3, it lacks a SAM-binding region and thus cannot bind to SAM. METTL14 is mainly responsible for the identification and localization of subunits, whereas METTL3 has catalytic activity (28). METTL3 and METTL14 interact at a 1:1 ratio to form a stable methyltransferase complex and catalyze the m6A modification of mRNA *in vivo* (29). Moreover, *in vitro* experiments have shown that METTL14 exhibits higher enzyme activity than METTL3, and their heterodimer exhibits markedly enhanced enzyme activity than either enzyme alone, which indicates that the two enzymes play a synergistic role in the methylation process (28, 30–32). WTAP is the third most important component of the methyltransferase complex. Similar to METTL14, WTAP lacks a SAM-binding region and has no catalytic activity. However, the knockdown of WTAP results in the absence of METTL3 and METTL14 at nuclear speckles and decreases the m6A level. Therefore, WTAP may colocalize at nuclear speckles by recruiting the METTL3-METTL14 heterodimer to promote the m6A modification of mRNA (33). In recent years, many new methyltransferase components, such as KIAA1429, RBM15/RBM15B, and METTL16, have been identified. KIAA1429 is mainly involved in mRNA 3′UTR and stop codon methylation, and its silencing reduces the m6A levels (34). Another study showed that interfering with the expression of KIAA1429 in lung cancer cells decreases the level of m6A, and the effect was more obvious than that observed with METTL3 or METTL14. Nevertheless, the role of KIAA1429 in the methyltransferase complex remains unclear (35). RBM15/RBM15B can interact with METTL3 and bind to the U-rich region near the m6A modification site to recruit methyltransferases to a methylation site, which requires the participation of WTAP (36, 37). METTL16, a newly discovered methyltransferase, correlates positively with m6A expression and is mainly involved in the methylation modification of U6 nucleolar RNA (U6 snRNA) and methionine adenosine transferase 2A (MAT2A) mRNA (7, 38).

m6A Erasers

The main m6A demethylases are FTO and AlkB homolog 5 (ALKBH5). FTO is a member of the Fe(II)- and α-ketoglutarate-dependent dioxygenase ALKB protein family, which is widely found in human tissues and primarily involved in the regulation of fat and energy metabolism (39). FTO also plays an important role in diabetes, cardiovascular diseases and tumors (40, 41). In 2011, FTO was proven to be a demethylase involved in the demethylation of m6A (23). Indeed, the knockdown of FTO increases the m6A level but does not affect the expression of METTL3, which indicates an independent modification of m6A by FTO. Overall, the m6A modification of mRNA is a reversible and dynamic process, and a new era of m6A research has begun. ALKBH5, the second discovered demethylase, also

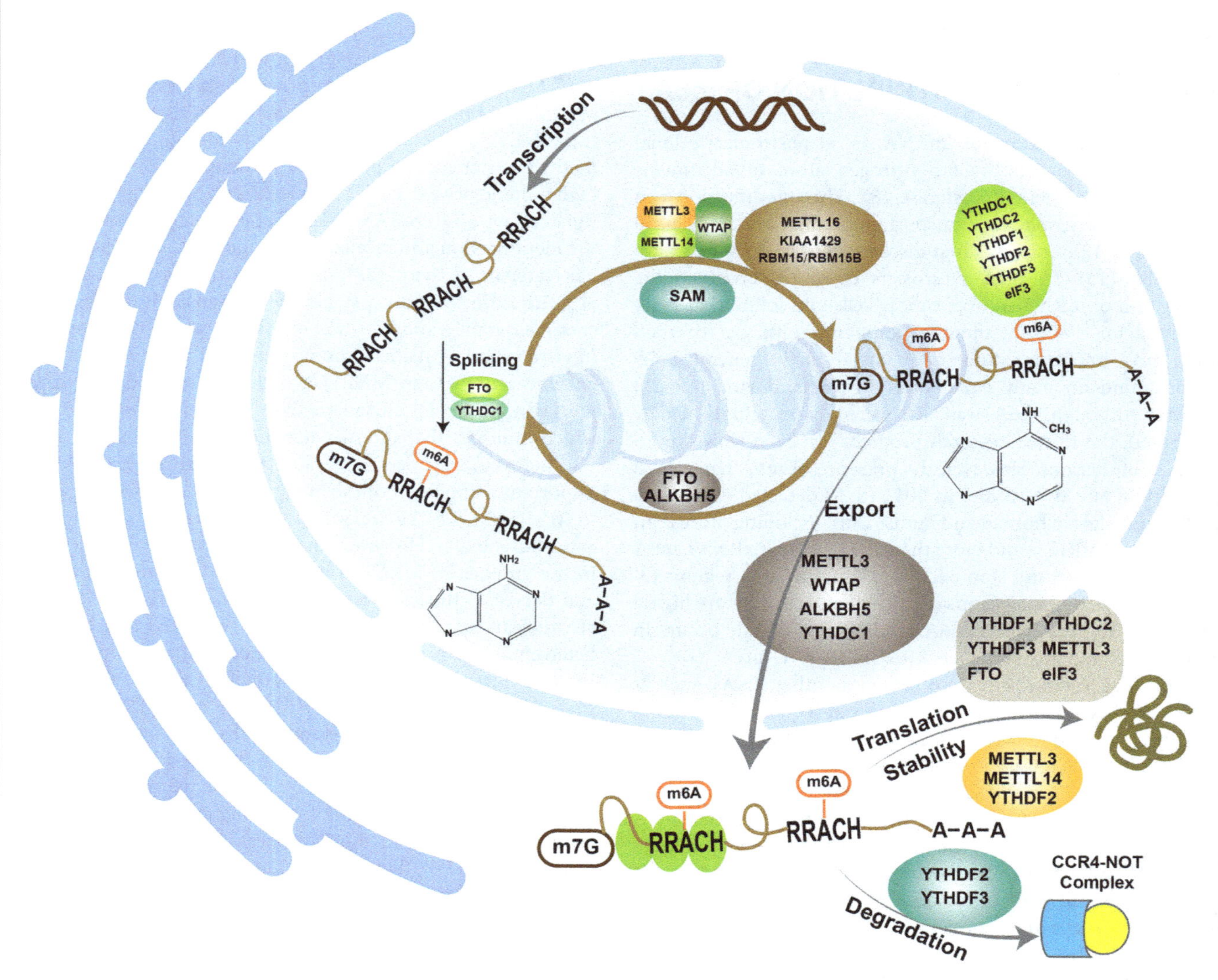

FIGURE 1 | m6A participates in various metabolic processes related to mRNAs.

belongs to the ALKB family, and its expression is negatively correlated with the m6A modification of mRNA (42). Unlike other members of the family, ALKBH5 only demethylates m6A on single-stranded RNA/DNA (43). Although ALKBH5 and FTO are homologous, they act independently, do not interfere with each other and exhibit some differences. ALKBH5 is mainly localized to the nucleus and can directly alter the m6A levels via demethylation. Most FTO is located in nuclear speckles, and hm6A and fm6A, which are known as intermediates, is needed for m6A demethylation by FTO (44). ALKBH5 is mainly expressed in the testis and is involved in sperm formation (42), whereas FTO exists in a wide range of human tissues but is mainly expressed in the brain. In addition to its effect on m6A, FTO demethylates m6Am, and its activity on m6Am is 100 times higher than that on m6A. The real substrate of FTO may be m6Am rather than m6A (45).

m6A Readers

In addition to methyltransferase and demethylase, the m6A modification of mRNA requires the involvement of methyl-binding proteins that recognize m6A sites. The readers identified to date mainly include YTH domain proteins, eukaryotic translation initiation factor 3 (eIF3) and human heterogeneous nuclear ribonucleoprotein A2B1 (HNRNPA2B1). The YTH domain proteins are further divided into the DC (YTHDC1 and YTHDC2) and DF (YTHDF1, YTHDF2, and YTHDF3) families. The three YTHDF proteins exhibit a similar structure, are mainly distributed in the cytoplasm, and can bind to all m6A sites on mRNA (9, 11). Among these proteins, YTHDF2 was the first reader found to degrade m6A RNA through the CCR4-NOT complex (46). YTHDF1 is involved in protein translation, but the process requires eIF3 and other factors (12). Although the regulatory function of YTHDF3 remains unclear, it has been reported to act in synergy with YTHDF1 to promote the translation of methylated RNA and synergizes with YTHDF2 to accelerate mRNA decay (47, 48). YTHDC is mainly distributed in the nucleus. YTHDC1 is involved in the modification of immature mRNA, and some nuclear non-coding RNAs regulate mRNA splicing and mediate the transfer of m6A mRNA from the nucleus to the cytoplasm (49, 50). YTHDC2 can improve the target translation efficiency and reduce the mRNA abundance (51). Studies have also shown that YTHDC2 can promote colon cancer metastasis through HIF-1 and is a potential diagnostic and therapeutic target of this tumor (52). eIF3 mediates translation initiation by binding to the 5′UTR of m6A mRNA in two ways: direct binding and indirect binding through YTHDF (12, 53). HNRNPA2B1, which is mainly located in the nucleus, recognizes m6A sites on precursor miRNAs through interaction with DGCR8, participates in the splicing and processing of precursor miRNAs and thus regulates the generation of mature miRNAs (54).

m6A AND mRNA

m6A is involved in mRNA metabolism (**Figure 1**).

m6A Influences mRNA Maturation

mRNA maturation includes 5′-capping, 3′-tailing and intron splicing. More m6A sites are found on premRNA than on mature mRNA, which indicates that introns also contain m6A sites. The m6A modification mainly occurs in the nucleus with the splicing of introns, which leads to a reduction in the number of m6A sites on mature mRNA (55). Many m6A modification-related proteins, writers (such as METTL3, METTL14, and WTAP), erasers (such as FTO and ALKBH5) and readers (YTHDC1), are primarily found in nuclear speckles (23, 33, 42, 49, 56). As mentioned above, the m6A modification may occur mainly in the nucleus, where m6A plays a role in mRNA splicing. The knockdown of METTL3 in mouse embryonic stem cells results in exon hopping and intron retention splicing abnormalities (27). Serine/arginine-rich splicing factor 2 (SRSF2) is an important splicing factor. Zhao et al. found that the knockdown of FTO in 3T3-L1 preadipocytes increases the m6A level in premRNA, which further promotes the binding ability to SRSF2 and results in an increase in target exons (57). FTO regulates differentiation by regulating the m6A levels around splice sites to control exon splicing of the adipogenic regulator RUNX1T1. YTHDC1 can block the binding of SRSF10 (SRp38) to mRNA by recruiting SRSF3 (SRp20), promoting an increase in the exons of targeted mRNA and thus aiding the selective splicing of mRNA (49). Dominissini et al. (9) found that the knockout of METTL3 reduces the level of m6A on mRNA and also decreases the level of gene expression through effects on the p53 signaling pathway and apoptosis. Thus, m6A plays an important role in mRNA splicing and promotes mRNA maturation through splicing.

m6A Affects mRNA Export

Gene expression involves transcription, i.e., mRNA synthesis, and translation, i.e., protein synthesis, which utilize DNA and mRNA as templates, respectively. The connection of the two processes requires the transfer of mRNA from the nucleus to the cytoplasm, which is a process termed export. Changes in export, including enhancement and suppression, alters gene expression. m6A can affect the export of mRNA. Fustin et al. found that silencing the m6A methylase METTL3 inhibits m6A methylation, which suppresses the export of mRNA and delays its processing (58). ALKBH5 also affects the export of mRNA, and its knockdown enhances the process (42).

m6A Affects mRNA Translation

There is no unified conclusion regarding the effect of m6A on mRNA translation: m6A can promote or inhibit translation or may have no effect. Earlier studies have suggested that the translational effect of m6A-containing mRNA is 1.5 times greater than that of m6A-free mRNA (59). METTL3 can improve the translation of a target mRNA by recruiting eIF3 to the translation initiation complex, and this process is independent of its methyltransferase activity (60). Additionally, YTHDF1 promotes mRNA translation with eIF3 participation (12), although m6A also reportedly decreases mRNA translation (61). Hess et al. found that the knockdown of FTO in mice lead to an increase in m6A and a significant increase in mRNA, and the corresponding protein levels increase, decrease or show no significant change (62). The reasons for these observations remain unclear but may be related to tissue specificity or m6A sites, and further study is needed.

m6A Regulates mRNA Stability

m6A can affect not only the splicing, translation and export of mRNA but also its stability. Dominissini et al. found that the knockdown of METTL3 decreased the m6A mRNA and gene expression levels, which indicates that m6A promotes the stability of mRNA (9). However, Wang et al. studied mouse embryonic stem cells and found that m6A is negatively correlated with mRNA stability (32). The knockdown of METTL3 and METTL14 decreases the level of mRNA m6A, which promotes the binding of human antigen R (HuR) to mRNA and thus increases its stability. Xie et al. (63) found that METTL3 could induce the downregulation of BATF2 expression in gastric cancer (GC) because METTL3 catalyzes the m6A modification of BATF2 mRNA, which reduces mRNA stability. Yan et al. (64) also reported that METTL3 can reduce the stability of PTEN mRNA and thus promotes the proliferation, migration and invasion of GC cells. Interestingly, METTL3 reportedly increases mRNA stability in GC. Wang et al. (65) found that H3K27 could acetylate METTL3 to increase its expression in GC, and this increased METTL3 level could induce the m6A modification of HDGF mRNA to increase its mRNA stability. HDGF promotes tumor growth and liver metastasis by promoting tumor angiogenesis. In addition, METTL3 can increase its stability through the m6A modification of ARHGAP5 mRNA in GC cells, which results in drug resistance (66). In colorectal cancer (CRC), Sec62 binds to β-catenin to inhibit its degradation and enhance WNT signaling, which leads to increased stemness and chemoresistance in CRC cells. The increase in Sec62 is caused by METTL3 increasing the stability of its mRNA (67). YTHDF2 also affects mRNA stability. Wang et al. reported that the C-terminal domain of YTHDF2 selectively binds to mRNA-containing m6A but that the N-terminal domain is responsible for binding to the YTHDF2-mRNA complex and directing it to the cellular RNA decay site for mRNA degradation (11). The knockdown of YTHDF2 increases the mRNA stability and prolongs the lifespan. Du et al. also confirmed that YTHDF2 can reduce the stability of m6A mRNA through the CCR4-NOT complex, which leads to its degradation (46). In CRC, YTHDF2 can increase the m6A modification of GSK3β mRNA, reduce the stability of GSK3β mRNA, and promote its degradation, which induces CRC cell proliferation and tumor progression (68). In addition, insulin-like growth factor 2 mRNA-binding proteins (IGF2BPs) dynamically promote RNA stability and/or increase mRNA storage under different physiological conditions (69). The above-mentioned studies indicate that the regulation of mRNA stability by m6A is not merely related to the cell type; that is, the same m6A-related protein may play opposite roles in different cells, and these different roles may also be related to external factors.

m6A AND GASTROINTESTINAL TRACT TUMORS

Hepatocellular Carcinoma and Cholangiocarcinoma

Digestive system tumors are the most common types of tumors, and many m6A-related proteins play important roles in the development and onset of these tumors. As the core component of the m6A methyltransferase complex, METTL3 is significantly increased in HCC tissues and associated with the clinical aspects of tumors (70). METTL3 inhibits the expression of SOCS2 through an m6A-YTHDF2-dependent mechanism and thus plays a role in HCC.

The knockdown of METTL3 inhibits HCC growth and metastasis, whereas its overexpression has the opposite effect. Interestingly, another study found that the m6A levels in normal liver tissues, adjacent normal liver tissues, and HCC tissues are successively reduced, which indicates that the m6A levels decrease from normal tissues to HCC tissues and that a low level of m6A is mainly associated with the downregulation of METTL14 (71). In addition to the occurrence of HCC, METTL14 downregulation is related to the downregulation of micRNA126 by interacting with DGCR8 to promote HCC metastasis. Cellular experiments have also demonstrated that METTL14 is negatively associated with HCC invasion and metastasis. This study also found that FTO is significantly downregulated in liver cancer tissues. A possible explanation is that METTL14 downregulation causes a decrease in the m6A levels and thereby leads to the downregulation of FTO to compensate for demethylation. Although m6A methylation appears to be a dynamic reversible process, there is no direct evidence. For the same tumor, two studies found that different m6A-related proteins play a major role, which may be due to sample error, and further investigation is thus needed. Another study found that YTHDF2 exhibits significantly higher expression in HCC tissues, whereas the change in YTHDF2 is negatively regulated by micRNA145 (72). In HepG2 cells, micRNA145 targets and binds to the 3′UTR of YTHDF2 mRNA, which causes a decrease in the YTHDF2 mRNA and protein levels and a decrease in the m6A levels. However, this study only found changes in the expression of the reading protein YTHDF2 in liver cancer and did not address the role of m6A in liver cancer. Moreover, only one liver cancer cell line, HepG2, was used, and no *in vivo* or *in vitro* experiments were performed. Regardless of these limitations, these two studies show that m6A-related proteins and miRNAs can interact and regulate each other and play a role in the occurrence and development of liver cancer. YTHDF1 has also been confirmed to be abnormally expressed in liver cancer, and its expression is upregulated in tumor tissues (73). Unfortunately, this study was based only on clinical data, and no *in vivo* and *in vitro* experiments were performed for verification; thus, the role of YTHDF1 in liver cancer needs to be further explored.

After primary liver cancer, CCA is the second most common malignant tumor of the hepatobiliary system, accounting for 10–15% of all hepatobiliary malignancies. Due to the absence of obvious symptoms at the early stage and the lack of specific diagnostic markers, most CCA cases are at an inoperable stage at the time of diagnosis (74). Although few studies have investigated m6A in CCA, a previous study showed that WTAP expression is increased in CCA tissues and that its overexpression or knockdown affects the metastatic ability of CCA. Nonetheless, this study failed to indicate whether the effect of WTAP on CCA is related to the m6A modification (75). The relationship between m6A and CCA is relatively clear with regard to FTO (76). FTO is significantly reduced in intrahepatic CCA and is associated with tumor differentiation and patient prognosis. The knockdown or overexpression of FTO decreases or increases the sensitivity of intrahepatic cholangiocarcinoma cells to cisplatin, respectively. FTO overexpression also inhibits tumor growth in mice. However, the study only examined intrahepatic CCA, excluded a large proportion of extrahepatic CCA cases, and did not elucidate the exact mechanism of action of FTO. Therefore, the role of m6A in cholangiocarcinoma remains unclear.

GC

In recent years, a number of studies have shown that m6A, particularly METTL3, is closely related to the occurrence and development of GC. Wang et al. found that the expression of METTL3 is significantly increased in GC tissues and associated with poor prognosis (65). Through a process mediated by P300, H3K27 acetylates METTL3 to increase its expression, and increased METTL3 promotes the m6A methylation of the mRNA of the downstream protein HDGF to enhance its stability. HDGF promotes tumor growth and liver metastasis by promoting tumor angiogenesis on the one hand and activating the expression of GLUT4 and ENO2 on the other hand, which results in promotion of glycolysis in GC cells. This study also comprises the first investigation that combines m6A with glucose metabolism to study its role in GC. Su et al. found that most m6A methylation-related proteins (METTL3, METTL14, WTAP, KIAA1429, RBM15, ZC3H13, YTHDC1, YTHDC2, YTHDF1, YTHDF2, HNRNPC, and FTO) are more highly expressed in GC tissues than in normal tissues and that patients with poor prognosis exhibit higher FTO expression (77). Yang et al.

observed higher levels of m6A in GC tissues than in adjacent tissues (78). Subsequently, these researchers detected methylases related to m6A and found that the mRNA levels of METTL3 and METTL14 are significantly increased but that WTAP, ALKBH5, and FTO did not exhibit significant changes. The role of METTL3 in the genesis and development of GC has been elucidated through its downstream targeting of the MYC pathway, and the results show that METTL3 acts as an oncogene in GC. However, both of these studies have shortcomings. The former study did not include any practical investigations, and all the results were based on database analysis and thus cannot be easily applied to clinical treatment. Although the latter study investigated the m6A modification of downstream targets, it did not specify which protein was regulated by m6A and did not evaluate the function of downstream targets. Liu et al. also confirmed that the m6A level is increased in GC tissues compared with adjacent tissues and found that METTL3 playa a major role among m6A-related proteins (79). METTL3 is elevated in tumor tissues and increases with progression of the tumor stage: a higher expression is associated with a worse prognosis. Cellular experiments have further demonstrated that METTL3 affects the proliferation and migration ability of GC cells by regulating the expression levels of GFI-1 and epithelial-mesenchymal transition (EMT). Xie et al. (63) found that BATF2 is a tumor suppressor in GC and exhibits significantly decreased mRNA and protein levels in GC tissues. However, the downregulation of BATF2 is due to the m6A modification of its mRNA by METTL3, which reduces its stability. This study combined the regulation of mRNA metabolism by m6A with its role in tumors and fundamentally illustrated the action of m6A in GC. In addition, Lin et al. (80) found that METTL3 can promote the proliferation, migration and invasion ability of GC cells by inhibiting apoptosis and activating the AKT pathway. Yue et al. (81) also reported that the expression of METTL3 is higher in GC tissues than in adjacent normal tissues and increases with progression of the tumor stage. Mechanistically, METTL3 affects the migration and invasion ability of GC cells by regulating the expression of zinc finger MYM-type containing 1 (ZMYM1) and promoting EMT. This process also involves the reader protein HuR. In addition to the role of m6A in GC through its effects on other factors, its related proteins themselves may also be regulated by non-coding RNAs and play a role in GC. Yan et al. (64) showed that the lncRNA LINC00470 is highly expressed in GC tissues. With involvement of the reader protein YTHDF2, the lncRNA LINC00470 affects the stability of PTEN by regulating the expression of METTL3, and this lncRNA also affects the proliferation, migration and invasion ability of GC cells. He et al. (82) confirmed that METTL3 affects the proliferation and apoptosis of GC cells by regulating SEC62, even though METTL3 itself is inhibited by miR-4429. These experiments all indicate that METTL3 expression is increased in GC but through different pathways, which indicates that the same m6A-related protein might play a role in the same tumor via different mechanisms. m6A is involved in the occurrence and development of GC and also plays an important role in the chemotherapy resistance of GC. METTL3 increases the stability of ARHGAP5 mRNA through the m6A modification and thereby causes drug resistance (66).

Pancreatic Cancer

The role of m6A in pancreatic cancer has also been probed. Studies have found that both the mRNA and protein levels of YTHDF2 in pancreatic cancer tissues are significantly higher than those in paratumor tissues, and the expression of YTHDF2 tends to increase as the stage of the disease advances (83). Interestingly, this study found that YTHDF2 plays a different role in the proliferation, invasion, metastasis and EMT of pancreatic cancer cells. The knockout of YTHDF2 inhibits the proliferative ability of pancreatic cancer cells, although the invasive and metastatic abilities and EMT are enhanced, possibly due to different modes of action. Nonetheless, the study had an obvious deficiency, namely, a lack of clinical specimens. The analysis of the clinical relationship between YTHDF2 and pancreatic cancer was based only on a database analysis without any actual verification, and no *in vivo* studies were performed. The role of the m6A demethylase ALKBH5 in pancreatic cancer has also been reported (84): the mRNA level of m6A in pancreatic cancer tissues is significantly increased due to a decrease in the demethylase ALKBH5. ALKBH5 acts as a tumor suppressor *in vitro* and *in vivo* in pancreatic cancer and can inhibit its growth and metastasis by targeting PER1. Moreover, Zhang et al. (85) found that the expression of miR-25-3p is significantly higher in tumor tissues than in adjacent tissues from patients with pancreatic cancer who smoke and that a higher expression was associated with a worse prognosis. This phenomenon may be related to m6A, i.e., cigarette smoke condensate (CSC)-induced promoter hypomethylation upregulates METTL3 expression, and METTL3 promotes the maturation of miR-25-3p by the m6A modification. In short, smoking plays a role in the development and progression of pancreatic cancer through the METTL3/miR-25-3p/PHLPP2/AKT regulatory axis. This study is very interesting because it links smoking with m6A, which not only highlights new directions for pancreatic cancer treatment but also provides evidence that smoking is a risk factor for pancreatic cancer. m6A can influence not only the occurrence and metastasis of pancreatic cancer but also its resistance to drugs (86). The knockdown of METTL3 in pancreatic cancer cell lines increases the sensitivity of the cells to gemcitabine, cisplatin and other drugs, even though the morphology and proliferative abilities of the cells did not change, providing a new potential target for the treatment of pancreatic cancer. However, this study has some shortcomings, such as too few cell types and no *in vivo* experiments. The study was only superficial and did not explain the mechanism through which METTL3 increases drug sensitivity. Further research is needed.

CRC

In addition to liver, stomach and pancreatic cancers, the clinical characteristics of CRC are also related to m6A. As the major m6A methyltransferase, METTL3 plays an important role in CRC (87–89). Peng et al. (87) found abnormal m6A modification in CRC. In normal tissues, paracancerous tissues and tumor tissues, the expression level of m6A exhibits a gradually increasing trend, and this change is mainly caused by increased expression of METTL3. Both *in vivo* and *in vitro* experiments have shown that the downregulation and upregulation of METTL3 reduces and

TABLE 1 | The roles and mechanisms of the m6A modification in digestive system tumors.

Cancer	m6A Regulator	Type	Role	Change	Mechanism	References
HCC	METTL14	Writer	Suppressor	Down	METTL14 downregulates micRNA126 by reacting with DGCR8.	(71)
	METTL3	Writer	Promoter	Up	METTL3 represses SOCS2 expression through an m6A/YTHDF2-dependent mechanism.	(70)
	YTHDF2	Reader	Promoter	Up	miR-145 modulates the m6A levels by targeting the 3'-UTR of YTHDF2 mRNA.	(72)
	YTHDF1	Reader	Promoter	Up	YTHDF1 regulates HCC cell cycle progression and metabolism.	(73)
CCA	WTAP	Writer	Promoter	Up	WTAP induces the expression of MMP7, MMP28, cathepsin H and Muc1.	(75)
	FTO	Eraser	Suppressor	Down	FTO regulates ICC progression through multiple key oncogenes and suppressors.	(76)
GC	METTL3	Writer	Promoter	Up	The METTL3-mediated m6A modification of HDGF mRNA promotes GC progression.	(65)
	FTO	Eraser	Promoter	Up	NA	(77)
	METTL3	Writer	Promoter	Up	METTL3 regulates the MYC pathway.	(78)
	METTL3	Writer	Promoter	Up	METTL3 affects the proliferation and migration abilities of GC cells by regulating the expression level of GFI-1 and EMT.	(79)
	METTL3	Writer	Promoter	Up	METTL3 regulates BATF2 mRNA and represses its expression.	(63)
	METTL3	Writer	Promoter	Up	METTL3 promotes the proliferation, migration and invasion of GC cells by activating the Akt pathway.	(80)
	METTL3	Writer	Promoter	Up	METTL3 enhances ZMYM1 mRNA expression through the m6A/HuR-dependent pathway.	(81)
	METTL3	Writer	Promoter	Up	LINC00470 promotes GC progression through the METTL3/PTEN axis.	(64)
	METTL3	Writer	Promoter	Up	miR-4429 inhibits GC progression through the METTL3/SEC62 axis.	(82)
	METTL3	Writer	Promoter	Up	ARHGAP5-AS1 recruits METTL3 for the m6A modification of ARHGAP5 mRNA.	(66)
Pancreatic cancer	YTHDF2	Reader	Promoter	Up	YTHDF2 regulates EMT probably via YAP signaling.	(83)
	ALKBH5	Eraser	Suppressor	Down	ALKBH5 loss downregulates the PER1 mRNA levels in a m6A/YTHDF2-dependent manner.	(84)
	METTL3	Writer	Promoter	UP	Cigarette smoke promotes the development and progression of pancreatic cancer via the METTL3/miR-25-3p/PHLPP2/AKT regulatory axis.	(85)
	METTL3	Writer	Promoter	Up	METTL3 influences the sensitivity of pancreatic cancer cells to anticancer reagents *via* a ubiquitin-dependent process, RNA splicing and the regulation of cellular processes.	(86)
CRC	METTL3	Writer	Promoter	Up	METTL3 promotes metastasis of CRC via the miR-1246/SPRED2/MAPK signaling pathway.	(87)
	METTL3	Writer	Promoter	Up	METTL3 facilitates CRC progression via a m6A/IGF2BP2-dependent mechanism.	(88)
	METTL3	Writer	Suppressor	Down	METTL3 suppresses CRC proliferation and migration through p38/ERK pathways.	(89)
	METTL3	Writer	Promoter	UP	β-catenin suppresses miR455-3p to increase the m6A modification of HSF1 mRNA.	(92)
	METTL3	Writer	Promoter	UP	m6A modification/Sec62/β-catenin molecular axis.	(67)
	YTHDF1	Reader	Promoter	Up	The oncogenic transcription factor c-Myc regulates YTHDF1 in CRC.	(90)
	YTHDF1	Reader	Promoter	Up	YTHDF1 inhibits Wnt/β-catenin pathway activity.	(68)
	YTHDF2	Reader	Promoter	Up	miR-6125/YTHDF2/GSK3β/β-catenin/cyclin D1 regulatory axis	(93)
Colon tumor	YTHDC2	Reader	Promoter	Up	YTHDC2 contributes to colon tumor metastasis by promoting the translation of HIF-1α.	(52)
	eIF3	Reader	Promoter	Up	NA	(91)

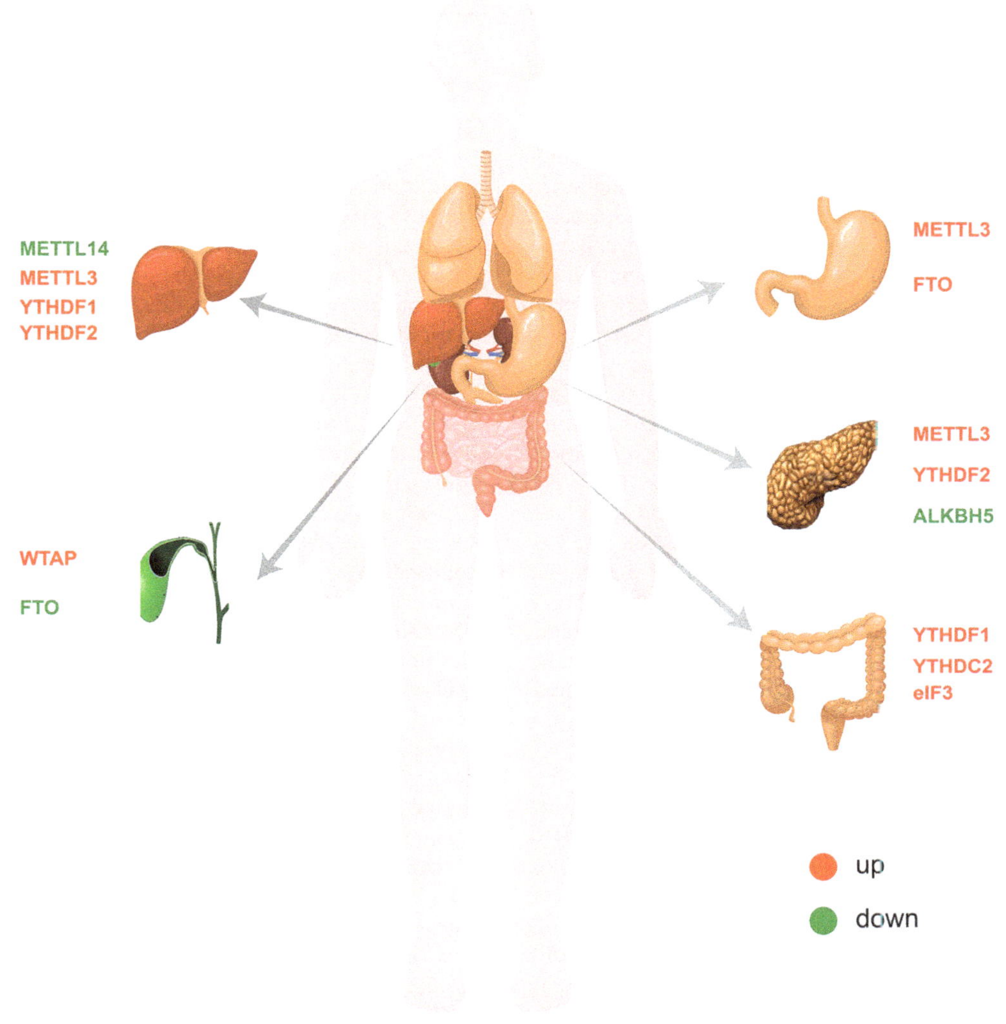

FIGURE 2 | Expression of m6A-related proteins in digestive system tumors.

enhances the metastatic ability of CRC, respectively, and this regulation is exerted through the METTL3/miR-1246/SPRED2 axis. Another study reached a similar conclusion. Li et al. (88) found that the expression of METTLE3 is significantly increased in primary CRC tissues compared with adjacent normal tissues and that METTL3 is significantly elevated in corresponding lymph node and liver metastatic foci. Patients with high METTL3 expression experience worse chemotherapy effects and shorter overall survival (OS) and disease-free survival (DFS) durations. As an oncogene, METTL3 plays a role by maintaining SOX2 expression in CRC cells through an m6A-IGF2BP2-dependent mechanism. However, there are contrasting conclusions regarding the role of METTL3 as a tumor suppressor in CRC (89). This study found that METTL3 expression is significantly negatively correlated with the tumor size and metastasis but positively correlated with patient prognosis; that is, a higher METTL3 expression in tumor is related to a better prognosis. This study further demonstrated that METTL3 plays a tumor-suppressive role in the proliferation, migration and invasion of CRC cells through the p38/ERK pathway. The reasons for the opposite conclusions reached for the same tumor and the same m6A protein may be due to sample problems, different transcripts of METTL3, or different risk factors that cause disease warrant further study. Nishizawa et al. found that YTHDF1 is an independent prognostic factor for CRC (90). YTHDF1 expression is significantly higher in CRC tissues than in normal tissues, and the YTHDF1 level is positively correlated with the depth of tumor invasion, lymph node metastasis, and clinical stage. The knockdown of YTHDF1 inhibits the proliferation of CRC cells and increases the sensitivity to oxaliplatin and other chemotherapeutic agents. However, this study had many limitations, such as too few clinical samples, incomprehensive experiments, no *in vivo* experiments, and no drug-resistant cell lines. Although YTHDF1 is an m6A reader, its downstream target was not identified in the study; that is, this target was not studied from the perspective of m6A. YTHDC2 also plays an important role in the metastasis of colon cancer (52). One study found a positive correlation between YTHDC2 and the clinical stage of colon cancer, including metastasis. The knockdown of YTHDC2 in colon cancer cells reduces the expression of metastasis-related proteins such as HIF-1α and inhibits tumor metastasis. The levels of eIF3 are also significantly higher in colon cancer tissues than in paratumor tissues, and the expression level of eIF3 is positively correlated with the tumor size, lymph node metastasis, distant metastasis, and vascular invasion, among others. The downregulation of eIF3 in colon cancer cells can inhibit cell proliferation and promote apoptosis (91). It should be noted that this study only collected data from patients at a single hospital for 2 years, and its limitations include a lack of representativeness, no *in vivo* experiments, a small number of experimental cells, and no mechanistic investigation. Therefore, this study has no practical reference value. The WNT signaling pathway plays a pivotal role in CRC, and m6A also reportedly plays a role through this pathway (67, 68, 92, 93). Song et al. (92) found that m6A is related to the occurrence of CRC, which is caused by METTL3 and related to the WNT signaling pathway. Increases in the expression of β-catenin increases METTL3 expression by inhibiting miR-455-3p and further increases the m6A modification of HSF1 to promote protein translation. The upregulation of β-catenin increases the HSF1 protein levels by promoting protein translation with no change in the mRNA levels or the protein half-life. In this study, the WNT signaling pathway, miRNAs and m6A were combined, and their relationship was described. Bai et al. (68) found that YTHDF1 can affect the stem cell-like activity of CRC cells and the proliferation ability of cells by affecting the cell cycle. A reduction in the expression of YTHDF1 will arrest cells at the G1 phase. Interestingly, the study found that YTHDF1 works by influencing the Wnt/β-catenin pathway rather than by being affected. However, this study also has some shortcomings, such as a small clinical sample size and many results from a database analysis. In addition to YTHDF1, YTHDF2 also affects the growth of CRC through the Wnt/β-catenin pathway (93). In CRC cells, increased protein levels of YTHDF2 are caused by decreased miR-6125. GSK3β mRNA can exhibit the M6A modification by increasing the YTHDF2 protein levels, which reduces the GSK3β mRNA stability and facilitates its degradation, and the levels of GSK3β protein and phosphorylated β-catenin are decreased. Abnormal accumulation of β-catenin activates cyclin D1 and thereby promotes CRC cell proliferation and tumor progression. This regulatory axis can be summarized as the miR-6125/YTHDF2/GSK3β/β-catenin/cyclin D1 regulatory pathway. In addition to clarifying the role of YTHDF2 in CRC, this study also noted the m6A modification site of GSK3β. m6A combined with the WNT signaling pathway not only plays a role in the occurrence and development of CRC but also leads to increases in the stemness of CRC cells and chemoresistance (67). Liu et al. found that Sec62 expression is increased in CRC. Elevated Sec62 binds to β-catenin to inhibit its degradation and enhance WNT signaling, which leads to increases in the stemness and chemoresistance of CRC cells. The elevation of Sec62 is caused by increased METTL3 expression. The m6A modification increases the stability of Sec62 mRNA.

m6A AND NON-NEOPLASTIC DISEASES OF THE GASTROINTESTINAL TRACT

In addition to playing a pivotal role in digestive system tumors, m6A also plays an important role in some non-tumor diseases. Wu et al. found that circRNAs are involved in important processes, such as the regulation of autophagy and protein digestion, in mouse models of severe acute pancreatitis. The observed changes in circRNA function are caused by increased ALKBH5 expression and decreased m6A levels (94). HBV infection is not only the main cause of chronic hepatitis but also closely related to cirrhosis and liver cancer (95). A recent study showed that the m6A modification of YTHDF2 and YTHDF3 can regulate the HBV lifecycle by decreasing HBV RNA stability and HBV protein expression or promoting the reverse transcription of pregenomic RNA (96). It has also been reported that the m6A modification can regulate the lifecycle of HCV, that METTL3 and METTL14 can negatively regulate HCV infection, and that FTO can positively regulate HCV infection. In addition, m6A does not regulate HCV translation or RNA replication but can regulate the production of infectious virus particles, which this process is negatively regulated by YTHDF proteins (97). This finding was also confirmed by Kim et al. (98). Although YTHDF proteins do not affect HCV translation and replication, YTHDC2 may be involved in the secondary structure of the HCV IRES region through its helicase domain to promote HCV IRES-mediated translation.

In addition to its roles in severe acute pancreatitis and viral hepatitis, the role of m6A in intestinal non-tumor diseases has also been studied. Wang et al. (99) found that ALKBH5 upregulates TAGLN expression by demethylating TAGLN mRNA and then inhibits the proliferation and migration of enteric neural crest cells, which results in promotion of the occurrence of Hirschsprung's disease. Lu et al. constructed a new model of METTL14 deletion-induced spontaneous colitis in mice and confirmed that METTL14 deficiency impairs the ability of naïve T cells to induce induced T_{reg} cells and thus promote the development of colitis (100). By studying the regulation of m6A on T cells, Li et al. found that METTL3 in mouse T cells could regulate T cell homeostasis by targeting the IL-7/STAT5/SOCS pathway and that the deletion of METTL3 destroys T cell homeostasis and differentiation. Naïve METTL3-deficient T cells are unable to undergo homeostatic expansion and remain significantly naïve for up to 12 weeks to prevent colitis in a lymphopenic mouse model of adoptive transfer (101). ALKBH5 plays an important role in gastric intestinal metaplasia caused by bile acid reflux (102). On the one hand, ALKBH5 abolishes YTHDF2-dependent mRNA degradation by the demethylation of ZNF333 mRNA and increases the expression of ZNF333, and on the other hand, ALKBH5 activates CDX2 by targeting the ZNF333/CYLD axis and activating NF-κB signaling. This study suggests that ALKBH5 is a promising therapeutic target for gastrointestinal metaplasia caused by bile reflux. Although the role of m6A in non-tumor diseases of the gastrointestinal tract has been studied, the research progress is limited mainly due to the following two reasons: too few types of diseases have been studied and the mechanism is unclear. The reasons for this phenomenon may be the following: First, the study of gastrointestinal non-tumor diseases mainly relies on the establishment of animal models, and the collection of sufficient clinical samples for analysis and cell experiments is difficult. Second, many diseases can be diagnosed by blood and imaging tests alone without any need for genetic testing. Third, most non-tumor diseases can be controlled or cured with medication or surgery alone.

m6A AND SMALL-MOLECULE INHIBITORS

The ultimate purpose of studying the role of m6A in tumors is to provide a new treatment direction. Many studies have reported small-molecule inhibitors of m6A, which mainly target METTL3 (103) and, in particular, FTO. A recent study reported that the small-molecule inhibitor STM2457 reduces the growth of acute myeloid leukemia (AML) and increases its differentiation and apoptosis (103). The pharmacological inhibition of METTL3 *in vivo* leads to impaired implantation and prolonged survival in a variety of mouse models of AML, particularly by targeting key stem cell subpopulations of AML. Overall, the small-molecule inhibition of METTL3 is not conducive to the maintenance of AML and exerts no significant or lasting effect on normal hematopoietic function. Qiao et al. (104) found that CHTB acts as an inhibitor of FTO and can specifically bind to it to increase the cellular m6A levels. However, the cells used in this study were not tumor cells, and whether the characteristics of the cells changed after the inhibition of FTO with CHTB is unclear. The natural compounds radicol and nafamostat mesilate inhibit FTO activity (105, 106), but these studies were not clinical studies and only demonstrated activity against FTO without any *in vivo* or *in vitro* analysis. It has also been reported that entacapone can directly bind to FTO to inhibit its activity (107). In mice with diet-induced obesity, the administration of entacapone reduces the body weight and fasting glucose concentrations, and entacapone affects gluconeogenesis in the liver and thermogenesis in adipose tissues of mice through the FTO/FOXO1 regulatory axis. Although this study was a clinical study, it was still a non-tumor study, and the results cannot be directly applied for the treatment of tumors, particularly gastrointestinal tumors. In addition to non-clinical studies, clinical studies of FTO inhibitors have been conducted. One study showed that meclofenamic acid can promote cisplatin-induced acute kidney injury by inhibiting FTO (108). *In vivo* and *in vitro* experiments have fully demonstrated that meclofenamic acid can affect the level of m6A by inhibiting FTO and increase the p53 mRNA and protein expression levels, which aggravates the acute kidney injury induced by cisplatin. Although meclofenamic acid does not affect the m6A level of mRNA, it can help clinicians avoid aggravation of but not treat the disease. Some studies have also investigated FTO inhibitors for tumors. Huang et al. (109) developed two promising FTO inhibitors, namely, FB23 and FB23-2, which can directly bind to FTO, selectively inhibit its m6A demethylase activity (particularly FB23-2), and thus play a role in AML. This study found that FB23-2 exhibits high selectivity for FTO and can significantly inhibit FTO expression to promote myeloid differentiation and apoptosis. *In vivo* experiments have also indicated that FB23-2 inhibits the progression of leukemia and improves the survival of leukemic mice. Most importantly, FB23-2 exhibits no toxicity or side effects in mice.

CONCLUSIONS AND OUTLOOK

The m6A modification, which is the most abundant epigenetic modification of mRNA in higher eukaryotes, is a process through which the genetic information of an organism can be changed without altering the genetic sequence. Similar to DNA methylation, mRNA m6A modification is a reversible and dynamic process that is performed by the interaction of writers, erasers and readers. Through methylation and demethylation, m6A can not only participate in the metabolic process of mRNA but also further affect the occurrence and development of tumors. Digestive tract tumors are the most common tumors in humans, and many studies have found that m6A plays an important role. In this review, we summarize the roles and mechanisms of the m6A modification in liver cancer (70–73), CCA (75, 76), GC (63–66, 77–82), pancreatic cancer (83–86) and CRC (87–91) (**Table 1** and **Figure 2**). These studies serve as good bases for the diagnosis and treatment of the corresponding tumors. However, the overall role of m6A in tumors remains not well-understood. In liver cancer, changes in the m6A levels are caused by increased METTL3 and/or METTL14 expression. In addition to writer proteins, reader proteins are altered in liver cancer, but their role is unclear (72, 73). For example, although many studies have confirmed that METTL3 expression is increased in GC, it plays different roles (63, 78). Thus, further details need to be revealed. Studies of the same tumor conducted by different researchers revealed that the m6A-related proteins METTL3 and FTO were important, although different results were obtained (77, 78). One study found that METTL3 but not FTO is significantly increased in cancer tissues, whereas the other study found that both were significantly increased. In CRC, different researchers even obtained completely opposite results for METTL3 expression (87–89). Moreover, the role of m6A in CCA remains unknown. Moreover, all the studies on m6A have many deficiencies, such as a lack of clinical samples, no *in vivo* or *in vitro* experiments, the inclusion of only superficial observations, no mechanistic investigation, and an inability to provide practical help for clinical application. Chemotherapy resistance has always been an important reason for poor therapeutic effects in cancer treatment, and the discovery of m6A provides a new direction to reduce chemotherapy resistance. Despite many studies in this direction, there remain limitations, and thus, the results do not provide any practical evidence for clinic application. In addition to tumors, m6A has also been studied in gastrointestinal non-tumor diseases, but the related research progress has been limited by the limitations of research methods and practical applications. The emergence of small-molecule inhibitors of m6A has provided new hope for the treatment of diseases, and many studies have explored the discovery and effects of such inhibitors. At present, the identified inhibitors mainly target two enzymes, METTL3 and in particular, FTO. Moreover, many inhibitors have only been shown to inhibit FTO, but their specific biological effects have not been explained. To date, the research on small-molecule inhibitors of m6A in tumors remains limited to AML, and studies on digestive tract tumors have not been reported. There are many difficulties regarding the application of small-molecule inhibitors of m6A to gastrointestinal malignancies. First, drugs that specifically bind to m6A-related proteins need to be identified or synthesized. Second, these drugs must act on m6A-related proteins by inhibiting their activity and not through other effects. Third, these small-molecule inhibitors must be more effective when used alone or in combination with clinically available antitumor agents. There is still a long way to go before small-molecule inhibitors can be used for the treatment of gastrointestinal malignancies. All of these problems need to be further addressed. The role of m6A in tumors is unquestionable, but there remain many issues to be resolved regarding not only gastrointestinal tumors but also other tumors. Further research will provide new directions for the diagnosis and treatment of tumors.

AUTHOR CONTRIBUTIONS

TC, WM, and YL involved in study design and drafting of the manuscript. TC and LA revised the manuscript. XZ, CH, MB, HM, CZ, WF, and LG reviewed and approved the manuscript. All authors contributed to the article and approved the submitted version.

REFERENCES

1. Sun WJ, Li JH, Liu S, Wu J, Zhou H, Qu LH, et al. RMBase: a resource for decoding the landscape of RNA modifications from high-throughput sequencing data. *Nucleic Acids Res.* (2016) 44:D259–65. doi: 10.1093/nar/gkv1036
2. Yue Y, Liu J, He C. RNA N6-methyladenosine methylation in post-transcriptional gene expression regulation. *Genes Dev.* (2015) 29:1343–55. doi: 10.1101/gad.262766.115
3. Desrosiers R, Friderici K, Rottman F. Identification of methylated nucleosides in messenger RNA from Novikoff hepatoma cells. *Proc Natl Acad Sci USA.* (1974) 71:3971–5. doi: 10.1073/pnas.71.10.3971
4. Berulava T, Rahmann S, Rademacher K, Klein-Hitpass L, Horsthemke B. N6-adenosine methylation in MiRNAs. *PLoS ONE.* (2015) 10:e0118438. doi: 10.1371/journal.pone.0118438
5. Yang Y, Fan X, Mao M, Song X, Wu P, Zhang Y, et al. Extensive translation of circular RNAs driven by N(6)-methyladenosine. *Cell Res.* (2017) 27:626–41. doi: 10.1038/cr.2017.31
6. Jacob R, Zander S, Gutschner T. The dark side of the epitranscriptome: chemical modifications in long non-coding rNAs. *Int J Mol Sci.* (2017) 182387. doi: 10.3390/ijms18112387
7. Warda AS, Kretschmer J, Hackert P, Lenz C, Urlaub H, Hobartner C, et al. Human METTL16 is a N(6)-methyladenosine (m(6)A) methyltransferase that targets pre-mRNAs and various non-coding RNAs. *EMBO Rep.* (2017) 18:2004–14. doi: 10.15252/embr.201744940
8. Meyer KD, Saletore Y, Zumbo P, Elemento O, Mason CE, Jaffrey SR. Comprehensive analysis of mRNA methylation reveals enrichment in 3′ UTRs and near stop codons. *Cell.* (2012) 149:1635–46. doi: 10.1016/j.cell.2012.05.003
9. Dominissini D, Moshitch-Moshkovitz S, Schwartz S, Salmon-Divon M, Ungar L, Osenberg S, et al. Topology of the human and mouse m6A RNA methylomes revealed by m6A-seq. *Nature.* (2012) 485:201–6. doi: 10.1038/nature11112
10. Roundtree IA, He C. Nuclear m(6)A Reader YTHDC1 Regulates mRNA Splicing. *Trends Genet.* (2016) 32:320–1. doi: 10.1016/j.tig.2016.03.006
11. Wang X, Lu Z, Gomez A, Hon GC, Yue Y, Han D, et al. N6-methyladenosine-dependent regulation of messenger RNA stability. *Nature.* (2014) 505:117–20. doi: 10.1038/nature12730
12. Wang X, Zhao BS, Roundtree IA, Lu Z, Han D, Ma H, et al. N(6)-methyladenosine modulates messenger RNA translation efficiency. *Cell.* (2015) 161:1388–99. doi: 10.1016/j.cell.2015.05.014
13. Dunn DB, Smith JD. Occurrence of a new base in the deoxyribonucleic acid of a strain of Bacterium coli. *Nature.* (1955) 175:336–7. doi: 10.1038/175336a0
14. Haugland RA, Cline MG. Post-transcriptional modifications of oat coleoptile ribonucleic acids. 5′-Terminal capping methylation of internal nucleosides in poly(A)-rich RNA. *Eur J Biochem.* (1980) 104:271–7. doi: 10.1111/j.1432-1033.1980.tb04425.x
15. Furuichi Y, Morgan M, Muthukrishnan S, Shatkin AJ. Reovirus messenger RNA contains a methylated, blocked 5′-terminal structure: m-7G(5′)ppp(5′)G-MpCp. *Proc Natl Acad Sci USA.* (1975) 72:362–6. doi: 10.1073/pnas.72.1.362
16. Desrosiers RC, Friderici KH, Rottman FM. Characterization of Novikoff hepatoma mRNA methylation and heterogeneity in the methylated 5′ terminus. *Biochemistry.* (1975) 14:4367–74. doi: 10.1021/bi00691a004
17. Perry RP, Kelley DE, Friderici K, Rottman F. The methylated constituents of L cell messenger RNA: evidence for an unusual cluster at the 5′ terminus. *Cell.* (1975) 4:387–94. doi: 10.1016/0092-8674(75)90159-2
18. Dubin DT, Taylor RH. The methylation state of poly A-containing messenger RNA from cultured hamster cells. *Nucleic Acids Res.* (1975) 2:1653–68. doi: 10.1093/nar/2.10.1653
19. Moss B, Gershowitz A, Stringer JR, Holland LE, Wagner EK. 5′-Terminal internal methylated nucleosides in herpes simplex virus type 1 mRNA. *J Virol.* (1977) 23:234–9. doi: 10.1128/jvi.23.2.234-239.1977
20. Beemon K, Keith J. Localization of N6-methyladenosine in the Rous sarcoma virus genome. *J Mol Biol.* (1977) 113:165–79. doi: 10.1016/0022-2836(77)90047-X
21. Chen-Kiang S, Nevins JR, Darnell JE. N-6-methyl-adenosine in adenovirus type 2 nuclear RNA is conserved in the formation of messenger RNA. *J Mol Biol.* (1979) 135:733–52. doi: 10.1016/0022-2836(79)90174-8
22. Cui Q, Shi H, Ye P, Li L, Qu Q, Sun G, et al. m(6)A RNA Methylation Regulates the Self-Renewal and Tumorigenesis of Glioblastoma Stem Cells. *Cell Rep.* (2017) 18:2622–34. doi: 10.1016/j.celrep.2017.02.059
23. Jia G, Fu Y, Zhao X, Dai Q, Zheng G, Yang Y, et al. N6-methyladenosine in nuclear RNA is a major substrate of the obesity-associated FTO. *Nat Chem Biol.* (2011) 7:885–7. doi: 10.1038/nchembio.687
24. Bokar JA, Rath-Shambaugh ME, Ludwiczak R, Narayan P, Rottman F. Characterization and partial purification of mRNA N6-adenosine methyltransferase from HeLa cell nuclei. Internal mRNA methylation requires a multisubunit complex. *J Biol Chem.* (1994) 269:17697–704. doi: 10.1016/S0021-9258(17)32497-3
25. Fu Y, Dominissini D, Rechavi G, He C. Gene expression regulation mediated through reversible m(6)A RNA methylation. *Nat Rev Genet.* (2014) 15:293–306. doi: 10.1038/nrg3724
26. Xiang W, Jing F, Yuan X, Zeyuan G, Delin Z, Zhu L, et al. Structural basis of N(6)-adenosine methylation by the METTL3-METTL14 complex. *Nature.* (2016) 534:18298. doi: 10.1038/nature18298
27. Geula S, Moshitch-Moshkovitz S, Dominissini D, Mansour AA, Kol N, Salmon-Divon M, et al. Stem cells. m6A mRNA methylation facilitates

resolution of naive pluripotency toward differentiation. *Science.* (2015) 347:1002–6. doi: 10.1126/science.1261417

28. Jianzhao L, Yanan Y, Dali H, Xiao W, Ye F, Liang Z, et al. A METTL3-METTL14 complex mediates mammalian nuclear RNA N6-adenosine methylation. *Nat Chem Biol.* (2014) 10:1432. doi: 10.1038/nchembio.1432
29. Wang X, Huang J, Zou T, Yin P. Human m(6)A writers: Two subunits, 2 roles. *RNA Biol.* (2017) 14:300–4. doi: 10.1080/15476286.2017.1282025
30. Wang P, Doxtader KA, Nam Y. Structural basis for cooperative function of Mettl3 and Mettl14 methyltransferases. *Mol Cell.* (2016) 63:306–17. doi: 10.1016/j.molcel.2016.05.041
31. Slobodin B, Han R, Calderone V, Vrielink J, Loayza-Puch F, Elkon R, et al. Transcription impacts the efficiency of mRNA translation via co-transcriptional N6-adenosine methylation. *Cell.* (2017) 169:326–37.e12. doi: 10.1016/j.cell.2017.03.031
32. Wang Y, Li Y, Toth JI, Petroski MD, Zhang Z, Zhao JC. N6-methyladenosine modification destabilizes developmental regulators in embryonic stem cells. *Nat Cell Biol.* (2014) 16:191–8. doi: 10.1038/ncb2902
33. Ping XL, Sun BF, Wang L, Xiao W, Yang X, Wang WJ, et al. Mammalian WTAP is a regulatory subunit of the RNA N6-methyladenosine methyltransferase. *Cell Res.* (2014) 24:177–89. doi: 10.1038/cr.2014.3
34. Yue Y, Liu J, Cui X, Cao J, Luo G, Zhang Z, et al. VIRMA mediates preferential m(6)A mRNA methylation in 3′UTR and near stop codon and associates with alternative polyadenylation. *Cell Discov.* (2018) 4:10. doi: 10.1038/s41421-018-0019-0
35. Schwartz S, Mumbach MR, Jovanovic M, Wang T, Maciag K, Bushkin GG, et al. Perturbation of m6A writers reveals two distinct classes of mRNA methylation at internal and 5′ sites. *Cell Rep.* (2014) 8:284–96. doi: 10.1016/j.celrep.2014.05.048
36. Patil DP, Chen CK, Pickering BF, Chow A, Jackson C, Guttman M, et al. m(6)A RNA methylation promotes XIST-mediated transcriptional repression. *Nature.* (2016) 537:369–73. doi: 10.1038/nature19342
37. Horiuchi K, Kawamura T, Iwanari H, Ohashi R, Naito M, Kodama T, et al. Identification of Wilms' tumor 1-associating protein complex and its role in alternative splicing and the cell cycle. *J Biol Chem.* (2013) 288:33292–302. doi: 10.1074/jbc.M113.500397
38. Pendleton KE, Chen B, Liu K, Hunter OV, Xie Y, Tu BP, et al. The U6 snRNA m(6)A methyltransferase METTL16 regulates SAM synthetase intron retention. *Cell.* (2017) 169:824–35.e14. doi: 10.1016/j.cell.2017.05.003
39. Gerken T, Girard CA, Tung YC, Webby CJ, Saudek V, Hewitson KS, et al. The obesity-associated FTO gene encodes a 2-oxoglutarate-dependent nucleic acid demethylase. *Science.* (2007) 318:1469–72. doi: 10.1126/science.1151710
40. Church C, Moir L, McMurray F, Girard C, Banks GT, Teboul L, et al. Overexpression of Fto leads to increased food intake and results in obesity. *Nat Genet.* (2010) 42:1086–92. doi: 10.1038/ng.713
41. Loos RJ, Yeo GS. The bigger picture of FTO: the first GWAS-identified obesity gene. *Nat Rev Endocrinol.* (2014) 10:51–61. doi: 10.1038/nrendo.2013.227
42. Zheng G, Dahl JA, Niu Y, Fedorcsak P, Huang CM, Li CJ, et al. ALKBH5 is a mammalian RNA demethylase that impacts RNA metabolism and mouse fertility. *Mol Cell.* (2013) 49:18–29. doi: 10.1016/j.molcel.2012.10.015
43. Tong J, Flavell RA, Li HB. RNA m(6)A modification and its function in diseases. *Front Med.* (2018) 12:481–9. doi: 10.1007/s11684-018-0654-8
44. Fu Y, Jia G, Pang X, Wang RN, Wang X, Li CJ, et al. FTO-mediated formation of N6-hydroxymethyladenosine and N6-formyladenosine in mammalian RNA. *Nat Commun.* (2013) 4:1798. doi: 10.1038/ncomms2822
45. Mauer J, Luo X, Blanjoie A, Jiao X, Grozhik AV, Patil DP, et al. Reversible methylation of m(6)Am in the 5′ cap controls mRNA stability. *Nature.* (2017) 541:371–5. doi: 10.1038/nature21022
46. Du H, Zhao Y, He J, Zhang Y, Xi H, Liu M, et al. YTHDF2 destabilizes m(6)A-containing RNA through direct recruitment of the CCR4-NOT deadenylase complex. *Nat Commun.* (2016) 7:12626. doi: 10.1038/ncomms12626
47. Li A, Chen YS, Ping XL, Yang X, Xiao W, Yang Y, et al. Cytoplasmic m(6)A reader YTHDF3 promotes mRNA translation. *Cell Res.* (2017) 27:444–7. doi: 10.1038/cr.2017.10
48. Shi H, Wang X, Lu Z, Zhao BS, Ma H, Hsu PJ, et al. YTHDF3 facilitates translation and decay of N(6)-methyladenosine-modified RNA. *Cell Res.* (2017) 27:315–28. doi: 10.1038/cr.2017.15
49. Xiao W, Adhikari S, Dahal U, Chen YS, Hao YJ, Sun BF, et al. Nuclear m(6)A reader YTHDC1 regulates mRNA splicing. *Mol Cell.* (2016) 61:507–19. doi: 10.1016/j.molcel.2016.01.012
50. Roundtree IA, Luo GZ, Zhang Z, Wang X, Zhou T, Cui Y, et al. YTHDC1 mediates nuclear export of N(6)-methyladenosine methylated mRNAs. *Elife.* (2017) 6:31311. doi: 10.7554/eLife.31311
51. Hsu PJ, Zhu Y, Ma H, Guo Y Shi X, Liu Y, et al. Ythdc2 is an N(6)-methyladenosine binding protein that regulates mammalian spermatogenesis. *Cell Res.* (2017) 27:1115–27. doi: 10.1038/cr.2017.99
52. Tanabe A, Tanikawa K, Tsunetomi M, Takai K, Ikeda H, Konno J, et al. RNA helicase YTHDC2 promotes cancer metastasis via the enhancement of the efficiency by which HIF-1alpha mRNA is translated. *Cancer Lett.* (2016) 376:34–42. doi: 10.1016/j.canlet.2016.02.022
53. Meyer KD, Patil DP, Zhou J, Zinoviev A, Skabkin MA, Elemento O, et al. 5′ UTR m(6)A promotes cap-independent translation. *Cell.* (2015) 163:999–1010. doi: 10.1016/j.cell.2015.10.012
54. Alarcon CR, Goodarzi H, Lee H Liu X, Tavazoie S, Tavazoie SF. HNRNPA2B1 is a mediator of m(6)A-dependent nuclear RNA processing events. *Cell.* (2015) 162:1299–308. doi: 10.1016/j.cell.2015.08.011
55. Salditt-Georgieff M, Jelinek W, Darnell JE, Furuichi Y, Morgan M, Shatkin A. Methyl labeling of HeLa cell hnRNA: a comparison with mRNA. *Cell.* (1976) 7:227–37. doi: 10.1016/0092-8674(76)90022-2
56. Sleeman JE, Trinkle-Mulcahy L. Nuclear bodies: new insights into assembly/dynamics and disease relevance. *Curr Opin Cell Biol.* (2014) 28:76–83. doi: 10.1016/j.ceb.2014.03.004
57. Zhao X, Yang Y, Sun BF, Shi Y, Yang X, Xiao W, et al. FTO-dependent demethylation of N6-methyladenosine regulates mRNA splicing and is required for adipogenesis. *Cell Res.* (2014) 24:1403–19. doi: 10.1038/cr.2014.151
58. Fustin JM, Doi M, Yamaguchi Y, Hida H, Nishimura S, Yoshida M, et al. RNA-methylation-dependent RNA processing controls the speed of the circadian clock. *Cell.* (2013) 155:793–806. doi: 10.1016/j.cell.2013.10.026
59. Heilman KL, Leach RA, Tuck MT. Internal 6-methyladenine residues increase the *in vitro* translation efficiency of dihydrofolate reductase messenger RNA. *Int J Biochem Cell Biol.* (1996) 28:823–9. doi: 10.1016/1357-2725(96)00014-3
60. Lin S, Choe J, Du P, Triboulet R, Gregory RI. The m(6)A methyltransferase METTL3 promotes translation in human cancer cells. *Mol Cell.* (2016) 62:335–45. doi: 10.1016/j.molcel.2016.03.021
61. Kariko K, Muramatsu H, Welsh FA, Ludwig J, Kato H, Akira S, et al. Incorporation of pseudouridine into mRNA yields superior nonimmunogenic vector with increased translational capacity and biological stability. *Mol Ther.* (2008) 16:1833–40. doi: 10.1038/mt.2008.200
62. Hess ME, Hess S, Meyer KD, Verhagen LA, Koch L, Bronneke HS, et al. The fat mass and obesity associated gene (Fto) regulates activity of the dopaminergic midbrain circuitry. *Nat Neurosci.* (2013) 16:1042–8. doi: 10.1038/nn.3449
63. Xie JW, Huang XB, Chen QY, Ma YB, Zhao YJ, Liu LC, et al. m(6)A modification-mediated BATF2 acts as a tumor suppressor in gastric cancer through inhibition of ERK signaling. *Mol Cancer.* (2020) 19:114. doi: 10.1186/s12943-020-01223-4
64. Yan J, Huang X, Zhang X, Chen Z, Ye C, Xiang W, et al. LncRNA LINC00470 promotes the degradation of PTEN mRNA to facilitate malignant behavior in gastric cancer cells. *Biochem Biophys Res Commun.* (2020) 521:887–93. doi: 10.1016/j.bbrc.2019.11.016
65. Wang Q, Chen C, Ding Q, Zhao Y, Wang Z, Chen J, et al. METTL3-mediated m(6)A modification of HDGF mRNA promotes gastric cancer progression and has prognostic significance. *Gut.* (2020) 69:1193–205. doi: 10.1136/gutjnl-2019-319639
66. Zhu L, Zhu Y, Han S, Chen M, Song P, Dai D, et al. Impaired autophagic degradation of lncRNA ARHGAP5-AS1 promotes chemoresistance in gastric cancer. *Cell Death Dis.* (2019) 10:383. doi: 10.1038/s41419-019-1585-2
67. Liu X, Su K, Sun X, Jiang Y, Wang L, Hu C, et al. Sec62 promotes stemness and chemoresistance of human colorectal cancer through activating Wnt/beta-catenin pathway. *J Exp Clin Cancer Res.* (2021) 40:132. doi: 10.1186/s13046-021-01934-6
68. Bai Y, Yang C, Wu R, Huang L, Song S, Li W, et al. YTHDF1 regulates

tumorigenicity and cancer stem cell-like activity in human colorectal carcinoma. *Front Oncol.* (2019) 9:332. doi: 10.3389/fonc.2019.00332

69. Huang H, Weng H, Sun W, Qin X, Shi H, Wu H, et al. Recognition of RNA N(6)-methyladenosine by IGF2BP proteins enhances mRNA stability and translation. *Nat Cell Biol.* (2018) 20:285–95. doi: 10.1038/s41556-018-0045-z
70. Chen M, Wei L, Law CT, Tsang FH, Shen J, Cheng CL, et al. RNA N6-methyladenosine methyltransferase-like 3 promotes liver cancer progression through YTHDF2-dependent posttranscriptional silencing of SOCS2. *Hepatology.* (2018) 67:2254–70. doi: 10.1002/hep.29683
71. Ma JZ, Yang F, Zhou CC, Liu F, Yuan JH, Wang F, et al. METTL14 suppresses the metastatic potential of hepatocellular carcinoma by modulating N(6) -methyladenosine-dependent primary MicroRNA processing. *Hepatology.* (2017) 65:529–43. doi: 10.1002/hep.28885
72. Yang Z, Li J, Feng G, Gao S, Wang Y, Zhang S, et al. MicroRNA-145 modulates N(6)-methyladenosine levels by targeting the 3′-untranslated mRNA region of the N(6)-methyladenosine binding YTH domain family 2 protein. *J Biol Chem.* (2017) 292:3614–23. doi: 10.1074/jbc.M116.749689
73. Zhao X, Chen Y, Mao Q, Jiang X, Jiang W, Chen J, et al. Overexpression of YTHDF1 is associated with poor prognosis in patients with hepatocellular carcinoma. *Cancer Biomark.* (2018) 21:859–68. doi: 10.3233/CBM-170791
74. Bergquist E. Epidemiology of cholangiocarcinoma. *Best Pract Res Clin Gastroenterol.* (2015) 29:221–32. doi: 10.1016/j.bpg.2015.02.003
75. Jo HJ, Shim HE, Han ME, Kim HJ, Kim KS, Baek S, et al. WTAP regulates migration and invasion of cholangiocarcinoma cells. *J Gastroenterol.* (2013) 48:1271–82. doi: 10.1007/s00535-013-0748-7
76. Rong ZX, Li Z, He JJ, Liu LY, Ren XX, Gao J, et al. Downregulation of Fat Mass and Obesity Associated (FTO) promotes the progression of intrahepatic cholangiocarcinoma. *Front Oncol.* (2019) 9:369. doi: 10.3389/fonc.2019.00369
77. Su Y, Huang J, Hu J. m(6)A RNA methylation regulators contribute to malignant progression and have clinical prognostic impact in gastric cancer. *Front Oncol.* (2019) 9:1038. doi: 10.3389/fonc.2019.01038
78. Yang DD, Chen ZH, Yu K, Lu JH, Wu QN, Wang Y, et al. mettl3 promotes the progression of gastric cancer via targeting the MYC pathway. *Front Oncol.* (2020) 10:115. doi: 10.3389/fonc.2020.00115
79. Liu T, Yang S, Sui J, Xu SY, Cheng YP, Shen B, et al. Dysregulated N6-methyladenosine methylation writer METTL3 contributes to the proliferation and migration of gastric cancer. *J Cell Physiol.* (2020) 235:548–62. doi: 10.1002/jcp.28994
80. Lin S, Liu J, Jiang W, Wang P, Sun C, Wang X, et al. METTL3 promotes the proliferation and mobility of gastric cancer cells. *Open Med (Wars).* (2019) 14:25–31. doi: 10.1515/med-2019-0005
81. Yue B, Song C, Yang L, Cui R, Cheng X, Zhang Z, et al. METTL3-mediated N6-methyladenosine modification is critical for epithelial-mesenchymal transition and metastasis of gastric cancer. *Mol Cancer.* (2019) 18:142. doi: 10.1186/s12943-019-1065-4
82. He H, Wu W, Sun Z, Chai L. MiR-4429 prevented gastric cancer progression through targeting METTL3 to inhibit m(6)A-caused stabilization of SEC62. *Biochem Biophys Res Commun.* (2019) 517:581–7. doi: 10.1016/j.bbrc.2019.07.058
83. Chen J, Sun Y, Xu X, Wang D, He J, Zhou H, et al. YTH domain family 2 orchestrates epithelial-mesenchymal transition/proliferation dichotomy in pancreatic cancer cells. *Cell Cycle.* (2017) 16:2259–71. doi: 10.1080/15384101.2017.1380125
84. Guo X, Li K, Jiang W, Hu Y, Xiao W, Huang Y, et al. RNA demethylase ALKBH5 prevents pancreatic cancer progression by posttranscriptional activation of PER1 in an m6A-YTHDF2-dependent manner. *Mol Cancer.* (2020) 19:91. doi: 10.1186/s12943-020-01158-w
85. Zhang J, Bai R, Li M, Ye H, Wu C, Wang C, et al. Excessive miR-25-3p maturation via N(6)-methyladenosine stimulated by cigarette smoke promotes pancreatic cancer progression. *Nat Commun.* (2019) 10:1858. doi: 10.1038/s41467-019-09712-x
86. Taketo K, Konno M, Asai A, Koseki J, Toratani M, Satoh T, et al. The epitranscriptome m6A writer METTL3 promotes chemo- and radioresistance in pancreatic cancer cells. *Int J Oncol.* (2018) 52:621–9. doi: 10.3892/ijo.2017.4219
87. Peng W, Li J, Chen R, Gu Q, Yang P, Qian W, et al. Upregulated METTL3 promotes metastasis of colorectal cancer via miR-1246/SPRED2/MAPK signaling pathway. *J Exp Clin Cancer Res.* (2019) 38:393. doi: 10.1186/s13046-019-1408-4
88. Li T, Hu PS, Zuo Z, Lin JF, Li X, Wu QN, et al. METTL3 facilitates tumor progression via an m(6)A-IGF2BP2-dependent mechanism in colorectal carcinoma. *Mol Cancer.* (2019) 18:112. doi: 10.1186/s12943-019-1038-7
89. Ru D, Yikan C, Shubiao Y, Jianwei Z, Runqing H, Peisi L, et al. m6A methyltransferase METTL3 suppresses colorectal cancer proliferation and migration through p38/ERK pathways. *OncoTargets Therapy.* (2019) 12:1052. doi: 10.2147/OTT.S201052
90. Nishizawa Y, Konno M, Asai A, Koseki J, Kawamoto K, Miyoshi N, et al. Oncogene c-Myc promotes epitranscriptome m(6)A reader YTHDF1 expression in colorectal cancer. *Oncotarget.* (2018) 9:7476–86. doi: 10.18632/oncotarget.23554
91. Li Z, Lin S, Jiang T, Wang J, Lu H, Tang H, et al. Overexpression of eIF3e is correlated with colon tumor development and poor prognosis. *Int J Clin Exp Pathol.* (2014) 7:6462–74.
92. Song P, Feng L, Li J, Dai D, Zhu L, Wang C, et al. beta-catenin represses miR455-3p to stimulate m6A modification of HSF1 mRNA and promote its translation in colorectal cancer. *Mol Cancer.* (2020) 19:129. doi: 10.1186/s12943-020-01244-z
93. Li H, Zhang N, Jiao X, Wang C, Sun W, He Y, et al. Downregulation of microRNA-6125 promotes colorectal cancer growth through YTHDF2-dependent recognition of N6-methyladenosine-modified GSK3beta. *Clin Transl Med.* (2021) 11:e602. doi: 10.1002/ctm2.602
94. Wu J, Yuan XH, Jiang W, Lu YC, Huang QL, Yang Y, et al. Genome-wide map of N(6)-methyladenosine circular RNAs identified in mice model of severe acute pancreatitis. *World J Gastroenterol.* (2021) 27:7530–45. doi: 10.3748/wjg.v27.i43.7530
95. Levrero M, Pollicino T, Petersen J, Belloni L, Raimondo G, Dandri M. Control of cccDNA function in hepatitis B virus infection. *J Hepatol.* (2009) 51:581–92. doi: 10.1016/j.jhep.2009.05.022
96. Imam H, Khan M, Gokhale NS, McIntyre ABR, Kim GW, Jang JY, et al. N6-methyladenosine modification of hepatitis B virus RNA differentially regulates the viral life cycle. *Proc Natl Acad Sci USA.* (2018) 115:8829–34. doi: 10.1073/pnas.1808319115
97. Gokhale NS, McIntyre ABR, McFadden MJ, Roder AE, Kennedy EM, Gandara JA, et al. N6-methyladenosine in flaviviridae viral RNA genomes regulates infection. *Cell Host Microbe.* (2016) 20:654–65. doi: 10.1016/j.chom.2016.09.015
98. Kim GW, Siddiqui A. N6-methyladenosine modification of HCV RNA genome regulates cap-independent IRES-mediated translation via YTHDC2 recognition. *Proc Natl Acad Sci USA.* (2021) 118:24118. doi: 10.1073/pnas.2022024118
99. Wang B, Fang X, Sun X, Du C, Zhou L, Lv X, et al. m(6)A demethylase ALKBH5 suppresses proliferation and migration of enteric neural crest cells by regulating TAGLN in Hirschsprung's disease. *Life Sci.* (2021) 278:119577. doi: 10.1016/j.lfs.2021.119577
100. Lu TX, Zheng Z, Zhang L, Sun HL, Bissonnette M, Huang H, et al. A new model of spontaneous colitis in mice induced by deletion of an RNA m(6)A methyltransferase component METTL14 in T cells. *Cell Mol Gastroenterol Hepatol.* (2020) 10:747–61. doi: 10.1016/j.jcmgh.2020.07.001
101. Li HB, Tong J, Zhu S, Batista PJ, Duffy EE, Zhao J, et al. m(6)A mRNA methylation controls T cell homeostasis by targeting the IL-7/STAT5/SOCS pathways. *Nature.* (2017) 548:338–42. doi: 10.1038/nature23450
102. Yue B, Cui R, Zheng R, Jin W, Song C, Bao T, et al. Essential role of ALKBH5-mediated RNA demethylation modification in bile acid-induced gastric intestinal metaplasia. *Mol Ther Nucleic Acids.* (2021) 26:458–72. doi: 10.1016/j.omtn.2021.08.019
103. Yankova E, Blackaby W, Albertella M, Rak J, De Braekeleer E, Tsagkogeorga G, et al. Small-molecule inhibition of METTL3 as a strategy against myeloid leukaemia. *Nature.* (2021) 593:597–601. doi: 10.1038/s41586-021-03536-w
104. Qiao Y, Zhou B, Zhang M, Liu W, Han Z, Song C, et al. A novel inhibitor of the obesity-related protein FTO. *Biochemistry.* (2016) 55:1516–22. doi: 10.1021/acs.biochem.6b00023
105. Wang R, Han Z, Liu B, Zhou B, Wang N, Jiang Q, et al. Identification of natural compound radicicol as a potent FTO inhibitor. *Mol Pharm.* (2018) 15:4092–8. doi: 10.1021/acs.molpharmaceut.8b00522

106. Han X, Wang N, Li J, Wang Y, Wang R, Chang J. Identification of nafamostat mesilate as an inhibitor of the fat mass and obesity-associated protein (FTO) demethylase activity. *Chem Biol Interact.* (2019) 297:80–4. doi: 10.1016/j.cbi.2018.10.023
107. Peng S, Xiao W, Ju D, Sun B, Hou N, Liu Q, et al. Identification of entacapone as a chemical inhibitor of FTO mediating metabolic regulation through FOXO1. *Sci Transl Med.* (2019) 11:7116. doi: 10.1126/scitranslmed.aau7116
108. Zhou P, Wu M, Ye C, Xu Q, Wang L. Meclofenamic acid promotes cisplatin-induced acute kidney injury by inhibiting fat mass and obesity-associated protein-mediated m(6)A abrogation in RNA. *J Biol Chem.* (2019) 294:16908–17. doi: 10.1074/jbc.RA119.011009
109. Huang Y, Su R, Sheng Y, Dong L, Dong Z, Xu H, et al. Small-molecule targeting of oncogenic FTO demethylase in acute myeloid leukemia. *Cancer Cell.* (2019) 35:677–91.e10. doi: 10.1016/j.ccell.2019.03.006

14

Serum STIP1, a Novel Indicator for Microvascular Invasion, Predicts Outcomes and Treatment Response in Hepatocellular Carcinoma

Xiao-Lu Ma[1,2†], Wei-Guo Tang[3,4†], Min-Jie Yang[5†], Su-Hong Xie[1,2], Min-Le Wu[6], Guo Lin[1,2] and Ren-Quan Lu[1,2*]*

[1] *Department of Clinical Laboratory, Shanghai Cancer Center, Fudan University, Shanghai, China,* [2] *Department of Oncology, Shanghai Medical School, Fudan University, Shanghai, China,* [3] *Department of Liver Surgery, Liver Cancer Institute, Zhongshan Hospital, Fudan University, Shanghai, China,* [4] *Department of Hepatobiliary and Pancreatic Surgery, Minhang Hospital, Fudan University, Shanghai, China,* [5] *Department of Interventional Radiology, Zhongshan Hospital, Fudan University and Shanghai Institute of Medical Imaging, Shanghai, China,* [6] *Department of Clinical Laboratory, Shanghai Public Health Clinical Center, Fudan University, Shanghai, China*

***Correspondence:**
Guo Lin
guolin500@hotmail.com
Ren-Quan Lu
lurenquan@126.com

† These authors have contributed equally to this work

Background: Previous studies reported that stress-induced phosphoprotein 1 (STIP1) can be secreted by hepatocellular carcinoma (HCC) cells and is increased in the serum of HCC patients. However, the therapy-monitoring and prognostic value of serum STIP1 in HCC remains unclear. Here, we aimed to systemically explore the prognostic significance of serum STIP1 in HCC.

Methods: A total of 340 HCC patients were recruited to this study; 161 underwent curative resection and 179 underwent transcatheter arterial chemoembolization (TACE). Serum STIP1 was detected by enzyme-linked immunosorbent assay (ELISA). Optimal cutoff values for serum STIP1 in resection and TACE groups were determined by receiver operating characteristic (ROC) analysis. Prognostic value was assessed by Kaplan-Meier, log-rank, and Cox regression analyses. Predictive values of STIP1 for objective response (OR) to TACE and MVI were evaluated by ROC curves and logistic regression.

Results: Serum STIP1 was significantly increased in HCC patients when compared with chronic hepatitis B patients or health donors (both $P < 0.05$). Optimal cutoff values for STIP1 in resection and TACE groups were 83.43 and 112.06 ng/ml, respectively. High pretreatment STIP1 was identified as an independent prognosticator. Dynamic changes in high STIP1 status were significantly associated with long-term prognosis, regardless of treatment approaches. Moreover, post-TACE STIP1 was identified as an independent predictor for OR, with a higher area under ROC curve (AUC-ROC) than other clinicopathological features. Specifically, pretreatment STIP1 was significantly increased in patients with microvascular invasion (MVI), and was confirmed as a novel, powerful predictor for MVI.

Conclusions: Serum STIP1 is a promising biomarker for outcome evaluation, therapeutic response assessment, and MVI prediction in HCC. Integration serum STIP1 detection into HCC management might facilitate early clinical decision making to improve the prognosis of HCC.

Keywords: hepatocellular carcinoma, resection, TACE, prognosis, STIP1, serum biomarker, microvascular invasion

INTRODUCTION

Hepatocellular carcinoma (HCC) is one of the most prevalent malignancies worldwide, with increasing incidence and mortality rates (1–3). Radical resection is considered the only curative approach for early-stage HCC. However, despite impressive innovations in surgical procedures, the overall survival (OS) of HCC patients remains unsatisfactory due to high incidence of recurrence or relapse after surgery (4–6). Nonetheless, for irresectable, intermediate-HCC patients, transcatheter arterial chemoembolization (TACE) has evolved as a recommended approach by the Barcelona Clinic Liver Cancer (BCLC) criteria to achieve stable clinical benefit in these patients (7, 8). Unfortunately, response rates are dramatically heterogeneous, and long-term prognosis also remains poor after TACE (9, 10). Therefore, identification of a reliable biomarker to assist pre-interventional stratification is urgently required.

Stress-induced phosphoprotein 1 (STIP1) was initially identified as an auxiliary partner for heat shock proteins (HSPs) 70 and 90 to modulate the function of HSPs by modulating their dimer structure (11). In addition to its role as a scaffold protein, STIP1 was also found to have a pivotal role in regulating transcription and intracellular signaling transduction, as well as cell proliferation and division (12–14). Consistently, accumulating evidences show that STIP1 is involved in several critical processes that mediate tumor progression including proliferation, migration, and invasion (15–18), indicating its necessity in the development of cancer. Conventionally, STIP1 was considered as a typical cytoplasmic protein due to its lack of transmembrane domain or trans-signal peptide (11). However, recent studies revealed that STIP1 could be secreted by several types of cancer cells, including HCC, and serves as a cytokine in regulating tumor progression (19–21), which strongly suggests serum STIP1 is a promising circulating biomarker for HCC. However, the clinical significance of serum STIP1 remains largely unknown.

Here, in the present study, we evaluated the prognostic value of pretreatment serum STIP1 and dynamic changes in STIP1 levels in HCC. In addition, we assessed the utility of serum STIP1 detection for predicting TACE response. Importantly, we also investigated the value of pretreatment STIP1 levels for predicting microvascular invasion (MVI).

METHODS AND MATERIALS

Patients

Two independent cohorts of HCC patients were enrolled in the present study. Cohort I was recruited from January 2011 to December 2012 and included 161 HCC patients who received curative resection at Zhongshan Hospital as the resection group. All patients in the resection group were Barcelona Clinic Liver Cancer (BCLC) stage 0 or A. Cohort II was recruited from January to December 2014 and included a total of 179 patients who received TACE as the TACE group. All patients in the TACE group were BCLC stage B. Enrollment criteria were as follows (22): (1) definitive HCC diagnosis; (2) no prior anti-HCC treatment; (3) complete resection of all tumor lesions with the cut surface being free of cancer; (4) TACE treatment targeting intrahepatic lesions; and (5) availability of complete clinicopathological and follow-up data. Exclusion criteria were as follows: (1) Child-Pugh C or severe liver dysfunction; (2) receiving any treatment before enrollment; (3) suffering intrahepatic or extrahepatic metastases; (4) having history of any malignancy other than HCC; and (5) insufficient available data. HCC diagnosis in the resection group was based on histopathology examination, while diagnosis was based on imaging scans according to the American Association for the Study of Liver Disease guidelines in the TACE group (22). MVI was defined according to a previous study and was examined by senior pathologists (23). In addition, a total of 122 HDs and 55 patients with CHB without any sign of malignancy were enrolled as negative controls. Approval for the use of human subjects was obtained from the Research Ethics Committee of Zhongshan Hospital. Importantly, informed consent was obtained from every individual who participated in the study.

Follow-Up and Prognosis Evaluations

Post-treatment surveillance was performed according to our previous studies. Follow-up ended on December 2018. Time to recurrence (TTR), time to progression (TTP), and overall survival (OS) were set as end points of follow-up in present study (24). TTR was defined as the time interval between resection and intrahepatic recurrence or the date of the last follow-up. TTP was defined as the time interval between TACE and disease progression according to mRECIST or the date of the last follow-up (25). OS was defined as the interval between treatment and the death of any cause or last observation date.

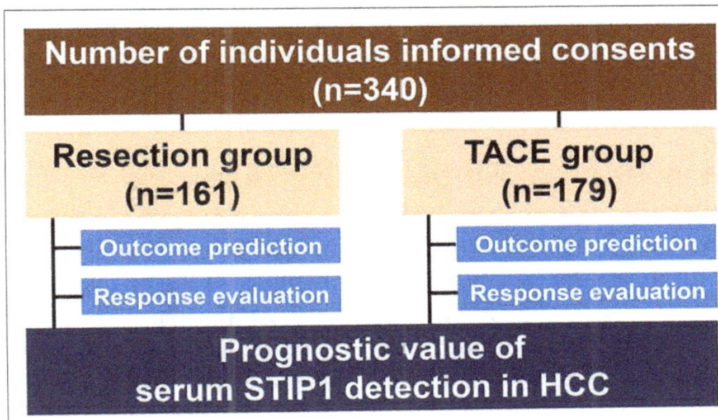

FIGURE 1 | Schematic diagram of present study.

Abbreviations: STIP1, stress-induced-phosphoprotein 1; HCC, hepatocellular carcinoma; TACE, transcatheter arterial chemoembolization; ELISA, enzyme-linked immunosorbent assay; ROC, receiver operating characteristic; OR, objective response; CHB, chronic hepatitis B; MVI, microvascular invasion; OS, overall survival; TTR, time to recurrence; TTP, time to progression; BCLC, Barcelona Clinic Liver Cancer; HSP, heat shock protein; CT, computed tomography; MRI, magnetic resonance imaging; CR, complete response; PR, partial response; SD, stable disease; PD, progressive disease.

TABLE 1 | Correlation between clinicopathological parameters of patients enrolled.

Variables		Resection ($n = 161$)			TACE ($n = 179$)		
		STIP1 ≤ 83.43 ng/ml	STIP1 > 83.43 ng/ml	*P*	STIP1 ≤ 112.06 ng/ml	STIP1 > 112.06 ng/ml	*P*
Sex	Female	10	16	0.365	6	15	0.206
	Male	65	70		68	90	
Age	≤50 year	29	36	0.680	30	52	0.235
	>50 year	46	50		44	53	
HBsAg	Negative	13	13	0.924	9	10	0.523
	Positive	62	73		65	95	
ALT	≤40 U/L	47	52	0.775	45	61	0.716
	>40 U/L	28	34		29	44	
AFP	≤400 ng/ml	60	61	0.184	46	58	0.355
	>400 ng/ml	15	25		28	47	
Cirrhosis	No	3	3	0.864	8	6	0.211
	Yes	72	83		66	99	
Tumor size	≤5 cm	60	52	0.012	21	25	0.491
	>5 cm	15	34		53	80	
Number	Single	63	76	0.420		Not applicable	
	Multiple	12	10				
MVI	Absent	57	38	<0.001		Not applicable	
	Present	18	48				
Encapsulation	Complete	60	51	0.005		Not applicable	
	Incomplete	15	35				
Differentiation	I–II	52	52	0.240		Not applicable	
	III–IV	23	34				

HR, hazard ratio; HBsAg, hepatitis B surface antigen; ALT, alanine aminotransferase; AFP, α-fetoprotein; STIP1, Stress Induced Phosphoprotein 1; MVI, microvascular invasion.

Sample Collection and STIP1 Level Determination

Serum samples were collected from all patients enrolled at baseline (1 or 2 days before interventions) and 1 month after treatments as we did previously (22). STIP1 concentrations were determined by enzyme-linked immunosorbent assay (ELISA) using the Human STIP1 ELISA Kit (Cat: LS-F7598, LifeSpan, USA), according to the manufacturer's instructions. Samples were 2-fold diluted by PBS to avoid exceeding detection limit (>100 ng/ml). The optimal cutoff values of STIP1 in resection and TACE groups were determined by receiver operating characteristics curve analysis, and were set as 83.43 and 112.06 ng/ml, respectively.

Evaluation of Single TACE Response

Single TACE response evaluation was conducted 1 month after initial treatment according to our previous study (26). Contrast-enhanced computed tomography (CT) or magnetic resonance imaging (MRI) scans were conducted, and results were interpreted by senior, experienced radiologists in imaging diagnosis. Treatment responses were assessed based on 1.1 modified RECIST and patients were stratified as follows: complete response (CR, $n = 0$); partial response (PR, $n = 136$); stable disease (SD, $n = 21$); and progressive disease (PD, $n = 22$). CR and PR were further defined as objective response (OR) according to previous studies (27, 28).

Statistical Analysis

Statistical analysis was performed with SPSS 21.0 software (IBM, USA). Continuous variables are shown as mean ± standard error of the mean, and chi-squared test, Fisher's exact probability test, and Student's *t*-tests were conducted to determine significant differences between the groups. If the data were not homogeneous, the non-parametric Mann-Whitney U test was applied. Receiver operating characteristic curve analysis was conducted to assess the value of STIP1 level for predicting response to TACE and MVI presence in HCC. Prognostic values were evaluated via Kaplan-Meier curve analysis, log-rank tests, and Cox proportional hazard ratio models. Logistic regression analysis was performed to evaluate the significance of STIP1 in predicting response to TACE. A *P*-value of <0.05 was considered statistically significant.

RESULTS

Baseline Characteristics of HCC Patients Enrolled

Overall, 517 individuals were recruited in the present study (HCC, 340; chronic hepatitis B, 55; healthy donors, 122,

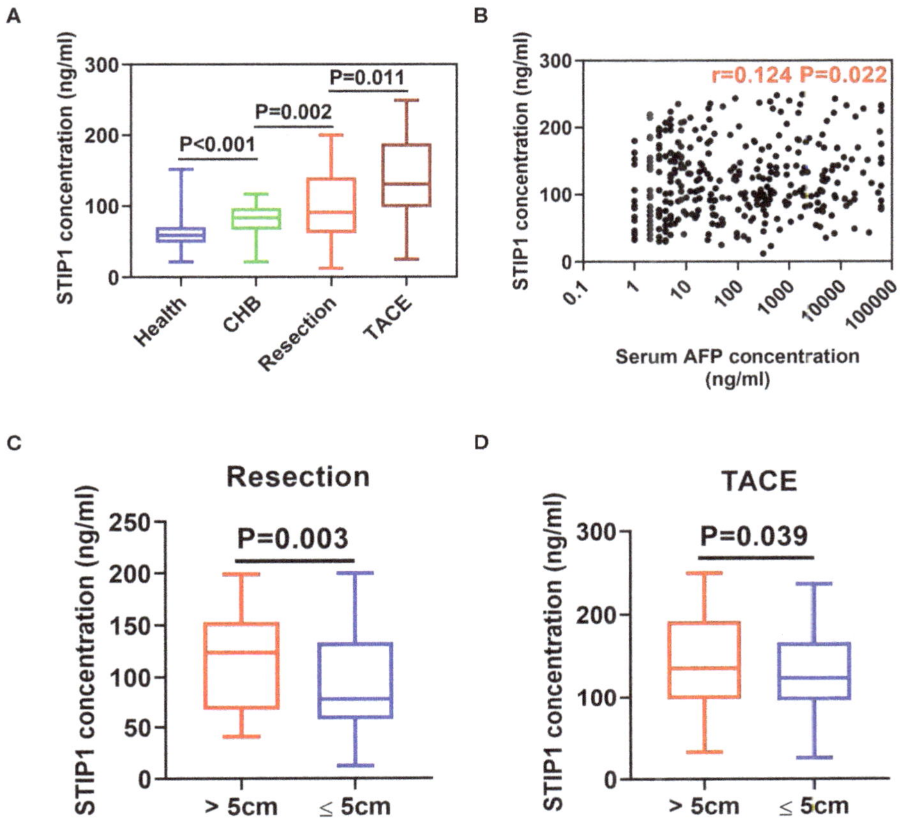

FIGURE 2 | Serum STIP1 was elevated in HCC and associated with tumor progression. **(A)** Distributions of serum STIP1 in HCC patients received curative resection ($n = 161$) and TACE ($n = 179$). Health donors ($n = 122$) and CHB patients ($n = 55$) was enrolled as controls. **(B)** Correlation between baseline serum STIP1 level and baseline serum AFP level. **(C)** Distribution of serum STIP1 of patients with distinct tumor size in resection group. **(D)** Distribution of serum STIP1 of patients with distinct tumor size in TACE group.

Figure 1). Baseline characteristics are illustrated in **Table 1**. Mean age was 53.38 years for the resection group and 50.25 years for the TACE group, and 16.15% of patients in the resection group were female while 11.73% of patients in the TACE group were female. HBsAg positivity was 83.85% in the resection group and 89.39% in the TACE group. According to BCLC staging criteria, all patients who underwent resection were BCLC stage 0 or A, while all patients undergoing TACE were BCLC stage B.

Serum STIP1 Was Elevated in HCC and Associated With Tumor Progression

Intermediate-HCC patients who received TACE showed the highest serum STIP1 levels, while early patients undergoing curative resection also had significantly higher STIP1 levels than CHB ($P = 0.002$) and HD ($P < 0.001$) individuals (**Figure 2A**). Interestingly, CHB patients also exhibited higher STIP1 levels than HDs. Further investigation indicated STIP1 levels showed a weak correlation with AFP level ($r = 0.124$, $P = 0.022$; **Figure 2B**). Moreover, we found patients with bigger tumor sizes (diameter over 5 cm) exhibited significantly higher serum STIP1 concentrations in both the resection ($P = 0.003$; **Figure 2C**) and TACE ($P = 0.039$; **Figure 2D**) groups. Together, our data demonstrated that serum STIP1 levels were elevated in HCC patients, and a higher concentration might indicate HCC progression.

Determination of Cutoff Value of Pretreatment Serum STIP1 for Predicting Prognosis in Resection and TACE Group

Pretreatment STIP1 levels were significantly higher in patients who encountered recurrence ($P < 0.001$) or death ($P = 0.001$, **Figure 3A**) in the resection group. Similarly, patients who experienced progression ($P < 0.001$) or death ($P = 0.002$) also exhibited significantly higher pretreatment STIP1 levels (**Figure 3B**). The above results indicated pretreatment STIP1 might act as a powerful tool for predicting prognosis in HCC. Because patients in the TACE group had significantly higher pretreatment STIP1 levels than the patients in the resection group, an independent cutoff value was set for these two groups to achieve the satisfactory performance of STIP1. Using receiver operating characteristic (ROC) curve analysis, 83.43 ng/ml was found to harbor the biggest Youden index

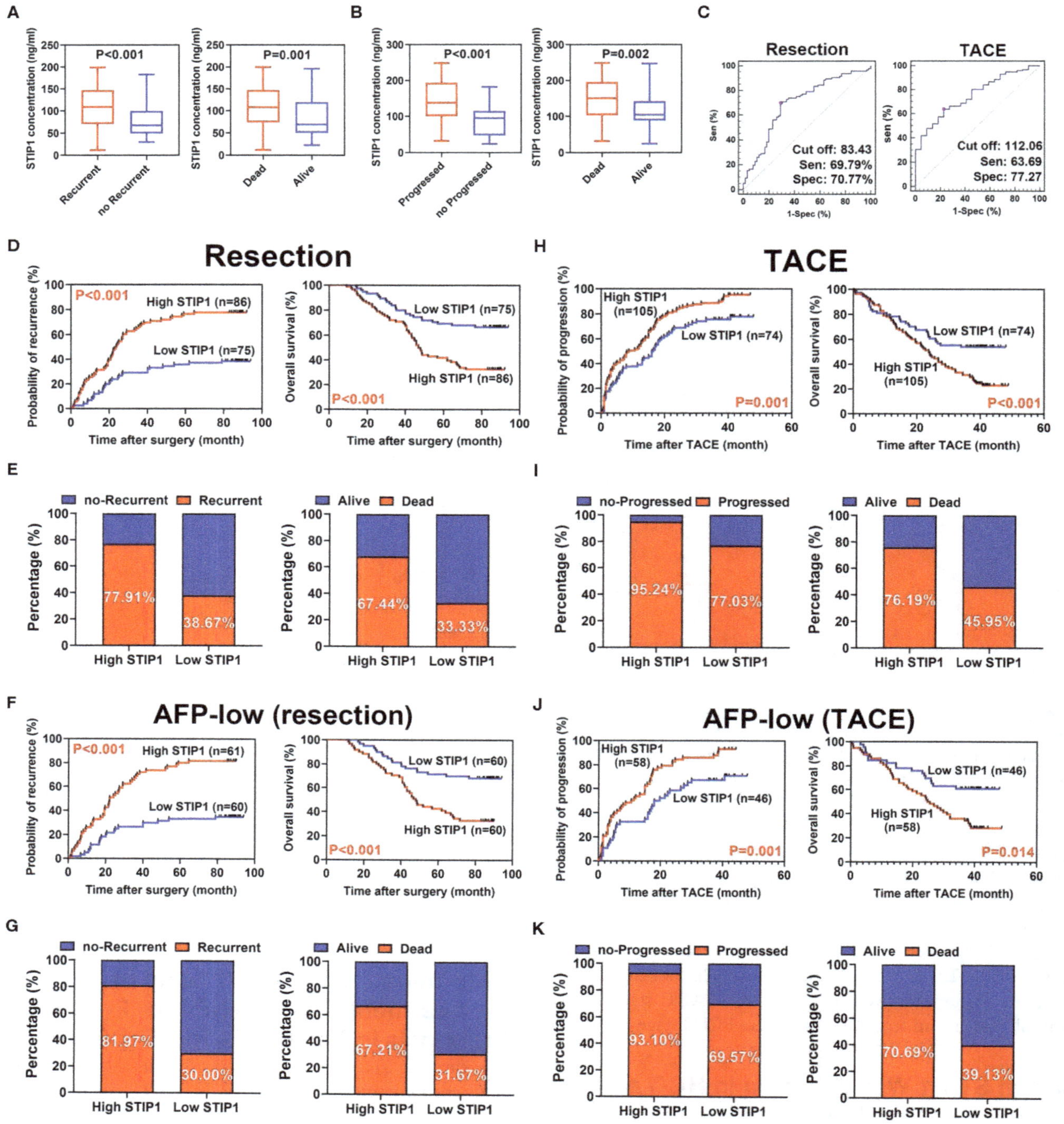

FIGURE 3 | Prognostic significance of pretreatment STIP1 in resectable and irresectable HCC. **(A)** Pretreatment STIP1 levels were significantly elevated in patients suffered recurrence or death in resection group. **(B)** Pretreatment STIP1 levels were significantly elevated in patients suffered progression or death in TACE group. **(C)** ROC curve analyses were conducted to determine the optimal cutoff values for patients received resection or TACE, respectively, via calculating Youden index. **(D)** Kaplan-Meier analyses of TTR (left) and OS (right) according to pretreatment STIP1 level in patients received curative resection. **(E)** Recurrence (left) and death (right) rates of patients with distinct pretreatment STIP1 levels in patients received curative resection. **(F)** Kaplan-Meier analyses of TTR (left) and OS (right) according to pretreatment STIP1 level in low-AFP (≤400 ng/ml) patients received curative resection. **(G)** Recurrence (left) and death (right) rates of patients with distinct pretreatment STIP1 levels in low-AFP patients received curative resection. **(H)** Kaplan-Meier analyses of TTP (left) and OS (right) according to pretreatment STIP1 level in patients received TACE. **(I)** Progression (left) and death (right) rates of patients with distinct pretreatment STIP1 levels in patients received TACE. **(J)** Kaplan-Meier analyses of TTP (left) and OS (right) according to pretreatment STIP1 level in low-AFP patients received TACE. **(K)** Progression (left) and death (right) rates of patients with distinct pretreatment STIP1 levels in low-AFP patients received TACE.

TABLE 2 | Univariate Cox proportional regression analysis of factors associated with recurrence and overall survival after curative resection.

Variables	Recurrence		Overall survival	
	HR (95% CI)	*P*	HR (95% CI)	*P*
Gender (male vs. female)	1.15 (0.66–1.99)	0.627	1.00 (0.56–1.78)	0.994
Age (>50 vs. ≤50 years)	0.82 (0.55–1.22)	0.319	0.85 (0.55–1.32)	0.471
HBsAg (positive vs. negative)	1.79 (0.99–3.21)	0.050	1.84 (0.97–3.50)	0.064
Cirrhosis (yes vs. no)	5.45 (0.76–39.13)	0.092	4.50 (0.63–32.34)	0.135
ALT (>40 vs. ≤40 U/L)	1.39 (0.91–2.14)	0.128	1.36 (0.87–2.10)	0.171
AFP (>400 vs. ≤400 ng/ml)	1.15 (0.73–1.81)	0.550	1.28 (0.79–2.07)	0.313
Tumor size (>5 vs. ≤5 cm)	1.04 (0.67–1.60)	0.871	0.94 (0.59–1.51)	0.803
Tumor number (multiple vs. single)	4.01 (2/48–6.53)	<0.001	3.71 (2.19–6.27)	<0.001
Microvascular invasion (present vs. absent)	4.59 (3.00–7.03)	<0.001	4.12 (2.60–6.53)	<0.001
Tumor encapsulation (incomplete vs. complete)	2.86 (1.92–4.29)	<0.001	2.24 (1.45–3.47)	<0.001
Tumor differentiation (III–IV vs. I–II)	2.30 (1.54–3.44)	<0.001	2.20 (1.43–3.39)	<0.001
Pretreatment serum STIP1 (>83.43 vs. ≤83.43 ng/ml)	2.97 (1.91–4.60)	<0.001	2.60 (1.62–4.16)	<0.001

HR, hazard ratio; HBsAg, hepatitis B surface antigen; ALT, alanine aminotransferase; AFP, α-fetoprotein; STIP1, Stress Induced Phosphoprotein 1.

TABLE 3 | Multivariate Cox proportional regression analysis of factors associated with recurrence and overall survival after curative resection.

Variables	Recurrence		Overall survival	
	HR (95% CI)	*P*	HR (95% CI)	*P*
Tumor number (multiple vs. single)	3.32 (1.92–5.72)	<0.001	2.45 (1.40–4.28)	0.002
Microvascular invasion (present vs. absent)	2.38 (1.49–3.80)	<0.001	1.91 (1.16–.13)	0.011
Tumor encapsulation (incomplete vs. complete)	1.43 (0.91–2.25)	0.123	1.19 (0.74–1.91)	0.483
Tumor differentiation (III–IV vs. I–II)	1.40 (0.91–2.17)	0.127	1.43 (0.90–2.27)	0.128
Pretreatment serum STIP1 (>83.43 vs. ≤83.43 ng/ml)	2.57 (1.58–4.17)	<0.001	2.48 (1.46–4.20)	0.001

HR, hazard ratio; HBsAg, hepatitis B surface antigen; ALT, alanine aminotransferase; AFP, α-fetoprotein; STIP1, Stress Induced Phosphoprotein 1.

TABLE 4 | Univariate Cox proportional regression analysis of factors associated with recurrence and overall survival after TACE.

Variables	Progression		Overall survival	
	HR (95% CI)	*P*	HR (95% CI)	*P*
Gender (male vs. female)	0.97 (0.60–1.55)	0.887	1.25 (0.68–2.27)	0.473
Age (>50 vs. ≤50 years)	0.79 (0.57–1.08)	0.134	0.65 (0.45–0.94)	0.023
HBsAg (positive vs. negative)	1.23 (0.76–2.00)	0.398	1.85 (0.93–3.70)	0.080
Cirrhosis (yes vs. no)	1.23 (0.68–2.21)	0.499	1.99 (0.88–4.54)	0.100
ALT (>40 vs. ≤40 U/L)	0.96 (0.70–1.32)	0.804	0.97 (0.66–1.41)	0.857
AFP (>400 vs. ≤400 ng/ml)	1.54 (1.12–2.11)	0.008	1.52 (1.05–2.20)	0.026
Tumor size (>5 vs. ≤5 cm)	1.25 (0.87–1.80)	0.231	1.18 (0.77–1.80)	0.456
Pretreatment serum STIP1 (>112.06 vs. ≤112.06 ng/ml)	1.69 (1.22–2.35)	0.002	1.95 (1.30–2.91)	0.001

HR, hazard ratio; HBsAg, hepatitis B surface antigen; ALT, alanine aminotransferase; AFP, α-fetoprotein; STIP1, Stress Induced Phosphoprotein 1.

when predicting recurrence in the resection group (sensitivity, 69.79%; specificity, 70.77%; **Figure 3C**), whereas 112.06 ng/ml was found to obtain the biggest Youden index when predicting progression in the TACE group (sensitivity, 63.69%; specificity, 77.27%). Therefore, these two values were set as cutoff values to stratify HCC patients into different pretreatment STIP1 states for subsequent investigations.

Prognostic Value of Pretreatment STIP1 Level in Resectable HCC

In the resection group, the median follow-up was 36.83 months (range, 1.0–94.0) for TTR and 68.45 months (range, 9.0–94.0) for OS. Patients with high pretreatment STIP1 (>83.43 ng/ml) had significantly shorter TTR (23.60 months vs. not reached, $P < 0.001$) and OS (47.33 months vs. not reached, $P < 0.001$) than patients with low pretreatment STIP1 (≤83.43 ng/ml) (**Figure 3D**). Consistently, patients with high pretreatment STIP1 had higher recurrence (77.91 vs. 38.67%) and death (67.44 vs. 33.33%) rates (**Figure 3E**). Cox regression analysis revealed that high pretreatment STIP1 level was an independent indicator for both TTR (hazard ratio [HR] 2.57, 95% CI 1.58–4.17, $P < 0.001$) and OS (HR 2.48, 95% CI 1.46–4.20, $P = 0.001$; **Tables 2, 3**). Moreover, in patients with low AFP levels (≤400 ng/ml), STIP1 was significantly correlated with both shorter TTR and OS (both $P < 0.001$; **Figure 3F**). Also, patients with high pretreatment STIP1 levels had higher recurrence (81.97 vs. 30.00%) and death (67.21 vs. 31.67%) rates in the low-AFP subgroup (**Figure 3G**). Pretreatment STIP1 retained its prognostic value in conventional low-risk subgroups such as single tumors, small tumor size, well differentiation, or complete encapsulation (all $P < 0.050$; **Figure S1**).

TABLE 5 | Multivariate Cox proportional regression analysis of factors associated with progression and overall survival after TACE.

Variables	Progression		Overall survival	
	HR (95% CI)	P	HR (95% CI)	P
Age (>50 vs. ≤50 years)	Not applicable		0.74 (0.51–1.08)	0.116
AFP (>400 vs. ≤400 ng/ml)	1.44 (1.05–1.98)	0.025	1.46 (1.10–2.12)	0.046
Pretreatment serum STIP1 (>112.06 vs. ≤112.06 ng/ml)	1.61 (1.16–2.24)	0.005	1.88 (1.25–2.82)	0.002

HR, hazard ratio; HBsAg, hepatitis B surface antigen; ALT, alanine aminotransferase; AFP, α-fetoprotein; STIP1, Stress Induced Phosphoprotein 1.

Prognostic Value of Pretreatment STIP1 Level in Irresectable HCC

In the TACE group, patients with high pretreatment STIP1 levels (>112.06 ng/ml) had significantly shorter TTP (median 8.23 vs. 16.27 months, $P = 0.001$) and OS (median 23.70 months vs. not reached, $P < 0.001$) than those who had low pretreatment STIP1 levels (≤112.06 ng/ml) (**Figure 3H**). In addition, patients with high pretreatment STIP1 had higher progression (95.24 vs. 77.03%) and death rates (76.19 vs. 45.85%; **Figure 3I**). Cox regression analysis revealed that high pretreatment STIP1 level was an independent indicator for both TTP (HR 1.61, 95% CI 1.16–2.24, $P = 0.005$) and OS (HR 1.88, 95% CI 1.25–2.82, $P = 0.002$; **Tables 4, 5**) in the TACE group. In addition, in patients with low AFP levels (≤400 ng/ml), STIP1 was significantly correlated with both shorter TTP ($P = 0.001$) and OS ($P = 0.014$; **Figure 3J**). Also, patients with high pretreatment STIP1 levels had higher progression (93.10 vs. 69.57%) and death (70.69 vs. 39.13%) rates in the low-AFP subgroup (**Figure 3K**). Additionally, high pretreatment STIP1 was significantly associated with MVI ($P < 0.001$) and incomplete tumor encapsulation ($P = 0.005$; **Table 1**).

Prognostic Value of Dynamic Changes of Serum STIP1 in Patients With Resectable HCC

We further explored the dynamic changes in STIP1 during the perioperative period in 169 patients who received curative resection. STIP1 levels were significantly decreased 1 month after surgery ($P < 0.001$; **Figure 4A**). Similarly, the percentage of patients with high STIP1 was also reduced after surgery (53.42 vs. 24.22%). These patients were further divided into four groups based on perioperative STIP1 levels: Group I, both high for pretreatment and post-treatment ($n = 25$); Group II, pretreatment high and post-treatment low ($n = 61$); Group III, pretreatment low and post-treatment high ($n = 13$); and Group IV, both low pretreatment and post-treatment ($n = 62$). Recurrence rates were 92.00, 72.13, 76.92, and 30.05%, respectively (**Figure 4B**). Median TTR was significantly shorter for Group I than for Group II ($P = 0.009$), Group III ($P = 0.041$), and Group IV ($P < 0.001$). Meanwhile, patients in Group II and Group III also had significantly shorter TTR than patients in Group IV (both $P < 0.001$). No significant difference in TTR between patients in Group II and Group III was observed ($P = 0.982$; **Figure 4B**). Death rates were 84.00, 60.66, 61.54, and 27.42%, respectively (**Figure 4C**). Median OS was significantly shorter for Group I than for Group II ($P < 0.001$), Group III ($P = 0.046$), and Group IV ($P < 0.001$). Also, patients in Group II and Group III had significantly shorter OS than patients in Group IV (both $P < 0.001$). No significant difference in OS between patients in Group II and Group III was observed ($P = 0.926$; **Figure 4C**).

Prognostic Value of Dynamic Changes of Serum STIP1 in Patients With Irresectable HCC

STIP1 levels showed a significant reduction after TACE ($P < 0.001$) and the percentage of patients with high STIP1 was also decreased after TACE (58.66 vs. 38.55%; **Figure 4D**). All 179 patients in the TACE group were divided into four groups based on their pre- and post-TACE STIP1 levels. Progression rates were 98.08, 92.45, 94.12, and 71.93% for these four groups, respectively (**Figure 4E**). Median TTP was significantly shorter in Group I than in Group II ($P = 0.016$) and Group IV ($P < 0.001$), and significantly shorter TTP was observed in Group III when compared with Group II and IV (both $P < 0.050$). Patients in Group II also had significantly shorter TTP than patients in Group IV ($P = 0.010$). Death rates were 82.69, 69.81, 76.47, and 36.84%, respectively. Median OS was significantly shorter in Group I than in Group II ($P = 0.016$) and Group IV ($P < 0.001$), and significantly shorter OS was observed in Group III when compared with Group II and IV (both $P < 0.050$; **Figure 4F**). Patients in Group II also had significantly shorter OS than patients in Group IV ($P = 0.005$).

Post-TACE but Not Pre-TACE STIP1 Level as a Promising Marker for Predicting Tumor Response to Single TACE Treatment

We first observed the single TACE response rate (defined as PR+CR according to the definition of objective response rate) in four groups stratified by peri-TACE STIP1 levels. Response rates were 57.69, 83.02, 29.14, and 78.95%, respectively (**Figure 5A**). Further investigations revealed that pre-TACE STIP1 levels showed no significant difference between responsive and non-responsive patients ($P = 0.669$), whereas post-TACE STIP1 levels were significantly decreased in responsive HCC patients ($P < 0.001$; **Figure 5B**). Multivariate logistic regression analysis indicated that post-TACE STIP1 level was the most powerful independent indicator for predicting response (odds ratio 21.09, 95% CI 7.37–60.23, $P < 0.001$; **Table S1**). Consistently, ROC curve analysis demonstrated post-TACE STIP1 had the largest AUC-ROC (AUC = 0.767) for predicting response among all variates investigated (**Figure 5C**). However, post-TACE STIP1 level showed no correlation with baseline AFP level or baseline total tumor size (both $P > 0.050$; **Figures 5D,E**).

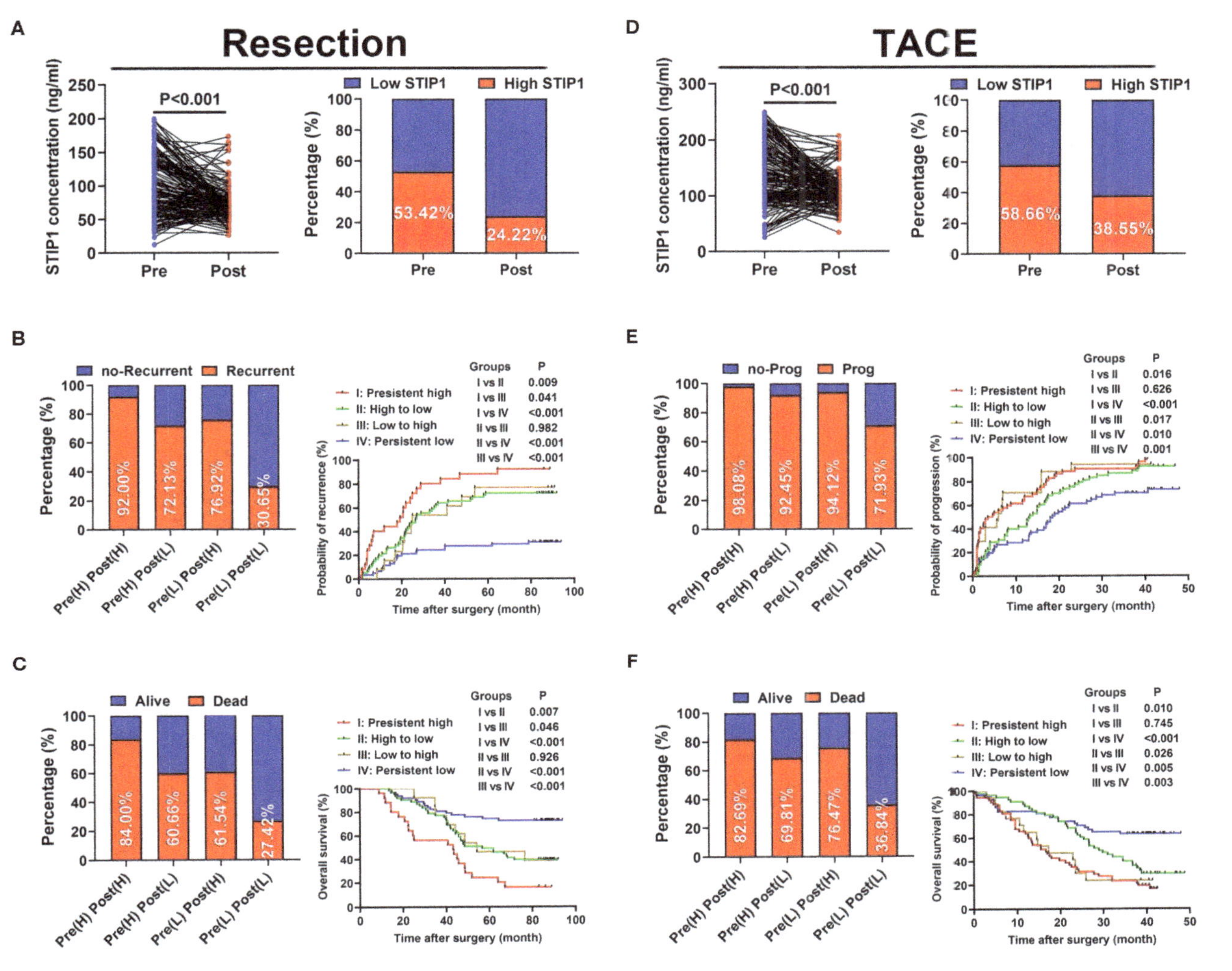

FIGURE 4 | Prognostic values of dynamic changes of serum STIP1 in patients with HCC. **(A)** Distribution of serum STIP1 level (left) and proportion of high STIP1 (right) during perioperative period in HCC patients received curative resection. **(B)** Recurrence rates (left) and Kaplan-Meier curve analyses of TTR (right) in HCC patients received curative resection according to their dynamic changes of serum STIP1 level. **(C)** Death rates (left) and Kaplan-Meier curve analyses of OS (right) in HCC patients received curative resection according to their dynamic changes of serum STIP1 level. **(D)** Distribution of serum STIP1 level (left) and proportion of high STIP1 (right) during peri-treatment period in HCC patients received TACE. **(E)** Progression rates (left) and Kaplan-Meier curve analyses of TTP (right) in HCC patients received TACE according to their dynamic changes of serum STIP1 level. **(F)** Death rates (left) and Kaplan-Meier curve analyses of OS (right) in HCC patients received TACE according to their dynamic changes of serum STIP1 level.

Pretreatment STIP1 Level as a Novel Indicator for Predicting MVI in HCC

Among all patients enrolled in the resection group, 66 (40.99%) patients encountered MVI. Pretreatment STIP1 levels were significantly increased in patients with MVI ($P < 0.001$; **Figure 6A**). Moreover, patients with high STIP1 had higher MVI-positive rates (55.81 vs. 24.00%; **Figure 6B**). ROC analysis revealed that pretreatment STIP1 exhibited the largest AUC (AUC = 0.644) among all variables explored (**Figure 6C** and **Table S2**). However, other involved predictors including AFP (AUC = 0.521), ALT (AUC = 0.456), differentiation (AUC = 0.611), tumor number (AUC = 0.602), and tumor size (AUC = 501) showed unsatisfactory performance. We further investigated the prognostic role of STIP1 in the MVI-absent subgroup. Similarly, pretreatment STIP1 was also significantly correlated with both shorter TTR ($P < 0.001$) and OS ($P = 0.012$; **Figure 6D**) in patients without MVI. Concordantly, MVI-absent patients with high pretreatment STIP1 levels had higher recurrence (60.53 vs. 22.81%) and death (44.74 vs. 21.57%) rates (**Figure 6E**).

DISCUSSION

Despite the great improvements made in last two decades, prognosis of HCC remains unsatisfactory (3). Such an embarrassing situation might be partially attributed to lack

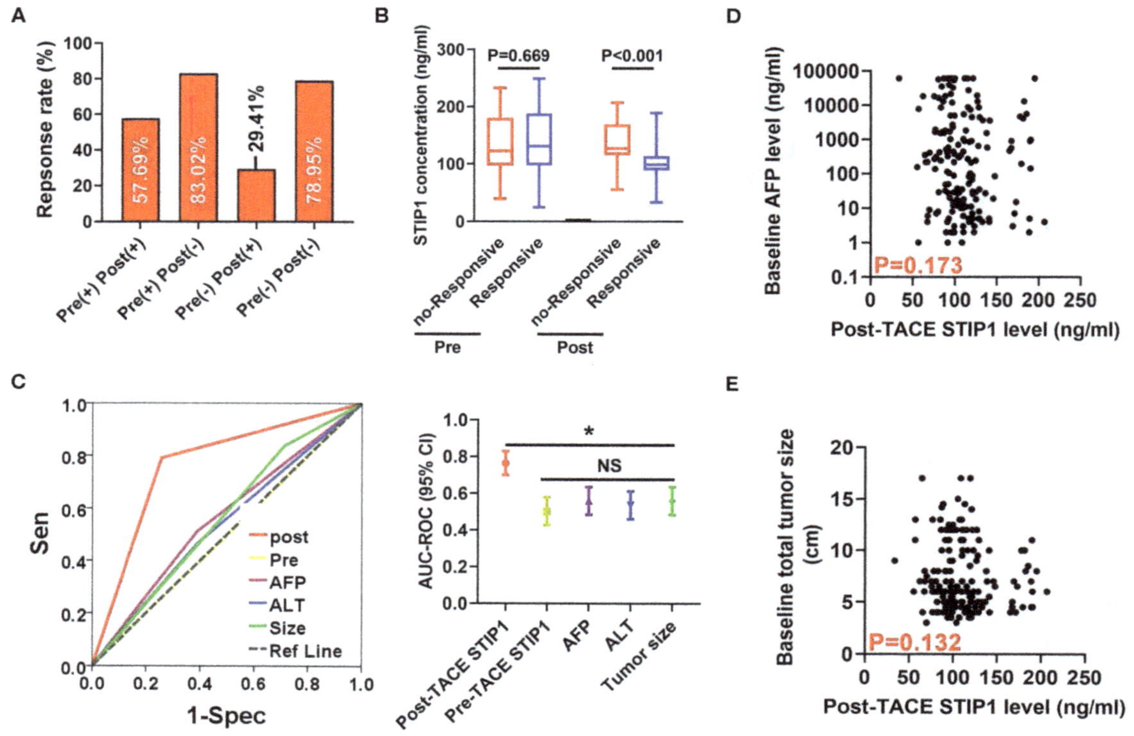

FIGURE 5 | Post-treatment STIP1 level as a novel indicator for predicting objective response after TACE. **(A)** Objective response (defined as CR+PR) rates in HCC patients received TACE according to their dynamic changes of serum STIP1 levels. **(B)** Distributions of pre- and post-TACE serum STIP1 levels in HCC patients with distinct response to TACE. **(C)** ROC curves of different variates for predicting OR after TACE. **(D)** Correlation between baseline AFP levels and post-TACE STIP1 levels. **(E)** Correlation between baseline AFP levels and post-TACE STIP1 levels. $^*P < 0.05$.

of a promising and reliable biomarker for outcome prediction and real-time surveillance of tumor progression. Here, we demonstrated serum STIP1 could serve as a novel biomarker to discriminate HCC patients with high risk of developing progression. Moreover, monitoring peri-treatment dynamic changes of STIP1 could provide useful information for predicting long-term prognosis after treatment. Importantly, post-TACE STIP1 level was identified as a powerful indicator to reflect the response to TACE. Specifically, our data also confirmed the clinical utility of STIP1 detection in predicting MVI.

As a crucial co-chaperone of HSP90 complex, STIP1 was reported to execute its elemental function with HSP90, resulting in rapid cancer progression (11). STIP1 was preferentially expressed in cancerous tissues of various solid tumors, including HCC, and high STIP1 expression was closely associated with dismal outcomes (11, 18, 21, 29). Moreover, functional assays confirmed STIP1 as a vital pro-oncogene during carcinogenesis process (30, 31). Interestingly, recent studies demonstrated STIP1 could be secreted by tumor cells and act as a critical cytokine to regulate malignant phenotype (17). STIP1 has been identified as crucial regulator of HCC progression. Previous studies have demonstrated that STIP1 promoted metastases foci formation via activating snail transcription and subsequently epithelial-to-mesenchymal transition in an HSP-dependent manner (31). Moreover, it could provoke HCC progression via interaction with Axin and DVL2 to activate beta-catenin signaling (29). Of note, secretory form STIP1 could stimulate HCC progression in an autocrine manner (21), which led us to raise the hypothesis that serum STIP1 might be a potential biomarker for predicting prognosis of HCC. Here, we showed that serum STIP levels were significantly elevated in HCC patients compared with either CHB patients or HDs. Intriguingly, STIP1 levels increased with HCC progression, suggesting the potential role of STIP1 in HCC diagnosis. Further investigation demonstrated pretreatment STIP1 level was an independent indicator for both tumor progression and survival, regardless of therapeutic approach. Clinically, AFP is currently the mostly widely used serum biomarker for evaluating prognosis. However, monitoring progression in low-AFP subgroups remains a challenge (22). We found serum STIP1 retained its prognostic value in low-AFP subgroups, suggesting STIP1 might be a useful supplement to AFP detection to achieve more accuracy in identifying patients with dismal outcomes. Together, our data indicated pretreatment STIP1 is a powerful and feasible biomarker for predicting prognosis in HCC.

Monitoring dynamic changes in tumor biomarkers during the peri-treatment period could provide critical information to reflect the disease status after treatment. Our data indicated serum STIP1 levels were dramatically decreased after treatment, and patients whose STIP1 level remained high or became high

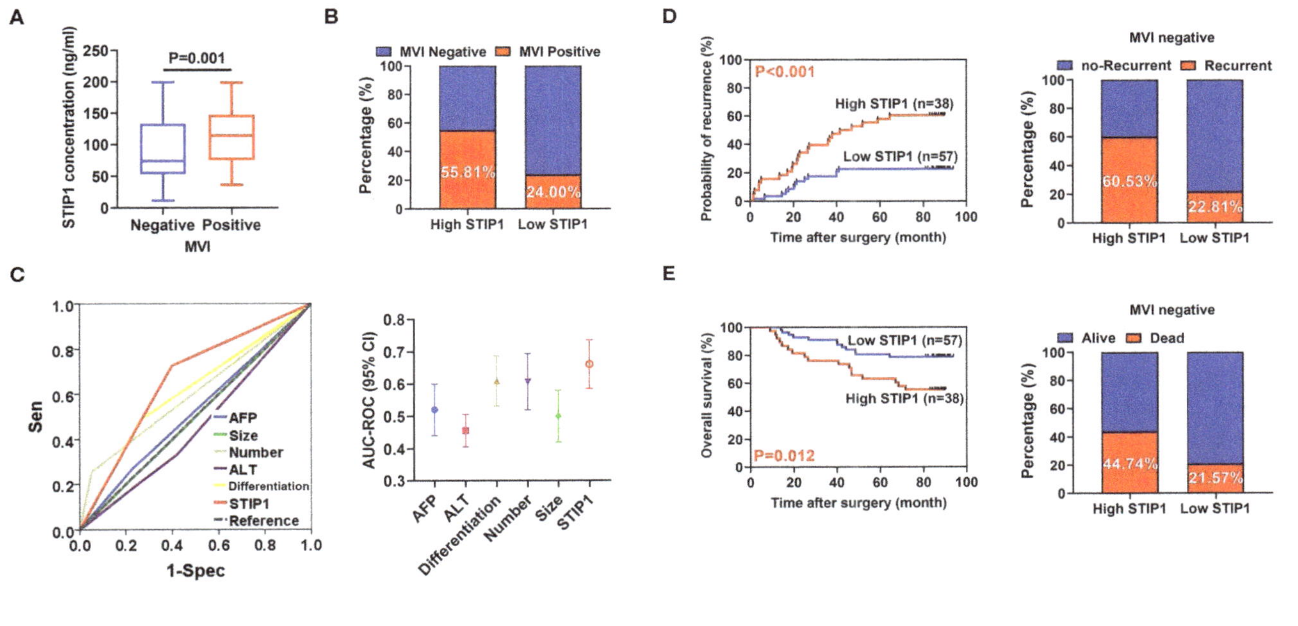

FIGURE 6 | Pretreatment serum STIP1 as a powerful predictor for MVI. **(A)** Comparison of pretreatment STIP1 levels between HCC patients with or without MVI. **(B)** MVI positive rates in HCC patients received curative resection according to pretreatment STIP1 levels. **(C)** ROC curves of various parameters for predicting MVI in HCC patients. **(D)** Kaplan-Meier curve of TTR (left) and recurrence rates (right) according to pretreatment STIP1 level in MVI-negative patients received curative resection. **(E)** Kaplan-Meier curve of OS (left) and recurrence rates (right) according to pretreatment STIP1 level in MVI-negative patients received curative resection.

after treatment suffered significantly worse long-term prognosis in both the resection and TACE groups. Because tumors were completely removed in patients who underwent curative resection, dynamic changes in STIP1 might reflect the micro-dissemination that could not be observed during operation. Thus, perioperative dynamic changes in STIP1 might be a valuable basis for the application of adjuvant interventions such as TACE or sorafenib after surgery. Meanwhile, for patients who received TACE, the predictive value of monitoring peri-TACE dynamic changes in STIP1 for long-term survival might reflect the intrinsic characteristics of HCC toward hypoxia and cytotoxicity. Thus, more importantly, our findings provide a more powerful and reliable basis to precisely predict the outcomes after TACE, as evidenced by greater AUC-ROC (**Figure S2**).

TACE is recommended as the first therapeutic approach for intermediate-HCC patients by BCLC criteria (32). However, heterogeneous responses to TACE were widely observed in clinical practice (33). Unfortunately, conventional pathological parameters for predicting treatment response were not available for patients in this study who received TACE due to difficulties in obtaining biopsy samples. Meanwhile, serum biomarkers are considered an ideal tool to monitor treatment response to TACE with the advantages of easy acquisition and noninvasiveness. Moreover, serum detection provides a safer and more convenient approach than imaging scans with the advantage of non-exposure to radiation. Here, we found post-TACE but not pre-TACE STIP1 levels were closely associated with the objective response rate after single TACE treatment. Further ROC curve analysis demonstrated the satisfactory performance of post-TACE STIP1 level for predicting OR. Notably, post-TACE STIP1 level showed no correlation with baseline tumor size or AFP level, suggesting the universal use of post-TACE STIP1 level in evaluating response to single TACE treatment, regardless of baseline HCC status. Together, our data indicated that post-TACE STIP1 detection was a promising non-invasive method with strong predictive power toward therapeutic response.

Accumulating clinical evidence confirmed the presence of MVI as a significant risk indicator for worse outcomes in HCC (34). Clinically, the presence of MVI acts as a crucial indicator for selecting appropriate therapeutic intervention for HCC patients (35). Unfortunately, most of the risk factors associated with MVI are pathological characteristics that can only be determined in resected samples or biopsy, posing a problem in routine clinical practice (36, 37). Therefore, identification of serum biomarkers for predicting MVI before treatment might improve HCC management. Here, we reported that patients with high pretreatment serum STIP1 levels had a high possibility of harboring MVI, and high STIP1 was confirmed as an independent predictor for MVI. Moreover, we found the predictive performance of STIP1 was stronger than other biomarkers such as AFP, tumor size, and tumor number. Thus, our findings demonstrate a powerful tool for providing accurate and useful information for MVI prediction in HCC, enabling early clinical decisions to tailor appropriate therapeutic approaches for individualized therapy in HCC.

There are several limitations in our present study. First, it was a single-centered, retrospective study. Therefore, prospective and external validations are further needed in the future. Second, most patients enrolled had HBV backgrounds, which greatly differed from the patients in United States or Europe (38). We could not exclude the possibility that the predictive value of serum STIP1 was not applicable in HCC patients with other etiology backgrounds, and further confirmation is also needed. Finally, despite the satisfactory performance of STIP1, more investigations should be conducted to optimize the best cutoff or generate novel index containing STIP1 and other serum biomarkers to improve the discrimination power.

CONCLUSIONS

In summary, our data demonstrated the prognostic significance of serum STIP1 in HCC. Importantly, dynamic changes in STIP1 were found to exert great significance in reflecting treatment response, especially in predicting objective response to single TACE intervention. Moreover, our data indicated STIP1 detection as a useful tool for predicting MVI before surgery with the advantages of convenience and accuracy. Integration of serum STIP1 detection into HCC management might facilitate early clinical decision-making to improve the prognosis of HCC patients in the future.

AUTHOR CONTRIBUTIONS

X-LM, GL, and R-QL: conceptualization. X-LM, S-HX, M-JY, M-LW, and W-GT: methodology. GL and R-QL: validation, visualization, supervision, and project administration. X-LM, M-LW, and M-JY: formal analysis. X-LM and M-JY: investigation. W-GT, GL, and R-QL: resources. X-LM, GL, and R-QL: data curation. X-LM: writing—original draft preparation. All authors: writing (review and editing). W-GT, GL, and R-QL: funding acquisition.

ACKNOWLEDGMENTS

We thank Prof. Ning Ren and Dr. Pei-Yao Fu from the Department of Liver Surgery, Zhongshan Hospital, Fudan University, for their help in evaluating objective response after TACE.

REFERENCES

1. Zhu XD, Sun HC. Emerging agents and regimens for hepatocellular carcinoma. *J Hematol Oncol.* (2019) 12:110. doi: 10.1186/s13045-019-0794-6
2. Hou J, Zhang H, Sun B, Karin M. The immunobiology of hepatocellular carcinoma in humans mice: basic concepts therapeutic implications. *J Hepatol.* (2019) 72:167–82. doi: 10.1016/j.jhep.2019.08.014
3. Yang JD, Hainaut P, Gores GJ, Amadou A, Plymoth A, Roberts LR. A global view of hepatocellular carcinoma: trends, risk, prevention and management. *Nat Rev Gastroenterol Hepatol.* (2019) 16:589–604. doi: 10.1038/s41575-019-0186-y
4. Toh TB, Lim JJ, Hooi L, Rashid MBMA, Chow EK. Targeting Jak/Stat pathway as a therapeutic strategy against SP/CD44+ tumorigenic cells in Akt/β-catenin-driven hepatocellular carcinoma. *J Hepatol.* (2019) 72:104–18. doi: 10.1016/j.jhep.2019.08.035
5. Bonnin M, Fares N, Testoni B, Estornes Y, Weber K, Vanbervliet B, et al. Toll-like receptor 3 downregulation is an escape mechanism from apoptosis during hepatocarcinogenesis. *J Hepatol.* (2019) 71:763–72. doi: 10.1016/j.jhep.2019.05.031
6. Yau T, Hsu C, Kim TY, Choo SP, Kang YK, Hou MM, et al. Nivolumab in advanced hepatocellular carcinoma: sorafenib-experienced Asian cohort analysis. *J Hepatol.* (2019) 71:543–52. doi: 10.1016/j.jhep.2019.05.014
7. Zhang XP, Liu YC, Chen ZH, Sun JX, Wang K, Chai ZT, et al. Postoperative adjuvant transarterial chemoembolization improves outcomes of hepatocellular carcinoma associated with hepatic vein invasion: a propensity score matching analysis. *Ann Surg Oncol.* (2019) 26:1465–73. doi: 10.1245/s10434-019-07223-z
8. Le Y, Shen JX, Zhang YF, He MK, Kan A, Chen HL, et al. Transarterial chemoembolization related to good survival for selected patients with advanced hepatocellular carcinoma. *J Cancer.* (2019) 10:665–71. doi: 10.7150/jca.28528
9. Wang Q, Xia D, Bai W, Wang E, Sun J, Huang M, et al. Development of a prognostic score for recommended TACE candidates with hepatocellular carcinoma: a multicentre observational study. *J Hepatol.* (2019) 70:893–903. doi: 10.1016/j.jhep.2019.01.013
10. Liu S, Li H, Guo L, Zhang B, Zhou B, Zhang W, et al. Tumor size affects efficacy of adjuvant transarterial chemoembolization in patients with hepatocellular carcinoma and microvascular invasion. *Oncologist.* (2019) 24:513–20. doi: 10.1634/theoncologist.2018-0305
11. Zhang S, Shao J, Su F. Prognostic significance of STIP1 expression in human cancer: a meta-analysis. *Clin Chim Acta.* (2018) 486:168–76. doi: 10.1016/j.cca.2018.07.037
12. Tsai CL, Chao A, Jung SM, Tsai CN, Lin CY, Chen SH, et al. Stress-induced phosphoprotein-1 maintains the stability of JAK2 in cancer cells. *Oncotarget.* (2016) 7:50548–63. doi: 10.18632/oncotarget.10500
13. Xu CP, Li X, Hu YJ, Cui Z, Wang L, Liang L, et al. Quantitative proteomics reveals ELP2 as a regulator to the inhibitory effect of TNF-α on osteoblast differentiation. *J Proteomics.* (2015) 114:234–46. doi: 10.1016/j.jprot.2014.11.002
14. Cho H, Kim S, Shin HY, Chung EJ, Kitano H, Hyon, et al. Expression of stress-induced phosphoprotein1 (STIP1) is associated with tumor progression and poor prognosis in epithelial ovarian cancer. *Genes Chromosomes Cancer.* (2014) 53:277–88. doi: 10.1002/gcc.22136
15. van Simaeys D, Turek D, Champanhac C, Vaizer J, Sefah K, Zhen J, et al. Identification of cell membrane protein stress-induced phosphoprotein 1 as a potential ovarian cancer biomarker using aptamers selected by cell systematic evolution of ligands by exponential enrichment. *Anal Chem.* (2014) 86:4521–7. doi: 10.1021/ac500466x
16. Tsai CL, Tsai CN, Lin CY, Chen HW, Lee YS, Chao A, et al. Secreted stress-induced phosphoprotein 1 activates the ALK2-SMAD signaling pathways and promotes cell proliferation of ovarian cancer cells. *Cell Rep.* (2012) 2:283–93. doi: 10.1016/j.celrep.2012.07.002
17. Wang TH, Chao A, Tsai CL, Chang CL, Chen SH, Lee YS, et al. Stress-induced phosphoprotein 1 as a secreted biomarker for human ovarian cancer promotes cancer cell proliferation. *Mol Cell Proteomics.* (2010) 9:1873–84. doi: 10.1074/mcp.M110.000802
18. Huang L, Zhai E, Cai S, Lin Y, Liao J, Jin H, et al. Stress-inducible Protein-1 promotes metastasis of gastric cancer via Wnt/β-catenin signaling pathway. *J Exp Clin Cancer Res.* (2018) 37:6. doi: 10.1186/s13046-018-0676-8
19. Krafft U, Tschirdewahn S, Hess J, Harke NN, Hadaschik BA, Nyirády P, et al. STIP1 tissue expression is associated with survival in chemotherapy-treated bladder cancer patients. *Pathol Oncol Res.* (2019). doi: 10.1007/s12253-019-00689-y. [Epub ahead of print].
20. Wang HS, Tsai CL, Chang PY, Chao A, Wu RC, Chen SH, et al. Positive associations between upregulated levels of stress-induced phosphoprotein 1 and matrix metalloproteinase-9 in endometriosis/adenomyosis. *PLoS ONE.* (2018) 13:e0190573. doi: 10.1371/journal.pone.0190573
21. Chen Z, Xu L, Su T, Ke Z, Peng Z, Zhang N, et al. Autocrine STIP1 signaling promotes tumor growth and is associated with disease outcome in

hepatocellular carcinoma. *Biochem Biophys Res Commun.* (2017) 493:365–72. doi: 10.1016/j.bbrc.2017.09.016
22. Ma XL, Jiang M, Zhao Y, Wang BL, Shen MN, Zhou Y, et al. Application of serum Annexin A3 in diagnosis, outcome prediction and therapeutic response evaluation for patients with hepatocellular carcinoma. *Ann Surg Oncol.* (2018) 25:1686–94. doi: 10.1245/s10434-018-6402-0
23. Zhang XP, Zhou TF, Wang ZH, Zhang F, Zhong CQ, Hu YR, et al. Association of preoperative hypercoagulability with poor prognosis in hepatocellular carcinoma patients with microvascular invasion after liver resection: a multicenter study. *Ann Surg Oncol.* (2019) 26:4117–25. doi: 10.1245/s10434-019-07504-7
24. Yoh T, Seo S, Taura K, Iguchi K, Ogiso S, Fukumitsu K, et al. Surgery for recurrent hepatocellular carcinoma: achieving long-term survival. *Ann Surg.* (2019). doi: 10.1097/SLA.0000000000003358. [Epub ahead of print].
25. Li J, Wang Q, Lei Z, Wu D, Si A, Wang K, et al. Adjuvant transarterial chemoembolization following liver resection for intrahepatic cholangiocarcinoma based on survival risk stratification. *Oncologist.* (2015) 20:640–7. doi: 10.1634/theoncologist.2014-0470
26. Guo W, Yang XR, Sun YF, Shen MN, Ma XL, Wu J, et al. Clinical significance of EpCAM mRNA-positive circulating tumor cells in hepatocellular carcinoma by an optimized negative enrichment and qRT-PCR-based platform. *Clin Cancer Res.* (2014) 20:4794–805. doi: 10.1158/1078-0432.CCR-14-0251
27. Loosen SH, Schulze-Hagen M, Leyh C, Benz F, Vucur M, Kuhl C, et al. IL-6 and IL-8 serum levels predict tumor response and overall survival after TACE for primary and secondary hepatic malignancies. *Int J Mol Sci.* (2018) 19:1766. doi: 10.3390/ijms19061766
28. Yoon SM, Ryoo BY, Lee SJ, Kim JH, Shin JH, An JH, et al. Efficacy and safety of transarterial chemoembolization plus external beam radiotherapy vs sorafenib in hepatocellular carcinoma with macroscopic vascular invasion: a randomized clinical trial. *JAMA Oncol.* (2018) 4:661–9. doi: 10.1001/jamaoncol.2017.5847
29. Luo X, Liu Y, Ma S, Liu L, Xie R, Li M, et al. STIP1 is over-expressed in hepatocellular carcinoma and promotes the growth and migration of cancer cells. *Gene.* (2018) 662:110–7. doi: 10.1016/j.gene.2018.03.076
30. Xu W, Rao Q, An Y, Li M, Zhang Z. Identification of biomarkers for Barcelona clinic liver Cancer staging and overall survival of patients with hepatocellular carcinoma. *PLoS ONE.* (2018) 13:e0202763. doi: 10.1371/journal.pone.0202763
31. Su T, Liao J, Dai Z, Xu L, Chen S, Wang Y, et al. Stress-induced phosphoprotein 1 mediates hepatocellular carcinoma metastasis after insufficient radiofrequency ablation. *Oncogene.* (2018) 37:3514–27. doi: 10.1038/s41388-018-0169-4
32. Llovet JM, Montal R, Sia D, Finn RS. Molecular therapies and precision medicine for hepatocellular carcinoma. *Nat Rev Clin Oncol.* (2018) 15:599–616. doi: 10.1038/s41571-018-0073-4
33. Raoul JL, Forner A, Bolondi L, Cheung TT, Kloeckner R, de Baere T. Updated use of TACE for hepatocellular carcinoma treatment: how and when to use it based on clinical evidence. *Cancer Treat Rev.* (2019) 72:28–36. doi: 10.1016/j.ctrv.2018.11.002
34. Finn RS, Zhu AX, Farah W, Almasri J, Zaiem F, Prokop LJ, et al. Therapies for advanced stage hepatocellular carcinoma with macrovascular invasion or metastatic disease: a systematic review and meta-analysis. *Hepatology.* (2018) 67:422–35. doi: 10.1002/hep.29486
35. Zhang X, Li J, Shen F, Lau WY. Significance of presence of microvascular invasion in specimens obtained after surgical treatment of hepatocellular carcinoma. *J Gastroenterol Hepatol.* (2018) 33:347–54. doi: 10.1111/jgh.13843
36. Hyun SH, Eo JS, Song BI, Lee JW, Na SJ, Hong IK, et al. Preoperative prediction of microvascular invasion of hepatocellular carcinoma using (18)F-FDG PET/CT: a multicenter retrospective cohort study. *Eur J Nucl Med Mol Imaging.* (2018) 45:720–6. doi: 10.1007/s00259-017-3880-4
37. Erstad DJ, Tanabe KK. Prognostic and therapeutic implications of microvascular invasion in hepatocellular carcinoma. *Ann Surg Oncol.* (2019) 26:1474–93. doi: 10.1245/s10434-019-07227-9
38. Hu B, Yang XR, Xu Y, Sun YF, Sun C, Guo W, et al. Systemic immune-inflammation index predicts prognosis of patients after curative resection for hepatocellular carcinoma. *Clin Cancer Res.* (2014) 20:6212–22. doi: 10.1158/1078-0432.CCR-14-0442

15

Liver Transplantation *versus* Liver Resection for Stage I and II Hepatocellular Carcinoma: Results of an Instrumental Variable Analysis

Wei Li[1†], Haitao Xiao[1†], Hong Wu[2], Xuewen Xu[1] and Yange Zhang[1*]*

[1] Department of Plastic and Burns Surgery, West China Hospital, Sichuan University, Chengdu, China, [2] Department of Liver Surgery & Liver Transplantation Center, West China Hospital, Sichuan University, Chengdu, China

Correspondence:
Yange Zhang
zhangyange7801@163.com
Xuewen Xu
xxw_0826@163.com

[†]These authors have contributed equally to this work

Background: This study aimed to compare the long-term outcomes of liver transplantation (LT) and liver resection (LR) among patients with stage I and II hepatocellular carcinoma (HCC).

Methods: SEER 18 registry from 2004 to 2015 was retrieved for this study. We included 1,765 and 1,746 cases with stage I–II (AJCC, 7th) HCC in the multivariable analyses and instrumental variable (IV) analyses, respectively. Propensity score matching (PSM) was further carried out to ensure comparability. Propensity score to receive LT was adjusted by stabilized inverse probability of treatment weighting (IPTW) and standardized mortality ratio weighting (SMRW) methods. In addition, IV analysis was performed to adjust both measured and unmeasured confounding factors.

Results: We identified 1,000 (56.7%) and 765 (43.3%) patients treated with LR and LT, respectively. In the multivariable adjusted cohort, after adjusting potential confounders, patients undergoing LT offered significant prognostic advantages over LR in overall survival (OS, $P < 0.001$) and disease-free survival (DSS, $P < 0.001$). The instrument variable in this study is LT rates in various Health Service Areas (HSAs). Results from the IV analysis showed that cases treated with LT had significantly longer OS ($P = 0.001$) and DSS ($P < 0.001$). In IV analysis stratified by clinicopathologic variables, the treatment effect of LT *vs.* LR in OS was consistent across all subgroups. Regarding DSS in IV analyses, the subgroup analyses observed that LT had better DSS across all subgroups, except for similar results in the older patients (interaction P value = 0.039) and the non-White patients (interaction P value = 0.041). In the propensity-matched cohort, patients with LT still had better OS ($P < 0.001$) and DSS ($P < 0.001$) in comparison to cases who underwent LR. In both IPTW and SMRW cohorts, patients who underwent LT had better OS (both P values < 0.001) and DSS (both P values < 0.001).

Conclusions: LT provided a survival benefit for cases with stage I–II HCC. These results indicated that if LT rate was to increase in the future, average long-term survival may also increase. However, for some special populations such as the elderly patients, owing to the similar outcomes between LT and LR, the selection of LT should be cautious.

Keywords: hepatocellular carcinoma, liver resection, liver transplantation, survival, instrumental variable analysis

INTRODUCTION

Liver cancer is the second most frequent cause of cancer death worldwide (1). Hepatocellular carcinoma (HCC) is the most common type of primary liver cancer globally (2). Liver resection (LR) is recommended as first-line treatment in HCC patients without liver cirrhosis (1). In contrast, for HCC cases with cirrhosis, indications for LR are generally based on the comprehensive evaluation of tumor burden, liver function, extent of resection, expected remnant liver volume, cases' comorbid conditions, and performance status (3, 4). Except for LR, liver transplantation (LT) is also an excellent radical therapy choice for HCC cases, eliminating both of the underlying liver cirrhosis and tumor. LT is a first-line therapeutic option for tumors meeting the Milan criteria but unsuitable for resection (1). Despite these recommendations, for early stage HCC patients with compensated liver function, in some situations (*e.g.*, patients with available liver donation), LT can also be utilized to achieve radical cure (5–7).

For cases with early stage HCC who are candidates for both LT and LR, there is no consensus on the eligibility criteria for LR or LT in the current data (5, 6, 8–11). Recent studies comparing LT with LR have demonstrated superior survival outcomes of LT in patients with early stage HCC (6, 12). However, owing to the significant heterogeneity among the included patients in these retrospective studies, it is still controversial with regard to which modality provides better long-term results. The aim of the present study was to compare the long-term outcomes of LT and LR in cases with early stage (stages I and II) HCC. To achieve it, instrumental variable (IV) analyses were used in this study. IV analysis is a statistical method that serves as an alternative to random assignment to treatment and addresses confounders owing to both known and unknown factors (13, 14).

PATIENTS AND METHODS

Patient Identification

Surveillance, Epidemiology, and End Results (SEER; seer.cancer.gov/about/overview.html) 18 database from 2004 to 2015 was retrieved for this study. Firstly, 68505 patients with pathological diagnosis as HCC were identified according to the International Classification of Diseases for Oncology, 3rd Edition [ICD-O-3] site code C22.0 and histologic type ICD-O-3 codes 8170-8175. All cases were treated between 2004 and 2015 from the SEER database. Flowchart of the patient selection process was presented in **Figure 1**. Patients with early-stage (stage I and II; AJCC, 7th) HCC matching the specified eligibility criteria were included in the multivariable analyses (n = 1765) and IV analyses (n = 1746), respectively. The codes in SEER database for HCC treatment included: LR: 20-25, 30, 36, 37, 50, 51, and 52; LT: 61.

Statistical Analysis

Overall survival (OS) was defined as the interval from the date of diagnosis to the date of death with any causes, and the disease-specific survival (DSS) was defined as the time until death attributed to HCC. Continuous variables were presented as mean ± SD (tested by t-test or Kruskal-Wallis H test) and categorical variables were expressed as number (%) (tested by Chi-square test or Fisher's exact test). Linear trends in the percentage of patients receiving each type of treatment was evaluated by Cochrane-Armitage trend test.

Survival curves were performed using the Kaplan-Meier method and the differences in the survival rates between two groups were compared via log-rank test. Multivariable Cox models were used to adjust for available confounding factors. Interaction tests were used to examine the influence of each stratified indicator on the relations between surgical modality and patient prognosis.

Propensity score-matched (PSM) analysis was done based on the following factors: race, sex, age, year of diagnosis, tumor size, fibrosis-score (Ishak; FS) and alpha-fetoprotein (AFP). Cases were matched with the closest estimated propensity score within 0.02, and we performed a 1:1 nearest-neighbor matching with the preset caliber. Univariable Cox regression was utilized to compare the survival outcomes of LR vs. LT in the cohort after PSM selection.

In addition, PS to receive LT was adjusted by a standardized mortality ratio weighting (SMRW) and stabilized inverse probability of treatment weighting (IPTW) methods. The IPTW assigned weights of 1/PS for patients receiving LT and 1/ (1-PS) for patients undergoing LR. The SMRW assigned a weight of 1 for LT patients and a weight of PS/ (1-PS) for cases with LR. OS and DSS of LT vs. LR were then compared (univariable Cox regression) using the PS-adjusted pseudopopulation created by these two statistical procedures.

In this study, the LT rate in different Health Service Areas (HSAs) was utilized as the instrumental variable. The IV approach depends on the assumption that LT rate was highly related to the selection of treatment methods (cases with higher HAS LR rates usually had a higher opportunity to receive LR), and the IV was not associated with patient survival except through its correlation with the treatment methods (15). In addition, the IV was unrelated to unmeasured risk factors affecting the outcome. Cases from HSAs with less than 10 cases were excluded, because the LT rates could not be

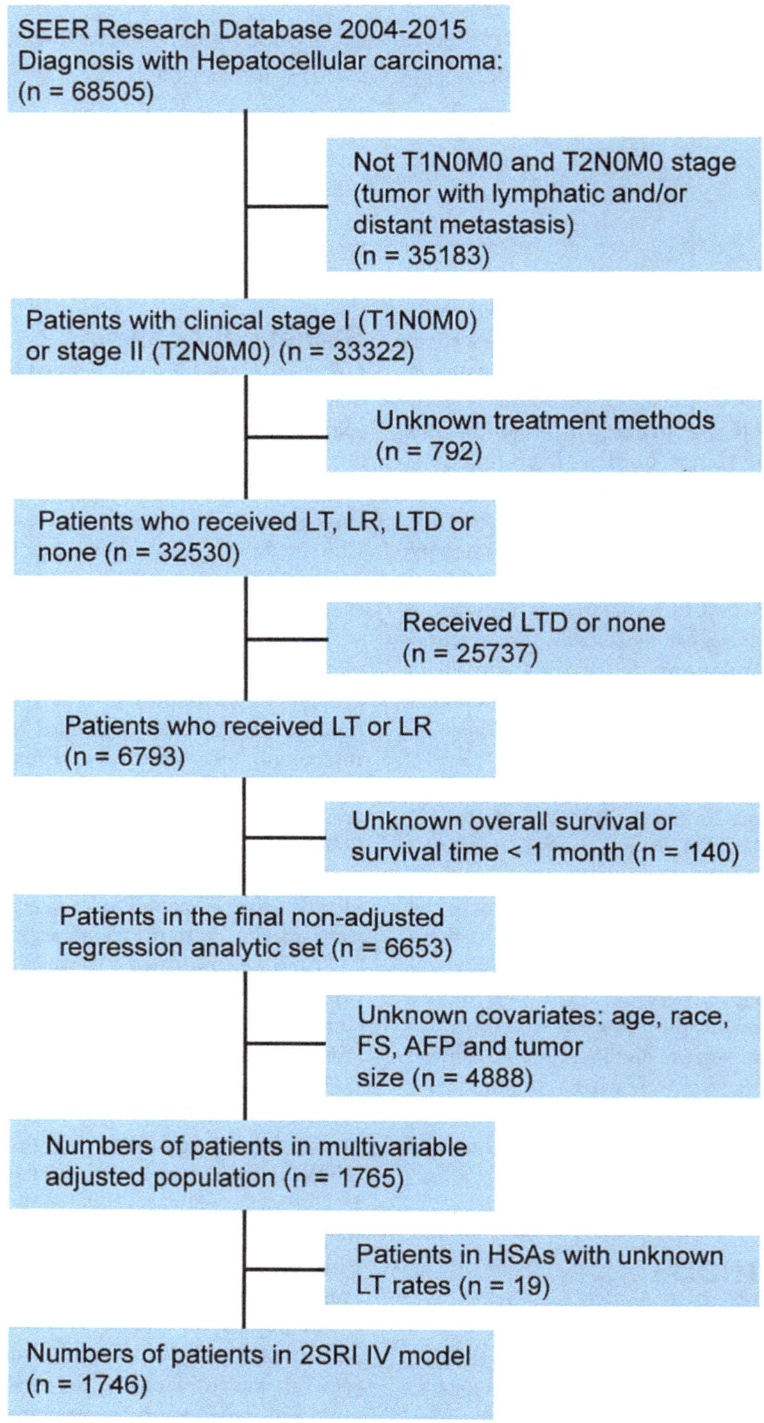

FIGURE 1 | Flowchart showing selection process of cases included in this study. SEER, Surveillance, Epidemiology, and End Results; LT, liver transplantation; LR, liver resection; LTD, local tumor destruction; FS, fibrosis score; AFP, alpha-fetoprotein; HAS, Health Service Area; 2SRI, two-stage residual inclusion; IV, instrumental variable.

confirmed accurately in those HSAs (16). To assess the validity of LT rates in HSAs as an IV, we verified that LT rate in a HSA was significantly associated with likelihood of treatment assignment (the F statistic exceeding 10 is suggestive of a strong instrument), while not associated with OS in the Multivariable regression analysis. Besides, covariate balance was examined across quintiles. We used a two-stage residual inclusion (2SRI) method in the instrumental variable analysis (17).

It is important to note that, rather than exploring the average treatment effects for a group of cases (as in a randomized trial), the IV analysis focuses on the treatment effect among those whose selection of therapy is affected by the instrumental variable (18). LT rates in HSAs was utilized as the IV, which indicates that our results are generalizable only to cases whose treatment assignment was influenced by the LT rates in different HSAs. In summary, this study analyzed the treatment effect among marginal patients. The marginal patients are those with early-stage HCC would receive LT in a areas with higher LR rates while not in HSAs with lower LR rates, (18, 19) because treatment method (LT or LR) for cases with a uncertain or borderline need for LT could be influenced by experience and preferences in different areas. P value < 0.05 was defined as statistically significant. Statistical analysis was carried out by R 3.6.3.

RESULTS

Demographics

Among 6653 patients treated surgically for stage I and II HCC, we identified 1000 (56.7%) and 765 (43.3%) patients treated with LR or LT, respectively. **Figure 2** showed the number and incidence of 6653 cases with stage I-II HCC (AJCC 7th) between 2004 and 2015 with LT or LR. Incidence rate of LT was decreased over time (P < 0 001), while incidence of cases undergoing LR was increased over time (P < 0.001). The general patient characteristics was shown in **Table 1**. The mean age of patients with LT and LR was 57.1 and 62.6 years, respectively. Cases undergoing LT were younger, more often male and the White, and more patients had stage II disease. When patients underwent LT, their tumors were more likely to measure < 3 cm (65.8%), and more cases had cirrhotic liver (88.9%). For cases

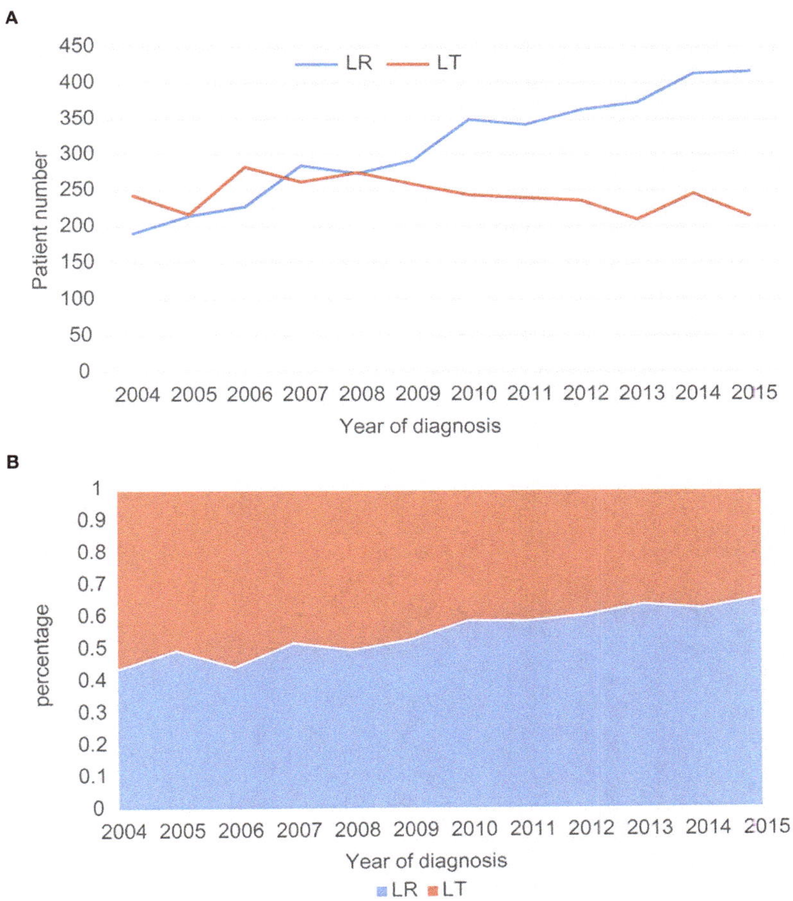

FIGURE 2 | **(A)** Number of cases with stage I-II HCC from 2004 to 2015 in the SEER cohort. **(B)** Incidence of cases with stage I-II HCC from 2004 to 2015 in the SEER cohort (both P trend values for LT and LR <0.001).

with LR, more cases had non-cirrhotic liver (FS in 53.5% of cases was between 0-4), and 35% of cases had tumors larger than 5 cm.

Multivariable Cox Regression

The current study included a total of 1765 cases with available data needed in survival analysis. The mean DSS for cases with LT or LR were 124.0 and 87.4 months, respectively. The mean OS for all of the cases receiving LT or LR were 106.6 and 77.8 months, respectively. In survival analysis, cases undergoing LT showed longer OS (P < 0.001) and DSS (P < 0.001) in comparison to cases receiving LR (**Figures 3A, C**).

The results in the multivariable adjusted cohort (OS: n = 1765; DSS: n = 1406) showed that cases receiving LT had a better DSS (HR 0.21, 95% CI 0.15 to 0.29, P < 0.001) and OS (HR 0.27, 95% CI 0.23 to 0.33, P < 0.001) compared to those undergoing LR.

Instrumental Variable Analyses

All cases were divided into quintiles based on the proportion of patients within each HSA undergoing LT (**Supplementary Table 1**). The average LT rate ranged from 3% (quintile 1) to 8% (quintile 5) among different HSAs. The F-statistic is 104.8 (P < 0.001), which confirmed the validity of this instrument. Besides, there was no significant relationship between the IV and OS in a standard Cox regression analysis (HR 1.12, 95% CI 0.94-1.34, P = 0.198). In summary, these observations indicated that LT rate in HSAs could be utilized as a valid instrument variable.

Finally, results in the IV analysis were consistent with those observed in the traditional regression analyses. Outcomes according to this instrument demonstrated that patients receiving LT had an obviously better DSS (HR 0.29, 95% CI 0.16-0.55, P < 0.001) and OS (HR 0.47, 95% CI 0.29-0.75, P = 0.001) after adjusting both measured and unmeasured confounders (**Table 2**).

Stratified Analyses

Based on multivariable Cox analyses, the **Figure 4** showed the relation of surgical modality and patient prognosis stratified by clinical parameters. In subgroup analyses, the salutary effect of LT vs. LR on overall survival was consistent in all subgroups, except for a similar outcome in the non-cirrhotic subgroup (HR 0.72, 95%CI 0.40-1.29, interaction P value = 0.017) (**Figure 4A**). The superior survival benefits of LT vs. LR on DSS were consistent across all subgroups with the exception of a similar outcome in the subgroup of age > 70 years (HR 0.40, 95%CI 0.08-2.03, interaction P value = 0.038) (**Figure 4B**).

In IV analyses stratified by clinical variables, we observed that the treatment effect of LT (OS) was consistent across all subgroups (all interaction P values > 0.05), as well as in those with a non-cirrhotic liver (**Figure 5A**). With regard to DSS, the exploratory subgroup analyses observed similar results in the older patients (> 60, <70 years: HR 0.33, 95%CI 0.10-1.10; ≥ 70 years: HR 1.32, 95%CI 0.16-11.25, interaction P value = 0.039) and the non-White population (Black: HR 0.10, 95%CI 0.01-1.23; Other: HR 0.31, 95% CI 0.07-1.41, interaction P value = 0.041), and LT had better DSS across the other subgroups (**Figure 5B**).

Results in Propensity Score Matched Cohort

As presented in **Supplementary Table 2**, in the matched cohort, most of the prognostic variables were well-balanced. After PSM, cases receiving LT showed better DSS and OS (both P values < 0.001) compared to patients undergoing LR (**Figures 3B, D**). In the PSM cohort, the univariable analysis demonstrated that

TABLE 1 | Characteristics of the entire study sample by treatment received.

	LR (n = 1,000)	LT (n = 765)	P value
Sex (female/male)	269/731	165/600	0.010
Age (years)			
≥18, <45	44 (4.4%)	29 (3.8%)	<0.001
≥45, <60	324 (32.4%)	427 (55.8%)	
≥60, <70	380 (38.0%)	286 (37.4%)	
>=70	252 (25.2%)	18 (2.4%)	
Marriage status (married/divorced or separated/single)	644/181/154	516/113/111	0.160
Insurance (yes/no)	867/14	593/2	0.037
Race (White/Black/other/unknown)	511/128/354/7	595/63/105/2	<0.001
Year of diagnosis (2004–2009/2010–2015)	307/693	341/424	<0.001
AFP (ng/ml negative/positive)	399/601	305/460	0.990
Tumor size (cm)			<0.001
<3	267 (26.7%)	503 (65.8%)	
≥3, <5	363 (36.3%)	225 (29.4%)	
≥5, <7	175 (17.5%)	32 (4.2%)	
≥7	195 (19.5%)	5 (0.7%)	
One lesion in one lobe (yes/no)	602/398	341/424	<0.001
Vascular invasion (no/yes)	766/234	548/217	0.018
AJCC-TNM stage (I/II/)	694/306	372/393	<0.001
Fibrosis score (0–4/5–6)	535/465	85/680	<0.001
Tumor differentiation (I/II/III/IV/unknown)	234/559/191/16/0	255/424/84/2/0	<0.001

Data are shown as mean ± SD or n (%). LR, liver resection; LT, liver transplantation; AFP, alpha-fetoprotein; AJCC, American Joint Committee on Cancer. Tumor differentiation: I, well-differentiated; II, moderate-differentiated; III, poor-differentiated; IV, un-differentiated.

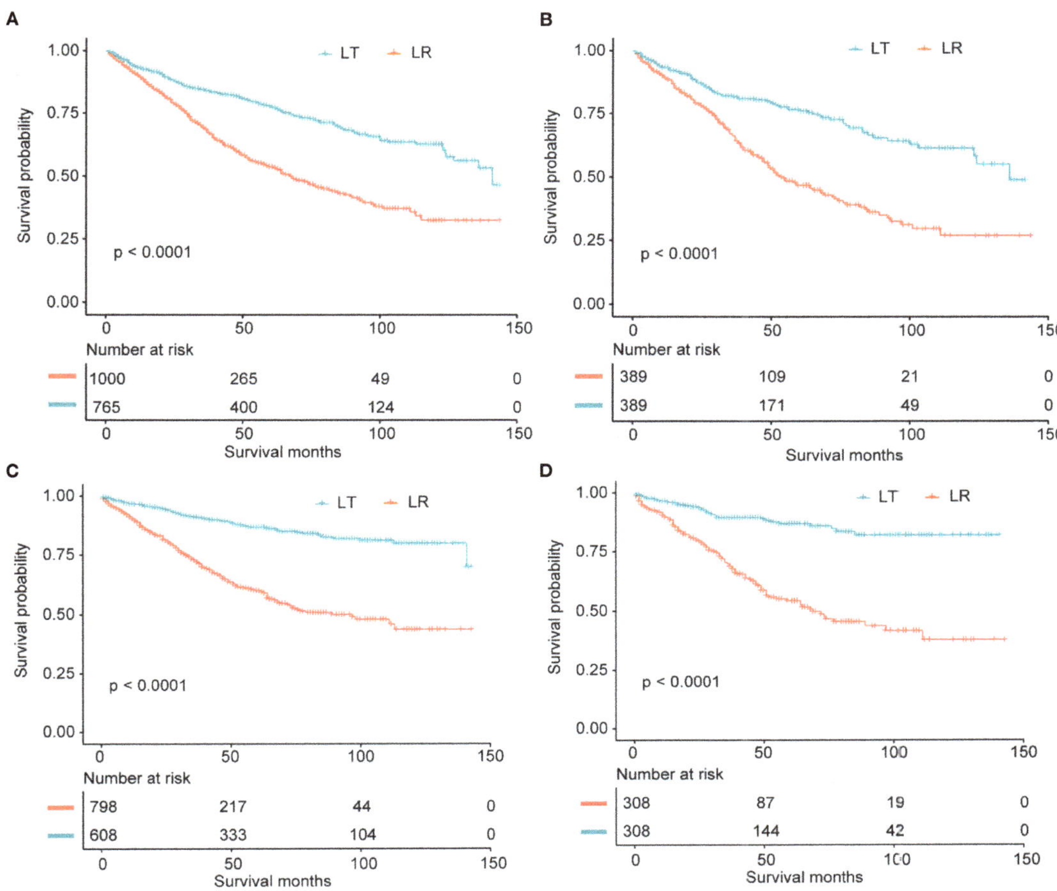

FIGURE 3 | **(A)** Overall survival analysis for patients who underwent LR and LT in non-adjusted population. **(B)** Overall survival analysis for patients after LR and LT in propensity score matched cohort. **(C)** Disease-specific survival analysis for cases receiving LR and LT in non-adjusted cohort. **(D)** Disease-specific survival analysis for cases after LR and LT in propensity score matched cohort.

TABLE 2 | Instrumental variable analysis of the impact of surgery methods (LT *vs.* LR) on survival for patients with hepatocellular carcinoma in 2SRI IV Model.

	All-cause survival			**Cancer-specific survival**		
	HR	**95% CI**	**P-value**	**HR**	**95% CI**	**P-value**
LT *vs.* LR	0.47	0.29–0.75	0.001	0.29	0.16–0.55	<0.001
Age, years	1.02	1.01–1.03	<0.001	1.02	1.00–1.03	0.017
Sex, male *vs.* female	1.05	0.86–1.28	0.656	0.17	0.89–1.53	0.268
Race						
Black *vs.* White	1.18	0.90–1.53	0.2315	1.39	0.99–1.94	0.056
Other *vs.* White	0.70	0.57–0.87	<0.001	0.67	0.51–0.88	0.004
AFP level ng/ml, positive *vs.* negative	1.30	1.08–1.57	0.005	1.22	0.96–1.55	0.111
Tumor size, cm	1.00	1.00–1.00	<0.001	1.00	1.00–1.01	<0.001
AJCC stage, II *vs.* I	1.21	1.01–1.45	0.034	1.50	1.19–1.89	0.001
Fibrosis score, 5–6 *vs.* 0–4	1.66	1.35–2.03	<0.001	1.65	1.28–2.14	<0.001
Tumor differentiation						
Moderate-differentiated *vs.* well-differentiated	1.18	0.96–1.47	0.120	1.28	0.94–1.73	0.116
Poor-differentiated *vs.* well-differentiated	1.56	1.22–2.10	<0.001	1.92	1.34–2.76	<0.001
Un-differentiated *vs.* well-differentiated	1.58	0.77–3.27	0.216	1.83	0.78–4.33	0.168
Year of diagnosis, 2010–2015 *vs.* 2004–2009	0.97	0.96–0.99	0.001	0.97	0.95–0.99	0.003

LR, liver resection; LT, liver transplantation; AFP, alpha-fetoprotein; AJCC, American Joint Committee on Cancer.

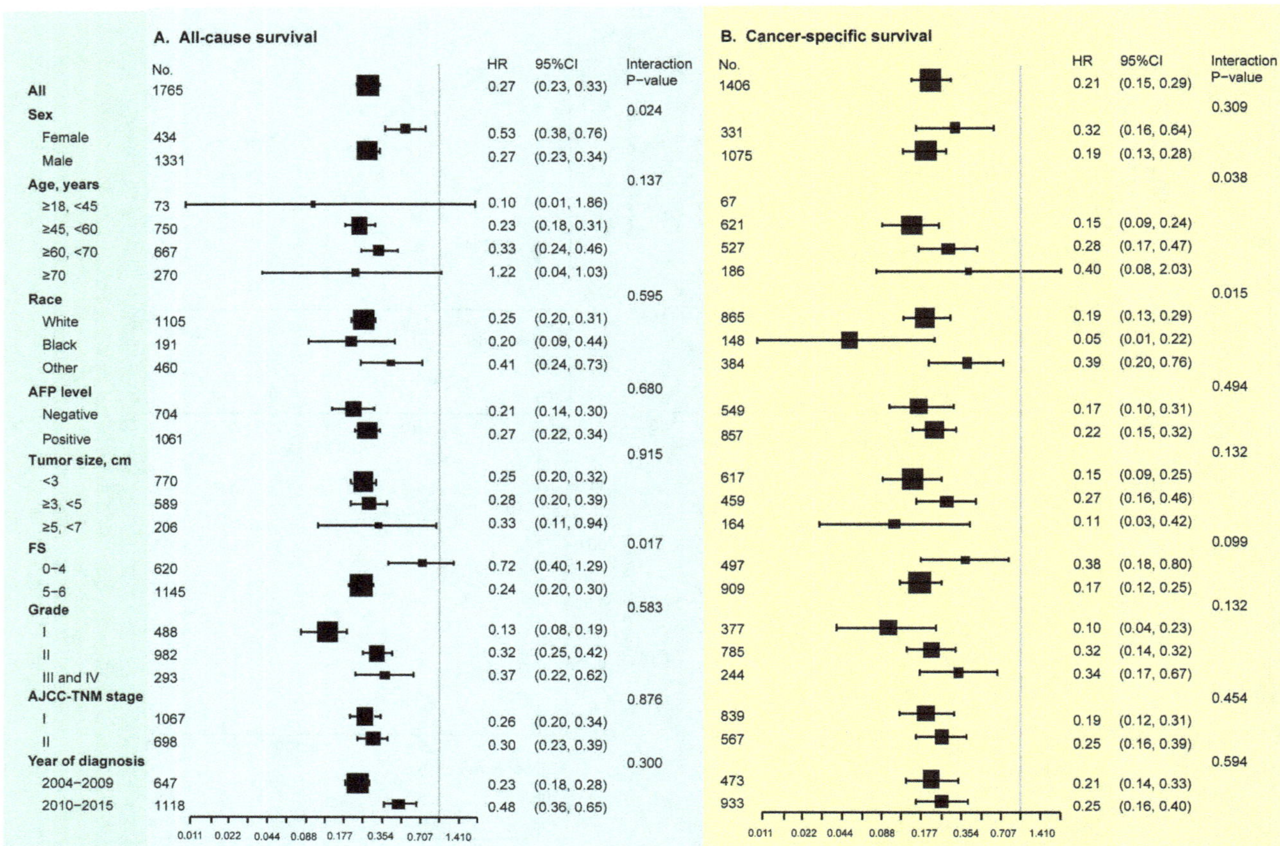

FIGURE 4 | Stratified analysis based on clinicopathologic features (multivariable COX analyses). **(A)** Results of LT vs. LR on overall survival. **(B)** Results of LT vs. LR on disease-specific survival. AFP, alpha-fetoprotein; FS, fibrosis score; AJCC, American Joint Committee on Cancer. Tumor grade: I, well-differentiated; II, moderate-differentiated; III, poor-differentiated; IV, un-differentiated. In subgroup analysis, all identified confounders were adjusted except for the factor that the subgroup was based on.

patients after LT still showed better DSS (HR 0.24, 95% CI 0.16-0.35, P < 0.001) and OS (HR 0.42, 95% CI 0.33-0.55, P < 0.001) in comparison to cases after LR (**Table 3**). In the Cox model only adjusting for propensity score, patients undergoing LT had both longer DSS (continuous: HR 0.23, 95% CI 0.17-0.32, P < 0.001; quintile: HR 0.26, 95% CI 0.18-0.36, P < 0.001) and OS (continuous: HR 0.41, 95% CI 0.32-0.52, P < 0.001; quintile: HR 0.43, 95% CI 0.34-0.54, P < 0.001) (**Table 3**).

Outcomes in IPTW and SMRW Analyses

After propensity score reweighting using the IPTW method, tumor size remained imbalanced. All other parameters were well-balanced in SMRW (data not shown). As shown in **Table 3**, in the IPTW cohort, patients who underwent LT showed better OS (HR 0.39, 95% CI 0.33-0.47, P < 0.001) and DSS (HR 0.25, 95% CI 0.20-0.33, P < 0.001) in comparison to cases with LR (**Table 3**). In the SMRW cohort, patients with LT showed better DSS (HR 0.21, 95% CI 0.16-0.27, P < 0.001) and CS (HR 0.33, 95% CI 0.28-0.39, P < 0.001) in comparison to those after LR.

DISCUSSION

In the present study, we aimed to explore the independent role of surgical modality (LT *vs.* LR) in long-term survival for cases with curable stage I and II HCC. Both conventional multivariable regression analyses and the propensity score reweighting methods indicated that cases after LT had better DSS and OS in comparison to cases after LR. Additionally, when accounting for both the known and unknown confounders by IV analyses, LT still showed significant survival benefit compared to LR, whereas the adjusted coefficients were increased (the survival benefits were decreased). In stratified IV analyses, we found that non-White patients and patients with age ≥60 years undergoing LT had similar DSS compared to patients after LR.

Previous studies which compared the effectiveness of LT *vs.* LR have increased in the past decade (5, 6, 8, 11, 12, 20). However, the majority of studies comparing LT and LR for HCC were single-institutional, descriptive or retrospective comparisons. Conventional observational studies have utilized multivariable regression analysis and propensity score methods to evaluate

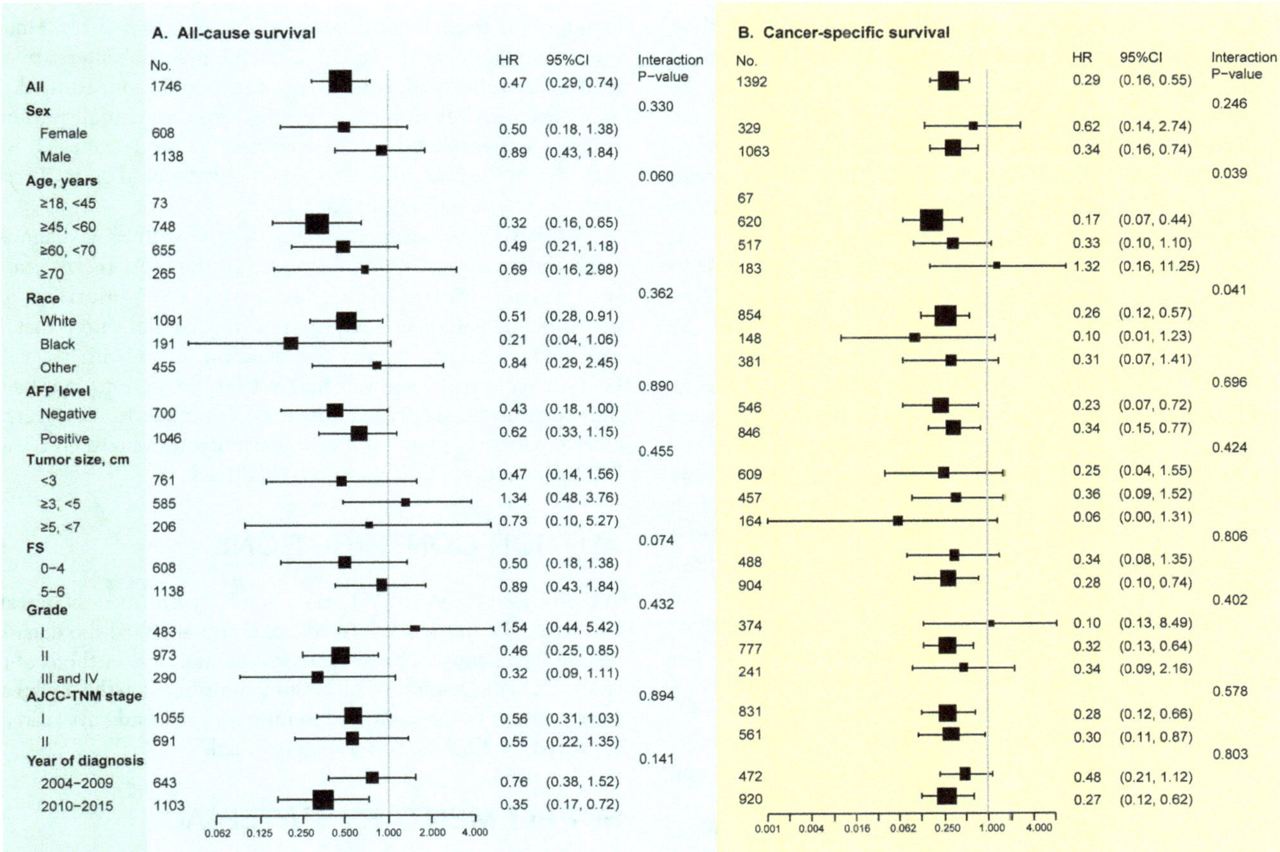

FIGURE 5 | Stratified analyses according to clinicopathologic parameters (instrumental variable analyses). **(A)** Results of LT vs. LR on overall survival. **(B)** Results of LT vs. LR on disease-specific survival. AFP, alpha-fetoprotein; FS, fibrosis score; AJCC, American Joint Committee on Cancer. Tumor grade: I, well-differentiated; II, moderate-differentiated; III, poor-differentiated; IV, un-differentiated. In subgroup analysis, all identified confounders were adjustec except for the factor that the subgroup was based on.

associations between surgical modality and patient prognosis. However, these analyses could not adjust unmeasured confounders (15). In contrast, IV analysis allowed for an unbiased estimation of the treatment effect in cases whose treatment option varied with the instrument variable. The instrumental variable analysis was a type of quasi-experimental and econometric modality using naturally existing variation to produce pseudorandomization. Outcomes from IV analysis were found to

TABLE 3 | Association of surgical methods with patient overall survival.

	All-cause survival			Cancer-specific survival		
	Number	HR (95% CI)	P-value	Number	HR (95% CI)	P-value
Non-adjusted	1765	0.45 (0.38, 0.54)	<0.001	1,406	0.28 (0.21, 0.36)	<0.001
Multivariable adjusted model*	1765	0.27 (0.23, 0.33)	<0.001	1,406	0.21 (0.15, 0.29)	<0.001
Matched on propensity score**	778	0.42 (0.33, 0.55)	<0.001	616	0.24 (0.16, 0.35)	<0.001
Regression adjusted with propensity score						
Propensity score, continuous	1765	0.41 (0.32, 0.52)	<0.001	1,406	0.23 (0.17, 0.32)	<0.001
Propensity score, quintile	1765	0.43 (0.34, 0.54)	<0.001	1,406	0.26 (0.18, 0.36)	<0.001
Weighted models						
SMRW	1765	0.33 (0.28, 0.39)	<0.001	1,406	0.21 (0.16, 0.27)	<0.001
IPTW	1765	0.39 (0.33, 0.47)	<0.001	1,406	0.25 (0.20, 0.33)	<0.001

*Data are shown as HR (95% CI) P value. *Adjusted model was adjusted for: race, age, sex, year of diagnosis, AFP level, tumor grade, fibrosis score, tumor size, and AJCC-TNM stage if available. **PSM model was based on the following variables: race, age, sex, year of diagnosis, AFP level, fibrosis score, tumor grade, tumor size, and AJCC-TNM stage. IPTW, inverse-probabilityof-treatment weighted; SMRW, standardized mortality ratio weighted.*

be more similar to results from randomized controlled trials (RCTs) (15). IV analysis calculated the treatment effect on the marginal patients, while not the average treatment effect of LT (13, 18) thus, the IV analysis did not need to define the specific clinical characteristics of the populations. Instead, it was based on the precondition that cases resided randomly around hospitals and some cases were treated differently in distinct hospitals.

Milan criteria are the benchmark for selection of cases with HCC for LT and the reference for comparison with other criteria (1). For patients within stages I and II, some of them had HCC beyond the Milan criterion (*e.g.*, tumor diameter >5 cm). In subgroup analyses, we found that patients with tumor of 5–7 cm undergoing LT still had better OS compared to those after LR, which was consistent with some expanded criteria such as the Up-to-seven criteria (21) and Hangzhou criteria (22). Specially, in stratified analyses, patients with age >60 years after LT were found to have a similar long-term prognosis compared to those after LR. It was possibly because older patients have more medical comorbidities and poorer performance status. Chen et al. showed that the risk of death increased with an increase in the age at transplantation, especially in dialysis patients (23). Sharma et al. showed that cases aged 70 years and older had obviously higher mortality following LT (24). These observations along with our results should make surgeons aware of the necessity for better risk classification in elderly LT candidates. Especially, in IV analyses, we found that Non-white patients cannot acquire a better survival benefit after LT, which may be caused by the differences in environmental, cultural, social, and genetic factors between the White and non-White patients.

Admittedly, the current study had several limitations. First, some clinicopathologic data including preoperative liver function, comorbidities, performance status, postoperative morbidities, and postoperative treatments were not available in the SEER registry, thus we could not evaluate the impact of these factors on patient survival in multivariable analyses. Second, the observations of this study should be interpreted cautiously, given that a number of cases were excluded from our main analysis owing to the unavailable covariates in the SEER registry. Finally, even though IV analysis was a useful practical alternative to RCTs, its validity depended on the population studied. IV analyses only evaluated the effect on marginal patients, whereas patients who would always or never receive LT were excluded in the marginal cases, and it only focused on HCC cases with uncertain indications for LT.

Despite the increasing incidence of cases with HCC diagnosed at an earlier stage, LT rate decreased in the most recent era. By integrating multivariable analysis, PSM method and instrumental variable analysis, our results indicated that LT provided a survival benefit for marginal cases with stage I-II HCC. These results showed that if LT rates were to increase in the future, average survival time may also increase. However, for elderly patients, owing to the similar outcomes between LT and LR, the selection of LT should be cautious.

AUTHOR CONTRIBUTIONS

WL proposed the study. WL, HW, and YZ performed the research and wrote the first draft. WL collected and analyzed the data. HX revised this manuscript and validated the statistical methods of this study. YZ is the guarantor. All authors contributed to the design and interpretation of the study and to further drafts, and have read and approved the final version to be published.

SUPPLEMENTARY MATERIAL

Supplementary Table 1 | Characteristics of patients by quintile of Health Services Area LT rates.

Supplementary Table 2 | Clinical features of the included patients with hepatocellular carcinoma after PSM.

REFERENCES

1. EASL Clinical Practice Guidelines: Management of hepatocellular carcinoma. *J Hepatol* (2018) 69(1):182–236. doi: 10.1016/j.jhep.2018.03.019
2. Akinyemiju T, Abera S, Ahmed M, Alam N, Alemayohu MA, Allen C, et al. The Burden of Primary Liver Cancer and Underlying Etiologies From 1990 to 2015 At the Global, Regional, and National Level: Results From the Global Burden of Disease Study 2015. *JAMA Oncol* (2017) 3:1683–91.
3. Fonseca AL, Cha CH. Hepatocellular Carcinoma: A Comprehensive Overview of Surgical Therapy. *J Surg Oncol* (2014) 110:712–9. doi: 10.1002/jso.23673
4. Forner A, Llovet JM, Bruix J. Hepatocellular Carcinoma. *Lancet* (2012) 379:1245–55. doi: 10.1016/S0140-6736(11)61347-0
5. Baccarani U, Isola M, Adani GL, Benzoni E, Avellini C, Lorenzin D, et al. Superiority of Transplantation Versus Resection for the Treatment of Small Hepatocellular Carcinoma. *Transplant Int Off J Eur Soc Organ Transplant* (2008) 21:247–54. doi: 10.1111/j.1432-2277.2007.00597.x
6. Seshadri RM, Besur S, Niemeyer DJ, Templin M, McKillop IH, Swan RZ, et al. Survival Analysis of Patients With Stage I and II Hepatocellular Carcinoma After a Liver Transplantation or Liver Resection. *HPB Off J Int Hepato Pancreato Biliary Assoc* (2014) 16:1102–9. doi: 10.1111/hpb.12300
7. Burman B, Helton WS. Disparities in Care for Patients With Curable Hepatocellular Carcinoma. *HPB Off J Int Hepato Pancreato Biliary Assoc* (2015) 17:745–6. doi: 10.1111/hpb.12477
8. Facciuto ME, Rochon C, Pandey M, Rodriguez-Davalos M, Samaniego S, Wolf DC, et al. Surgical Dilemma: Liver Resection or Liver Transplantation for Hepatocellular Carcinoma and Cirrhosis. Intention-to-treat Analysis in Patients Within and Outwith Milan Criteria. *HPB Off J Int Hepato Pancreato Biliary Assoc* (2009) 11:398–404. doi: 10.1111/j.1477-2574.2009.00073.x
9. Moon DB, Lee SG, Hwang S. Liver Transplantation for Hepatocellular Carcinoma: Single Nodule With Child-Pugh Class A Sized Less Than 3 Cm. *Digest Dis (Basel Switzerland)* (2007) 25:320–8. doi: 10.1159/000106912
10. Huang X, Lu S. A Meta-analysis Comparing the Effect of Anatomical Resection vs. non-Anatomical Resection on the Long-Term Outcomes for Patients Undergoing Hepatic Resection for Hepatocellular Carcinoma. *HPB Off J Int Hepato Pancreato Biliary Assoc* (2017) 19:843–9. doi: 10.1016/j.hpb.2017.06.003
11. Menahem B, Lubrano J, Duvoux C, Mulliri A, Alves A, Costentin C. Liver Transplantation Versus Liver Resection for Hepatocellular Carcinoma in Intention to Treat: An Attempt to Perform an Ideal Meta-Analysis. (2017) 23:836–44. doi: 10.1002/lt.24758
12. Benjamin AJ, Baker TB, Talamonti MS, Bodzin AS, Schneider AB, Winschester DJ, et al. Liver Transplant Offers a Survival Benefit Over Margin Negative Resection in Patients With Small Unifocal Hepatocellular Carcinoma and Preserved Liver Function. *Surgery* (2018) 163:582–6. doi: 10.1016/j.surg.2017.12.005

13. McDowell BD, Chapman CG, Smith BJ, Button AM, Chrischilles EA, Mezhir JJ. Pancreatectomy Predicts Improved Survival for Pancreatic Adenocarcinoma: Results of an Instrumental Variable Analysis. *Ann Surg* (2015) 261:740–5. doi: 10.1097/SLA.0000000000000796
14. Baiocchi M, Cheng J, Small DS. Instrumental Variable Methods for Causal Inference. *Stat Med* (2014) 33:2297–340. doi: 10.1002/sim.6128
15. Terza JV, Basu A, Rathouz PJ. Two-Stage Residual Inclusion Estimation: Addressing Endogeneity in Health Econometric Modeling. *J Health Economics* (2008) 27:531–43. doi: 10.1016/j.jhealeco.2007.09.009
16. Xu H, Xia Z, Jia X, Chen K, Li D, Dai Y, et al. Primary Tumor Resection Is Associated With Improved Survival in Stage Iv Colorectal Cancer: An Instrumental Variable Analysis. *Sci Rep* (2015) 5:16516. doi: 10.1038/srep16516
17. Gore JL, Litwin MS, Lai J, Yano EM, Madison R, Setodji C, et al. Use of Radical Cystectomy for Patients With Invasive Bladder Cancer. *J Natl Cancer Inst* (2010) 102:802–11. doi: 10.1093/jnci/djq121
18. Valley TS, Sjoding MW, Ryan AM, Iwashyna TJ, Cooke CR. Association of Intensive Care Unit Admission With Mortality Among Older Patients With Pneumonia. *Jama* (2015) 314:1272–9. doi: 10.1001/jama.2015.11068
19. Tan HJ, Norton EC, Ye Z, Hafez KS, Gore JL, Miller DC. Long-Term Survival Following Partial vs Radical Nephrectomy Among Older Patients With Early-Stage Kidney Cancer. *Jama* (2012) 307:1629–35. doi: 10.1001/jama.2012.475
20. Kutlu OC, Chan JA, Aloia TA, Chun YS, Kaseb AO, Passot G, et al. Comparative Effectiveness of First-Line Radiofrequency Ablation Versus Surgical Resection and Transplantation for Patients With Early Hepatocellular Carcinoma. *Cancer* (2017) 123:1817–27. doi: 10.1002/cncr.30531
21. Mazzaferro V, Llovet JM, Miceli R, Bhoori S, Schiavo M, Mariani L, et al. Predicting Survival After Liver Transplantation in Patients With Hepatocellular Carcinoma Beyond the Milan Criteria: A Retrospective, Exploratory Analysis. *Lancet Oncol* (2009) 10:35–43. doi: 10.1016/S0739-5930(09)79300-6
22. Zheng SS, Xu X, Wu J, Chen J, Wang WL, Zhang M, et al. Liver Transplantation for Hepatocellular Carcinoma: Hangzhou Experiences. *Transplantation* (2008) 85:1726–32. doi: 10.1097/TP.0b013e31816b67e4
23. Chen HP, Tsai YF, Lin JR, Liu FC, Yu HP. Recipient Age and Mortality Risk After Liver Transplantation: A Population-Based Cohort Study. *PloS One* (2016) 11:e0152324. doi: 10.1371/journal.pone.0152324
24. Sharma M, Ahmed A, Wong RJ. Significantly Higher Mortality Following Liver Transplantation Among Patients Aged 70 Years and Older. (2017) 27:225–31. doi: 10.1177/1526924817715468

16

Immunohistochemical Signature Add Prognostic Value in Patients with Early and Intermediate Hepatocellular Carcinoma Underwent Curative Liver Resection

Yannan Bai[1†], Yuane Lian[2†], Xiaoping Chen[3†], Jiayi Wu[1], Jianlin Lai[1], Funan Qiu[1], Songqiang Zhou[1], Zijing Zhu[3], Yifeng Tian[1], Yaodong Wang[1], Yinghong Yang[2*] and Maolin Yan[1*]*

[1] Department of Hepatobiliopancreatic Surgery, Fujian Provincial Hospital, Shengli Clinical Medical College of Fujian Medical University, Fuzhou, China, [2] Department of Pathology, Fujian Medical University Union Hospital, Fuzhou, China, [3] Department of Statistics, College of Mathematics and Informatics & FJKLMAA, Fujian Normal University, Fuzhou, China

***Correspondence:**
Yaodong Wang
fjslgdy@dingtalk.com
Yinghong Yang
xhyyhsci@163.com
Maolin Yan
yanmaolin74@163.com

[†]These authors have contributed equally to this work

Hepatocellular carcinoma (HCC) is the third most lethal cancer worldwide; however, accurate prognostic tools are still lacking. We aimed to identify immunohistochemistry (IHC)-based signature as a prognostic classifier to predict recurrence and survival in patients with HCC at Barcelona Clinic Liver Cancer (BCLC) early- and immediate-stage. In total, 567 patients who underwent curative liver resection at two independent centers were enrolled. The least absolute shrinkage and selection operator regression model was used to identify significant IHC features, and penalized Cox regression was used to further narrow down the features in the training cohort (n = 201). The candidate IHC features were validated in internal (n = 101) and external validation cohorts (n = 265). Three IHC features, hepatocyte paraffin antigen 1, CD34, and Ki-67, were identified as candidate predictors for recurrence-free survival (RFS), and were used to categorize patients into low- and high-risk recurrence groups in the training cohort ($P < 0.001$). The discriminative performance of the 3-IHC_based classifier was validated using internal and external cohorts ($P < 0.001$). Furthermore, we developed a 3-IHC_based nomogram integrating the BCLC stage, microvascular invasion, and 3-IHC_based classifier to predict 2- and 5-year RFS in the training cohort; this nomogram exhibited acceptable area under the curve values for the training, internal validation, and external validation cohorts (2-year: 0.817, 0.787, and 0.810; 5-year: 0.726, 0.662, and 0.715; respectively). The newly developed 3-IHC_based classifier can effectively predict recurrence and survival in patients with early- and intermediate-stage HCC after curative liver resection.

Keywords: hepatocellular carcinoma, immunohistochemistry, prognostic marker, classifier, prognosis

INTRODUCTION

Hepatocellular carcinoma (HCC) is the third most lethal cancer worldwide, with 780,000 annual deaths recorded globally (1). Although hepatic resection remains the treatment of choice to achieve a cure in patients with HCC, a high recurrence rate after curative resection is still a major cause of death (2–4). Conventional HCC staging systems, such as the Barcelona Clinic Liver Cancer (BCLC) (5), Japan Integrated Staging (JIS) (6), and Tumor-Node-Metastasis (TNM) systems (7), use conventional clinicopathological features (liver function, tumor size, number, and vascular invasion) for prognostic stratification. However, HCC is a heterogeneous entity, with considerable variation in clinical outcomes, even for identical tumor stages. There is an ongoing pursuit for prognostic biomarkers for cancer. Clinicopathological parameters, and integrative and comprehensive genomic alterations have been analyzed and used to stratify patients into various groups with different prognoses (8–18), none of these stratification tools have been routinely employed in staging systems for predicting recurrence and survival after surgical resection.

As an inexpensive and easy-to-use pathological technique, immunohistochemistry (IHC) is routinely used for analyzing HCC carcinogenesis, development, and invasiveness. Despite the development of IHC markers with diagnostic value, prognostic markers are not well-established. Previous studies have investigated the value of IHC-based classifiers as predictors of overall survival (OS), but not of recurrence-free survival (RFS) (10, 19). It should be noted that OS is mainly determined by the status of liver function and post-recurrence treatment, yet RFS reflects the biological heterogeneity of HCC. A panel of common IHC markers was selected—including hepatocyte markers hepatocyte paraffin antigen 1 (HepPar-1) and Glypian-3, cytokeratin (CK) proteins CK18 and CK19, angiogenesis-related CD34, canalicular staining marker CD10, epithelial-mesenchymal transition markers vimentin (VIM), melanocyte marker HMB45, and tumor proliferation and aggressiveness marker Ki-67—based on its diagnostic value with respect to carcinogenesis, development, and invasiveness of HCC. We hypothesize that a combination of IHC markers could have greater prognostic value than each of the markers alone when considering tumor recurrence and long-term survival.

The aim of this study was to develop a recurrence-related IHC-based classifier. We used a cohort of 201 patients with HCC after curative liver resection using the least absolute shrinkage and selection operator (LASSO) Cox regression model and validated the classifier using an internal, and an external cohort of 101, and 265 patients, respectively. We then developed a prognostic nomogram incorporating the BCLC stage, microvascular invasion (MVI), and the 3-IHC_based classifier to improve the predictive power. This study may contribute to early detection of recurrence in patients with HCC who underwent curative resection, thereby possibly improving patient outcome.

METHODS

Patients and Samples

Between March 2010 and December 2014, a total of 1,436 consecutive patients who had undergone curative-intent liver resection for HCC from two tertiary Chinese centers were retrospectively screened. The following inclusion criteria were used: HCC at BCLC early- or intermediate-stage, without extrahepatic metastasis or other homochromous malignancies, and without any anticancer treatment before surgery. A total of 302 HCC patients during surgical resection were included at Fujian Provincial Hospital (FPH) and 265 patients at Fujian Medical University Union Hospital (FMUUH). Patients were excluded when the tumor specimen or clinicopathological data were missing. This retrospective study was approved by the Institutional Review Board of FPH and FMUUH and was performed in accordance with the Declaration of Helsinki. Written informed consent for tissue collection was obtained from each patient prior to the study. Patients at FPH were further randomly stratified into a training cohort (201 patients) and an internal validation cohort (101 patients) at a 2:1 ratio.

The data were censored on December 31, 2019. Patients were followed up at 2-month intervals in the first year after surgery and at 3-month intervals thereafter. The clinicopathological data are presented in **Table 1**. The computation of Child-Turcotte-Pugh (CTP) functional class, albumin-bilirubin (ALBI) grade, and BCLC stage were determined as per standard published methodologies (5, 20). The severity of liver fibrosis and tumor differentiation was defined using the Ishak scoring system and Edmondson grading system, respectively (21, 22). MVI was defined as the presence of tumor emboli in a portal vein, hepatic vein, or within a vascular space lined by endothelial cells that was visible only on microscopy (23). The primary clinical endpoints were RFS, calculated from the date of resection to the date of recurrence, metastasis, or last follow-up, and OS, calculated from the date of resection to the date of death or last follow-up.

Immunohistochemistry

Formalin-fixed and paraffin-embedded tissue sections (5-μm thick) were obtained. Rabbit monoclonal anti-bodies against HepPar-1, Glypian-3, CK18, CK19, CD10, CD34, VIM, HMB45, and Ki-67 were used (MXB Biotechnologies, Inc., Fuzhou, China). The IHC outcomes for each marker were semiquantitative evaluated by two independent and trained pathologists who were blind to the clinical outcomes (LY AND YY). HepPar-1, Glypian-3, CK18, CK19, CD10, CD34, VIM, and HMB45 were localized in the cytoplasm of HCC cells, while Ki-67 was localized in the nuclei. The immunoreaction was recorded as the percentage of positively stained cells and cell staining intensity (absent, weak, moderate or strong) in 3 respective areas at ×200 magnification, and the mean value was adopted. Dichotomization as negative (absent/weak staining) or positive (moderate/strong staining) was then determined based on the

TABLE 1 | Clinicopathological factors of patients in training and validation cohort.

Baseline characteristics	Number/Median [IQR]*		
	Internal cohort (n = 201) (n = 101)	**Training cohort**	**External cohort (n = 265)**
Gender			
M: F	175: 26	87: 14	233: 32
Age (year)	61 [50, 68]	59 [51, 67]	56 [48, 62]
≥60: <60	111: 90	49:52	93: 172
HBsAg			
Pos: Neg	169: 32	85: 32	239: 26
HCV			
Pos: Neg	**9:192**	**6:95**	**11:254**
ALB (g/l)	43.9 [40.9, 46.6]	44.4 [40.7, 46.7]	40.2 [37.8, 43.0]
TB (umol/l)	13.8 [10.8, 18.7]	14.0 [11.0, 18.1]	13.2 [9.6, 17.4]
ALT (U/l)	37 [27, 50]	37 [25, 53]	32 [22, 44]
AST (U/l)	34 [26, 50]	31 [25, 46]	29 [23, 41]
plt (10^(9)/l)	175 [133, 231]	175 [137, 223]	161 [127, 197]
AFP (ug/l)			
<20: ≥20	91: 110	50: 51	111: 154
CTP score			
A5: A6: B7	169: 22: 10	84: 13: 4	233: 27: 5
ALBI	-2.96 [-3.23, -2.70]	-3.01 [-3.24, -2.65]	-2.69 [-2.92, -2.46]
Size (cm)	4.0[3.0, 8.0]	4.5[3.0, 7.0]	4.0[2.8, 5.5]
Number			
1: 2-3: >3	173: 22: 6	88: 11: 2	218: 38: 9
MVI			
Abs: Pre	149: 52	72: 29	216: 49
Ishak classification			
F0: F1	51: 150	24: 77	63: 202
Grade			
I-II: III-IV	168: 33	85: 16	98: 167
BCLC classification			
early: intermediate	117: 84	59: 42	166: 99
3-IHC-based classifier			
Low: high	156: 45	79: 22	182: 83
RFS (month)	42[12, 55]	41[16, 59]	48[20, 60]
OS (month)	55[43, 68]	53[39, 67]	53[41, 62]

M, male; F, female; HbsAg, hepatitis B virus surface antigen; AFP, α-fetoprotein; CTP, Child-Turcotte-Pugh score; ALBI, albumin-bilirubin; MVI, microvascular invasion; F0: Ishak F0-F4; F1: Ishak F5-F6; BCLC, Barcelona Clinic Liver Cancer; IHC, Immunohistochemistry; RFS, recurrence-free survival; OS, overall survival; Pos, positive; Neg, negative; Abs, absence; Pre, presence; IQR, interquartile range.

**Median with interquartile range are shown for quantitative variables, whereas counts are shown for categorical variables.*

reactivity of IHC markers (10, 24). Representative expressions of HepPar-1, CD34 and Ki-67 are shown in **Figure S1**.

Statistical Analysis

Initially, a LASSO Cox regression model with penalty parameter tuning (10-fold cross-validation) was used to identify the most useful prognostic IHC-based markers. An L1 penalized Cox analysis was performed to further narrow down markers in the training cohort. A multi-marker classifier, derived from the prognostic score for each selected marker, was constructed based on RFS. Cumulative OS and RFS were evaluated using the Kaplan–Meier method and compared using the log-rank test, followed by multivariate Cox regression to identify significant variables. A nomogram was constructed based on the results of the Cox regression models. A decision curve analysis (DCA) was used to assess the clinical utility of the nomogram.

All statistical analyses were performed using R version 3.6.1 with the packages glmnet, pROC, and rms. A two-sided P-value <0.05 was considered significant.

RESULTS

Patient Characteristics

A total of 567 patients was included in the study, including 201 in the training cohort, 101 in the internal validation cohort, and 265 in the external validation cohort. Characteristics of the studied populations in the training, internal validation, and external validation cohorts are presented in **Table 1** and **Figure 1**. The median follow-up time for 567 patients with HCC was 53.0 months (range, 3.0 to 84.0 months). During the follow-up, 53.6% of the patients (304 of 567) exhibited recurrence, and 33.9% of the patients (192 of 567) died. For patients who had not been diagnosed with HCC recurrence, adjuvant transarterial chemoembolization (TACE), at the interval of 2 months from surgery, was routinely recommended for patients with high risk factors (tumor size larger than 5 cm, multiple tumors, MVI, poor-differentiation grade, and so on) after completely informing the potential benefits and risks of this treatment. Among 304 patients with recurrence, 107 (35.2%) underwent a repeated resection or ablation, 92 (30.3%) received TACE, 51 (16.8%)

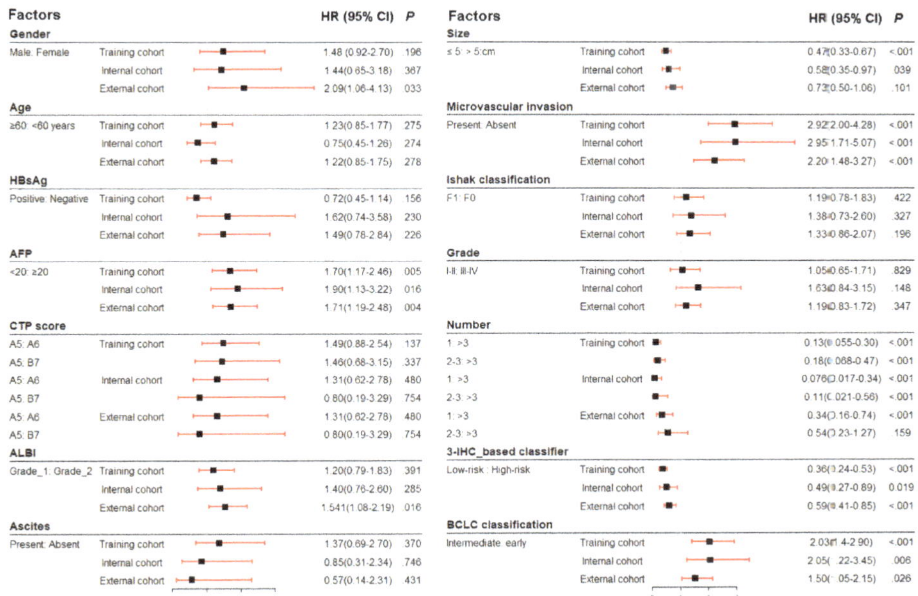

FIGURE 1 | Association of clinicopathologic characteristics with recurrence-free survival in three cohorts. HBsAg, hepatitis B virus surface antigen; AFP, α-fetoprotein; ALBI, albumin-bilirubin; CTP, Child-Turcotte-Pugh score; IHC, immunohistochemistry; BCLC, Barcelona Clinic Liver Cancer; HR, hazard ratio.

received targeted therapy, and 54 (17.8%) received no further treatment. For the entire cohort, the 2- and 5- year RFS rates were 66.5% and 48.7%, respectively, and the 2- and 5-year OS rates were 85.0% and 69.0%, respectively.

Feature Selection and Predictive Immunohistochemistry-Based Signature Building

We identified potential IHC features for RFS prediction from among a set of markers (HepPar-1, Glypian-3, CK18, CK19, CD10, CD34, VIM, HMB45, and Ki-67) using the LASSO Cox regression model. The nine features were reduced to three prognostic markers (HepPar-1, CD34, and Ki-67) in the training cohort and features with penalized Cox coefficients were included in the regression model (**Figure 2**). To better understand the performance of the IHC signature for predicting recurrence, a 3-IHC_based risk score for each patient was derived as follows: risk score = (0.7280 × Ki-67) - (0.4495 × CD34) - (0.6027 × HepPar-1). The status of each IHC marker was categorized as negative (equals 0) and positive (equals 1).

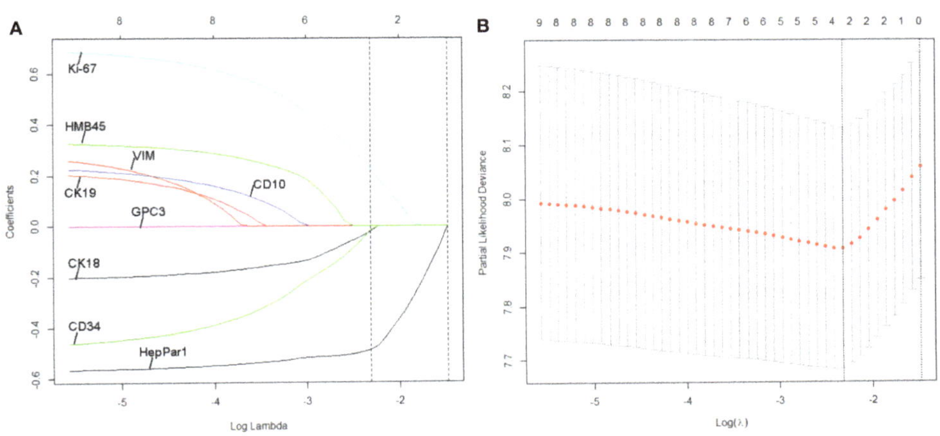

FIGURE 2 | Least absolute shrinkage and selection operator (LASSO) coefficient profiles of the three selected IHC signatures. **(A)** Tuning parameter (selection by 10-fold cross-validation *via* minimum criteria. Partial likelihood deviance was plotted versus log(Lamda). **(B)** Coefficient profile of the IHC markers associated with recurrence-free survival (RFS) of patients with HCC patients at early- and intermediate-stage. Vertical line is shown at the optimal value with three nonzero coefficients.

The optimum cut-off value for the risk score was defined as −0.613 based on the training cohort. We assigned patients with a risk score exceeding −0.613 to the high-risk group (n = 45) and others to the low-risk group (n = 156). On applying the cutoff, the low-risk group had a better RFS (hazard ratio [HR], 0.359; 95% CI, 0.242–0.533; P < 0.001; **Figure 3A**) than the high-risk group in the training cohort.

Validation of the Predictive Immunohistochemistry Signature

To assess the robustness of the 3-IHC_based classifier, validation analyses were performed using in both the internal and external validation cohorts. In the internal validation cohort, the 3-IHC_based classifier categorized 79 patients (78.2%) into the low-risk group and 22 patients (21.8%) into the high-risk group with a significant difference in RFS (HR, 0.492; 95% CI, 0.272–0.890; P = 0.016; **Figure 3B**). Similar analyses indicated that 182 low-risk patients (68.7%) had a better RFS than 83 high-risk patients (31.3%) in the external validation cohort (HR, 0.592; 95% CI, 0.413–0.850; P = 0.004; **Figure 3C**). In the combined cohort containing 567 patients, recurrence occurred at a later time point in the low-risk group than in the high-risk group (median time, 22.0 [range, 1.0–84.0] versus 9.0 [range, 1.0–84.0] months; P < 0.001; **Figure S2**).

We also investigated the performance of the 3-IHC_based classifier for predicting OS and effectively stratified patients into low- and high-risk groups with respect to long-term prognosis in all three cohorts (training cohort: HR, 0.362; 95% CI, 0.222–0.592; P < 0.001; internal validation cohort: HR, 0.471; 95% CI, 0.224–0.991; P = 0.042; external validation: HR, 0.427; 95% CI, 0.281–0.650; P < 0.001; **Figure S3**). Upon setting 2 years post-hepatectomy as the threshold for early recurrence (ER, representing true recurrence from the primary HCC) or late recurrence of HCC (LR, representing *de novo* HCC recurrence) (25), we assigned 304 patients with recurrence to an ER group (190 patients) and an LR group (114 patients). In our study, the 3-IHC_based classifier maintained its discriminative ability for predicting OS in patients with ER (HR, 0.717; 95% CI, 0.517–0.996; P = 0.047) but not for patients with LR (**Figure S4**).

Furthermore, the Area Under the Receiver Operating Characteristics (AUC) curve analysis for the 3-IHC_based classifier was performed. As shown in **Figure 4**, the AUC values of the 3-IHC_based classifier for 2- and 5-year RFS prediction in the training cohort (0.711, 95% CI: 0.638–0.784; 0.671, 95% CI: 0.599–0.742; respectively) indicated significantly better discrimination ability than that of the individual IHC markers. Similar discrimination ability was observed in case of the internal (AUC for 2- and 5-year RFS, 0.694, 95% CI: 0.583–0.804; 0.581, 95% CI: 0.472–0.691) and external validation cohort (0.741, 95% CI: 0.674–0.809; 0.656, 95% CI: 0.591–0.721). Moreover, AUC value for the combination of the BCLC stage and 3-IHC_based classifier exhibited better performance for predicting RFS than those for the BCLC stage alone (2-year: 0.817, 0.787, and 0.810; 5-year: 0.726, 0.662, and 0.715; P < 0.001, for the training, internal validation, and external validation cohorts, respectively), indicating that the 3-IHC_based classifier has better prognostic value than that of the conventional BCLC stage for predicting RFS in HCC (**Figure 4**).

Nomogram Construction and Clinical Usage

Prior to the development of a clinically useful prognostic algorithm for predicting individual recurrence probabilities, we evaluated common clinicopathological features by multivariate Cox regression analyses based on RFS using a combination of significant variables and 3-IHC_based classifier (**Figure 1** and **Table 2**). Based on the significant predictors in multivariate analysis (BCLC stage, MVI, and 3-IHC_based classifier), we constructed a nomogram to predict 2- or 5-year RFS in the training cohort (**Figure 5A**). The Calibration curves showed good correspondence between the predicted and actual probability of 2- or 5-year RFS for all three cohorts (**Figures 5B–D**). Furthermore, a DCA was used to compare the 3-IHC_based nomogram and each predictor alone (BCLC stage, MVI, and 3-IHC_based classifier, respectively). DCA graphically showed that the 3-IHC_based nomogram provided a net benefit over the range of threshold probabilities for 2- or 5-year RFS when compared with each individual predictor (**Figure S5**).

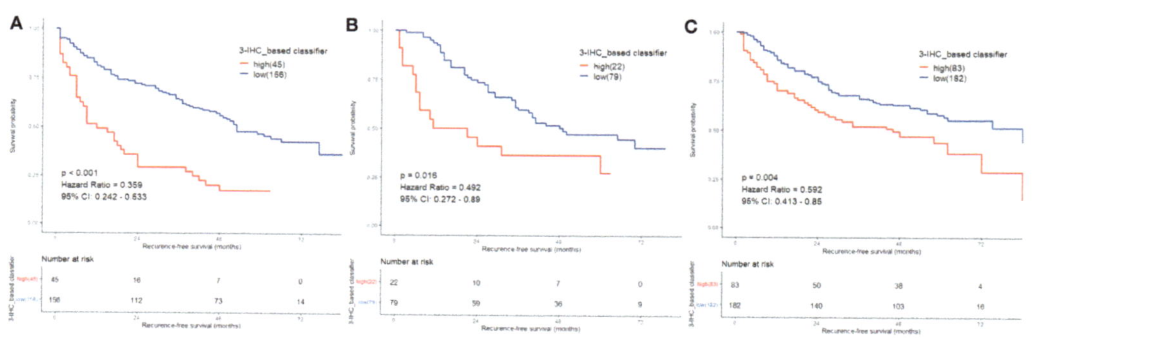

FIGURE 3 | Comparison of recurrence-free survival (RFS) in low-risk vs. high-risk patients stratified by 3-IHC_based classifier. **(A)** Training cohort; **(B)** internal validation cohort; **(C)** external validation cohort.

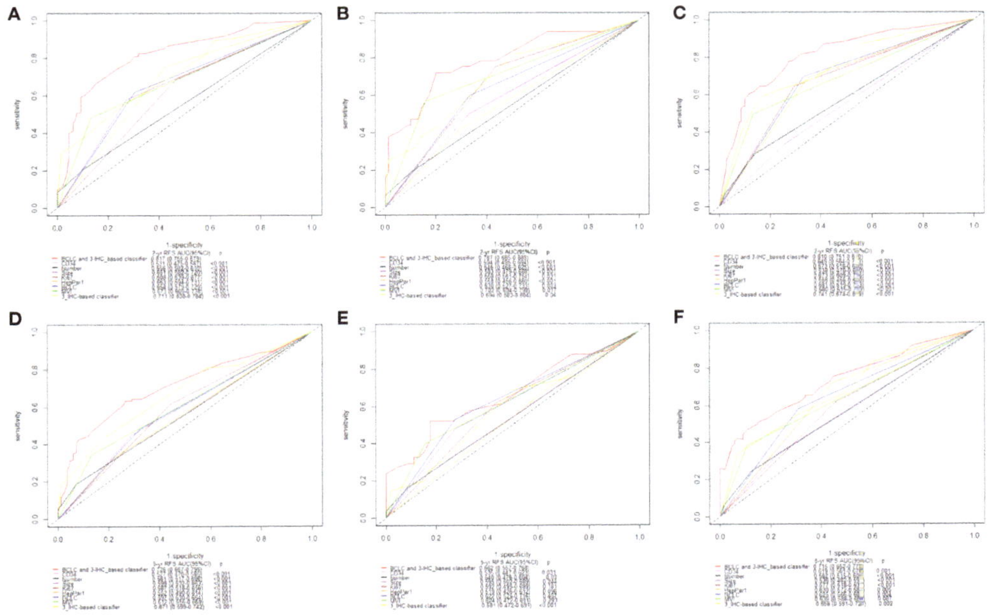

FIGURE 4 | Time-dependent receiver operating characteristic (ROC) analysis on basis of recurrence-free survival (RFS) [2-year, **(A–C)**; and 5-year, **(D–F)**; respectively] was used to compare performance of 3-IHC_based classifier with the clinicopathological factors and three single immunohistochemistry (IHC) features alone. Training cohort **(A, D)**; Internal validation cohort **(B, E)**; External validation cohort **(C, F)**. BCLC, Barcelona Clinic Liver Cancer; MVI, microvascular invasion.

DISCUSSION

In this study, we used IHC to screen the expression status of routinely available markers in resected HCC samples from an FPH cohort. By using the LASSO Cox regression algorithm, we reduced the features to a set of three candidates and developed an IHC signature (i.e., a 3-IHC_based classifier) in the training cohort, which was then validated using internal and external validation cohorts. Based on the classifier, patients with HCC could be stratified into two distinct subgroups with low and high probabilities of recurrence and OS. Interestingly, nearly half of the patients in the high-risk group experienced ER, while recurrent HCC was observed in less than one-quarter in the low-risk group (**Data Supplement**), suggesting that patients in the high-risk group require more intensive medical surveillance within 2 years after curative liver resection. Furthermore, among patients with ER, the 3-IHC_based classifier was able to discriminate between patients with different OS, suggesting the practical predictive value of our classifier in ER entity, which was considered as true recurrence from the primary HCC (25). Finally, to improve management decisions for individualized follow-up and treatment strategies, we integrated the BCLC stage and MVI into a prognostic nomogram to predict the 2- and 5-year RFS in patients with HCC after curative liver resection. Calibration curves showed a good consistency between the predicted and actual RFS. The DCA further supported the prognostic value of the nomogram for clinical application.

TABLE 2 | Multivariate Cox Analysis of Clinicopathologic Factors and 3_IHC-based classifier with Recurrence-Free Survival in the Entire Cohort.

Factor	Multivariate Analysis	
	HR (95% CI)	P
AFP (<20/≥20 ug/l)	1.272 (0.846-1.913)	0.248
BCLC (intermediate/early)	1.723 (1.193-2.487)	0.004
MVI (present/absent)	2.179 (1.454-3.266)	<0.001
3_IHC-based classifier (low-risk/high-risk)	0.512 (0.327-0.799)	0.003

AFP, α-fetoprotein; MVI, microvascular invasion; BCLC, Barcelona Clinic Liver Cancer; IHC, Immunohistochemistry.

In our study, we developed a 3-IHC_based classifier based on IHC markers that are routinely used in clinical pathology. Each candidate IHC marker has an established biological and diagnostic role in the carcinogenesis, development, and invasiveness of HCC. HepPar-1 and Glypian-3 are hepatocyte functional markers associated with the degree of tumor differentiation (with different sensitivities) (26). CK18 and CK19 are widely used to distinguish between HCC and biliary-derived carcinoma (27). CD34 is used to determine the degree of tumor angiogenesis (28). CD10 and HMB45 are used for the differential diagnosis of HCC from exogenous metastases and other liver mesenchymal tumors (29, 30). VIM is a marker of tumor epithelial-mesenchymal transition and HCC metastasis (31); and Ki-67 is a marker of proliferation (32). It should be noted that some of these IHC markers or combinations of markers have been identified as risk factors with prognostic value for predicting recurrence or long-term survival in HCC after surgery. For example, High-level Ki-67 expression in HCC tumor was associated with more rapid ER (32). HepPar-1, as a

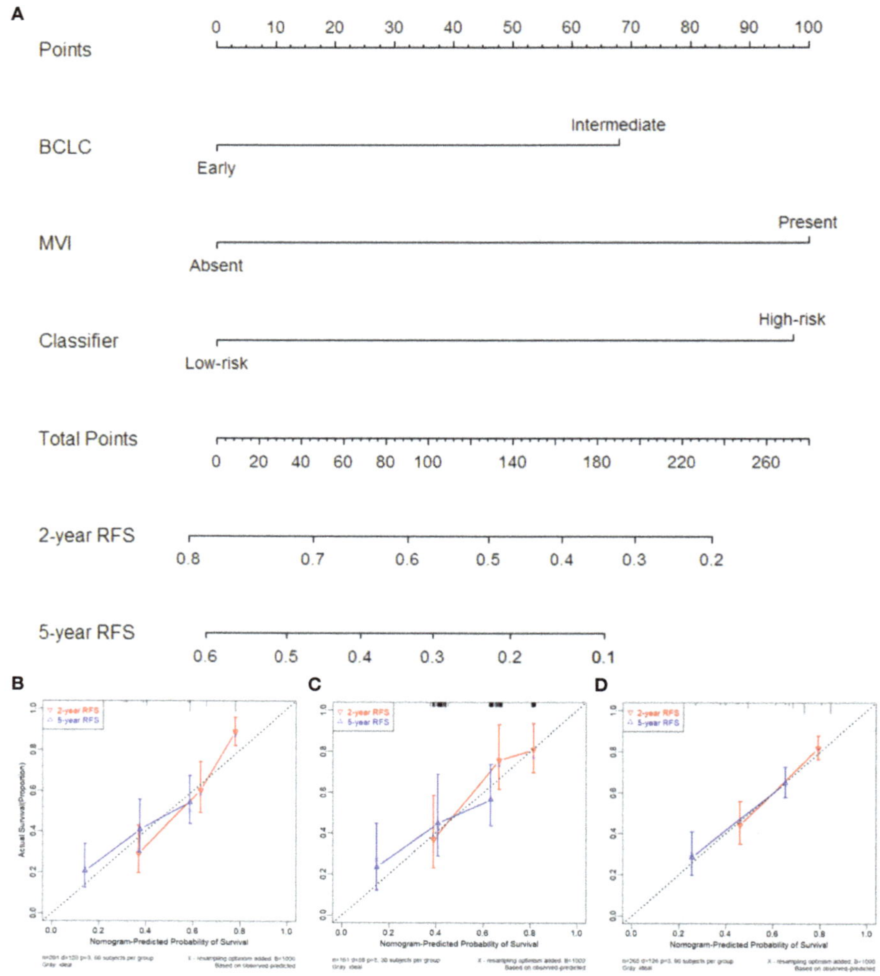

FIGURE 5 | **(A)** Nomogram to predict the 2- and 5-year recurrence-free survival (RFS). Calibration curve for RFS nomogram in training cohort **(B)**, internal validation cohort **(C)**, and external validation cohort **(D)**.

hepatocyte specific antigen, its data of prognostic significance in HCC was limited and inconsistent. However, combination with CK19 might increase the prognostic power for predicting OS in HCC (33). A previous study developed a morpho-molecular prognosticator of patients with HCC based on the combination of several clinicopathological features and IHC markers (10). The prognosticator was able to classify subgroups with different OS and RFS, however, risk score for predicting RFS was identical to the one for predicting OS which calculated using Cox regression model based on OS outcomes. In fact, only two IHC features (P53 and CD31) were identified as independent risk factors for tumor recurrence. Recently, another study proposed a prognostic and a recurrent classifier separately to predict OS and RFS for patients with HCC based on a set of 29 IHC features (19). The study showed a favorable prognostic model with high prediction accuracy for 3-year recurrence in all three cohorts (95% CI: 0.734, 0.693–0.710; 0.749, 95% CI: 0.677–0.812; 0.730, 95% CI: 0.635–0.812; respectively). The AUC value for the prognostic classifier developed was slightly lower than the one developed in our study when considering 2-year recurrence (0.817, 95% CI: 0.755–0.879; 0.787, 95% CI: 0.685–0.888; and 0.810, 0.751–0.870; respectively) and 5-year recurrence in all three cohorts (0.726, 95% CI: 0.657–0.795; 0.662, 95% CI: 0.557–0.768; 0.715, 95% CI: 0.652–0.778; respectively). Besides, MVI was not included and assessed as an important clinicopathological feature. To further improve the prognostic accuracy and to identify the most effective IHC signature, nine markers were reduced to three prognostic features using the LASSO method for variable selection in the Cox model (34). As indicated in our study, the proposed signature showed substantial prognostic ability with a higher AUC value than that of predictors evaluated in previous studies.

Several strengths of this study should be noted. First, a 3-IHC_based signature was identified as prognostic classifier to stratify HCC risk groups based on the recurrence probability. This is important because RFS is a more accurate representation of the biological characteristics of HCC than OS, which is mainly influenced by liver function and post-recurrence treatment. Second, compared with previous studies—based on high-throughput genetic profiles—we focused on clinically available IHC-based markers, which are characterized by the following features: potential for easy, inexpensive, and reliable results. These pathological diagnosis-based markers are expected to have substantial prognostic value. Third, patients with advanced HCC were not included in our study to exclude highly unfavorable factors, such as macrovascular invasion and end-stage liver failure. We included patients classified as BCLC early-stage and intermediate-stage and validated the features in samples from two-centers, considering that the classifications and therapeutic modalities for BCLC early- and intermediate-stage HCC remain controversial (2–6).

Although the 3-IHC_based nomogram showed substantial power for tumor recurrence and survival in patients with HCC after curative liver resection, several limitations should be noted. First, we used retrospective data from two centers. Second, only nine IHC markers were assessed in this study. This might explain the failure of the 3-IHC_based classifier in stratifying patients with LR based on OS. The assessment of additional IHC markers related to cell cycle regulation, angiogenesis, invasiveness, immunoreactivity, tumor microenvironment, etc., will provide more comprehensive data in the future. Third, prospective studies using multiple cohorts are required to verify our findings.

In summary, our study shows that the newly developed 3-IHC_based classifier is a feasible prognostic tool for predicting recurrence and survival in patients with HCC classified as BCLC early- and intermediate-stage after curative liver resection. By integrating the classifier with the BCLC stage and MVI, the nomogram might improve personized prognostic assessments and aid in management decisions and development of treatment strategies.

AUTHOR CONTRIBUTIONS

BY and LY conceptualized the study. CX and ZZ contributed to the methodology. WJ, LJ, QF, ZS, and TY contributed to the data curation. BY and LY wrote and prepared the the original draft. WY, YY, and YM wrote, reviewed, and edited the manuscript. BY, LY, and CX contributed to the project administration. All authors contributed to the article and approved the submitted version.

REFERENCES

1. Bray F, Ferlay J, Soerjomataram I, Siegel RL, Torre LA, Jemal A. Global cancer statistics 2018: GLOBOCAN estimates of incidence and mortality worldwide for 36 cancers in 185 countries. *CA Cancer J Clin* (2018) 68:394–424. doi: 10.3322/caac.21492
2. Forner A, Reig M, Bruix J. Hepatocellular carcinoma. *Lancet (Lond Engl)* (2018) 391:1301–14. doi: 10.1016/S0140-6736(18)30010-2
3. Heimbach JK, Kulik LM, Finn RS, Sirlin CB, Abecassis MM, Roberts LR, et al. AASLD guidelines for the treatment of hepatocellular carcinoma. *Hepatology* (2018) 67:358–80. doi: 10.1002/hep.29086
4. European Association for the Study of the Liver. Electronic address eee, European Association for the Study of the L. EASL Clinical Practice Guidelines: Management of hepatocellular carcinoma. *J Hepatol* (2018) 69:182–236. doi: 10.1016/j.jhep.2018.03.019
5. Llovet JM, Bru C, Bruix J. Prognosis of hepatocellular carcinoma: the BCLC staging classification. *Semin Liver Dis* (1999) 19:329–38. doi: 10.1055/s-2007-1007122
6. Kudo M, Chung H, Osaki Y. Prognostic staging system for hepatocellular carcinoma (CLIP score): its value and limitations, and a proposal for a new staging system, the Japan Integrated Staging Score (JIS score). *J Gastroenterol* (2003) 38:207–15. doi: 10.1007/s005350300038
7. Chun YS, Pawlik TM, Vauthey JN. 8th Edition of the AJCC Cancer Staging Manual: Pancreas and Hepatobiliary Cancers. *Ann Surg Oncol* (2018) 25:845–7. doi: 10.1245/s10434-017-6025-x
8. Hoshida Y, Villanueva A, Kobayashi M, Peix J, Chiang DY, Camargo A, et al. Gene expression in fixed tissues and outcome in hepatocellular carcinoma. *N Engl J Med* (2008) 359:1995–2004. doi: 10.1056/NEJMoa0804525
9. Wang SM, Ooi LL, Hui KM. Identification and validation of a novel gene signature associated with the recurrence of human hepatocellular carcinoma. *Clin Cancer Res* (2007) 13:6275–83. doi: 10.1158/1078-0432.CCR-06-2236
10. Srivastava S, Wong KF, Ong CW, Huak CY, Yeoh KG, Teh M, et al. A morpho-molecular prognostic model for hepatocellular carcinoma. *Br J Cancer* (2012) 107:334–9. doi: 10.1038/bjc.2012.230
11. Totoki Y, Tatsuno K, Covington KR, Ueda H, Creighton CJ, Kato M, et al. Trans-ancestry mutational landscape of hepatocellular carcinoma genomes. *Nat Genet* (2014) 46:1267–73. doi: 10.1038/ng.3126
12. Schulze K, Imbeaud S, Letouze E, Alexandrov LB, Calderaro J, Rebouissou S, et al. Exome sequencing of hepatocellular carcinomas identifies new mutational signatures and potential therapeutic targets. *Nat Genet* (2015) 47:505–11. doi: 10.1038/ng.3252
13. Villanueva A, Portela A, Sayols S, Battiston C, Hoshida Y, Mendez-Gonzalez J, et al. DNA methylation-based prognosis and epidrivers in hepatocellular carcinoma. *Hepatology* (2015) 61:1945–56. doi: 10.1002/hep.27732
14. Tan PS, Nakagawa S, Goossens N, Venkatesh A, Huang T, Ward SC, et al. Clinicopathological indices to predict hepatocellular carcinoma molecular classification. *Liver Int* (2016) 36:108–18. doi: 10.1111/liv.12889
15. Qiu J, Peng B, Tang Y, Qian Y, Guo P, Li M, et al. CpG Methylation Signature Predicts Recurrence in Early-Stage Hepatocellular Carcinoma: Results From a Multicenter Study. *J Clin Oncol* (2017) 35:734–42. doi: 10.1200/JCO.2016.68.2153
16. Cancer Genome Atlas Research Network. Electronic address wbe, Cancer Genome Atlas Research N. Comprehensive and Integrative Genomic Characterization of Hepatocellular Carcinoma. *Cell* (2017) 169:1327–41.e1323. doi: 10.1016/j.cell.2017.05.046
17. Fang F, Wang X, Song T. Five-CpG-based prognostic signature for predicting survival in hepatocellular carcinoma patients. *Cancer Biol Med* (2018) 15:425–33. doi: 10.20892/j.issn.2095-3941.2018.0027
18. Long J, Chen P, Lin J, Bai Y, Yang X, Bian J, et al. DNA methylation-driven genes for constructing diagnostic, prognostic, and recurrence models for hepatocellular carcinoma. *Theranostics* (2019) 9:7251–67. doi: 10.7150/thno.31155
19. Zhang X, Bai Y, Xu L, Zhang B, Feng S, Xu L, et al. Clinical and morpho-molecular classifiers for prediction of hepatocellular carcinoma prognosis and recurrence after surgical resection. *Hepatol Int* (2019) 13:715–25. doi: 10.1007/s12072-019-09978-9
20. Pinato DJ, Sharma R, Allara E, Yen C, Arizumi T, Kubota K, et al. The ALBI grade provides objective hepatic reserve estimation across each BCLC stage of hepatocellular carcinoma. *J Hepatol* (2017) 66:338–46. doi: 10.1016/j.jhep.2016.09.008
21. Frederick LG, Page DL, Fleming ID, Fritz AG, Balch CM, Haller DG, et al. *AJCC Cancer Staging Manual*. New York: Springer (2013).
22. Edmondson HA, Steiner PE. Primary carcinoma of the liver: a study of 100 cases among 48,900 necropsies. *Cancer* (1954) 7:462–503. doi: 10.1002/1097-0142(195405)7:3<462::aid-cncr2820070308>3.0.co;2-e
23. Roayaie S, Blume IN, Thung SN, Guido M, Fiel MI, Hiotis S, et al. A system of classifying microvascular invasion to predict outcome after resection in patients with hepatocellular carcinoma. *Gastroenterology* (2009) 137:850–5. doi: 10.1053/j.gastro.2009.06.003
24. Tatrai P, Somoracz A, Batmunkh E, Schirmacher P, Kiss A, Schaff Z, et al. Agrin and CD34 immunohistochemistry for the discrimination of benign

versus malignant hepatocellular lesions. *Am J Surg Pathol* (2009) 33:874–85. doi: 10.1097/PAS.0b013e318194b3ea

25. Portolani N, Coniglio A, Ghidoni S, Giovanelli M, Benetti A, Tiberio GA, et al. Early and late recurrence after liver resection for hepatocellular carcinoma: prognostic and therapeutic implications. *Ann Surg* (2006) 243:229–35. doi: 10.1097/01.sla.0000197706.21803.a1
26. Shafizadeh N, Ferrell LD, Kakar S. Utility and limitations of glypican-3 expression for the diagnosis of hepatocellular carcinoma at both ends of the differentiation spectrum. *Mod Pathol* (2008) 21:1011–8. doi: 10.1038/modpathol.2008.85
27. Johnson DE, Herndier BG, Medeiros LJ, Warnke RA, Rouse RV. The diagnostic utility of the keratin profiles of hepatocellular carcinoma and cholangiocarcinoma. *Am J Surg Pathol* (1988) 12:187–97. doi: 10.1097/00000478-198803000-00004
28. Kimura H, Nakajima T, Kagawa K, Deguchi T, Kakusui M, Katagishi T, et al. Angiogenesis in hepatocellular carcinoma as evaluated by CD34 immunohistochemistry. *Liver* (1998) 18:14–9. doi: 10.1111/j.1600-0676.1998.tb00121.x
29. Saad RS, Luckasevic TM, Noga CM, Johnson DR, Silverman JF, Liu YL. Diagnostic value of HepParl, pCEA, CD10, and CD34 expression in separating hepatocellular carcinoma from metastatic carcinoma in fine-needle aspiration cytology. *Diagn Cytopathol* (2004) 30:1–6. doi: 10.1002/dc.10345
30. Tsui WM, Colombari R, Portmann BC, Bonetti F, Thung SN, Ferrell LD, et al. Hepatic angiomyolipoma: a clinicopathologic study of 30 cases and delineation of unusual morphologic variants. *Am J Surg Pathol* (1999) 23:34–48. doi: 10.1097/00000478-199901000-00004
31. Hu L, Lau SH, Tzang CH, Wen JM, Wang W, Xie D, et al. Association of Vimentin overexpression and hepatocellular carcinoma metastasis. *Oncogene* (2004) 23:298–302. doi: 10.1038/sj.onc.1206483
32. Guzman G, Alagiozian-Angelova V, Layden-Almer JE, Layden TJ, Testa G, Benedetti E, et al. p53, Ki-67, and serum alpha feto-protein as predictors of hepatocellular carcinoma recurrence in liver transplant patients. *Mod Pathol* (2005) 18:1498–503. doi: 10.1038/modpathol.3800458
33. Jin Y, Liang ZY, Zhou WX, Zhou L. Combination with CK19 Might Increase the Prognostic Power of Hep Par 1 in Hepatocellular Carcinoma after Curative Resection. *J Invest Surg* (2018) 31:412–9. doi: 10.1080/08941939.2017.1347218
34. Tibshirani R. The lasso method for variable selection in the Cox model. *Stat Med* (1997) 16:385–95. doi: 10.1002/(sici)1097-0258(19970228)16:4<385::aid-sim380>3.0.co;2-3

17

Transarterial Chemoembolization Combined with Hepatectomy for the Treatment of Intermediate-Stage Hepatocellular Carcinoma

Qunfang Zhou[1], Fei Tuo[2], Ruixia Li[1], Xiaohui Wang[3], Juncheng Wang[3], Zhimei Huang[1], Minshan Chen[3*] and Jinhua Huang[1*]*

[1] *Department of Minimally Invasive Interventional Therapy, Sun Yat-sen University Cancer Center, Guangzhou, China,*
[2] *Department of Ultrasound Diagnose, The First Hospital of Hunan University of Chinese Medicine, Changsha, China,*
[3] *Department of Hepatobiliary Oncology, Sun Yat-sen University Cancer Center, Sun Yat-sen University, Guangzhou, China*

Correspondence:
Xiaohui Wang
wangxh2@sysucc.org.cn
Minshan Chen
chenmsh@sysucc.org.cn
Jinhua Huang
huangjh@sysucc.org.cn

Background: Transarterial chemoembolization (TACE) is currently the recommended treatment for intermediate-stage hepatocellular carcinoma (HCC). Liver resection (LR) may be an effective option, although recurrences are not uncommon. TACE prior to LR has been proposed as an even better alternative.

Methods: Patients with intermediate-stage HCC who underwent curative resection were enrolled between January 2007 and December 2015. We compared overall survival (OS) and recurrence-free survival (RFS) for the 2 groups using the Kaplan-Meier method, and we determined independent risk factors for death and recurrence using multivariate regression analyses.

Results: A total of 488 patients with HCC at BCLC B (265 patients with LR, 223 patients with TACE+LR) enrolled from our center. Mean follow-up was 40.2 (range, 3.0–128.7) months. For patients receiving TACE+LR and LR, estimated 1-, 3-, and 5-year OS rates were 90.6% and 73.3%, 61.7% and 43.5%, and 52.9% and 33.8%, respectively (all $P <$ 0.001) and estimated 1-, 2-, and 3-year RFS rates were 54.6% and 39.4%, 41.4% and 29.4%, and 36.3% and 26.3%, respectively ($P < 0.001$, $P = 0.002$, and $P = 0.008$, respectively). Significant independent predictors of poor OS were more than 3 (vs. 3 or fewer) tumors (HR=2.19, 95% CI 1.69–2.84), non-anatomical (vs. anatomical) hepatectomy (HR=1.29, 95% CI 1.01–1.66), microscopic vascular invasion (HR=1.46, 95% CI 1.15–.90), cirrhosis (HR=2.41, 95%CI 1.88–3.01), and intraoperative blood transfusion (HR=1.29, 95% CI 1.01–1.66).

Conclusion: Preoperative TACE with LR may result in better oncological outcomes than either TACE or LR alone, without a substantial increase in morbidity, and could be considered an effective combination treatment for intermediate-stage HCC.

Keywords: combination therapy, hepatectomy, intermediate hepatocellular carcinoma, overall survival, transarterial chemoembolization

INTRODUCTION

Hepatocellular carcinoma (HCC) is one of the most common cancers in the world, ranked as the sixth most common neoplasm and the third leading cause of cancer-related mortality worldwide (1). Advances in diagnostic imaging and widespread application of screening programs in high-risk populations have allowed detection of HCC at earlier stages, but some patients with HCC still continue to present in intermediate or even advanced stages. According to the Barcelona Clinic Liver Cancer (BCLC) algorithm for the treatment of HCC, intermediate-stage HCC (stage B) is defined as extensive multifocal disease without vascular invasion in patients with preserved liver function and the absence of cancer-related symptoms (2).

However, intermediate-stage HCC actually involves a heterogeneous group of patients, encompassing those with a wide range of tumor sizes (larger than 3 cm to over 10 cm) and numbers (2 to over 20), provided that patients have good liver function (Child-Pugh classes A or B) (3). Likewise, the prognosis of patients with intermediate-stage HCC varies (4). According to the BCLC algorithm, transarterial chemoembolization (TACE) is the recommended treatment for patients with intermediate-stage HCC (5). Whereas TACE has been reported to extend the survival of groups of patients with intermediate-stage HCC, the outcomes for individual patients treated with TACE for intermediate-stage HCC have remained mixed (6). At the present time, it remains controversial whether there is enough evidence supporting TACE, particularly relative to liver resection (LR), as the best treatment for patients with intermediate-stage HCC (7).

In fact, multiple recent reports have suggested that LR, when compared to TACE, might provide a survival benefit to patients with intermediate-stage HCC (8–10). Historically, LR has been reserved for the treatment of patients with early–stage HCC who have good liver function (11). Yet with improvements in surgical techniques and perioperative care, the surgical mortality rate for LR in patients with HCC has been reduced to less than 1% (12, 13). In addition, the complete surgical removal of the tumor may offer the best chance for long-term survival in patients with HCC. Nevertheless, patients who have LR for HCC larger than 5 cm often relapse after a short recurrence-free interval, especially those patients with huge (10 cm or larger) HCC (14, 15).

At the same time, TACE has been used successfully as a neoadjuvant therapy for large HCC prior to LR (16). A 2018 systematic review demonstrated that TACE can feasibly be combined with other modalities to improve the resectability rate for HCC (17). Along these lines, the use of preoperative TACE followed by LR has been shown to improve survival outcomes for some patients with large HCC (18).

Over the years, our Cancer Center has treated a relatively large population of patients with intermediate-stage HCC. Provided that liver function reserve was adequate and complete resection of the tumor appeared feasible, we offered LR to these patients. For some, we also recommended preoperative TACE, with the belief that this might potentially reduce postoperative recurrences and improve long-term survival. Our hypothesis has been that some patients with BCLC stage B may benefit from not only LR but also preoperative TACE. The aim of this retrospective study was to identify patients at our Cancer Center with intermediate-stage HCC who had LR and others who had TACE prior to LR, to compare the outcomes of each approach using survival rates, and to determine the prognostic factors for recurrence and death in these patients.

METHODS

This study was conducted in accordance with the principles of the Declaration of Helsinki (19), and the study protocol was approved by the Ethics Committee of the Sun Yat-sen University Cancer Center.

Study Population

We retrospectively reviewed the medical records of patients who received a diagnosis of HCC from January 2007 to December 2015 at our Cancer Center. The diagnosis of HCC was made using criteria defined by the American Association for the Study of Liver Disease and the European Association for the Study of the Liver, and was based either on positive liver biopsy or characteristic findings on imaging (multiphasic CT or dynamic contrast-enhanced MRI) combined with serum Alpha-fetoprotein (AFP) levels (20, 21). The clinical stage of HCC was determined according to the BCLC guidelines (22).

The inclusion criteria for this study included: (a) age 18 to 75 years; (b) Eastern Cooperative Oncology Group (ECOG) performance status score of 0 or 1; (c) HCC with 2 or more tumors, at least one of which with a diameter greater than 3 cm, confirmed on postoperative pathological examination; (d) no macrovascular invasion or extrahepatic metastasis; (e) adequate liver function (i.e., Child–Pugh class A or B liver function); (f) adequate renal function (i.e., serum creatinine concentration no higher than 1.5 times the upper limit of normal); and (g) adequate coagulation function (i.e., prothrombin activity > 40%, international normalized ratio [INR] < 1.26, and platelet count > 50×10^9/L). Patients were excluded from the analysis for any of the following reasons: (1) under 18 years or over 75 years of age; (2) recurrent HCC; (3) only a single HCC tumor of any size, or multiple HCC tumors but all with diameters of 3 cm or less; (4) received previous systematic chemotherapy, targeted (Sorafenib) therapy, or radiofrequency ablation (RFA) for HCC; (5) lost to follow-up within 90 days after LR; or (6) information about prognostic variables or follow-up could not be obtained.

Demographic and Clinicopathological Characteristics

We collected data about each patient's demographic and clinical characteristics, including sex, age, body mass index (BMI), Child-Pugh grade (severity of liver disease, based on 5 clinical factors: PT or INR, albumin, bilirubin, ascites, and hepatic encephalopathy), diameter of largest HCC tumor, number of tumors, preoperative hepatitis (based on history of chronic HBV infection and/or positive hepatitis B virus RNA testing), preoperative portal hypertension (defined as esophageal varices and/or splenomegaly on imaging studies, combined with a decreased platelet count [100 × $10^3/\mu L$ or less]), and preoperative blood testing (including AFP, liver and renal function tests, prothrombin time [PT] and international normalized ratio [INR], and complete blood count).

We also collected data for each patient about their histopathological findings from LR (microvascular invasion and cirrhosis [of the noncancerous part of the resected specimen]), volumes of intraoperative blood loss and intraoperative blood transfusion, and postoperative complications (large pleural effusion, pneumonia, portal vein thrombosis, cholestasis, and/or ascites).

TACE Procedure

The decision to utilize TACE before LR was made by the treating physician and was based on the patient's liver function as well as the number, size, and degree of enhancement of HCC tumors observed in imaging studies. Patients receiving TACE had it administered within 3 months of LR. TACE was carried out under the guidance of digital subtraction angiography (DSA) (Allura Xper FD 20, Philips), and it was performed through the left or right hepatic artery, and directly through a tumor-feeding artery when technically possible. Hepatic artery angiography, which was performed using a 5 Fr (RH or Yashiro) catheter, was first used to assess the location, number, size, and blood supply of the target tumors. The embolization emulsion was a mixture of Epirubicin (Farmorubicin; Pharmacia, Tokyo, Japan) 30 mg to 60 mg, Lobaplatin (Chang'an International Pharmaceutical, Hainan, China) 30 mg to 50 mg, and Lipiodol (Laboratorie Guerbet, Aulnay-sous-Bois, France) 10 mL to 30 mL, and it was infused into tumor-feeding arteries *via* a 2.7/2.8 Fr micro-catheter. The doses of the agents contained in the embolization emulsion were selected based on patient age, weight, comorbidity, tumor size, tumor number, and anticipated tolerance. The endpoint of the TACE procedure was reached when there was no flow in the tumor-feeding vessels.

Liver Resection

Liver resection was performed by experienced surgeons. We developed a surgical plan based on tumor size, tumor location, and liver function. The hepatectomy method contains anatomical resection and non-anatomical resection, and the extent was defined using the Brisbane 2000 Terminology of Liver Anatomy and Resections (23). We applied Pringle's maneuver with cycles of clamping and unclamping times of 1 to 10 and 5 min each time, respectively, and controlled central venous pressure below 4 mmHg during parenchyma dissection to control intraoperative bleeding. Complete hepatic resection was defined as the complete removal of all detected tumors without involving any major branch of the portal or hepatic veins, without invasion of adjacent organs and without lymph node or distant metastasis, and tumor-free margins confirmed by histopathology.

Propensity Score Matching (PSM)

A PSM method was used to balance the potential biases between two groups. The propensity score was estimated using a multivariate logistic regression by using variables of diameter of largest HCC tumor, number of tumors, serum AFP level, microvascular invasion, tumor encapsulation, resection margin, and type of hepatectomy. Patients were matched 1:1 using the nearest neighbor method with a caliber of 0.05; the matching process has been described in a previous study (24).

Follow-Up

The follow-up period for this study was terminated on September 30, 2019. Patients were followed at least once every 3 months after LR; the visits involved checking serum AFP levels and performing screening abdominal imaging (e.g., abdominal CT and/or MRI and/or ultrasound scans). HCC recurrence was suspected when there was a progressive elevation of serum AFP levels, a new showing contrast enhancement in the arterial phase and washout in the venous phase on CT and/or MRI, and/or hypervascularity on hepatic angiography.

The dates of tumor recurrence, last follow-up, and death were recorded. The primary endpoint was overall survival (OS), and the secondary endpoint was recurrence-free survival (RFS). OS was defined as the time from LR to death or last follow-up, and RFS was defined as the time from LR to tumor progression, death, or last follow-up (whichever came first). Tumor progression was defined as the local tumor recurrence or the occurrence of new lesions in the liver or elsewhere, based on imaging.

Statistical Methods

For the study, the patients were divided into 2 groups, with those having TACE prior to LR placed in the TACE+LR group, and those having only LR placed in the LR group. The demographic and clinicopathological characteristics of the groups were summarized using frequencies and percentages for categorical covariates and means and standard deviation (SD) for continuous covariates. The Fisher exact test was used to compare categorical covariates, while the Wilcoxon rank-sum test was used to compare continuous covariates. The cutoffs for continuous variables were chosen to allow for easy interpretation. OS and RFS rates were calculated using the Kaplan–Meier method. Univariate and multivariate Cox regression analyses were used to determine the impact of risk factors on recurrence (using RFS) and death (using OS). Variables with *P*-values less than 0.10 in the univariate analysis were subjected to the multivariate Cox regression model using a forward stepwise variable selection; results were reported as hazards ratios (HR) and 95% confidence intervals (CI). A 2-tailed *P*-value less than 0.05 was considered statistically significant for all of the tests. Statistical analyses were performed using SPSS version 25.0 (IBM).

RESULTS

Demographic and Clinicopathological Characteristics

A total of 488 patients met the inclusion criteria for the study. The mean follow-up period was 40.2 (range, 3.0 to 128.7) months. Of these, 223 (45.7%) were in the TACE+LR group and 265 (54.3%) were in the LR group (**Table 1**). When

TABLE 1 | Demographic and clinicopathological characteristics of patients with BCLC stage B hepatocellular carcinoma (HCC) before and after propensity score matching (PSM), by treatment (TACE+LR vs. LR), January 2007 to December 2015.

Characteristics	**Before PSM**		**P**	**After PSM**		**P**
	TACE+LRN (%)	**LRN (%)**		**TACE+LRN (%)**	**LRN (%)**	
Total patients	223 (100)	265 (100)	-	189	189	
Sex						
Male	197 (88.3)	238 (89.8)	0.60	169(89.4)	171(90.5)	0.73
Female	26 (12.7)	27 (10.2)	20(10.6)	18(9.5)		
Age, *years*						
<60	179 (80.2)	215 (81.3)	0.81	150(79.4)	155(82)	0.515
≥60	44 (19.8)	50 (18.7)	39(20.6)	34(28)		
Largest HCC tumor diameter, *cm*						
<10	150 (67.2)	199 (75.1)	0.056	137(72.5)	133(70.4)	0.65
≥10	73 (28.2)	66 (24.9)	52(37.5)	56(29.6)		
HCC tumors, *n*						
≤3	172 (77.1)	193 (72.8)	0.28	141(74.6)	143(75.7)	0.81
>3	51 (22.9)	72 (27.2)	48(25.4)	46(24.3)		
Hepatitis[a]	174 (78.0)	203 (76.6)	0.71	142(75.1)	147(77.8)	0.51
Portal hypertension[b]	18 (8.1)	11 (4.2)	0.07	12(6.3)	8(4.2)	0.36
Comorbidity[c]	25 (11.2)	27 (10.2)	0.72	21(11.1)	18(9.5)	0.61
Alpha-fetoprotein (AFP) level, *ng/ml*						
≤400	127 (57.0)	134 (50.6)	0.16	101(53.4)	103(54.5)	0.84
>400	96 (43.0)	131 (49.4)	88(46.6)	86(55.5)		
Type of hepatectomy[d]						
Anatomical	64 (28.7)	79 (35.4)	0.79	53(28)	60(31.7)	0.43
Non-anatomical	159 (71.3)	186 (64.6)	136(72)	129(68.3)		
Resection margin[e], *cm*						
≤1	200 (89.7)	203 (76.6)	**<0.001**	166(87.8)	164(86.8)	0.76
>1	23 (10.3)	62 (24.3)	23(12.2)	25(13.2)		
Tumor encapsulation[f]	156 (70.0)	161 (60.8)	**0.03**	122(64.6)	119(63)	0.75
Microvascular invasion[g]	61 (27.4)	110 (41.5)	**0.001**	61(32.3)	59(31.2)	0.83
Cirrhosis[g]	117(52.5)	147(55.5)	0.507	107(56.6)	116(61.4)	0.347
Postoperative complication[h]	13 (6.0)	21 (8.0)	0.37	11(6)	16(8.5)	0.32
Characteristics	**Before PSM**		***P***	**After PSM**		***P***
	TACE+LR Mean ± SD	**LR Mean ± SD**		**TACE+LR Mean ± SD**	**LR Mean ± SD**	
Body Mass Index (BMI), *kg/m²*	22.2 ± 3.1	22.4 ± 3.1	0.61	22.2 ± 3.1	22.1 ± 2.7	0.65
Alanine aminotransferase (ALT), *IU/L*	56.1 ± 54.9	53.9 ± 49.4	0.63	58.7 ± 58.4	57.4 ± 55.2	0.65
Albumin (ALB), *g/L*	39.9 ± 6	40.7 ± 4.5	0.083	39.9 ± 6.5	40.6 ± 4.7	0.27
Total bilirubin (TBIL), *μmol/L*	13.8 ± 6.7	14.5 ± 6.5	0.22	13.9 ± 7.1	13.9 ± 5.4	0.98
White blood count (WBC), *x* 10^9*/L*	6.4 ± 2.0	6.8 ± 3.1	0.08	6.4 ± 1.9	6.8 ± 3.2	0.075
Platelet count (PLT), *x* 10^9*/L*	194.2 ± 85.1	195.9 ± 76.3	0.82	196.3 ± 84.4	200.3 ± 77.8	0.63
Prothrombin time (PT), *seconds*	12.1 ± 1.1	12.2 ± 1.1	0.43	12.1 ± 1.1	12.2 ± 1.1	0.74
International normalized ratio (INR)	1.1 ± 0.1	1.1 ± 0.1	0.70	1.1 ± 0.1	1.1 ± 0.1	0.51
Intraoperative blood loss, *mL*	651.6 ± 639.8	567.0 ± 794.2	0.20	673.3 ± 677.1	571.2 ± 637.2	0.13
Intraoperative blood transfusion, *mL*	176.5 ± 356.2	148.7 ± 378.8	0.41	177 ± 359.5	156.6 ± 379.3	0.59

[a]*Hepatitis defined preoperatively as a history of chronic HBV infection and/or positive hepatitis C virus RNA test.*
[b]*Portal hypertension defined preoperatively as esophageal varices and/or splenomegaly on imaging studies combined with a decreased platelet count [100 ×* 10^3*/μL or less]).*
[c]*Comorbidity defined as preoperative hypertension, diabetes, coronary disease, and/or severe anemia.*
[d]*Determined by surgeon intraoperatively, anatomical approach based on the Brisbane 2000 nomenclature of liver anatomy, whereas non-anatomical approach consisted of wedge or limited resection.*
[e]*Based on intraoperative surgeon estimation.*
[f]*Based on intraoperative surgeon description of tumor appearing encapsulated or infiltrating (not encapsulated).*
[g]*Based on postoperative histopathology report.*
[h]*Postoperative large pleural effusion, pneumonia, portal vein thrombosis, and/or cholestasis.*
BCLC, Barcelona Clinic Liver Cancer; TACE, transarterial chemoembolization; LR, liver resection (hepatectomy).
All bold P value were represented the significance (P < 0.05).

compared to the patients in the LR group, significantly more of those in the TACE+LR group had resection margins of 1 cm or less (89.7% vs. 76.6%, $P < 0.001$) and tumor encapsulation (70.0% vs. 60.8%, $P = 0.03$), and significantly less had microvascular invasion (27.4% vs. 51.5%, $P = 0.001$). Conversely, there were no significant differences between the 2 groups with regards to sex, age, BMI, tumor size, number of tumors, hepatitis, portal hypertension, comorbidity, AFP and all other biochemical blood tests, type of hepatectomy, cirrhosis, intraoperative blood loss and transfusion, and postoperative complications.

A PSM model was established to balance the bias of clinicopathological characteristics between the two groups. As shown in **Table 1**, total of 378 patients were enrolled and 189 in each group. Resection margins, tumor encapsulation, and microvascular invasion presented no difference between the two groups after PSM, and other characteristics also showed no significance.

Overall Survival (OS)

By the last follow-up, 107 (48%) patients in the TACE+LR group and 181 (68.3%) patients in the LR group had died. The 90-day mortality rate for patients in the TACE+LR group was 1.3% (3 patients) and for patients in the LR group was 4.2% (11 patients). Over the entire study period, patients in the TACE+LR group had significantly higher OS than patients in the LR group before PSM (P < 0.001) (**Figure 1A**). After PSM, the OS curve of patients in TACE+LR group showed better survival rate than LR group (P < 0.001) (**Figure 1B**). The estimated 1-, 3-, and 5-year OS rates for patients receiving TACE+LR were 90.6%, 61.7%, and 52.9%, respectively, whereas the rates for those receiving LR were 73.3%, 43.5%, and 33.8%, respectively (all P < 0.001) (**Table 2**).

Based on multivariate analysis, LR (vs. TACE+LR) as treatment (HR=1.94, 95% CI 1.52–2.48, P < 0.001), more than 3 (vs. 3 or fewer) tumors (HR=2.19, 95% CI 1.69–2.84, P < 0.001), non-anatomical (vs. anatomical) hepatectomy (HR=1.29, 95% CI 1.01–1.66, P = 0.046), microscopic vascular invasion (HR=1.46, 95% CI 1.15–1.90, P = 0.002), cirrhosis (HR=2.41, 95% CI 1.88–3.01, P < 0.001), and intraoperative blood transfusion (HR=1.29, 95% CI 1.01–1.66, P = 0.004) were all significantly independently associated with OS (**Table 3**).

Recurrence-Free Survival (RFS)

By the last follow-up, 158 (70.9%) patients in the TACE+LR group and 213 (80.4%) patients in the LR group had experienced recurrence. Over the entire study period, patients in the TACE+LR group had significantly higher RFS than patients in the LR group (P = 0.001) (**Figure 2A**). After PSM, patients in TACE+LR group had obvious longer RFS than the LR group (P = 0.01) (**Figure 2B**). The median RFS in the TACE+LR group (15.4 months, 95% CI 10.2–20.6 months) was 7 months longer than in the LR group (8.3 months, 95% CI 8.6–12.2 months). The estimated 1-, 2-, and 3-year RFS rates for patients receiving TACE +LR were 54.6%, 41.4%, and 36.3%, respectively, whereas the rates for those receiving LR were 39.4%, 29.4%, and 26.3%, respectively (P < 0.001, P = 0.002, and P = 0.008, respectively) (**Table 2**).

Based on multivariate analysis, LR (vs. TACE+LR) as treatment (HR=1.55, 95% CI 1.26–1.91, P < 0.001), tumor size of 10 cm or more (vs. less than 10 cm) (HR=1.39, 95% CI 1.11–1.75, P = 0.005), more than 3 (vs. 3 or fewer) tumors (HR=2.98, 95% CI 2.35–3.79, P < 0.001), microscopic vascular invasion (HR=1.45, 95% CI 1.16–1.81, P = 0.001), and cirrhosis (HR=1.74, 95% CI 1.41–2.15, P < 0.001) were all significant independent predictors of recurrence (**Table 4**).

DISCUSSION

Patients with intermediate-stage HCC have large and multifocal HCCs and do not have evidence of intrahepatic macrovascular invasion or extrahepatic metastases (25). Progression after treatment continues to be a substantial challenge in the clinical management of patients with large HCC and is associated with poor survival outcomes. Currently, the most common treatment for intermediate-stage HCC is TACE (26). TACE concludes with

TABLE 2 | Overall survival (OS) and recurrence-free survival (RFS) rates in 488 patients with BCLC stage B hepatocellular carcinoma (HCC), by treatment (TACE +LR vs. LR), January 2007 to December 2015.

Rates	Treatment		P
	TACE+LR (n = 223) %	LR (n = 265) %	
1-year OS	90.6	73.3	**<0.001**
3-year OS	61.7	43.5	**<0.001**
5-year OS	52.9	33.8	**<0.001**
1-year RFS	54.6	39.4	**<0.001**
2-year RFS	41.4	29.4	**0.002**
3-year RFS	36.3	26.3	**0.008**

BCLC, Barcelona Clinic Liver Cancer; TACE, transarterial chemoembolization; LR, liver resection (hepatectomy).
Bold values provided in this table was that P value < 0.05, there was significant difference between the two groups.

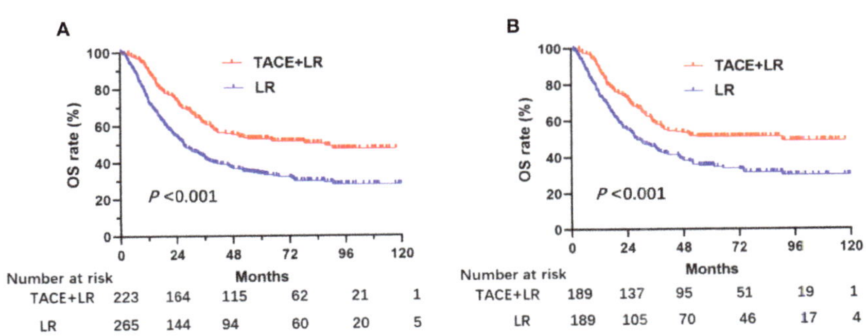

FIGURE 1 | Kaplan–Meier overall survival (OS) rate curves for patients underwent TACE+LR and LR for BCLC stage B hepatocellular carcinoma (HCC) before and after PSM, January 2007 to December 2015. **(A)** the OS rate of patients before PSM, **(B)** the OS rate of patients after PSM. OS rates of the patients who received TACE+LR were significantly higher than OS rates of those who received only LR both before and after PSM (P < 0.001).

TABLE 3 | Univariate and multivariate analyses of demographic and clinicopathological prognostic factors for overall survival (OS) in 488 patients with BCLC stage B hepatocellular carcinoma (HCC), January 2007 to December 2015.

Characteristics	Variables	Univariate Analysis		Multivariate Analysis	
		Hazard Ratio (95% CI)	*P*	Hazard Ratio (95% CI)	*P*
Type of treatment	LR vs. TACE+LR	1.80 (1.42–2.29)	**<0.001**	1.94 (1.52–2.48)	**<0.001**
Age, *years*	>60 vs. ≤60	1.00 (0.75–1.34)	0.99	–	–
Sex	Male vs. female	0.94 (0.64–1.37)	0.73	–	–
Largest HCC tumor diameter, *cm*	≥10 vs. < 10	1.32 (1.03–1.7)	0.03	NS	0.30
HCC tumors, *n*	>3 vs. ≤3	2.52 (1.97–3.23)	**<0.001**	2.19 (1.69–2.84)	**<0.001**
Portal hypertension[a]	Yes vs. no	0.97 (0.60–1.59)	0.91	–	–
Alpha-fetoprotein (AFP), *ng/mL*	>400 vs. ≤400	1.46 (1.16–1.84)	**0.001**	NS	0.15
Type of hepatectomy[b]	Non-anatomical vs. anatomical	1.35 (1.05–1.73)	**0.02**	1.29 (1.01–1.66)	**0.046**
Resection margin[c], *cm*	>1 vs. ≤1	1.09 (0.81–1.47)	0.56	–	–
Tumor encapsulation[d]	Yes vs. no	0.84 (0.66–1.06)	0.15	–	–
Microscopic vascular invasion[e]	Yes vs. no	1.94 (1.53–2.45)	**<0.001**	1.48 (1.15–1.90)	**0.002**
Cirrhosis[e]	Yes vs. no	2.67 (2.09–3.41)	**<0.001**	2.41 (1.88–3.01)	**<0.001**
Intraoperative blood transfusion	Yes vs. no	1.71 (1.33–2.20)	**<0.001**	1.45 (1.13–1.93)	**0.004**

[a]*Portal hypertension defined preoperatively as esophageal varices and/or splenomegaly on imaging studies combined with a decreased platelet count [100 × 10^3/μL or less]).*
[b]*Determined by surgeon intraoperatively, anatomical approach based on the Brisbane 2000 nomenclature of liver anatomy, whereas non-anatomical approach consisted of wedge or limited resection.*
[c]*Based on intraoperative surgeon estimation.*
[d]*Based on intraoperative surgeon description of tumor appearing encapsulated or infiltrating (not encapsulated).*
[e]*Based on postoperative histopathology report.*
BCLC, Barcelona Clinic Liver Cancer; CI, confidence interval; TACE, transarterial chemoembolization; LR, liver resection (hepatectomy); NS, not significant.
Bold values provided in this table was that P value < 0.05, there was significant difference between the two groups.

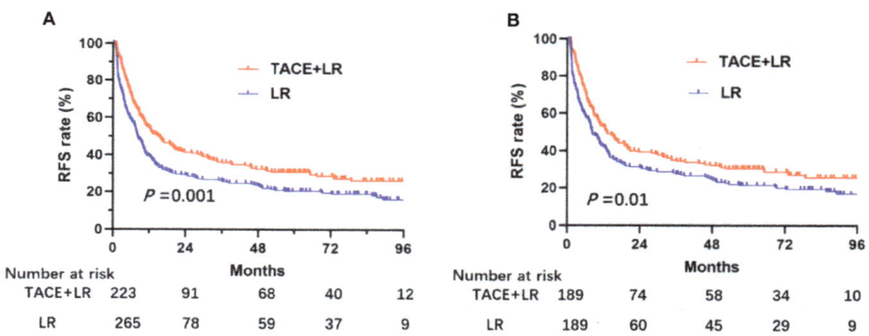

FIGURE 2 | Kaplan–Meier recurrence-free survival (RFS) rate curves for patients underwent TACE+LR and LR for BCLC stage B hepatocellular carcinoma (HCC) before and after PSM, January 2007 to December 2015. **(A)** the RFS rate of patients before PSM, **(B)** the RFS rate of patients after PSM. Patients who received TACE+LR were significantly higher than RFS rates of those who received only LR both before and after PSM (*P* < 0.05).

selective embolization of HCC tumors. However, before that, the procedure involves the intra-arterial infusion of a chemotherapy agent embedded in lipiodol, which tends to accumulate in the blood and lymph vessels of tumors, and serves as a vehicle for prolonging tumor exposure to the agent, yet does not adversely affect normal liver cells (8) (27).

Some researchers suggest that the evidence supporting TACE as first-line treatment for intermediate-stage HCC may not be strong enough, and they suggest that because LR may result in better outcomes than TACE, it should be considered first-line treatment for most patients with intermediate-stage disease (28). Others have echoed this, suggesting that treatments more aggressive than TACE, such as LR or energy ablation, should be considered first-line treatment for intermediate-stage HCC (29, 30). Some may argue that the high number and large size of tumors in some patients with intermediate-stage HCC make LR an inferior option. However, several large studies have demonstrated that the number and size of HCC tumors should not be used as a selection criterion for LR, provided that tumor location and liver function would otherwise allow resection (31–34). The results of these studies suggest that patients with multiple HCCs and Child-Pugh classes A or B should be considered for LR. Furthermore, recent advances in surgical technique, perioperative care, and accurate patient selection have gradually reduced the morbidity and mortality of LR, and encouraging postoperative results and oncological outcomes are being reported in patients with intermediate-stage HCC (10, 35, 36).

In this retrospective clinical study, we looked not only at 256 patients who had received LR for intermediate-stage HCC but also

TABLE 4 | Univariate and multivariate analyses of demographic and clinicopathological prognostic factors for recurrence-free survival in 488 patients with BCLC stage B hepatocellular carcinoma (HCC), January 2007 to December 2015.

Characteristics	Variables	Univariate Analysis		Multivariate Analysis	
		Hazard Ratio (95% CI)	*P*	Hazard Ratio (95% CI)	*P*
Type of treatment	LR vs TACE+LR	1.44 (1.17–1.76)	**0.001**	1.55 (1.26–1.91)	**<0.001**
Age, *years*	>60 vs. ≤60	0.97 (0.75–1.25)	0.80	–	–
Sex	Male vs. female	0.85 (0.60–1.20)	0.85	–	–
Largest HCC tumor diameter, *cm*	≥10 vs. < 10	1.51 (1.21–1.88)	**<0.001**	1.39 (1.11–1.75)	**0.005**
HCC tumors, *n*	>3 vs. ≤3	3.43 (2.73–4.32)	**<0.001**	2.98 (2.35–3.79)	**<0.001**
Portal hypertension[a]	Yes vs. no	1.00 (0.66–1.53)	0.99	–	–
Alpha-fetoprotein (AFP), *ng/mL*	>400 vs. ≤400	1.35 (1.10–1.65)	**0.004**	NS	0.12
Type of hepatectomy[b]	Non-anatomical vs. anatomical	1.31 (1.05–1.64)	**0.02**	NS	0.09
Resection margin[c], *cm*	>1 vs. ≤1	0.97 (0.74–1.27)	0.83	–	–
Tumor encapsulation[d]	Yes vs. no	0.86 (0.70–1.07)	0.18	–	–
Microscopic vascular Invasion[e]	Yes vs. no	1.79 (1.45–2.21)	**<0.001**	1.45 (1.16–1.81)	**0.001**
Cirrhosis[e]	Yes vs. no	1.91 (1.55–2.36)	**<0.001**	1.74 (1.41–2.15)	**<0.001**
Intraoperative blood transfusion	Yes vs. no	0.92 (0.74–1.27)	0.83	–	–

[a]*Portal hypertension defined preoperatively as esophageal varices and/or splenomegaly on imaging studies combined with a decreased platelet count [100 × $10^3/\mu L$ or less]).*

[b]*Determined by surgeon intraoperatively, anatomical approach based on the Brisbane 2000 nomenclature of liver anatomy, whereas non-anatomical approach consisted of wedge or limited resection.*

[c]*Based on intraoperative surgeon estimation.*

[d]*Based on intraoperative surgeon description of tumor appearing encapsulated or infiltrating (not encapsulated).*

[e]*Based on postoperative histopathology report.*

BCLC, Barcelona Clinic Liver Cancer; CI, confidence interval; TACE, transarterial chemoembolization; LR, liver resection (hepatectomy); NS, not significant.

Bold values provided in this table was that P value < 0.05, there was significant difference between the two groups.

at 223 patients who underwent LR preceded by TACE, over a 9-year period, with a mean duration of follow-up of 40.2 months. When we compared the 2 groups in the study, we found them to be well-matched, with no significant differences in demographic or preoperative clinical characteristics (including tumor size or number, as well as baseline hepatitis, comorbidity, or AFP levels), or in type of hepatectomy performed, histopathological evidence of cirrhosis, or postoperative complications.

However, we did find that relative to the group that underwent LR alone, a significantly higher proportion of patients in the group that received TACE+LR had intraoperative findings of narrow resection margins, and a significantly lower proportion in that group had postoperative histopathological evidence of microvascular invasion. These observations suggest that by exposing the disease to cytotoxic agents and then blocking tumor vessels, TACE may have created a strong cytotoxic effect and caused substantial tumor necrosis prior to surgery, resulting in tumor contraction, narrower margins, and eradication of some of the microvascular invasion. These findings and potential mechanisms are consistent with those reported by others (24). They conflict with a 1995 study from Wu et al., which suggested that TACE should be avoided prior to LR because it did not provide complete necrosis in large tumors (though it did result in a mean 42.8% reduction in tumor volume) and it resulted in delayed surgery (37). However, their study differed from ours in that most of their patients in the TACE+LR group had multiple TACE treatments, administered every 4 to 6 weeks, and the overall survival for their patients who received TACE+LR was worse than for those who received only LR.

When we compared survival outcomes, patients having TACE+LR showed significantly longer OS and RFS than those having only LR. For example, the 5-year OS rate for the TACE+LR group was 52.9%, whereas that for the LR group was 33.8%. Likewise, the 3-year RFS rate for the TACE+LR group was 36.3%, whereas that for the LR group was 26.3%. Our OS and RFS results for patients having TACE+LR were markedly better than those reported by Zhao et al. for patients with intermediate-stage HCC having TACE alone. The 5-year OS rate was 12% and the 3-year RFS rate was 25% for the patients treated with only TACE, despite the vast majority of their patients having only a solitary tumor (8). Taken together, these observations and our results suggest that the combination of TACE and LR could offer more effective tumor eradication than either TACE or LR alone for patients with intermediate-stage HCC, particularly among those with multifocal HCC.

As noted above, some authors in the past have suggested that doing TACE before LR may increase the risk of perioperative morbidity. However, in our study there was no significant difference in the proportion of patients having postoperative complications, when comparing those having LR with those having TACE before LR. Similarly, Li et al. showed not only that the addition of preoperative TACE to LR for huge HCC (10 cm or larger) was associated with an improved OS and RFS, but also that this combination therapy did not increase perioperative morbidity or mortality (24).

Compared to the group of patients in our study who had LR alone, those who received TACE before LR exhibited higher numerical mean volumes of intraoperative blood loss (652 mL vs. 567 mL) and intraoperative blood transfusion (177 mL vs. 149 mL), but these differences were not statistically significant. Some have suggested that patients with hepatitis who undergo preoperative TACE before LR might suffer more intraoperative bleeding and present more operative challenges than those who do not have TACE before LR (38). In our study, the proportion of patients with hepatitis in each group was not significantly different. This, combined with a lack of significant differences in blood loss and transfusion, may provide additional evidence that cirrhosis should not be considered a contraindication to TACE before LR. Some authors have reported that TACE had little influence on subsequent surgery if the interval between the last TACE and LR was long enough (39). The patients in our study who received preoperative TACE had an interval between the last TACE and LR of at least 4 weeks; this suggests the possibility that waiting at least 4 weeks between TACE and LR may result in a risk for bleeding and a need for transfusion that is closer to the risks for LR alone. Finally, the results of our study may provide some support for the proposal that the amount of intraoperative blood loss and blood transfusion during LR may more likely be a function of tumor size (40). The TACE+LR group in our study, which had numerically higher volumes of blood loss and transfusion, also had a higher proportion of patients with huge (10 cm or greater) HCC when compared to the LR group (28.2% vs. 24.9%, respectively), though once again these differences were not statistically significant.

On multivariate analyses, confirming our results based on Kaplan-Meier estimates, we observed that LR alone was independently associated with HCC recurrence and death. Furthermore, we observed that more than 3 HCC tumors, non-anatomical hepatectomy, microscopic vascular invasion, cirrhosis, and intraoperative blood transfusion were all independent predictors of poor OS. Most of these results echo the findings from several other studies of patients who have had LR for intermediate-stage HCC (1, 25, 41). However, the influence of intraoperative blood transfusion on post-LR outcomes continues to be debated. Several studies have observed that intraoperative transfusion had no influence on the OS of patients with HCC after LR (1, 24, 41). In contrast, Mori et al. reported that perioperative blood transfusion was an independent risk factor for poor prognosis after curative surgery for primary HCC in a multi–center study (42). Similarly, Maehara et al. reported that the presence of intraoperative transfusion was an independent poor prognostic factor for OS in patients having LR for HCC of 5 cm or larger (16). Our findings are in line with the studies from Mori et al. and Maehara et al.

This study has several limitations. First, this was a retrospective, single-center study that lacked randomization. The fact that the choice of treatment was made at the discretion of the treating physician may have introduced selection bias. Second, this study does not address which patients might benefit most from the addition of TACE prior to LR. It would be worthwhile to conduct an additional study to develop clinical prediction models (including with the possible use of radiomics) to identify the population that would be best served by the addition of TACE to LR for intermediate-stage HCC.

CONCLUSION

In this large retrospective study of patients with intermediate-stage HCC, the addition of TACE 1 to 3 months prior to LR resulted in significantly longer OS and RFS compared to LR alone. These results and comparisons with findings from other studies suggest that preoperative TACE with LR may result in better oncological outcomes than either TACE or LR alone, without a substantial increase in morbidity, and that this approach could be considered an effective combination treatment for intermediate-stage HCC.

AUTHOR CONTRIBUTIONS

Conceptualization: MC, JH. Data curation: QZ, JW, ZH, FT. Formal analysis: QZ, XW, RL. Data analysis: RL, QZ. Funding acquisition: JH, QZ. Investigation: QZ, JW, ZH. Methodology: QZ, XW, ZH. Project administration: QZ, XW, JH, MC. Resources: QZ, MC, JH. Original draft: QZ, XW. Writing—review and editing: QZ, MC, JH. All authors contributed to the article and approved the submitted version.

REFERENCES

1. Xu XF, Xing H, Han J, Li ZL, Lau WY, Zhou YH, et al. Risk Factors, Patterns, and Outcomes of Late Recurrence After Liver Resection for Hepatocellular Carcinoma: A Multicenter Study From China. *JAMA Surg* (2019) 154:209–17. doi: 10.1001/jamasurg.2018.4334
2. Elshaarawy O, Gomaa A, Omar H, Rewisha E, Waked I. Intermediate stage hepatocellular carcinoma: a summary review. *J Hepatocell Carcinoma* (2019) 6:105–17. doi: 10.2147/JHC.S168682
3. Llovet JM, Zucman-Rossi J, Pikarsky E, Sangro B, Schwartz M, Sherman M, et al. Hepatocellular carcinoma. *Nat Rev Dis Primers* (2016) 2:16018. doi: 10.1038/nrdp.2016.18
4. Di Costanzo GG, Tortora R. Intermediate hepatocellular carcinoma: How to choose the best treatment modality? *World J Hepatol* (2015) 7:1184–91. doi: 10.4254/wjh.v7.i9.1184
5. Chen RX, Gan YH, Ge NL, Chen Y, Ma M, Zhang BH, et al. A new prediction model for prognosis of patients with intermediate-stage HCC after conventional transarterial chemoembolization: an internally validated study. *J Cancer* (2019) 10:6535–42. doi: 10.7150/jca.34064
6. Llovet JM, Bruix J. Systematic review of randomized trials for unresectable hepatocellular carcinoma: Chemoembolization improves survival. *Hepatology* (2003) 37:429–42. doi: 10.1053/jhep.2003.50047
7. Yang B, Zheng B, Yang M, Zeng Z, Yang F, Pu J, et al. Liver resection versus transarterial chemoembolization for the initial treatment of Barcelona Clinic Liver Cancer stage B hepatocellular carcinoma. *Hepatol Int* (2018) 12:417–28. doi: 10.1007/s12072-018-9888-4
8. Zhao YN, Zhang YQ, Ye JZ, Liu X, Yang HZ, Cong FY, et al. Hepatic resection versus transarterial chemoembolization for patients with Barcelona Clinic Liver Cancer intermediate stage Child-Pugh A hepatocellular carcinoma. *Exp Ther Med* (2016) 12:3813–9. doi: 10.3892/etm.2016.3810
9. Kim JY, Sinn DH, Gwak GY, Choi GS, Saleh AM, Joh JW, et al. Transarterial chemoembolization versus resection for intermediate-stage (BCLC B) hepatocellular carcinoma. *Clin Mol Hepatol* (2016) 22:250–8. doi: 10.3350/cmh.2016.0015
10. Ho MC, Huang GT, Tsang YM, Lee PH, Chen DS, Sheu JC, et al. Liver resection improves the survival of patients with multiple hepatocellular carcinomas. *Ann Surg Oncol* (2009) 16:848–55. doi: 10.1245/s10434-008-0282-7
11. Villa E, Colantoni A, Camma C, Grottola A, Buttafoco P, Gelmini R, et al. Estrogen receptor classification for hepatocellular carcinoma: comparison with clinical staging systems. *J Clin Oncol* (2003) 21:441–6. doi: 10.1200/JCO.2003.11.051
12. Fan ST, Lo CM, Liu CL, Lam CM, Yuen WK, Yeung C, et al. Hepatectomy for hepatocellular carcinoma: toward zero hospital deaths. *Ann Surg* (1999) 229:322–30. doi: 10.1097/00000658-199903000-00004

13. Bruix J, Sherman M. Management of hepatocellular carcinoma. *Hepatology* (2005) 42:1208–36. doi: 10.1002/hep.20933
14. Wakayama K, Kamiyama T, Yokoo H, Orimo T, Shimada S, Einama T, et al. Huge hepatocellular carcinoma greater than 10 cm in diameter worsens prognosis by causing distant recurrence after curative resection. *J Surg Oncol* (2017) 115:324–9. doi: 10.1002/jso.24501
15. Hwang S, Lee YJ, Kim KH, Ahn CS, Moon DB, Ha TY, et al. Long-Term Outcome After Resection of Huge Hepatocellular Carcinoma ≥ 10 cm: Single-Institution Experience with 471 Patients. *World J Surg* (2015) 39:2519–28. doi: 10.1007/s00268-015-3129-y
16. Yamashita Y, Takeishi K, Tsuijita E, Yoshiya S, Morita K, Kayashima H, et al. Beneficial effects of preoperative lipiodolization for resectable large hepatocellular carcinoma (≥ 5 cm in diameter). *J Surg Oncol* (2012) 106:498–503. doi: 10.1002/jso.23098
17. Tustumi F, Ernani L, Coelho FF, Bernardo WM, Junior SS, Kruger JAP, et al. Preoperative strategies to improve resectability for hepatocellular carcinoma: a systematic review and meta-analysis. *HPB (Oxford)* (2018) 20:1109–18. doi: 10.1016/j.hpb.2018.06.1798
18. Zhang YF, Guo RP, Zou RH, Shen JX, Wei W, Li SH, et al. Efficacy and safety of preoperative chemoembolization for resectable hepatocellular carcinoma with portal vein invasion: a prospective comparative study. *Eur Radiol* (2016) 26:2078–88. doi: 10.1007/s00330-015-4021-8
19. Bray F, Ferlay J, Soerjomataram I, Siegel RL, Torre LA, Jemal A. Global cancer statistics 2018: GLOBOCAN estimates of incidence and mortality worldwide for 36 cancers in 185 countries. *CA Cancer J Clin* (2018) 68:394–424. doi: 10.3322/caac.21492
20. Marrero JA, Kulik LM, Sirlin CB, Zhu AX, Finn RS, Abecassis MM, et al. Diagnosis, Staging, and Management of Hepatocellular Carcinoma: 2018 Practice Guidance by the American Association for the Study of Liver Diseases. *Hepatology* (2018) 68:723–50. doi: 10.1002/hep.29913
21. EASL Clinical Practice Guidelines. Management of hepatocellular carcinoma. *J Hepatol* (2018) 69:182–236. doi: 10.1016/j.jhep.2018.03.019
22. Bruix J, Gores GJ, Mazzaferro V. Hepatocellular carcinoma: clinical frontiers and perspectives. *Gut* (2014) 63:844–55. doi: 10.1136/gutjnl-2013-306627
23. Strasberg SM. Nomenclature of hepatic anatomy and resections: a review of the Brisbane 2000 system. *J Hepatobiliary Pancreat Surg* (2005) 12:351–5. doi: 10.1007/s00534-005-0999-7
24. Li C, Wang MD, Lu L, Wu H, Yu JJ, Zhang WG, et al. Preoperative transcatheter arterial chemoembolization for surgical resection of huge hepatocellular carcinoma (>/= 10 cm): a multicenter propensity matching analysis. *Hepatol Int* (2019) 13:736–47. doi: 10.1007/s12072-019-09981-0
25. Lin CW, Chen YS, Lo GH, Hsu YC, Hsu CC, Wu TC, et al. Comparison of overall survival on surgical resection versus transarterial chemoembolization with or without radiofrequency ablation in intermediate stage hepatocellular carcinoma: a propensity score matching analysis. *BMC Gastroenterol* (2020) 20:99. doi: 10.1186/s12876-020-01235-w
26. Heimbach JK, Kulik LM, Finn RS, Sirlin CB, Abecassis MM, Roberts LR, et al. AASLD guidelines for the treatment of hepatocellular carcinoma. *Hepatology* (2018) 67:358–80. doi: 10.1002/hep.29086
27. Raoul JL, Forner A, Bolondi L, Cheung TT, Kloeckner R, de Baere T. Updated use of TACE for hepatocellular carcinoma treatment: How and when to use it based on clinical evidence. *Cancer Treat Rev* (2019) 72:28–36. doi: 10.1016/j.ctrv.2018.11.002
28. Zhong JH, Lu SD, Wang YY, Ma L, Li LQ. Intermediate-stage HCC–upfront resection can be feasible. *Nat Rev Clin Oncol* (2015) 12:122-c3. doi: 10.1038/nrclinonc
29. Yin L, Li H, Li AJ, Lau WY, Pan ZY, Lai EC, et al. Partial hepatectomy vs. transcatheter arterial chemoembolization for resectable multiple hepatocellular carcinoma beyond Milan Criteria: a RCT. *J Hepatol* (2014) 61:82–8. doi: 10.1016/j.jhep.2014.03.012
30. Kariyama K, Nouso K, Wakuta A, Oonishi A, Toyoda H, Tada T, et al. Treatment of Intermediate-Stage Hepatocellular Carcinoma in Japan: Position of Curative Therapies. *Liver Cancer* (2020) 9:41–9. doi: 10.1159/000502479
31. Zhong JH, Wu FX, Li H. Hepatic resection associated with good survival for selected patients with multinodular hepatocellular carcinoma. *Tumour Biol* (2014) 35:8355–8. doi: 10.1007/s13277-014-2571-z
32. Zhong JH, Ke Y, Gong WF, Xiang BD, Ma L, Ye XP, et al. Hepatic resection associated with good survival for selected patients with intermediate and advanced-stage hepatocellular carcinoma. *Ann Surg* (2014) 260:329–40. doi: 10.1097/SLA.0000000000000236
33. Omata M, Lesmana LA, Tateishi R, Chen PJ, Lin SM, Yoshida H, et al. Asian Pacific Association for the Study of the Liver consensus recommendations on hepatocellular carcinoma. *Hepatol Int* (2010) 4:439–74. doi: 10.1007/s12072-010-9165-7
34. Kudo M, Matsui O, Izumi N, Iijima H, Kadoya M, Imai Y, et al. JSH Consensus-Based Clinical Practice Guidelines for the Management of Hepatocellular Carcinoma: 2014 Update by the Liver Cancer Study Group of Japan. *Liver Cancer* (2014) 3:458–68. doi: 10.1159/000343875
35. Day RW, Brudvik KW, Vauthey JN, Conrad C, Gottumukkala V, Chun YS, et al. Advances in hepatectomy technique: Toward zero transfusions in the modern era of liver surgery. *Surgery* (2016) 159:793–801. doi: 10.1016/j.surg.2015.10.006
36. Sharma R, Gibbs JF. Recent advances in the management of primary hepatic tumors refinement of surgical techniques and effect on outcome. *J Surg Oncol* (2010) 101:745–54. doi: 10.1002/jso.21506
37. Wu CC, Ho YZ, Ho WL, Wu TC, Liu TJ, P'Eng FK. Preoperative transcatheter arterial chemoembolization for resectable large hepatocellular carcinoma: a reappraisal. *Br J Surg* (1995) 82:122–6. doi: 10.1002/bjs.1800820141
38. Paye F, Jagot P, Vilgrain V, Farges O, Borie D, Belghiti J. Preoperative chemoembolization of hepatocellular carcinoma: a comparative study. *Arch Surg* (1998) 133:767–72. doi: 10.1001/archsurg.133.7.767
39. Nagasue N, Galizia G, Kohno H, Chang YC, Hayashi T, Yamanoi A, et al. Adverse effects of preoperative hepatic artery chemoembolization for resectable hepatocellular carcinoma: a retrospective comparison of 138 liver resections. *Surgery* (1989) 106:81–6. doi: 10.1002/bjs.1800760836
40. Pawlik TM, Poon RT, Abdalla EK, Zorzi D, Ikai I, Curley SA, et al. Critical appraisal of the clinical and pathologic predictors of survival after resection of large hepatocellular carcinoma. *Arch Surg* (2005) 140:450–7; discussion 457-458. doi: 10.1001/archsurg.140.5.450
41. Wang Z, Ren Z, Chen Y, Hu J, Yang G, Yu L, et al. Adjuvant Transarterial Chemoembolization for HBV-Related Hepatocellular Carcinoma After Resection: A Randomized Controlled Study. *Clin Cancer Res* (2018) 24:2074–81. doi: 10.1158/1078-0432.CCR-17-2899
42. Wada H, Eguchi H, Nagano H, Kubo S, Nakai T, Kaibori M, et al. Perioperative allogenic blood transfusion is a poor prognostic factor after hepatocellular carcinoma surgery: a multi-center analysis. *Surg Today* (2018) 48:73–9. doi: 10.1007/s00595-017-1553-3

18

Complications of Radiofrequency Ablation for Hepatic Hemangioma: A Multicenter Retrospective Analysis on 291 Cases

Shilun Wu[1†], Ruize Gao[1†], Tao Yin[2†], Ruhang Zhu[1], Shigang Guo[3], Zonghai Xin[4], Aolei Li[5], Xinliang Kong[6], Jun Gao[1] and Wenbing Sun[1*]*

[1] Department of Hepatobiliary Surgery, Beijing Chaoyang Hospital Affiliated to Capital Medical University, Beijing, China, [2] Department of General Surgery, Affiliated Hospital of Chifeng University, Chifeng, China, [3] Department of General Surgery, Chaoyang Central Hospital, Chaoyang, China, [4] Department of General Surgery, Binzhou Second People's Hospital, Binzhou, China, [5] Department of General Surgery, Chaoyang Second Hospital, Chaoyang, China, [6] Department of Hepatobiliary Surgery, Rizhao Central Hospital, Rizhao, China

***Correspondence:**
Jun Gao
gaojun8430@163.com
Wenbing Sun
sunwenbing@bjcyh.com

[†]These authors have contributed equally to this work and share first authorship

Purpose: To report the complications of radiofrequency ablation (RFA) for hepatic hemangioma.

Patients and Methods: Investigators from six centers performed RFA for hepatic hemangioma and used a standardized follow-up protocol. Data were collected from 291 patients, including 253 patients with hepatic hemangioma 5 to 9.9 cm in diameter (group A) and 38 with hepatic hemangioma ≥ 10 cm (group B). Technical success, complete ablation, and complications attributed to the RFA procedure were reported. Analysis of variance was used to determine whether the major complication rate was related to tumor size or clinical experience.

Results: A total of 304 lesions were treated in 291 patients. Technical success was achieved without adverse events in all cases. A total of 301 lesions were completely ablated, including 265 of 265 (100%) lesions in group A, and 36 of 39 (92.31%) in group B. The rate of technology-related complications was similar in groups A and B (5.14% (13/253) and 13.16% (5/38), respectively; $P = 0.121$). Moreover, all technology-related complications occurred during the early learning curve period. The rate of hemolysis-related complications in two groups were 83.40% (211/253) and 100% (38/38) ($P = 0.007$) and the systemic inflammatory response syndrome-related complications in two groups were 33.99% (86/253) and 86.84% (33/38) ($P < 0.001$). There were no delayed complications in either group.

Conclusion: RFA is minimally invasive, safe, and effective for hepatic hemangiomas 5 to 9.9 cm in diameter. More clinical data are needed to confirm the safety of RFA for hepatic hemangiomas ≥ 10 cm.

Keywords: hepatic hemangioma, complication, safety, radiofrequency ablation (RFA), multicenter

INTRODUCTION

Hepatic hemangioma is the most common benign tumor of the liver. Hepatic hemangioma is divided into three categories based on diameter: small (< 5 cm), huge (5–9.9 cm), and giant (≥ 10 cm). Most incidentally identified and asymptomatic hepatic hemangiomas do not need medical interventions. However, hepatic hemangiomas ≥ 5 cm likely will continue to grow and cause symptoms. Moreover, the peripherally located hemangiomas posing the risk of life-threatening spontaneous rupture and hemorrhage. Active treatments for the symptomatic-enlarging hemangiomas need to be considered to relieve the symptoms and prevent the lesions from growth (1–4).

In recent years, radiofrequency ablation (RFA) ablation has been increasingly accepted to treat hepatic hemangioma because of its unique advantages, including minimal invasiveness, definite efficacy, high degree of safety, fast recovery, and wide applicability (1). Although preliminary reports suggest that RFA is safe and effective (5–8), these studies included samples that are too small to allow clinicians to clearly establish the true complication rate, especially for rare but potentially serious complications. For every new intervention, it is essential to evaluate the safety and efficacy to obtain an accurate assessment of the risks and benefits and to determine its relative and absolute contraindications.

To permit an objective assessment of the risks and benefits of RFA, we report the complications encountered by members of a large collaborative group from six centers who have performed RFA in a large number of patients with hepatic hemangiomas (291 patients in total).

MATERIALS AND METHODS

Patient Cohort

We retrospectively reviewed the data of consecutive patients with hepatic hemangioma treated by RFA from June 2009 to July 2019. Data were collected from the clinical databases of six hospitals in China: Beijing Chaoyang Hospital affiliated with Capital Medical University, Beijing, China; Rizhao Central Hospital, Shandong, China; Binzhou Second People's Hospital, Shandong, China; Chaoyang Central Hospital, Liaoning, China; Affiliated Hospital of Chifeng University, Inner Mongolia Autonomous Region, China; Chaoyang Second Hospital, Liaoning, China. This study was approved by the ethics committee of each participating hospital and complied with the Declaration of Helsinki. All patients provided informed consent for review and analysis of their preoperative medical records.

The diagnosis of the hepatic hemangioma was based on two coincidental radiologic findings on contrast-enhanced ultrasound (US), contrast-enhanced computed tomography (CT), or magnetic resonance imaging (MRI). On US images, hepatic hemangiomas present as a homogeneous, round, or oval lesion with well-defined hyperechogenicity, and the likelihood of posterior acoustic enhancement. Other imaging techniques, such as contrast-enhanced CT or MRI, are recommended for confirmation in case of inconclusive ultrasonographic results, or if a giant hemangioma requires treatment. The typical hemangioma appears on CT or MRI scans as a hypointense, well-defined lesion, which after contrast injection shows peripheral nodular enhancement with progressive homogeneous centripetal filling (1).

Inclusion criteria: maximum diameter of the hemangioma > 5 cm; regular follow-up imaging showing tumor enlargement of more than 1 cm on regular follow-up imaging studies within at least 2 years' observation; persistent hemangioma-related abdominal pain or discomfort with the definite exclusion of other gastrointestinal diseases *via* gastroscopic examination; patients who declined surgical treatment but consented to RFA.

Exclusion criteria: severe coagulopathy (international normalized ratio > 1.5); infection, especially biliary system inflammation; severe failure of a primary organ such as the liver, kidney, heart, lung, and/or brain; concomitant malignant tumors.

Traditionally, hepatic hemangioma is divided into huge (5–9.9 cm) and giant (≥ 10 cm) based on diameter. Moreover, with larger hepatic hemangiomas, the risk of complications is greater. In our study, we classified the hepatic hemangiomas into two groups (5–9.9 cm as group A and ≥ 10 cm as group B) according to tumor size and severity of complications.

RFA System

Before 2011, the RITA StarBurst Xli-enhanced RF electrode with RF generator (Radiofrequency Interstitial Thermal Ablation Medical System) was used. The RITA system can achieve maximal ablation zones of 7 cm with a single placement of electrodes, with a maximum power of 250 W. After 2011, the internally cooled cluster electrodes Cool-tip ACTC2025 or ACTC1525 electrodes (COVIDIEN, USA) and RF generator (Covidien Healthcare, Ireland) were used for the RFA procedure. With a 2.5 cm exposed tip, the Cool-tip electrodes can produce ablation zones of 4.5 cm with a single placement of electrodes and a maximum power of 200 W. The power and time of ablation were set based on the tumor size and location according to the manufacturer's instructions.

RFA Procedure

All patients were fitted with a tracheal tube or laryngeal mask airway while under intravenous anesthesia to control their respiration. Grounding was achieved by attaching two pads to patient's thighs. Hepatic hemangiomas deeply located in the liver parenchyma were treated by the percutaneous CT-guided approach, whereas subcapsular hepatic hemangiomas were treated by the laparoscopic approach under intraoperative ultrasound guidance. The procedures and strategies of ablation used has been described previously (1, 4). RFA for hepatic hemangiomas does not require an ablative margin of the normal hepatic parenchyma surrounding the tumor. Therefore, the target scope of ablation for hepatic hemangioma is definite and clear, unlike that for malignant neoplasms. Visualization of hepatic vein is easy for the CT-guided approach. And intraoperative US was used routinely in conjunction with the laparoscopic approach to increase the ability to guide the RF electrode placement and avoid vascular injury.

Perioperative Data

Preoperatively, we collected the following biographical data of the patients: age, sex, medical history, liver function, and the location, size, and number of hepatic hemangiomas on imaging. Intraoperatively, we recorded the operation path, ablation time, total operation time, vital signs, and urine output and color. Postoperatively, we recorded the length of hospital stay, complications, and laboratory examination results.

Post-Treatment Evaluation

The primary endpoint was safety (complications related to RFA), technical success, which was defined as correct placement of the ablation device into tumors with completion of the planned ablation protocol, and confirmed complete ablation. Secondary endpoints were improvement of symptoms, change in the size of the ablation zone, recurrence of the residual tumor. Complication of treatment was described using the Clavien-Dindo Classification (9).

All patients underwent follow-up contrast-enhanced CT or MRI 1 month after RFA. Complete ablation was defined as the absence of nodular or irregular enhancement adjacent to the ablation zone. Incomplete ablation was defined as the presence of irregular, peripherally enhanced foci in the ablation zone. In cases of complete ablation, CT or MRI examinations were repeated at 6-month intervals as part of the follow-up protocol. In cases of incomplete ablation, repeated RFA procedures were not performed unless progression of the residual tumor was seen on follow-up imaging performed at 6-month intervals.

Data Analysis

Continuous data were expressed as mean ± SD and compared between groups using the Student's t-test and analysis of variance. Differences in categorical data were analyzed by the χ^2 test or Fisher's exact test. Two-tailed P values < 0.05 were deemed significant. Statistical analysis was performed using SPSS version 26.0. Receiver operating characteristic (ROC) curve was conducted by R 3.5.3 software.

RESULTS

All six centers responded. The number of patients treated in each center ranged from 12 to 167, and a total of 304 lesions were treated in 291 patients (**Table 1**). Patients were divided into groups based on the diameter of the hepatic hemangioma. Group A contained 253 (86.94%) patients with 265 hepatic hemangiomas 5 to 9.9 cm in diameter, whereas group B contained 38 (13.06%) patients with 39 hepatic hemangiomas ≥ 10 cm in diameter. Of the 291 patients, 278 (95.53%) patients had a single lesion and 13 (4.47%) had two lesions. The patients' demographic characteristics are provided in **Table 2**.

Outcome data for the RFA treatment are given in **Table 3**. A total of 198 hemangiomas underwent laparoscopic RFA, whereas 106 hemangiomas located in the deeper liver parenchyma underwent CT-guided percutaneous RFA. RFA was performed successfully in all patients. No technical failure occurred.

Of the 304 lesions, 265 of 265 (100%) lesions in group A received only a single RFA session, whereas seven of 38 (18.42%) lesions in group B (single lesions 13–20 cm in diameter) received two RFA sessions to minimize the risk of complications attributable to the RFA procedure. Group A had a significantly shorter ablation time than group B (43.07 ± 26.79 min *vs.* 85.82 ± 34.64 min, P < 0.001) (**Table 3**).

Effectiveness of RFA

Of the 304 hepatic hemangiomas, 301 were ablated completely, including 265 of 265 (100%) lesions in group A and 36 of 39 (92.31%) lesions in group B. Three hepatic hemangiomas were incompletely ablated; the diameters of these lesions were 10.4 cm, 12.5 cm, and 12.6 cm, respectively.

Complications

The perioperative complications and delayed complications during follow-up are summarized in **Table 4**. In accordance with the cause of complications, we classified the perioperative complications into technology-related complications, hemolysis-related complications, systemic inflammatory response (SIR) syndrome-related complications, and others complications.

Technology-Related Complications

The rates of technology-related complications in groups A and B were 5.14% (13/253) and 13.16% (5/38), respectively (P = 0.121). All technology-related complications occurred during the early learning curve period of every clinical research center.

Bleeding at the puncture site (Grade III) occurred in four of 291 (1.38%) patients during laparoscopic RFA. The strategy of simultaneously pressing on the bleeding point and managing the bleeding site was adopted, resulting in no conversion to laparotomy.

Tumor rupture occurred (Grade III) in three of 291 (1.03%) patients; these patients had undergone laparoscopic RFA for hepatic hemangiomas located on the surface of the liver. Hemostasis was achieved by blocking the hepatic hilum combined with RFA under laparoscopy. The blood loss in two of the patients with tumor rupture was 600 ml and 900 ml, respectively. Another patient with a 12 cm

TABLE 1 | Summary of patients and lesions treated with RFA according to location and center.

Location and Center	No. of patients	No. of lesions	5–9.9 cm		≥ 10 cm	
			CT - guide	Laparoscopy	CT - guide	Laparoscopy
Chaoyang Hospital, Beijing BeijingBeijing	167	176	54	93	3	26
Peoples Hospital, Binzhou	40	41	21	13	3	4
Central Hospital, Rizhao	16	16	4	12	0	0
Central Hospital, Chaoyang	23	23	6	16	0	1
Second Hospital, Chaoyang	12	12	8	4	0	0
Affiliated Hospital, Chifeng	33	36	6	28	1	1
Total	291	304	99	166	7	32

RFA, radiofrequency ablation.

TABLE 2 | The demographic characteristics of 291 patients in the study.

Variables	Size of tumor		*P*-Value
	5–9.9 cm (n = 253)	≥ 10 cm (n = 38)	
Age (y)	49.20 ± 11.16	48.75 ± 10.45	0.943
Gender			0.570
Male	85 (33.60%)	11 (28.95%)	
Female	168 (66.40%)	27 (71.05%)	
Comorbidities, *N* (%)			
Gallbladder polyps	12 (4.74%)	3 (7.89%)	0.670
Hypertension	44 (17.39%)	9 (23.68%)	0.349
Type 2 diabetes mellitus	10 (3.95%)	2 (5.26%)	1.000
Hepatitis B/C	10 (3.95%)	3 (7.89%)	0.499
Hepatic cysts	11 (4.35%)	3 (7.89%)	0.577
Child-Pugh grading, *N* (%)			1.000
Glass A	246 (97.23%)	37 (97.37%)	
Glass B	7 (2.77%)	1 (2.63%)	
No. of tumor			0.868
Single lesion	241 (95.26%)	37 (97.37%)	
Two lesion	12 (4.74%)	1 (2.63%)	
Distribution of lesion, *N* (%)			0.074
Right lobe	134 (52.96%)	25 (65.79%)	
Left lobe	78 (30.83%)	12 (31.58%)	
Both	41 (16.21%)	1 (2.63%)	
Reason for RFA, *N* (%)			0.003
Abdominal pain	73 (28.85%)	21 (55.26%)	
Enlargement of hemangioma	101 (39.92%)	7 (18.42%)	
Abdominal pain and enlargement hemangioma	79 (31.23%)	10 (26.32%)	
Laboratory findings			
Hb (g/L)	135.13 ± 15.87	130.55 ± 14.81	0.097
ALT (U/L)	21.42 ± 20.91	17.72 ± 8.10	0.289
AST (U/L)	23.78 ± 40.15	18.23 ± 4.14	0.659
TBil (μmol/L)	12.53 ± 5.20	13.90 ± 6.91	0.247
BUN (mmol/L)	4.95 ± 1.47	4.84 ± 1.23	0.614
Creatinine (μmol/L)	70.57 ± 36.30	65.33 ± 12.51	0.484
PT (s)	12.18 ± 1.33	12.87 ± 4.38	0.376
APTT (s)	31.38 ± 4.32	32.85 ± 6.65	0.074

Continuous variables are expressed by median ± standard deviation.
Hb, hemoglobin; TBil, total bilirubin; ALT, alanine aminotransferase; AST, aspartate transaminase; BUN, blood urea nitrogen.
PT, prothrombin time; APTT, activated partial thromboplastin time.
For the patients with multiple hepatic hemangiomas, the hepatic hemangiomas not managed were not included statistical range.

TABLE 3 | RFA for 304 hepatic hemangiomas.

Variables	Size of tumor		*P*-Value
	5 - 9.9 cm (n = 265)	≥ 10 cm (n = 39)	
Mean diameter before RFA, (cm)	6.72 ± 1.48	12.56 ± 2.28	<0.001
Approach of RFA			0.019
CT-guided approach	99 (37.36%)	7 (17.95%)	
Laparoscopic approach	166 (62.64%)	32 (82.05%)	
Ablation time, (mins)	43.07 ± 26.79	85.82 ± 34.65	<0.001
RFA session			<0.001
Single session	265 (100.00%)	32 (82.05%)	
Two session	0	7 (17.95%)	
Postoperative length of stay (d)	5.73 ± 3.86	9.04 ± 6.44	<0.001
Mean diameter in 1 month follow-up, (cm)	4.05 ± 1.36	8.71 ± 2.13	<0.001

Continuous variables are expressed by median ± standard deviation.
RFA, radiofrequency ablation.

hepatic hemangioma developed tumor rupture and was converted to open RFA because of a rapid blood loss of 1,400 ml under laparoscopy. After intra- and postoperative transfusion and rehydration therapy, all three patients recovered well.

Five of 291 (1.72%) patients experienced lung injury (Grade I), and four of 291 (1.38%) patients experienced diaphragmatic injury (Grade II-III). All nine of these patients had a hepatic hemangioma near the dome of the right liver lobe and had undergone CT-guided

TABLE 4 | Complications after RFA for hepatic hemangiomas of 291 patients.

Complications	Glavien Grade	Size of tumor		*P*-Value
		5 - 9.9 cm (n = 253)	≥10 cm (n = 38)	
Perioperative complications				
Technology-related, *N* (%) (Time)		13 (5.14%) (2009 - 2015)	5 (13.16%) (2010 - 2012)	0.121
1 Bleeding at the electrode entry site	III	3 (1.19%) (2009 - 2012)	1 (2.63%) (2011)	0.430
2 Rupture of hepatic hemangioma	III	2 (0.79%) (2011 - 2012)	1 (2.63%) (2010)	0.344
3 Damage of adjacent organs				
Lung injury	I	4 (1.58%) (2011 - 2015)	1 (2.63%) (2012)	0.506
Diaphragmatic injury	II - III	3 (1.19%) (2010 - 2015)	1 (2.63%) (2011)	0.430
Esophageal injury	II	0	1 (2.63%) (2010)	0.272
Symptomatic pleural effusion	III	1 (0.40%) (2011)	0	1.000
Hemolysis-related, *N* (%) (Time)		211 (83.40%) (2009 - 2019)	38 (100%) (2009 - 2019)	0.007
1. Hemoglobinuria	I	211 (83.40%) (2009 - 2019)	38 (100%) (2009 - 2019)	0.007
2. Anemia[a]	I	26 (10.28%) (2009 - 2019)	14 (36.84%) (2009 - 2019)	<0.001
3. AKI	II - III	0	3 (7.89%) (2011 - 2018)	0.002
SIR syndrome-related, N (%) (Time)		86 (33.99%) (2009 - 2019)	33 (86.84%) (2009 - 2019)	<0.001
1. SIR syndrome	I	86 (33.99%) (2009 - 2019)	33 (86.84%) (2009 - 2019)	<0.001
2. Organ dysfunction				
Myocardial dysfunction	II	0	1 (2.63%) (2019)	0.272
ARDS	IV	0	1 (2.63%) (2012)	0.272
Others, *N* (%) (Time)				
1 Postprocedural pain	I	15 (5.93%) (2009 - 2019)	7 (18.42%) (2011 - 2019)	0.017
2 Transient hepatic injury[b]	I	37 (14.62%) (2009 - 2019)	12 (31.58%) (2010 - 2019)	0.009
3 Asymptomatic pleural effusion	I	12 (4.74%) (2009 - 2019)	6 (15.79%) (2010 - 2018)	0.023
4 Skin burn	I	1 (0.40%) (2009)	2 (5.26%) (2009 - 2010)	0.046
Delayed complications, *N* (%) (Time)				
1. Liver abscess		0	0	–
2. Biliary damages		0	0	–
3. Tumor progression		0	0	–

AKI, acute kidney injury; SIR, systemic inflammatory response; ARDS, acute respiratory distress syndrome.
[a]*Hemoglobin < 100 g/L and hemoglobin was normal before surgery.*
[b]*Glutamate pyruvate transaminase > 80 U/L.*

percutaneous RFA. One patient with a 7.5 cm hemangioma underwent thoracoscopic surgery to insert two chest tubes into the pleural space, which were removed 1 week later. The other eight patients were cured by conservative treatment.

One of 291 (0.34%) patients with an 11.0 cm hemangioma in the left lateral liver lobe developed a lower esophageal fistula (Grade II) caused by direct puncture from one of the radiated arrays and the subsequent ablation, but recovered with conservative treatment.

One patient with a 9.8 cm hepatic hemangioma diagnosed with moderate pleural effusion (Grade III) developed obvious chest tightness and suffocation after RFA, and chest radiography revealed right pulmonary pleural effusion associated with lung compression. The symptoms disappeared after pleural puncture drainage and diuretic therapy.

Hemolysis-Related Complications

The rates of hemolysis-related complications in groups A and B were 83.40% (211/253) and 100% (38 of 38) ($P = 0.007$), respectively. The typical manifestation of hemolysis was hemoglobinuria. In the present study, hemoglobinuria was diagnosed by the results of Hemoglobin (Hb) positive and red blood cells (RBCs) negative, using urine routine analysis (10). Mild hemolysis subsided within 72 h when managed with adequate hydration, whereas severe hemolysis induced other complications, such as anemia and acute kidney injury (AKI).

In group B, three patients with hemoglobinuria developed AKI (Grade II-III). Two patients (with a 13.6- and 13.7-cm hepatic hemangioma, respectively) presented with obvious hemoglobinuria and progressive elevation of creatinine after RFA. After 1 week of symptomatic treatment comprising the administration of adequate fluids, urine alkalizer, and diuretics, the hemoglobinuria disappeared and the renal function and urine volume of these two patients returned to normal. One patient experienced hemoglobinuria after RFA of a 14.8 cm hepatic hemangioma and subsequently developed oliguria and anhelation, indicating AKI. After 15 days of hemodialysis, the patient's kidney function returned to normal and he was discharged 27 days after the operation.

Of the patients with hemoglobinuria (Grade I), anemia (Grade I) occurred in 26 of 198 (13.13%) in group A and 14 of 38 (36.84%) in group B. In group A, all 26 patients had slight anemia with no obvious clinical symptoms and did not need treatment. In group B, four of 14 patients had moderate anemia, which was successfully treated with rehydration.

SIR Syndrome-Related Complications

SIR syndrome has been described in previous articles (9, 11). SIR syndrome (Grade I) was identified in 83 (33.99%) patients in group A and 33 (86.64%) patients in group B ($P < 0.01$). In group B, one patient with SIR syndrome developed myocardial dysfunction (Grade II) and another developed acute respiratory distress syndrome (ARDS) (Grade IV) immediately after RFA. Moreover, we further constructed the ROC curve (**Figure S1**) and detected the cutoff value for tumor size in predicting the presence of SIR syndrome. Optimal cutoff value for tumor size is 7.450 cm

($P < 0.001$, specificity = 0.892, sensitivity = 0.817, area under the ROC curve is 0.887).

Other Complications

The other complications are reported in **Table 4**. Twenty-two of 291 (7.56%) patients developed postoperative pain (Grade I) that lasted more than 3 days; the pain was mild, and was relieved after the application of common analgesic drugs and antibiotics, without causing serious physical or psychological discomfort. Eighteen of 291 (6.19%) patients developed pleural effusion (Grade I); all patients were asymptomatic, and the pleural effusion was absorbed within 1 week after conservative treatment. Three patients in group B had skin burns (Grade I) at the edge of the grounding pads; these burns healed spontaneously. Transient hepatic injury (Grade I) after ablation was documented in 37 of 253 (14.62%) patients in group A and 12 of 38 (31.58%) in group B; the liver function recovered spontaneously within 1 week.

Follow-Up

The mean follow-up period was 35 ± 29 months (range 6–120 months). There was no mortality related to RFA, no recurrence, and no delayed complications, such as local tumor progression, biliary damage, or liver abscess formation. No patient developed new symptoms attributed to hepatic hemangioma. The subjective health status and quality of life were rated as good to excellent by 100% of the patients at final follow-up.

DISCUSSION

In recent years, minimally invasive, local ablation therapies have been increasingly used as an effective alternative treatment for hepatic hemangioma, among which RFA is the most widely utilized treatment modality. Regardless of the resulting benefits, new treatments are always accompanied by unpredictable risks. It is important to characterize these risks and determine methods with which to avoid complications. Hence, multicenter experience of several years is required to characterize special and rare complications and to objectively quantify the expected complication rate. Although the complications caused by needle placement in RFA for hepatic hemangioma are expected to be similar to those of RFA for hepatocellular carcinoma, the complications specific to thermal ablation of hepatic hemangioma still require evaluation in a large population. Significantly, in this study, complications of hepatic hemangioma treated with RFA were recorded and evaluated from the initial development of technology to maturity, which is expected to provide reference for the other research teams to carry out and optimize the RFA techniques.

RFA is a complicated procedure, and substantial experience is required for it to be performed safely. However, in this study, some of the participating centers with less practical experience reported no serious complications. Many of the serious complications mainly occurred at the largest participating centers, which may be attributed to the fact that the center with the most experience was the first to perform RFA and so reported a greater number of complications during a learning curve period in which many of the relative contraindications were identified. Furthermore, with the exception of the first center to perform RFA for hepatic hemangioma, all investigators were required to observe RFA performed in a minimum of 10 patients at a center with more experience prior to commencing RFA at their own institution, which may provide the critical threshold knowledge to master the RFA technique. In addition, many of the smaller centers performed RFA only in straightforward cases, and referred more difficult cases to the larger centers.

A few rare complications were observed in the present study. Hence, we think that the large number of patients analyzed in the present study is almost certainly sufficient to determine the relative risks of RFA for hepatic hemangioma. In accordance with the cause of complications, we classified the main complications into three categories: technology-related, hemolysis-related, and SIR syndrome-related. Technology-related complications mainly comprised bleeding at the electrode entry site, rupture of the hepatic hemangioma, and damage of adjacent organs, such as the esophagus, diaphragm, and lung. All technology-related complications occurred in the early learning curve period. In the later period, technology-related complications can be largely avoided by upgrading ablation equipment, improving techniques, and optimizing ablation strategies (1, 4, 11, 12). For instance, we employed internally cooled cluster electrodes instead of multitined expandable electrodes after 2011. The internally cooled cluster electrode was proved to be more suitable for RFA of hemangioma because of its efficiency and more concentrated release of heat. Besides, internally cooled cluster electrodes keep a steady high temperature in the tumor while limiting vascular cooling. This characteristic increases the effectiveness of perivascular ablation. Moreover, the design of internally cooled cluster electrodes permits their ready placement into target lesions without risk of accidental injury to adjacent organs (13).

The nearly unavoidable hemolysis after RFA, attributable to the generous blood supply of hepatic hemangiomas, especially for those ≥ 10 cm is a major disadvantage of RFA. The hemolysis-related complications, mainly including hemoglobinuria, anemia, and mild renal failure, were the direct results of hemolysis and their severity was directly proportional to the extent of hemolysis. Hb is released upon erythrocyte destruction and is filtered by the glomerulus into the urinary space. In the urinary space, hemoglobin is degraded and releases heme pigments, which can cause tubular injury. Furthermore, volume depletion enhances both vasoconstriction and the formation of obstructing casts, and is of critical importance for the development of hemolysis-induced AKI (14). In the present study, we used strict diagnostic criteria to accurately evaluate hemoglobinuria (10). Therefore, the incidence of hemoglobinuria in this study was relatively high. However, in most cases, hemoglobinuria was minor and disappeared within 3 days. For the hepatic hemangioma 5–9.9 cm in diameter, all the hemolysis-related complications are minor (Grade I).

SIR syndrome-related complications mainly included cases of SIR syndrome and subsequent myocardial dysfunction and organ dysfunction. In the early study period, we thought that postoperative fever was related to the amount of tissue necrosis. However, with the occurrence of some serious complications, such as ARDS and myocardial dysfunction, we found that SIR syndrome played an important role in the occurrence of complications. SIR syndrome is the body's excessive defensive stress response to inflammatory cytokines, which eventually transforms into a clinical syndrome of pathological systemic inflammation. Mild cases of SIR syndrome are mainly manifested as fever, tachycardia, and tachypnea, whereas severe cases often lead to multiple organ dysfunctions (8). According to experimental study (15), damage to RBCs caused by RFA not only leads to hemoglobinuria but also releases heme to the peripheral circulation, which induced the production of inflammatory factors that contribute to SIR syndrome. So, recognition of hemolytic processes during this treatment will likely serve as a foundation for developing new approaches, to diminish or neutralize the effects of the extracellular Hb and heme. For hemangiomas 5-9.9 cm, using a more effective RFA system can help reduce the RBC damage. In addition, the power and time of ablation are supposed to be based on the tumor size and location according to the manufacturer's instructions. Patients with hepatic hemangiomas ≥ 10 cm should be sufficiently hydrated to decrease the Hb concentration in the circulation system before and during RFA procedure. When any signs or symptoms indicating hemolysis emerge in the course of RFA, such as rising body temperature and hemoglobinuria, the procedure should be terminated and a repeat RFA treatment may need to be rescheduled based on a comprehensive evaluation of the tumor.

The other complications of RFA for hepatic hemangioma included mild pain, liver damage, asymptomatic pleural effusion, and skin burn injury at the site where the grounding pad was attached. Most patients experienced postoperative pain, mainly from percutaneous puncture and trocar port insertion. Delayed pain that occurred more than 3 days after the procedure was uncommon, and suggested the possibility of more serious underlying complications. Skin burns were noted particularly early in the study period when insufficient grounding pads were used. To prevent such burn injury, patients receiving prolonged RFA require multiple grounding pads or the application of an ice pad to cool the skin in contact with the grounding pad. For superficial lesions, it is important to ensure that the entire active electrode tip is well embedded in the liver and does not course through the skin, muscle, or diaphragm.

It should be emphasized that the morbidity rate patients with hemangiomas 5 to 9.9 cm could be regarded as being acceptable with consideration of the composition of the complications and the benefit of minimal invasiveness patients gained. In view of the present data with high rate of complication, even though with no mortality, we have recognized that RFA for hepatic hemangiomas ≥ 10 cm, be it percutaneous or laparoscopic, is inappropriate. The present study showed that RFA was safe and effective for hepatic hemangiomas less than 10 cm in diameter. More clinical cases and evidence are needed to prove the safety of RFA for hepatic hemangiomas ≥ 10 cm because of the relatively high incidence and severity of hemolysis-related and SIR syndrome-related complications. Many problems associated with RFA of hepatic hemangiomas ≥ 10 cm need further study, such as the optimization of ablation strategies to reduce the incidence of ablation-related complications, the mechanism of some serious complications, and a comparison of the efficacy of RFA *versus* microwave ablation for hepatic hemangiomas ≥ 10 cm.

CONCLUSION

The present study supports the use of RFA as an alternative treatment for symptomatic hepatic hemangioma with a diameter of 5 to 9.9 cm because of the low risk of complications and high likelihood of complete ablation. More clinical data are needed to confirm the safety of RFA for hepatic hemangiomas ≥ 10 cm.

AUTHOR CONTRIBUTIONS

SW and RG: wrote the manuscript and prepared the tables. TY, RZ, SG, ZX, AL, and XK modified the manuscript. JG and WS designed the manuscript. All authors contributed to the article and approved the submitted version.

ACKNOWLEDGMENTS

We thank Kelly Zammit, BVSc, from Liwen Bianji, Edanz Editing China (www.liwenbianji.cn/ac), for editing the English text of a draft of this manuscript.

SUPPLEMENTARY MATERIAL

Supplementary Figure 1 | ROC curve for tumor size in predicting the presence of SIR syndrome. Optimal cutoff value for tumor size is 7.450 cm ($P < 0.001$, specificity = 0.892, sensitivity = 0.817, area under the ROC curve is 0.887).

REFERENCES

1. Gao J, Fan R-F, Yang J-Y, Cui Y, Ji J-S, Ma K-S, et al. Radiofrequency Ablation for Hepatic Hemangiomas: A Consensus From a Chinese Panel of Experts. *World J Gastroenterol* (2017) 23(39):7077–86. doi: 10.3748/wjg.v23.i39.7077
2. Leon M, Chavez L, Surani S. Hepatic Hemangioma: What Internists Need to Know. *World J Gastroenterol* (2020) 26(1):11–20. doi: 10.3748/wjg.v26.i1.11
3. Jing L, Liang H, Caifeng L, Jianjun Y, Feng X, Mengchao W, et al. New Recognition of the Natural History and Growth Pattern of Hepatic Hemangioma in Adults. *Hepatol Res* (2016) 46(8):727–33. doi: 10.1111/hepr.12610
4. Gao J, Ke S, Ding X-m, Zhou Y-m, Qian X-j, Sun W-b. Radiofrequency Ablation for Large Hepatic Hemangiomas: Initial Experience and Lessons. *Surgery* (2013) 153(1):78–85. doi: 10.1016/j.surg.2012.06.004
5. Qu C, Liu H, Li X-Q, Feng K, Ma K. Percutaneous Ultrasound-Guided 'Three-Step' Radiofrequency Ablation for Giant Hepatic Hemangioma (5-15 Cm): A Safe and Effective New Technique. *Int J Hyperthermia* (2020) 37(1):212–9. doi: 10.1080/02656736.2020.1732484
6. Zhang X, Yan L, Li B, Wen T, Wang W, Xu M, et al. Comparison of Laparoscopic Radiofrequency Ablation Versus Open Resection in the Treatment of Symptomatic-Enlarging Hepatic Hemangiomas: A Prospective Study. *Surg Endosc* (2016) 30(2):756–63. doi: 10.1007/s00464-015-4274-y

7. Wen S-Q, Wan M, Len K-M, Hu Q-H, Xie X-Y, Wu Q, et al. Safety and Efficacy of Laparoscopic Radiofrequency Ablation for Hepatic Hemangiomas: A Multicenter Retrospective Study. *Ann Hepatol* (2018) 17(2):268–73. doi: 10.5604/01.3001.0010.8653
8. Gao J, Ji J-S, Ding X-M, Ke S, Xin Z-H, Ning C-M, et al. Laparoscopic Radiofrequency Ablation for Large Subcapsular Hepatic Hemangiomas: Technical and Clinical Outcomes. *PloS One* (2016) 11(2):e0149755. doi: 10.1371/journal.pone.0149755
9. Clavien PA, Barkun J, de Oliveira ML, Vauthey JN, Dindo D, Schulick RD, et al. The Clavien-Dindo Classification of Surgical Complications: Five-Year Experience. *Ann Surg* (2009) 250(2):187–96. doi: 10.1097/SLA.0b013e3181b13ca2
10. Liu F, Yu X, Cheng Z, Han Z, Dou J, Yu J, et al. Risk Factors for Hemoglobinuria After Ultrasonography-Guided Percutaneous Microwave Ablation for Large Hepatic Cavernous Hemangiomas. *Oncotarget* (2018) 9 (39):25708–13. doi: 10.18632/oncotarget.25379
11. Maitra S, Som A, Bhattacharjee S. Accuracy of Quick Sequential Organ Failure Assessment (qSOFA) Score and Systemic Inflammatory Response Syndrome (SIRS) Criteria for Predicting Mortality in Hospitalized Patients With Suspected Infection: A Meta-Analysis of Observational Studies. *Clin Microbiol Infect* (2018) 24(11):1123–9. doi: 10.1016/j.cmi.2018.03.032
12. Gao J, Kong J, Ding X-M, Ke S, Niu H-G, Xin Z-H, et al. Laparoscopic vs Computerized Tomography-Guided Radiofrequency Ablation for Large Hepatic Hemangiomas Abutting the Diaphragm. *World J Gastroenterol* (2015) 21(19):5941–9. doi: 10.3748/wjg.v21.i19.5941
13. Gao J, Ding X, Ke S, Xin Z, Ning C, Sha Q, et al. Radiofrequency Ablation in the Treatment of Large Hepatic Hemangiomas: A Comparison of Multitined and Internally Cooled Electrodes. *J Clin Gastroenterol* (2014) 48(6):540–7. doi: 10.1097/MCG.0b013e31829ef037
14. van Tilborg AAJM, Dresselaars HF, Scheffer HJ, Nielsen K, Sietses C, van den Tol PM, et al. RF Ablation of Giant Hemangiomas Inducing Acute Renal Failure: A Report of Two Cases. *Cardiovasc Interventional Radiol* (2016) 39 (11):1644–8. doi: 10.1007/s00270-016-1415-1
15. Yang X, Liu J, Yang M-M, Wang S-H, Xu L, Ke S, et al. Heme Is Involved in the Systemic Inflammatory Response Following Radiofrequency Ablation of Hepatic Hemangiomas. *Eur J Gastroenterol Hepatol* (2020) 32(9):1200–6. doi: 10.1097/MEG.0000000000001636

19

Development of Models to Predict Postoperative Complications for Hepatitis B Virus-Related Hepatocellular Carcinoma

Mingyang Bao[1†], Qiuyu Zhu[2,3†], Tuerganaili Aji[4†], Shuyao Wei[5†], Talaiti Tuergan[4], Xiaoqin Ha[6], Alimu Tulahong[4], Xiaoyi Hu[2] and Yueqing Hu[1,7*]*

[1] State Key Laboratory of Genetic Engineering, Institute of Biostatistics, School of Life Sciences, Fudan University, Shanghai, China, [2] Division of Hepatobiliary and Pancreatic Surgery, Department of Surgery, The First Affiliated Hospital, Zhejiang University School of Medicine, Hangzhou, China, [3] Department of Surgery, Shanghai Jiaotong University School of Medicine, Shanghai, China, [4] Department of Hepatobiliary and Hydatid Surgery, The First Affiliated Hospital of Xinjiang Medical University, Urumqi, China, [5] Clinical Laboratory Diagnostics, School of Public Health, Gansu University of Chinese Medicine, Lanzhou, China, [6] Department of Clinical Laboratory, The 940th Hospital of Joint Logistics Support Force of Chinese People's Liberation Army, Lanzhou, China, [7] Shanghai Center for Mathematical Sciences, Fudan University, Shanghai, China

***Correspondence:**
Xiaoyi Hu
21818140@zju.edu.cn
Yueqing Hu
yuehu@fudan.edu.cn

†These authors have contributed equally to this work

Background: Surgical treatment remains the best option for patients with hepatocellular carcinoma (HCC) caused by chronic hepatitis B virus (HBV) infection. However, there is no optimal tool based on readily accessible clinical parameters to predict postoperative complications. Herein, our study aimed to develop models that permitted risk of severe complications to be assessed before and after liver resection based on conventional variables.

Methods: A total of 1,047 patients treated by hepatectomy for HCC with HBV infection at three different centers were recruited retrospectively between July 1, 2014, and July 1, 2018. All surgical complications were recorded and scored by the Comprehensive Complication Index (CCI). A CCI ≥26.2 was used as a threshold to define patients with severe complications. We built two models for the CCI, one using preoperative and one using preoperative and postoperative data. Besides, CCI and other potentially relevant factors were evaluated for their ability to predict early recurrence and metastasis. All the findings were internally validated in the Hangzhou cohort and then externally validated in the Lanzhou and Urumqi cohorts.

Results: Multivariable analysis identified National Nosocomial Infections Surveillance (NNIS) index, tumor number, gamma-glutamyltransferase (GGT), total cholesterol (TC), potassium, and thrombin time as the key preoperative parameters related to perioperative complications. The nomogram based on the preoperative model [preoperative CCI After Surgery for Liver tumor (CCIASL-pre)] showed good discriminatory performance internally and externally. A more accurate model [postoperative CCI After Surgery for Liver tumor (CCIASL-post)] was established, combined with the other four postoperative predictors including leukocyte count, basophil count, erythrocyte count, and total bilirubin level. No significant association was observed between CCI and long-term complications.

Conclusion: Based on the widely available clinical data, statistical models were established to predict the complications after hepatectomy in patients with HBV infection. All the findings were extensively validated and shown to be applicable nationwide. Such models could be used as guidelines for surveillance follow-up and the design of post-resection adjuvant therapy.

Keywords: modeling, hepatocellular carcinoma, complications, liver resection, comprehensive complication index

INTRODUCTION

Hepatocellular carcinoma (HCC) is the most common primary liver tumor and the third leading cause of cancer-related deaths around the world. China alone accounts for more than half of the global HCC cases (1, 2). Hepatitis B virus (HBV) infection is one of the main etiologies of HCC around the world, especially in hepatitis B-prevalent regions such as sub-Saharan Africa and East Asia (3, 4). For patients suffering from chronic hepatitis B infection, the treatment of HCC is more difficult, the prognosis is worse, and the recurrence is earlier. Nevertheless, surgical treatment still remains the best option for patients with preserved liver function among a variety of treatments (5, 6).

Currently, there is no consensus regarding the optimal tool for risk stratification derived from surgically managed patients with HBV infection. Suboptimal management of perioperative period may partially lead to severe postoperative complications such as post-hepatectomy liver failure (PHLF) (7), post-hepatectomy hemorrhage (PHH), and postoperative death. For a long time, Child–Pugh scoring system, albumin–bilirubin (ALBI) grading system, and end-stage liver disease (MELD) score were the traditional basic indices of preoperative liver functions (8–10). In recent years, many novel approaches to assessing total liver function and functional remnant liver have emerged, such as indocyanine green (ICG) clearance test (10–13), liver scintigraphy, and liver stiffness measurement (LSM) by transient elastography (TE) (14–18). However, few people have access to these latest liver-specific evaluations in developing countries due to the lack of detection equipment. Hence, a prediction model that only consists of readily accessible clinical and pathological parameters is more practical to help surgeons to identify patients at risk of severe complications.

Clavien–Dindo classification was a traditional widely used grading system of surgical complications (19). On this basis, the Comprehensive Complication Index (CCI) has been proposed recently. The index integrates all recorded complications after surgery in a single formula weighted by severity and shows more sensitivity than the traditional one (20, 21).

CCI is a comprehensive measurement of short-term complications during perioperative period. In addition, tumor recurrence, a major long-term complication, deserves attention as well. Two-year duration is generally used as the cutoff to determine early or late recurrence (22, 23). Early recurrence (i.e., within 2 years after surgery) accounts for more than 70% of tumor recurrence and is considered a "real recurrence" (24). Furthermore, metastasis is also a long-term complication and an important manifestation of recurrence. Different metastatic targets represent different tumor development trends (25). However, no clear relationship has been found between short- and long-term complications after operation. In particular, prediction of tumor metastasis and correlations of metastatic sites were rarely taken into account regarding HBV-related HCC in the previous analysis.

In this study, we recruited a large number of surgically treated patients for HCC with HBV infection from different provinces in China. Comprehensive common clinical, imaging, and pathological parameters were retrospectively reviewed in order to develop and validate models of complication prediction. Two models were first developed: one included parameters available before surgery for prediction of perioperative complications measured by CCI preoperatively, and the other included all accessible variables to enhance the accuracy of prediction. Moreover, risk factors for early recurrence and metastasis were identified from all variables as well as CCI.

METHODS

Patient Recruitment

In this national retrospective cohort study, patients were recruited from three centers in different provinces. These centers comprise Hangzhou (the First Affiliated Hospital of Zhejiang University School of Medicine, Hangzhou), Lanzhou (the 940th Hospital of Joint Logistics Support Force of Chinese People's Liberation Army, Lanzhou), and Urumqi (the First Affiliated Hospital of Xinjiang Medical University, Urumqi).

The inclusion criteria were as follows: 1) patients undergoing liver resection for HCC diagnosed pathologically; 2) HBV surface antigen (HBsAg)- and/or HBV core antibody (HBcAb)-positive patients; 3) Child–Pugh class A or B (score ≤7) patients; 4) patients performing preoperative abdominal contrast-enhanced magnetic resonance imaging (MRI) and/or contrast-enhanced computed tomography (CT) scan; 5) anatomical and non-anatomical hepatectomies before July 1, 2018. The following exclusion criteria were also met: 1) patients undergoing more than one additional procedure in the liver; 2) patients with a history of tumors; 3) HCV-positive patients; 4) patients with incomplete clinical data; 5) patients receiving antitumor therapy before operation [i.e., transarterial chemoembolization (TACE), radiotherapy, or chemotherapy].

Through strict selection and careful data record, 1,047 eligible patients were included in total, 675 of whom were from Hangzhou (415 available survival data), 252 from Lanzhou, and 120 from Urumqi. The study obeyed the ethical guidelines of the 1975 Declaration of Helsinki and was approved by the institutional ethics committee. Informed consent was obtained from each patient before surgery.

Data Collection

The information of patients was prospectively collected into electronic spreadsheets by each center and then retrospectively reviewed. Demographics and comorbidities of patients were obtained from detailed consultation records. Preoperative and postoperative blood was taken from the patients for laboratory tests, including marks related to HBV, a complete blood count, blood chemical analysis, and coagulation testing; all the postoperative laboratory examinations were performed 3–5 days after surgery. Serum tumor markers were also investigated, such as α-fetoprotein (AFP), carbohydrate antigen 199 (CA199), and carcinoembryonic antigen (CEA). Tumor classification and characteristics relied on imaging examination reports and pathologic results of the resected specimens. The imaging data included tumor number, diameter, capsule status, location, lymphadenectasis, esophageal varices, ascites, and cirrhosis based on preoperative contrast-enhanced MRI and/or CT. The presence of arterial enhancement and washout of lesions on each of the dynamic imaging phases were also recorded. Arterial enhancement was defined as lesions exhibiting higher signal intensity on arterial phase images (26–28). Washout was defined as lesions with higher intensity compared with the surrounding liver on any late dynamic images except the arterial phase images (26–28). The pathologic results included the microvascular invasion, tumor giant cell, status of surrounding liver tissue, and differentiation and encapsulation of tumor. In addition, pathological immunohistochemistry tests for cytokeratin 19 (CK19), cytokeratin 7 (CK7), glypican 3, and CD34 were carried out. For both imaging and pathological data, two experienced specialists independently evaluated all results respectively. Any controversies in findings between the specialists were settled by discussion and generated a unified answer. Perioperative data were derived from operative recordings. Patients were followed up in the first 2 years after surgery to observe postoperative complications and early oncological outcomes. Information collection ended on July 1, 2020.

Measurement of Postoperative Complications and Clinical Outcomes

All surgical complications, defined as any deviation from the normal postoperative course that occurred before discharge, were recorded and scored using the CCI, ranging from 0 (uneventful course) to 100 (death). The threshold for defining patients with at least one grade III (major) complication was CCI ≥26.2 according to Clavien–Dindo classification (19, 29). This cutoff also takes into account the weight of multiple low-grade complications (e.g., grades I–II). Although these complications are not usually regarded as endpoints, they are considered to increase the postoperative experience of patients longer than a grade III complication in the CCI model. The CCI was used as the primary endpoint to assess the postoperative situation of patients.

Early recurrence of HCC was defined as the appearance of a newly detected tumor confirmed on two radiologic images within 2 years (30, 31). Relapse-free survival (RFS), the interval between liver resection and recurrence, was measured as the secondary endpoint. Among all kinds of recurrence, new tumor not located as the same as the primary one was diagnosed as metastasis. The metastasis was further divided into six categories depending on the location where tumor was newly discovered (lung, liver, abdomen, bone, lymph nodes, and brain).

Statistical Analyses

Continuous variables were described as medians with interquartile range (IQR), and nonparametric Mann–Whitney U tests were applied for statistical significance between high CCI (≥26.2) group and low CCI (<26.2) group. For categorical variables, we expressed the numbers and percentages of patients in each category. Proportions were compared using the χ^2 test, with Yates' correction or Fisher's exact test. Serum HBV DNA, AFP, CA199, CA125, and ferritin were natural log transformed due to high skewness to the right.

The preoperative and postoperative CCI After Surgery for Liver tumor (CCIASL) models were built to predict the risk of developing high CCI on the Hangzhou dataset and then internally validated through bootstrap resampling. Subsequently, external validation of the two models was conducted on datasets from Lanzhou and Urumqi. One of the models, CCIASL-pre model, was based on preoperative predictors available before surgery; the other model, CCIASL-post model, was constructed on all available parameters.

Univariable logistic regression analyses were performed to screen potentially relevant variables. Those that reached $p < 0.05$ at univariable analysis were included in the multivariable logistic regression, and two-way stepwise strategy was applied for predictor selection. A number of potentially clinically plausible interactions were also taken into account during this process. The candidate multivariable regression model was built when Akaike information criterion (AIC) reached the minimum. We retained the statistically significant predictors in the final model. The risk score for prediction of high CCI was defined as the weight sum of the value of those significant parameters, and the weights were model β-estimates. The samples from each cohort were cut to high-risk and low-risk groups based on the median of risk score. Boxplots were drawn to compare risk differences between the two groups. The discrimination performance of the two models in the derivation and validation sets was then measured by the Harrell's concordance index (C-index) and the receiver operating characteristic (ROC) curves. A relatively corrected C-index was also calculated by 1,000 bootstrap resampling for internal validation. Moreover, we made comparisons between two models. Net reclassification improvement (NRI) and integrated discrimination improvement (IDI) were computed using the category-free approach with 1,000 bootstrap replications to estimate the 95% confidence interval (CI) (32). The significant factors related to high CCI in the two models were used to construct nomograms. Calibration curves were subsequently drawn to assess the Hosmer–Lemeshow goodness of fit (33). Bootstrapping was used for each model to get bias-corrected (overfitting-corrected) estimates of predicted vs. observed values. As a reference line, the diagonal represents the best prediction. We also performed a decision curve analysis to determine whether our established nomogram was suitable for clinical utility by estimating the net benefits at different threshold probabilities.

Moreover, univariable Cox regression was applied to identify the association between CCI and early recurrence of HCC. The samples were stratified into various subgroups based on a number of important HCC-related markers, surgical factors, and tumor characteristics. Subgroup analysis was then conducted to explore possible correlations in each specific group of HCC patients. To identify more predictive factors for RFS, significant variables at univariable analysis were included to build a multivariable Cox regression model by both-direction stepwise selection. The proportional hazards assumption of the models was tested by examining the plots of scaled Schoenfeld residuals against time for each variable in the models. The patients were grouped into high risk and low risk according to median of the risk score, which was computed similar to the logistic regression described above. Kaplan–Meier (KM) survival analysis was performed to estimate the prediction value of the model. Survival nomogram was then constructed based on the significant factors in the multivariable Cox regression model. The predictive accuracy of the models was quantified through the concordance index (C-index) and time-dependent ROC curves with area under the curve (AUC). The level of agreement between the predicted probabilities and the actual possibility of early recurrence was measured by calibration plots. Model discrimination was performed both in the derivation cohort and in the validation cohorts.

To further explore the association between CCI and metastasis of HCC, univariable generalized linear model (GLM, here was logistic regression) was used. To identify more factors related to metastasis, significant variables at univariable analysis were included to build a multivariable GLM by both forward and backward stepwise selection. Given that tumor metastasis involved multiple locations, generalized estimation equation (GEE) was established to obtain more robust coefficients of the variables chosen by GLM selection and explore the correlations between different metastasis sites. The unstructured working correlation matrix was adopted due to the uncertainty of associations between various metastasis sites. The external validation set in this part was composed of Lanzhou and Urumqi cohorts.

All statistical tests were two-tailed, and differences were considered significant at a p-value <0.05. All statistical analyses were performed using R 3.6.1 software (R Foundation for Statistical Computing, Vienna, Austria) and SPSS 24.0 (SPSS, Chicago, USA).

RESULTS

Patient Characteristics

Baseline features and postoperative complications were collected from 675 patients who were infected with HBV and received liver section for HCC in the Hangzhou cohort (**Table 1**). The median age was 56 years (IQR: 48–63), and the majority of patients were male (81.19%). Nearly all of the patients were Child–Pugh A (98.8%) and had positive HBsAg and HBcAb (99.4%). A total of 92 patients was considered high CCI (≥26.2), accounting for 13.6% of the whole population. Perioperative complications of patients with high CCI in the Hangzhou cohort were shown in detail in **Table 2**. This proportion was 13.3% in the Urumqi cohort and 7.9% in the Lanzhou cohort. Compared with patients with low CCI, those with high CCI were more likely from the worse physical condition and higher surgery risk according to the National Nosocomial Infections Surveillance (NNIS) index ($p < 0.001$), American Society of Anesthesiologists (ASA) score ($p = 0.009$), and Barcelona Clinic Liver Cancer (BCLC) stage ($p < 0.001$). Patients with high CCI had a longer hospital stay and a larger amount of ascites than those with low CCI. The median HBV-DNA level of all patients was 11.13 IU/ml (after natural log transformation), and insignificantly level increase was observed in high CCI group. High CCI patients also showed numerous differences in preoperative laboratory results, such as proportion of various blood cells, levels of bilirubin and enzymes, and coagulation time. Moreover, these differences became more significant after surgery. Based on imaging examination and pathological analysis, we discovered that tumor number, maximum tumor size, and conditions of hepatic capsule and surrounding satellite nodules were significantly different between the two groups. Of 415 patients with survival data, nearly half relapsed within 2 years and 65 metastasized. The average RFS of all was 16.29 months. No significant differences in clinical outcomes between the two groups of patients were observed. More detailed information of patients was shown in **Table S1**.

Construction of the Model Predicting Severe Perioperative Complications

The result of univariable logistic regression analysis revealed that NNIS index, ASA score (III *vs.* I), BCLC stage (A4 *vs.* 0 and A4 *vs.* 0), tumor number, hepatic capsule (invaded *vs.* normal), surrounding satellite nodules, surgical approach, postoperative day (POD) 1 ascites volume, and intraoperative blood loss were significantly relevant with high CCI (**Table 3**). From the results of laboratory tests, erythrocyte count, total protein (TP), alkaline phosphatase (ALP), gamma-glutamyltransferase (GGT), and total cholesterol (TC) were discovered to be significantly associated with high CCI both before and after operation. Notably, the correlation between proportion of basophils in leukocytes and high CCI became significant in those experiencing surgery. The change of significance was observed in the relation of total bilirubin and high CCI as well.

After a multistep selection of significant variables at univariable analysis available before surgery, six of them were employed for building CCIASL-pre model, including NNIS index, tumor number, GGT, TC, potassium, and thrombin time (TT) (**Figure 1A**). The risk score formula was shown at the bottom of **Table 3**. As shown in the boxplot, patients with high CCI were scored significantly higher (**Figure 1B**). Based on the independent predictors in the final multivariable model, a nomogram was constructed to visualize the relationship with probability of high CCI (**Figure 1C**). In addition, another multivariable logistic regression model was developed based on all variables significant at univariable analysis to construct

TABLE 1 | Characteristics of study population and grouped by comprehensive complication index (CCI).

Variables	All patients (n=675)	CCI≥26.2 (n=92)	CCI<26.2 (n=583)	P
Baseline features				
Age, years, median [IQR]	56.00 [48.00, 63.00]	57.50 [48.00, 64.25]	56.00 [48.00, 63.00]	0.326
Male, n (%)	548 (81.19)	469 (80.45)	79 (85.87)	0.274
NNIS index, n (%)				<0.001
0	196 (29.0)	11 (12.0)	185 (31.7)	
1	462 (68.4)	75 (81.5)	387 (66.4)	
2	17 (2.5)	6 (6.5)	11 (1.9)	
Antivirus treatment, n (%)	168 (24.9)	23 (25.0)	145 (24.9)	>0.999
Child Pugh, n (%)				0.299
A	667 (98.8)	90 (97.8)	577 (99.0)	
B	8 (1.2)	2 (2.2)	6 (1.0)	
BCLC stage, n (%)				<0.001
0	424 (62.8)	46 (50.0)	378 (64.8)	
A1	153 (22.7)	20 (21.7)	133 (22.8)	
A2	12 (1.8)	2 (2.2)	10 (1.7)	
A3	65 (9.6)	15 (16.3)	50 (8.6)	
A4	21 (3.1)	9 (9.8)	12 (2.1)	
Hepatitis B marks				
Hepatitis B Virus DNA, IU/mL, median [IQR]	11.13 [0.00, 16.71]	12.33 [0.00, 17.99]	11.03 [0.00, 16.45]	0.187
Hepatitis B core antibody, S/CO, median [IQR]	10.62 [9.41, 11.73]	10.70 [9.40, 11.94]	10.60 [9.42, 11.70]	0.626
Hepatitis B surface antigen positive, n (%)	671 (99.4)	579 (99.3)	92 (100.0)	>0.999
Hepatitis B e antigen positive, n (%)	154 (22.8)	129 (22.1)	25 (27.2)	0.287
Hepatitis B e antibody positive, n (%)	191 (28.3)	167 (28.6)	24 (26.1)	0.709
Hepatitis B surface antibody positive, n (%)	190 (28.1)	160 (27.4)	30 (32.6)	0.319
Radiology findings				
Multiple lesions, n (%)	86 (12.8)	24 (26.1)	62 (10.7)	<0.001
Maximum tumor size, cm, median [IQR]	5.00 [3.50, 7.50]	6.00 [4.38, 8.00]	5.00 [3.50, 7.50]	0.041
Hepatic capsule, n (%)				0.042
Normal	526 (78.2)	66 (71.7)	460 (79.2)	
Invaded	89 (13.2)	20 (21.7)	69 (11.9)	
Attached	58 (8.6)	6 (6.5)	52 (9.0)	
Cirrhosis, n (%)	389 (57.9)	51 (55.4)	338 (58.3)	0.650
Ascites, n (%)				0.110
No	555 (83.0)	74 (81.3)	481 (83.2)	
Mild	107 (16.0)	14 (15.4)	93 (16.1)	
Moderate	6 (0.9)	3 (3.3)	3 (0.5)	
Surrounding satellite nodules, n (%)	98 (14.6)	22 (23.9)	76 (13.1)	0.010
Preoperative laboratory findings (median [IQR])				
Leukocyte, 10^9/L	6.90 [5.30, 8.70]	7.35 [5.12, 9.54]	6.78 [5.22, 8.77]	0.097
Basophil, %	0.30 [0.20, 0.50]	0.30 [0.20, 0.50]	0.30 [0.20, 0.50]	0.331
Erythrocyte, 10^12/L	4.64 [4.27, 5.00]	4.46 [4.20, 4.85]	4.66 [4.30, 5.01]	0.015
Albumin-globulin ratio	1.60 [1.30, 1.80]	1.50 [1.30, 1.80]	1.60 [1.40, 1.80]	0.478
Alanine aminotransferase, U/L	29.00 [20.00, 45.00]	29.00 [19.00, 46.00]	29.00 [21.00, 45.00]	0.862
Aspartate aminotransferase, U/L	32.00 [25.00, 44.00]	30.50 [25.00, 47.00]	32.50 [25.00, 44.00]	0.730
Total bilirubin, μmol/L	13.00 [10.00, 17.00]	14.00 [10.50, 17.50]	13.00 [10.00, 17.00]	0.168
Gamma-glutamyltransferase, U/L	59.00 [34.00, 109.00]	82.50 [40.50, 155.25]	57.00 [34.00, 105.00]	0.004
Total cholesterol, mmol/L	3.91 [3.45, 4.57]	3.71 [3.11, 4.50]	3.96 [3.51, 4.58]	0.010
Potassium, mmol/L	4.16 [3.92, 4.40]	4.04 [3.88, 4.31]	4.18 [3.94, 4.41]	0.005
Thrombin time, s	18.60 [17.60, 19.70]	18.30 [17.30, 19.20]	18.70 [17.60, 19.70]	0.031
Surgical features				
Laparoscopy surgery, n (%)	98 (14.6)	6 (6.5)	92 (15.8)	0.017
Open surgery, n (%)	577 (85.7)	87 (94.6)	490 (84.3)	0.006
Minor hepatectomy, n (%)	522 (77.6)	66 (71.7)	456 (78.5)	0.178
Major hepatectomy, n (%)	149 (22.1)	26 (28.3)	123 (21.2)	0.138
Pringle Maneuver, n (%)	76 (11.3)	11 (12.0)	65 (11.2)	0.859
Intraoperative blood transfusion, n (%)	44 (6.6)	10 (11.0)	34 (5.9)	0.107
Intraoperative blood loss, mL, median [IQR]	200.00 [100.00, 400.00]	300.00 [200.00, 500.00]	200.00 [100.00, 400.00]	<0.001
Pathologic characteristics				
Tumor differentiation, n (%)				0.734
Well	6 (0.9)	0 (0.0)	6 (1.0)	
Moderate	32 (4.8)	6 (6.5)	26 (4.5)	
Moderate to Poor	568 (84.9)	78 (84.8)	490 (84.9)	
Poor	63 (9.4)	8 (8.7)	55 (9.5)	

(Continued)

TABLE 1 | Continued

Variables	All patients (n=675)	CCI≥26.2 (n=92)	CCI<26.2 (n=583)	P
Satellites, n (%)	62 (9.2)	8 (8.7)	54 (9.3)	>0.999
Microvascular invasion, n (%)	215 (31.9)	31 (33.7)	184 (31.7)	0.719
CD34, n (%)	479 (97.8)	66 (100.0)	413 (97.4)	0.374
Cytokeratin 19, n (%)	198 (33.6)	27 (35.5)	171 (33.3)	0.698
Postoperative laboratory findings (median [IQR])				
Leukocyte, 10^9/L	7.10 [5.50, 9.20]	7.75 [5.47, 10.45]	7.00 [5.50, 9.00]	0.033
Basophil, %	0.30 [0.20, 0.40]	0.30 [0.20, 0.50]	0.20 [0.20, 0.40]	0.022
Erythrocyte, 10^12/L	3.65 [3.23, 4.05]	3.44 [3.02, 3.82]	3.68 [3.30, 4.07]	0.001
Alanine aminotransferase, U/L	65.00 [45.00, 96.50]	59.00 [42.50, 98.50]	67.00 [45.00, 96.25]	0.337
Aspartate aminotransferase, U/L	34.00 [26.00, 48.00]	36.00 [26.00, 50.00]	33.50 [26.00, 47.00]	0.723
Total bilirubin, μmol/L	19.00 [14.00, 26.00]	22.60 [15.00, 36.00]	19.00 [14.00, 25.00]	<0.001
Gamma-glutamyltransferase, U/L	72.00 [43.00, 116.00]	89.00 [46.50, 142.75]	71.00 [43.00, 114.00]	0.031
Total cholesterol, mmol/L	2.61 [2.11, 3.15]	2.42 [1.90, 2.96]	2.62 [2.15, 3.16]	0.034
Perioperative situation (median [IQR])				
POD 1 ascites volume, mL	150.00 [80.00, 250.00]	200.00 [100.00, 300.00]	130.00 [80.00, 220.00]	0.001
Hospital stay, days	19.00 [16.00, 24.00]	27.00 [22.00, 32.00]	19.00 [15.00, 23.00]	<0.001
Postoperative hospital stay, days	10.00 [8.00, 13.00]	16.00 [13.00, 20.00]	10.00 [8.00, 12.00]	<0.001
Clinical outcomes **				
Recurrence within 2 years, n (%)	199 (47.95)	24 (43.64)	175 (48.61)	0.587
Recurrence-free survival, months (mean±SD)	16.29±8.93	17.15±8.94	16.16±8.93	0.447
Metastasis, n (%)	65 (15.66)	7 (12.73)	58 (16.11)	0.657

*NNIS, National Nosocomial Infection Surveillance; ASA, American Society of Anesthesiologists; BCLC, Barcelona Clinic Liver Cancer; POD, postoperative day; IQR, interquartile range; SD, standard deviation. * data was natural log transformed; ** the total number of patients available to survival data was 415.*

CCIASL-post. Five parameters of the CCIASL-pre model, namely, NNIS index, tumor number, GGT, TC, and potassium, maintained independence. On this basis, another four postoperative laboratory findings were identified, including leukocyte count, basophil, erythrocyte count, and total bilirubin (**Figure 2A**). Similar to the CCIASL-pre model, postoperative model formula of risk score was shown at the bottom of **Table 3**, and boxplot was drawn to display risk differences between two groups classified by the median risk score (**Figure 2B**). Nine independent predictors of CCIASL-post model were integrated in the nomogram (**Figure 2C**).

Internal and External Assessment of the CCIASL Model

Both CCIASL models were first assessed internally in the Hangzhou cohort. As to CCIASL-pre model, the Hosmer–Lemeshow test did not indicate evidence of poor fit (p = 0.769), and the calibration plot also showed a good prediction capability (**Figure 1D**). The Harrell's C-index, equivalent to AUC on ROC curves, was 0.757 (95% CI: 0.704–0.810) and corrected to be 0.767 (95% CI: 0.715–0.817) through bootstrapping validation, which indicated good discriminatory performance of the model (**Figure 1E** and **Table 4**). Additionally, the decision curve showed that making use of this model for predicting the probability of high CCI would gain more net benefits than an all-or-none patient intervention scheme if the threshold probability was less than 88%, which suggested a high potential for clinical application (**Figure 1F**). In the external validation cohorts, good discrimination and prediction ability were also observed, although calibration plots showed a slight deterioration, which was most pronounced in the Urumqi cohort (**Figure S1**). In terms of clinical usefulness, the Lanzhou cohort displayed better if threshold probability was more than 60%, while the Urumqi cohort performed better if threshold probability was less than 60%.

A better result was obtained regarding discriminatory performance of CCIASL-post model (**Figures 2D, E**).

TABLE 2 | Postoperative complications of patients with comprehensive complication index (CCI) ≥26.2 and their grade of severity.

Grading of complications (CCI≥26.2)	No. of complications	Details of complications
Grade I	64	abdominal infection=9; electrolytes=2; fever=1; pneumonia=45; wound infection=7
Grade II	57	abdominal abscess=1; ascites=7; atrial fibrillation=3; biliary leak=7; blood oozing=5; blood transfusion=24; delirium=1; gastroplegia=1; hemoperitoneum=1; ileus=2; pleural effusion=1; thrombosis=3
Grade IIIa	79	abdominal abscess=1; ascites=13; bleeding=1; bleeding/hematoma=1; perihepatic ascites=8; pleural effusion=51; thrombosis=2; wound infection=2
Grade IIIb	4	hemoperitoneum=3; bleeding/hematoma=1
Grade IVa	9	acute liver failure=3; pulmonary embolism=3; respiratory insufficiency=3
Grade IVb	1	shock=1
Grade V	2	MOF=2

MOF, multi-organ failure.

TABLE 3 | Uni- and multivariate logistics regression analysis of predictors for high Comprehensive Complication Index (CCI≥26.2).

	Univariate analysis			Multivariate analysis					
				Without postoperative results			*With postoperative results*		
Variables	**OR**	**95% CI**	**P**	**OR**	**95% CI**	**P**	**OR**	**95% CI**	**P**
Baseline factors									
Sex (male vs female)	1.477	0.794-2.749	0.218						
Age (years)	1.008	0.988-1.029	0.448						
NNIS index									
1 vs 0	3.259	1.690-6.285	<0.001	2.727	1.369-5.433	0.004	2.243	1.103-4.559	0.026
2 vs 0	9.174	2.859-29.44	<0.001	7.322	2.099-25.54	0.002	4.903	1.269-18.94	0.021
ASA score									
II vs I	1.312	0.759-2.268	0.331						
III vs I	3.576	1.601-7.984	0.002						
Child Pugh (B vs A)	2.137	0.425-10.75	0.357						
BCLC stage									
A1 vs 0	1.236	0.705-2.165	0.460						
A2 vs 0	1.643	0.349-7.734	0.530						
A3 vs 0	2.465	1.283-4.737	0.007						
A4 vs 0	6.163	2.464-15.42	<0.001						
Tumor characteristics									
Tumor number (multiple vs solitary)	2.943	1.724-5.024	<0.001	2.827	1.583-5.049	<0.001	2.855	1.571-5.188	0.001
Hepatic capsule									
Invaded vs Normal	2.020	1.153-3.539	0.014						
Attached vs Normal	0.804	0.332-1.946	0.629						
Surrounding satellite nodules (present vs absent)	2.088	1.221-3.570	0.007						
Perioperative situation									
Laparoscopy surgery (yes vs no)	0.371	0.157-0.874	0.023						
Open surgery (yes vs no)	3.231	1.277-8.179	0.013						
POD 1 ascites volume (mL)	1.002	1.001-1.003	0.001						
Intraoperative blood loss (mL)	1.001	1.000-1.001	0.003						
Preoperative laboratory results									
Leukocyte (10^9/L)	1.068	0.936-1.136	0.074						
Basophil (%)	1.443	0.678-3.071	0.342						
Erythrocyte (10^12/L)	0.623	0.419-0.929	0.020						
Total protein (g/L)	0.959	0.926-0.992	0.016						
Alkaline phosphatase (U/L)	1.007	1.003-1.012	0.001						
Total bilirubin (μmol/L)	1.016	0.981-1.052	0.379						
Gamma-glutamyltransferase (U/L)	1.004	1.002-1.006	<0.001	1.005	1.003-1.007	<0.001	1.005	1.003-1.007	<0.001
Total cholesterol (mmol/L)	0.735	0.566-0.954	0.021	0.681	0.513-0.905	0.008	0.670	0.498-0.901	0.008
Potassium (mmol/L)	0.465	0.257-0.839	0.011	0.404	0.209-0.780	0.007	0.292	0.145-0.590	0.001
Thrombin time (s)	0.853	0.738-0.986	0.032	0.848	0.727-0.989	0.036			
Carbohydrate antigen199 (kU/L)	1.160	1.018-1.323	0.026						
Postoperative laboratory results									
Leukocyte (10^9/L)	1.098	1.026-1.175	0.007				1.154	1.065-1.249	<0.001
Basophil (%)	4.553	1.742-11.90	0.002				7.273	2.459-21.51	<0.001
Erythrocyte (10^12/L)	0.570	0.391-0.832	0.004				0.565	0.367-0.870	0.009
Total protein (g/L)	0.946	0.910-0.983	0.005						
Alkaline phosphatase (U/L)	1.007	1.003-1.012	0.002						
Total bilirubin (μmol/L)	1.020	1.010-1.029	<0.001				1.020	1.009-1.031	<0.001
Gamma-glutamyltransferase (U/L)	1.003	1.001-1.005	0.003						
Total cholesterol (mmol/L)	0.687	0.495-0.954	0.025						

CCIASL-pre score = 1.013 × NNIS index (=1) or 1.002 × NNIS index (=2) + 0.005 × Gamma-glutamyltransferase (U/L) − 0.382 × Total cholesterol (mmol/L) − 0.920 × Potassium (mmol/L) − 0.172 × Thrombin time (s) + 1.037 × Tumor number (0: solitary; 1: multiple) + 4.775

CCIASL-post score = 0.847 × NNIS (=1) or 0.824 × NNIS (=2) + 0.005 × Gamma-glutamyltransferase (U/L) − 0.407 ×Total cholesterol (mmol/L) + 0.132 × Leukocyte (10^9/L)* + 2.015 × Basophil (%)* − 0.497 ×Erythrocyte (10^12/L)* + 0.0019 × Total bilirubin (μmol/L)* + 1.063 × Tumor number (0: solitary; 1: multiple) +3.150

*NNIS, National Nosocomial Infection Surveillance; ASA, American Society of Anesthesiologists; BCLC, Barcelona Clinic Liver Cancer; POD, postoperative day; OR, odds ratio; CI, confidence interval; CCIASL, CCI After Surgery for Liver tumor. *postoperative data.*

The C-indices reached around 0.8 in both the derivation cohort and validation cohorts. As shown in **Figure 2F**, the CCIASL-post model performed better in the validation cohorts, suggesting that its clinical practice was wider than that of the CCIASL-pre model, although the postoperative model would only gain more benefits if the threshold probability was less than 70% in the Hangzhou cohort. However, the results of reclassification analyses detected no significant differences between performance of the two models in all cohorts.

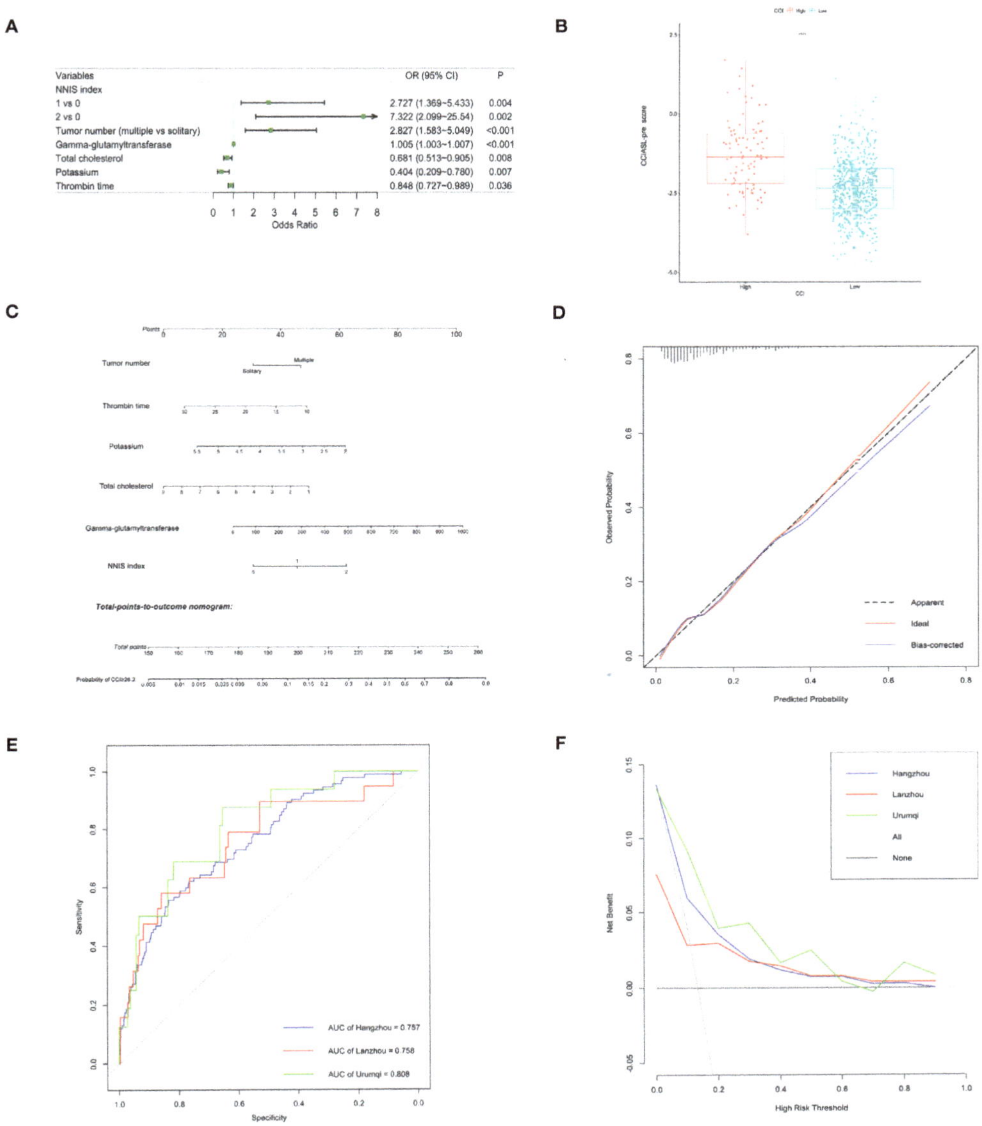

FIGURE 1 | Construction and validation of the CCIASL-pre model. **(A)** Forest plot of predictors for CCI≥26.2 based on the result of multivariate analysis. **(B)** Boxplot of the CCIASL-pre risk score between high CCI group and low CCI group. Significant difference was observed. ****: P<0.0001. **(C)** Nomogram to predict probability of CCI≥26.2 in HCC patients. **(D)** Calibration curve for the nomogram to predict probability of CCI≥26.2 in the derivation cohort. The x-axis represents the predicted CCI≥26.2 probability and the y-axis denotes the actual proportion of CCI≥26.2. The black diagonal line indicates the best prediction. The red ideal line represents the uncorrected performance of the nomogram while the blue line shows the bias-corrected performance. **(E)** Receiver operating characteristic (ROC) curves in the derivation and validation cohorts. Corresponding area under curves (AUC) in the Hangzhou, Lanzhou and Urumqi were 0.757, 0.758 and 0.808, respectively. **(F)** Decision curve for the predictive nomogram. The net benefits were measured at different threshold probabilities. The blue, red and green lines represent the predictive ability of nomogram in the Hangzhou, Lanzhou and Urumqi cohorts, respectively. The gray line represents the assumption that all patients have severe complications. The black line represents the assumption that no patients have severe complications.

Prediction for Early Recurrence and Metastasis

Among all variables analyzed, CCI (high *vs.* low) was found not to be potentially relevant with early recurrence in the univariable analysis (hazard ratio = 0.862, 95% CI: 0.563–1.321, p = 0.496) (**Table S2**). The result was consistent in subgroup analysis, which demonstrated that perioperative complications after liver resection in patients with HBV infection had little association with the prediction for early relapse (**Table S3**). Nevertheless, by stepwise analysis, independent parameters were identified to be correlated with early recurrence, including HBV DNA, arterial phase, surrounding satellite nodules, microvascular invasion, preoperative TP, preoperative direct bilirubin, postoperative platelets, and postoperative ALP (**Figure 3A**). We did not

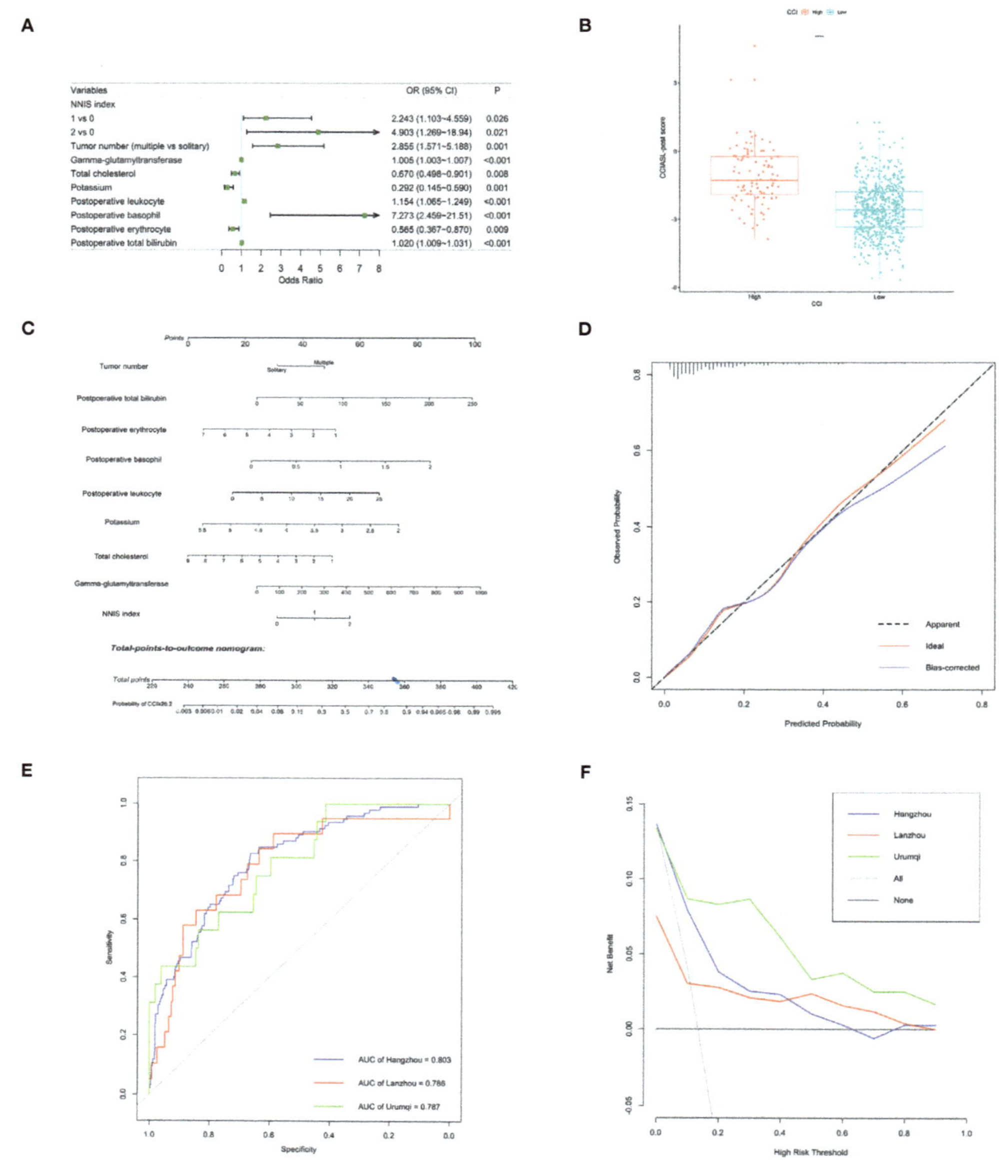

FIGURE 2 | Construction and validation of the CCIASL-post model. **(A)** Forest plot of predictors for CCI≥26.2 based on the result of multivariate analysis. **(B)** Boxplot of the CCIASL-post risk score between high CCI group and low CCI group. Significant difference was observed. ****: P<0.0001. **(C)** Nomogram to predict probability of CCI≥26.2 in HCC patients. **(D)** Calibration curve for the nomogram to predict probability of CCI≥26.2 in the derivation cohort. The x-axis represents the predicted CCI≥26.2 probability and the y-axis denotes the actual proportion of CCI≥26.2. The black diagonal line indicates the best prediction. The red ideal line represents the uncorrected performance of the nomogram while the blue line shows the bias-corrected performance. **(E)** Receiver operating characteristic (ROC) curves for severe complications in the derivation and validation cohorts. Corresponding area under curves (AUC) in the Hangzhou, Lanzhou and Urumqi were 0.803, 0.786 and 0.787, respectively. **(F)** Decision curve for the predictive nomogram. The net benefits were measured at different threshold probabilities. The blue, red and green lines represent the predictive ability of nomogram in the Hangzhou, Lanzhou and Urumqi cohorts, respectively. The gray line represents the assumption that all patients have severe complications. The black line represents the assumption that no patients have severe complications.

detect any significant violation of the proportional hazard assumption, assessed by scaled Schoenfeld residuals on functions of time. The prognostic nomogram for early recurrence was shown in **Figure 3B**, which had a good prediction capability with a C-index of 0.701 (95% CI: 0.672–0.740) and the bootstrap estimate of C-index was 0.710 (95% CI: 0.649–0.776). The estimator in the validation cohort reached around 0.7, indicating that the prediction performance of the model was stable. The calibration plot showed an overall good agreement between the nomogram-predicted RFS and observed outcome (**Figure 3C**). This was also the case for the Lanzhou validation sets, but the deviation was larger in the Urumqi cohort

TABLE 4 | Performance measurement and comparison of the CCIASL models.

Measure of discrimination	Cohort	CCIASL-pre	95% CI	CCIASL-post	95% CI	P
Harrell's c-index	Hangzhou	0.757	0.704-0.810	0.803	0.756-0.850	
	Hangzhou (bootstrap) *	0.767	0.715-0.817	0.811	0.764-0.859	
	Lanzhou	0.758	0.632-0.884	0.786	0.671-0.901	
	Urumqi	0.808	0.698-0.919	0.787	0.670-0.905	
Net reclassification improvement	Hangzhou	Reference		-0.006	-0.061-0.048	0.820
	Lanzhou	Reference		-0.011	-0.107-0.084	0.814
	Urumqi	Reference		0.154	-0.086-0.393	0.208
Integrated discrimination improvement	Hangzhou	Reference		0.005	-0.019-0.028	0.688
	Lanzhou	Reference		-0.006	-0.018-0.006	0.342
	Urumqi	Reference		0.024	-0.103-0.151	0.712

*CCIASL, Comprehensive Complication Index After Surgery for Liver tumor. *The Harrell's c-index was internally validated by 1000 bootstrap resampling.*

(**Figures S2A, B**). Furthermore, time-dependent ROC analysis indicated that the prediction accuracies exceeded 0.7 in all cohorts (**Figure 3E**). KM survival curves displayed significantly poorer RFS of high-risk group categorized by the median risk score in the derivation and validation sets ($p < 0.0001$; **Figure 3D**; **Figures S2C, D**).

To analyze impact factors on early relapse in more detail, we identified 65 patients with tumor metastasis from those experiencing recurrence in the internal cohort. The locations of metastasis in more than two cases were lung, liver, abdomen, bone, lymph nodes, and brain. Lung was the most common metastatic site, accounting for 7.23% of the entire population (**Table S4**). In the univariable analysis, CCI showed no relationship with metastasis (odds ratio = 0.759, 95% CI: 0.327–1.761, p = 0.521), which was consistent with previous findings. However, a total of 20 features were identified to be found potentially associated with metastasis (**Table S5**). These variables were then included in the multivariable model to select independent factors. As a result, fasting blood glucose (FBG) and TT decreased the odds of metastasis, while postoperative TP, intraoperative blood loss, maximum tumor size, surrounding satellite nodules, and tumor encapsulation increased the odds. In the external set, GEE analysis revealed that TT was a protective factor for metastasis, and absence of tumor encapsulation increased the risk of metastasis (**Table 5**). The correlations between the locations of tumor metastasis were uncertain according to working correlation matrix (**Table S6**), but whether negative or positive, the correlation was weak.

DISCUSSION

Two models (CCIASL-pre and CCIASL-post) that enable risk assessment of perioperative complications before and after surgery have been derived and validated in a large national multicenter study of patients who underwent liver resection for HCC. Considering China is a hepatitis B-prevalent region, the models were constructed based on patients infected with HBV. Correspondingly, two predictive nomograms made assessments of complications more accurate by quantitatively establishing the relationship between values of predictors and probability of high CCI in a personalized way. This is a user-friendly tool for surgeons in clinical decision-making. The models are also suitable for simple application by stratifying surgical candidates into different risk levels based on risk scores.

Attentive postoperative management forms a core element in speeding recovery and reducing the chance of complications after hepatectomy, especially in cirrhotic livers with HBV infection. Postoperative bile leakage, ascites, hemorrhage, liver failure, and intra-abdominal abscesses were major short-term complications after liver resection, and the incidence of hepatectomy-related PHLF ranged from 0% to 43.1% that was frequently associated with mortality (34). In recent studies, LSM by emerging imaging examination, especially transient elastography and magnetic resonance elastography (35, 36), has been demonstrated to quantify the status of fibrosis and reflect the liver function in patients with HCC in order to promote perioperative management. Serenari et al. (18) reported a preoperative prediction of high CCI in patients with resectable HCC mainly based on LSM values. However, the accuracy of this transient elastography (FibroScan®) has been challenged by the risk of overestimating LSM. Actually, LSM is influenced by several other confounding factors such as age, obesity or high body mass index (BMI) and serum alanine aminotransferase (ALT), and total bilirubin levels (18, 37). Furthermore, recent studies showed that both acute hepatitis B (38) and chronic HBV infection (39) could increase the LSM value without significant fibrosis, indicating its less diagnostic accuracy in patients with HBV infection. Moreover, these measurements have not been easily accessible in developed countries, suggesting restricted practice in the clinics. Notably, our models are the first to be built solely on simple and readily available clinicopathological parameters. NNIS index, GGT, TC, potassium, and tumor number were identified to be significantly associated with severe complications in both models, indicating that these five preoperative variables possessed strong predictive capabilities for severe complications.

The NNIS system was first proposed by the Centers for Disease Control and Prevention (CDC), Atlanta, in the 1970s to predict surgical site infections (SSIs), which were considered to be the third most frequent nosocomial infection, occurring in 14%–16% of hospital inpatients (40, 41). A total of three risk factors have been evaluated in the NNIS system containing the status of surgical wound, the anesthesia score, and the procedure duration. As a nosocomial infection surveillance system, NNIS index is also an essential component in the Study of the Efficacy of

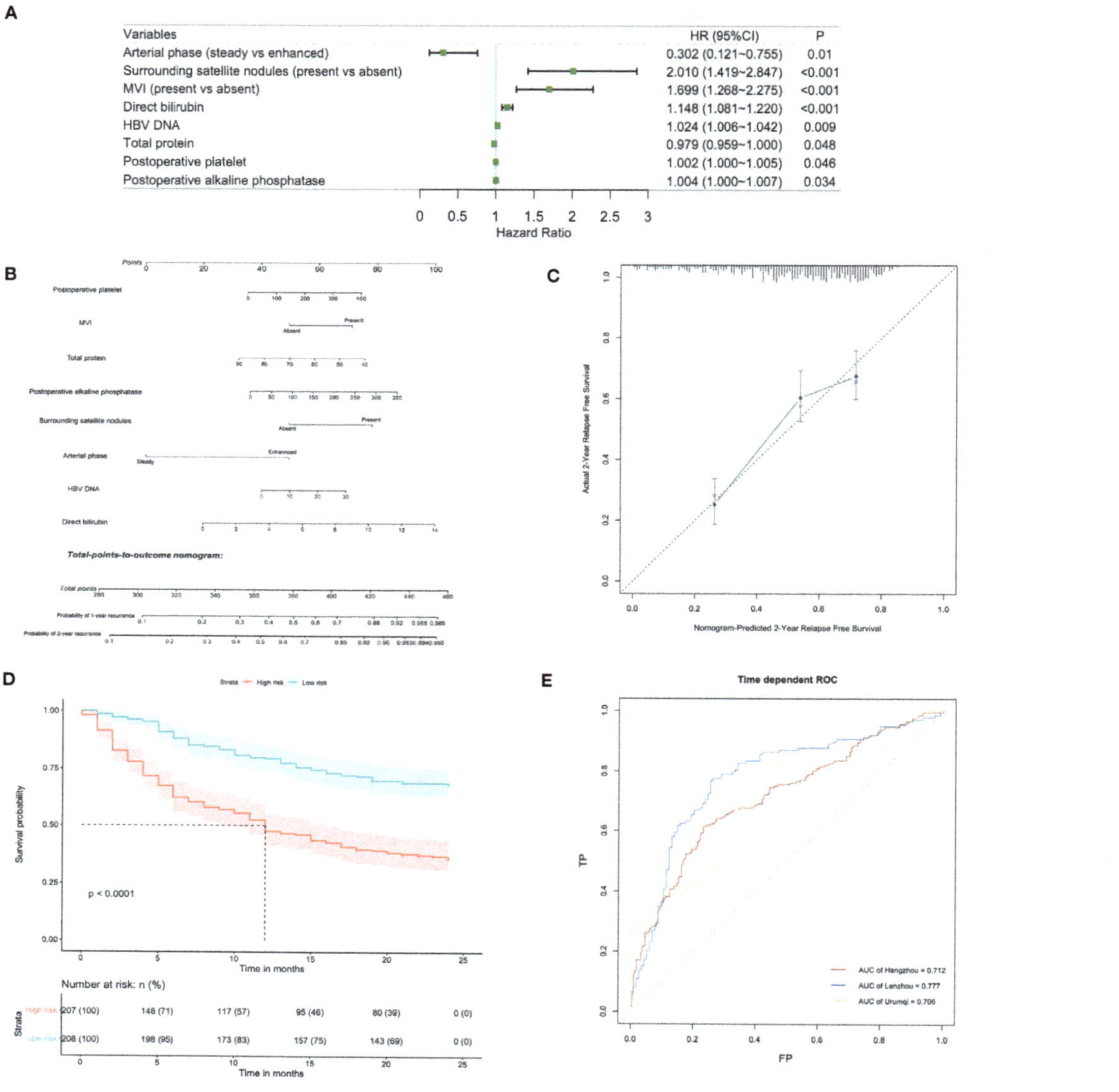

FIGURE 3 | Identification and validation of risk factors for early recurrence. **(A)** Forest plot of predictors for early recurrence based on the result of multivariate analysis. **(B)** Nomogram to predict probability of early recurrence. **(C)** Calibration curve for the nomogram to predict probability of early recurrence in the derivation cohort. **(D)** Kaplan-Meier survival curve (high-risk vs low-risk patients) for relapse-free survival in the derivation cohort. **(E)** Time-dependent receiver operating characteristic (ROC) curves for relapse-free survival at 2 years in the derivation and validation cohorts. Corresponding area under curves (AUC) in the Hangzhou, Lanzhou and Urumqi were 0.712, 0.777 and 0.706, respectively.

Nosocomial Infection Control (SENIC) index (41) and can be used in different predictive models for postsurgical complications (42, 43). Additionally, coagulation parameters in cancer patients that represent hemostatic and fibrinolytic systems have been proven to have association with tumor progression and dissemination (44). It has been reported that the decreased pretreatment TT was associated with the shorter esophageal squamous cell carcinoma (ESCC) and HCC survival (45, 46). Meanwhile, conventional coagulation tests after liver surgery are frequently prolonged by postoperative hypercoagulability (47), and prolonged TT before surgery indicated hyper-fibrinogenolysis, suggested as a factor that prevents the occurrence of thromboembolic complications. Other parameters that might influence perioperative complications have also been added to our models including tumor number, potassium, GGT, and TC. Although the CCIASL-pre model is applicable solely on the basis of preoperative parameters, it still appears comparable to the existing model. Despite a minor degree of discrepancy in the validation cohorts, good discriminatory performance was maintained in general. Furthermore, CCIASL-post model provides a more accurate prediction for clinicians when all postoperative indicators are available several days after

TABLE 5 | Selection of variables associated with tumor metastasis.

Variables	Multivariate GLM Selection				GEE Internal Validation				GEE External Validation			
	Coefficient	Standard Error	OR (95% CI)	P	Coefficient	Standard Error	OR (95% CI)	P	Coefficient	Standard Error	OR (95% CI)	P
Fasting blood glucose (mmol/L)	-0.387	0.166	0.679 (0.490-0.940)	0.020	-0.363	0.151	0.696 (0.518-0.934)	0.016				
Thrombin time (s)	-0.262	0.11	0.769 (0.620-0.954)	0.017	-0.261	0.109	0.771 (0.623-0.953)	0.016	-0.113	0.032	0.893 (0.839-0.951)	<0.001
Postoperative total protein (g/L)	0.079	0.025	1.082 (1.031-1.136)	0.001	0.076	0.038	1.079 (1.002-1.163)	0.045				
Intraoperative blood loss (mL)	0.001	<0.001	1.001 (1.000-1.002)	0.003								
Maximum tumor size (cm)	0.122	0.043	1.130 (1.038-1.229)	0.005								
Surrounding satellite nodules (yes vs no)	0.938	0.345	2.555 (1.299-5.026)	0.007	0.674	0.314	1.962 (1.060-3.630)	0.032				
Tumor encapsulation (absent vs complete)	1.156	0.442	3.178 (1.336-7.557)	0.009	1.414	0.388	4.111 (1.921-8.795)	<0.001	0.359	0.174	1.432 (1.019-2.013)	0.039

GLM, Generalized linear model; GEE, Generalized estimation equation; OR, Odds ratio; CI, Confidence interval.

operation. The CCIASL models are quite reliable because of external validation in different geographic regions.

Although the prediction models for early recurrence after liver resection of HCC had been built a lot (48–50), they are seldom derived from comprehensive candidate variables potentially relevant to HBV-related HCC. In our study, the third model for prediction of early recurrence of HCC was constructed by incorporating eight parameters from HBV-related marks, surgical conditions, pathological examination, preoperative and postoperative laboratory results. A high HBV-DNA load was identified to be an independent hepatitis-related risk for early recurrence (51, 52). In addition to HBV-related marks, the capability of laboratory findings and tumor characteristics was also evaluated in predicting early recurrence. An approach to risk stratification for early recurrence of HBV-related HCC was developed by incorporating serum AFP, tumor number, and largest tumor diameter based on the Chinese population (53). From a broader perspective of HCC studies, there is a consensus that microvascular invasion is a well-known independent prognostic factor associated with more advanced tumor stage, tumor progression, and poorer clinical outcome (54). Microvascular invasion is an essential component in the majority of current prediction models (55, 56). However, associations between these predictors were detected as well. A high HBV DNA level was an independent risk factor of microvascular invasion, and HBcAb-positive HCC was much bigger, more often involved with vascular invasion and elevated AFP (50, 56). In this case, if all possible clinical variables are not included in the candidates, it is impossible to determine the truly independent predictors. The predictive factors included in the model we built on the basis of comprehensive candidate variables are more likely to avoid this problem.

Another highlight of this article is that we discovered two significant risk factors for early metastasis, namely, short TT and absence of tumor encapsulation. Thrombin is a serine protease that performs a multifaceted role in coagulation. Previous analysis has revealed that the coagulation system has an effect on solid tumors, such as ESCC and HCC (45, 46). Zhu et al. (57) also reported that the abnormal coagulation system was an independent prognostic factor for brain metastases of non-small cell lung cancer, which is consistent with our findings in HCC. The potential mechanism may refer to the damage of liver cells, the secretion of tumor cells, and the involvement of inflammation (58, 59). Notably, capsulation of tumor was first discovered to be relevant with tumor migration.

There are still three points worth further discussion. First of all, no significant association was observed between CCI and early recurrence. Some variables included in the CCIASL models have been identified in the prediction for long-term complications but never short-term ones. In this setting, the effect of short-term complications on long-term complications still remains inconclusive. Our results provide an exploration for this topic, and no certain relationship is a preliminary conclusion. Secondly, the difference of discrimination performance between preoperative and postoperative model was insignificant according to reclassification analyses. The improvement of prediction accuracy based on postoperative data did not live up to the expectation. However, the C-index of the CCIASL-post model is much higher than that of the pre-model. Better performance is likely to be found in larger samples. Thirdly, antiviral treatment was excluded at univariable analysis of predicting high CCI, suggesting that reduction of HBV load seemed not to be helpful for prevention of severe complications. Despite a lot of evidence that long-term survival is correlated with antiviral therapy (51, 60), the association of short-term complications has never been discovered. Hence, antiviral treatment is likely to be difficult to improve clinical perioperative complications.

In summary, CCI is a well-performed measurement of postoperative complications. Our CCIASL models are clinically relevant, externally validated, and powerful tools to predict severe perioperative complications in patients with HBV-related HCC. Further prospective studies are required to explore the clinical applicability of CCIASL models in patient allocation for more frequent follow-up and clinical trials for adjuvant therapy.

AUTHOR CONTRIBUTIONS

MB and QZ contributed to the conceptualization, data curation and software, formal analysis, visualization, investigation, and writing-original draft. YH contributed to funding acquisition and project administration. XyH, TA, and SW contributed to the methodology. TT, XqH, and AT contributed to the resources and validation. MB contributed to the supervision. MB and YH contributed to the writing-review and editing. All authors contributed to the article and approved the submitted version.

REFERENCES

1. Sung H, Ferlay J, Siegel RL, Laversanne M, Soerjomataram I, Jemal A, et al. Global Cancer Statistics 2020: GLOBOCAN Estimates of Incidence and Mortality Worldwide for 36 Cancers in 185 Countries. *CA Cancer J Clin* (2021) 71(3):209–249. doi: 10.3322/caac.21660
2. Chen W, Zheng R, Baade PD, Zhang S, Zeng H, Bray F, et al. Cancer Statistics in China, 2015. *CA Cancer J Clin* (2016) 66(2):115–32. doi: 10.3322/caac.21338
3. Li M, Li J, Li P, Li H, Su T, Zhu R, et al. Hepatitis B Virus Infection Increases the Risk of Cholangiocarcinoma: A Meta-Analysis and Systematic Review. *J Gastroenterol Hepatol* (2012) 27(10):1561–8. doi: 10.1111/j.1440-1746.2012.07207.x
4. Zhou Y, Zhao Y, Li B, Huang J, Wu L, Xu D, et al. Hepatitis Viruses Infection and Risk of Intrahepatic Cholangiocarcinoma: Evidence From a Meta-Analysis. *BMC Cancer* (2012) 12:289. doi: 10.1186/1471-2407-12-289
5. Bruix J, Sherman M. Management of Hepatocellular Carcinoma: An Update. *Hepatology* (2011) 53(3):1020–2. doi: 10.1002/hep.24199
6. Bellissimo F, Pinzone MR, Cacopardo B, Nunnari G. Diagnostic and Therapeutic Management of Hepatocellular Carcinoma. *World J Gastroenterol* (2015) 21(42):12003–21. doi: 10.3748/wjg.v21.i42.12003
7. Rahbari NN, Garden OJ, Padbury R, Brooke-Smith M, Crawford M, Adam R, et al. Posthepatectomy Liver Failure: A Definition and Grading by the International Study Group of Liver Surgery (ISGLS). *Surgery* (2011) 149 (5):713–24. doi: 10.1016/j.surg.2010.10.001
8. Child CG, Turcotte JG. Surgery and Portal Hypertension. *Major Probl Clin Surg* (1964) 1:1–85.
9. Vauthey JN, Chaoui A, Do KA, Bilimoria MM, Fenstermacher MJ, Charnsangavej C, et al. Standardized Measurement of the Future Liver Remnant Prior to Extended Liver Resection: Methodology and Clinical Associations. *Surgery* (2000) 127(5):512–9. doi: 10.1067/msy.2000.105294
10. Cholongitas E, Marelli L, Shusang V, Senzolo M, Rolles K, Patch D, et al. A Systematic Review of the Performance of the Model for End-Stage Liver Disease (MELD) in the Setting of Liver Transplantation. *Liver Transpl* (2006) 12(7):1049–61. doi: 10.1002/lt.20824
11. Hiraoka A, Kumada T, Michitaka K, Kudo M. Newly Proposed ALBI Grade and ALBI-T Score as Tools for Assessment of Hepatic Function and Prognosis in Hepatocellular Carcinoma Patients. *Liver Cancer* (2019) 8(5):312–25. doi: 10.1159/000494844
12. Johnson PJ, Berhane S, Kagebayashi C, Satomura S, Teng M, Reeves HL, et al. Assessment of Liver Function in Patients With Hepatocellular Carcinoma: A New Evidence-Based Approach-the ALBI Grade. *J Clin Oncol* (2015) 33 (6):550–8. doi: 10.1200/JCO.2014.57.9151
13. Huo TI, Lin HC, Huo SC, Lee PC, Wu JC, Lee FY, et al. Comparison of Four Model for End-Stage Liver Disease-Based Prognostic Systems for Cirrhosis. *Liver Transpl* (2008) 14(6):837–44. doi: 10.1002/lt.21439
14. Dinant S, de Graaf W, Verwer BJ, Bennink RJ, van Lienden KP, Gouma DJ, et al. Risk Assessment of Posthepatectomy Liver Failure Using Hepatobiliary Scintigraphy and CT Volumetry. *J Nucl Med* (2007) 48(5):685–92. doi: 10.2967/jnumed.106.038430
15. Hirai I, Kimura W, Fuse A, Suto K, Urayama M. Evaluation of Preoperative Portal Embolization for Safe Hepatectomy, With Special Reference to Assessment of Nonembolized Lobe Function With 99mtc-GSA SPECT Scintigraphy. *Surgery* (2003) 133(5):495–506. doi: 10.1067/msy.2003.138
16. Marasco G, Colecchia A, Colli A, Ravaioli F, Casazza G, Bacchi Reggiani ML, et al. Role of Liver and Spleen Stiffness in Predicting the Recurrence of Hepatocellular Carcinoma After Resection. *J Hepatol* (2019) 70(3):440–8. doi: 10.1016/j.jhep.2018.10.022
17. Rajakannu M, Cherqui D, Ciacio O, Golse N, Pittau G, Allard MA, et al. Liver Stiffness Measurement by Transient Elastography Predicts Late Posthepatectomy Outcomes in Patients Undergoing Resection for Hepatocellular Carcinoma. *Surgery* (2017) 162(4):766–74. doi: 10.1016/j.surg.2017.06.006
18. Serenari M, Han KH, Ravaioli F, Kim SU, Cucchetti A, Han DH, et al. A Nomogram Based on Liver Stiffness Predicts Postoperative Complications in Patients With Hepatocellular Carcinoma. *J Hepatol* (2020) 73(4):855–62. doi: 10.1016/j.jhep.2020.04.032
19. Clavien PA, Barkun J, de Oliveira ML, Vauthey JN, Dindo D, Schulick RD, et al. The Clavien-Dindo Classification of Surgical Complications: Five-Year Experience. *Ann Surg* (2009) 250(2):187–96. doi: 10.1097/SLA.0b013e3181b13ca2
20. Slankamenac K, Graf R, Barkun J, Puhan MA, Clavien PA. The Comprehensive Complication Index: A Novel Continuous Scale to Measure Surgical Morbidity. *Ann Surg* (2013) 258(1):1–7. doi: 10.1097/SLA.0b013e318296c732
21. Clavien PA, Vetter D, Staiger RD, Slankamenac K, Mehra T, Graf R, et al. The Comprehensive Complication Index (CCI®): Added Value and Clinical Perspectives 3 Years "Down the Line". *Ann Surg* (2017) 265(6):1045–50. doi: 10.1097/SLA.0000000000002132
22. Cucchetti A, Piscaglia F, Caturelli E, Benvegnù L, Vivarelli M, Ercolani G, et al. Comparison of Recurrence of Hepatocellular Carcinoma After Resection in Patients With Cirrhosis to Its Occurrence in a Surveilled Cirrhotic Population. *Ann Surg Oncol* (2009) 16(2):413–22. doi: 10.1245/s10434-008-0232-4
23. European Association For The Study Of The Liver, European Organisation For Research And Treatment Of Cancer. EASL-EORTC Clinical Practice Guidelines: Management of Hepatocellular Carcinoma. *J Hepatol* (2012) 56 (4):908–43. doi: 10.1016/j.jhep.2011.12.001
24. Chan AW, Chan SL, Wong GL, Wong VW, Chong CC, Lai PB, et al. Prognostic Nutritional Index (PNI) Predicts Tumor Recurrence of Very Early/Early Stage Hepatocellular Carcinoma After Surgical Resection. *Ann Surg Oncol* (2015) 22(13):4138–48. doi: 10.1245/s10434-015-4516-1
25. Gupta GP, Massagué J. Cancer Metastasis: Building a Framework. *Cell* (2006) 127(4):679–95. doi: 10.1016/j.cell.2006.11.001
26. Witjes CD, Willemssen FE, Verheij J, van der Veer SJ, Hansen BE, Verhoef C, et al. Histological Differentiation Grade and Microvascular Invasion of Hepatocellular Carcinoma Predicted by Dynamic Contrast-Enhanced MRI. *J Magn Reson Imaging* (2012) 36(3):641–7. doi: 10.1002/jmri.23681
27. Kim MJ, Lee M, Choi JY, Park YN. Imaging Features of Small Hepatocellular Carcinomas With Microvascular Invasion on Gadoxetic Acid-Enhanced MR Imaging. *Eur J Radiol* (2012) 81(10):2507–12. doi: 10.1016/j.ejrad.2011.11.014
28. Choi YS, Rhee H, Choi JY, Chung YE, Park YN, Kim KW, et al. Histological Characteristics of Small Hepatocellular Carcinomas Showing Atypical Enhancement Patterns on Gadoxetic Acid-Enhanced MR Imaging. *J Magn Reson Imaging* (2013) 37(6):1384–91. doi: 10.1002/jmri.23940
29. Yamashita S, Sheth RA, Niekamp AS, Aloia TA, Chun YS, Lee JE, et al. Comprehensive Complication Index Predicts Cancer-Specific Survival After Resection of Colorectal Metastases Independent of RAS Mutational Status. *Ann Surg* (2017) 266(6):1045–54. doi: 10.1097/SLA.0000000000002018
30. Chan AWH, Zhong J, Berhane S, Toyoda H, Cucchetti A, Shi K, et al. Development of Pre and Post-Operative Models to Predict Early Recurrence of Hepatocellular Carcinoma After Surgical Resection. *J Hepatol* (2018) 69(6):1284–93. doi: 10.1016/j.jhep.2018.08.027

31. European Association for the Study of the Liver. EASL Clinical Practice Guidelines: Management of Hepatocellular Carcinoma. *J Hepatol* (2018) 69 (1):182–236. doi: 10.1016/j.jhep.2018.03.019
32. Pencina MJ, D'Agostino RBR, Steyerberg EW. Extensions of Net Reclassification Improvement Calculations to Measure Usefulness of New Biomarkers. *Stat Med* (2011) 30(1):11–21. doi: 10.1002/sim.4085
33. Hosmer DW, Hosmer T, Le Cessie S, Lemeshow S. A Comparison of Goodness-of-Fit Tests for the Logistic Regression Model. *Stat Med* (1997) 16(9):965–80. doi: 10.1002/(SICI)1097-0258(19970515)16:9<965::AID-SIM509>3.0.CO;2-O
34. Mehrabi A, Golriz M, Khajeh E, Ghamarnejad O, Probst P, Fonouni H, et al. Meta-Analysis of the Prognostic Role of Perioperative Platelet Count in Posthepatectomy Liver Failure and Mortality. *Br J Surg* (2018) 105 (10):1254–61. doi: 10.1002/bjs.10906
35. Singh S, Muir AJ, Dieterich DT, Falck-Ytter YT. American Gastroenterological Association Institute Technical Review on the Role of Elastography in Chronic Liver Diseases. *Gastroenterology* (2017) 152 (6):1544–77. doi: 10.1053/j.gastro.2017.03.016
36. Bae JS, Lee DH, Yi NJ, Lee KW, Suh KS, Kim H, et al. Magnetic Resonance Elastography Versus Transient Elastography in the Prediction of Complications After Resection for Hepatocellular Carcinoma. *Ann Surg* (2020). doi: 10.1097/SLA.0000000000004576
37. European Association for Study of Liver, Asociacion Latinoamericana para el Estudio del Higado. EASL-ALEH Clinical Practice Guidelines: Non-Invasive Tests for Evaluation of Liver Disease Severity and Prognosis. *J Hepatol* (2015) 63(1):237–64. doi: 10.1016/j.jhep.2015.04.006
38. Wong GL, Chan HL, Choi PC, Chan AW, Lo AO, Chim AM, et al. Association Between Anthropometric Parameters and Measurements of Liver Stiffness by Transient Elastography. *Clin Gastroenterol Hepatol* (2013) 11(3):295–302.e1-3. doi: 10.1016/j.cgh.2012.09.025
39. Viganò M, Massironi S, Lampertico P, Iavarone M, Paggi S, Pozzi R, et al. Transient Elastography Assessment of the Liver Stiffness Dynamics During Acute Hepatitis B. *Eur J Gastroenterol Hepatol* (2010) 22(2):180–4. doi: 10.1097/MEG.0b013e328332d2fa
40. Horan TC, Gaynes RP, Martone WJ, Jarvis WR, Emori TG. CDC Definitions of Nosocomial Surgical Site Infections, 1992: A Modification of CDC Definitions of Surgical Wound Infections. *Am J Infect Control* (1992) 20 (5):271–4. doi: 10.1016/S0196-6553(05)80201-9
41. Emori TG, Culver DH, Horan TC, Jarvis WR, White JW, Olson DR, et al. National Nosocomial Infections Surveillance System (NNIS): Description of Surveillance Methods. *Am J Infect Control* (1991) 19(1):19–35. doi: 10.1016/0196-6553(91)90157-8
42. Del Toro MD, Peñas C, Conde-Albarracín A, Palomino J, Brun F, Sánchez S, et al. Development and Validation of Baseline, Perioperative and at-Discharge Predictive Models for Postsurgical Prosthetic Joint Infection. *Clin Microbiol Infect* (2019) 25(2):196–202. doi: 10.1016/j.cmi.2018.04.023
43. Shen Z, Lin Y, Ye Y, Jiang K, Xie Q, Gao Z, et al. The Development and Validation of a Novel Model for Predicting Surgical Complications in Colorectal Cancer of Elderly Patients: Results From 1008 Cases. *Eur J Surg Oncol* (2018) 44(4):490–5. doi: 10.1016/j.ejso.2018.01.007
44. McAlister RK, Ito S. Minimal Prolongation of Prothrombin Time With Extended Exposure to Argatroban. *Pharmacotherapy* (2015) 35(7):e122–6. doi: 10.1002/phar.1613
45. Li XH, Wang XP, Gu WS, Lin JH, Huang H, Kang T, et al. Clinical Significance of Preoperative Thrombin Time in Patients With Esophageal Squamous Cell Carcinoma Following Surgical Resection. *PLoS One* (2015) 10 (10):e0140323. doi: 10.1371/journal.pone.0140323
46. Wang XP, Mao MJ, He ZL, Zhang L, Chi PD, Su JR, et al. A Retrospective Discussion of the Prognostic Value of Combining Prothrombin Time(PT) and Fibrinogen(Fbg) in Patients With Hepatocellular Carcinoma. *J Cancer* (2017) 8 (11):2079–87. doi: 10.7150/jca.19181
47. Mahla E, Lang T, Vicenzi MN, Werkgartner G, Maier R, Probst C, et al. Thromboelastography for Monitoring Prolonged Hypercoagulability After Major Abdominal Surgery. *Anesth Analg* (2001) 92(3):572–7. doi: 10.1213/00000539-200103000-00004
48. Zhang Z, Jiang H, Chen J, Wei Y, Cao L, Ye Z, et al. Hepatocellular Carcinoma: Radiomics Nomogram on Gadoxetic Acid-Enhanced MR Imaging for Early Postoperative Recurrence Prediction. *Cancer Imaging* (2019) 19(1):22. doi: 10.1186/s40644-019-0209-5
49. Xing H, Zhang WG, Cescon M, Liang L, Li C, Wang MD, et al. Defining and Predicting Early Recurrence After Liver Resection of Hepatocellular Carcinoma: A Multi-Institutional Study. *HPB (Oxford)* (2020) 22(5):677–89. doi: 10.1016/j.hpb.2019.09.006
50. Saito A, Toyoda H, Kobayashi M, Koiwa Y, Fujii H, Fujita K, et al. Prediction of Early Recurrence of Hepatocellular Carcinoma After Resection Using Digital Pathology Images Assessed by Machine Learning. *Mod Pathol* (2021) 34(2):417–25. doi: 10.1038/s41379-020-00671-z
51. Li Z, Lei Z, Xia Y, Li J, Wang K, Zhang H, et al. Association of Preoperative Antiviral Treatment With Incidences of Microvascular Invasion and Early Tumor Recurrence in Hepatitis B Virus-Related Hepatocellular Carcinoma. *JAMA Surg* (2018) 153(10):e182721. doi: 10.1001/jamasurg.2018.2721
52. Sohn W, Paik YH, Kim JM, Kwon CH, Joh JW, Cho JY, et al. HBV DNA and HBsAg Levels as Risk Predictors of Early and Late Recurrence After Curative Resection of HBV-Related Hepatocellular Carcinoma. *Ann Surg Oncol* (2014) 21(7):2429–35. doi: 10.1245/s10434-014-3621-x
53. Al-Ameri AAM, Wei X, Lin L, Shao Z, Guo H, Xie H, et al. Preoperative Risk Stratification for Early Recurrence of HBV-Related Hepatocellular Carcinoma After Deceased Donor Liver Transplantation: A Five-Eight Model Development and Validation. *BMC Cancer* (2019) 19(1):1136. doi: 10.1186/s12885-019-6343-4
54. Zhang X, Li J, Shen F, Lau WY. Significance of Presence of Microvascular Invasion in Specimens Obtained After Surgical Treatment of Hepatocellular Carcinoma. *J Gastroenterol Hepatol* (2018) 33(2):347–54. doi: 10.1111/jgh.13843
55. Lei Z, Li J, Wu D, Xia Y, Wang Q, Si A, et al. Nomogram for Preoperative Estimation of Microvascular Invasion Risk in Hepatitis B Virus-Related Hepatocellular Carcinoma Within the Milan Criteria. *JAMA Surg* (2016) 151(4):356–63. doi: 10.1001/jamasurg.2015.4257
56. Shim JH, Jun MJ, Han S, Lee YJ, Lee SG, Kim KM, et al. Prognostic Nomograms for Prediction of Recurrence and Survival After Curative Liver Resection for Hepatocellular Carcinoma. *Ann Surg* (2015) 261(5):939–46. doi: 10.1097/SLA.0000000000000747
57. Zhu JF, Cai L, Zhang XW, Wen YS, Su XD, Rong TH, et al. High Plasma Fibrinogen Concentration and Platelet Count Unfavorably Impact Survival in Non-Small Cell Lung Cancer Patients With Brain Metastases. *Chin J Cancer* (2014) 33(2):96–104. doi: 10.5732/cjc.012.10307
58. Aytac S, Turkay C, Bavbek N, Kosar A. Hemostasis and Global Fibrinolytic Capacity in Chronic Liver Disease. *Blood Coagul Fibrinolysis* (2007) 18 (7):623–6. doi: 10.1097/MBC.0b013e328285d80e
59. Rak J, Milsom C, May L, Klement P, Yu J. Tissue Factor in Cancer and Angiogenesis: The Molecular Link Between Genetic Tumor Progression, Tumor Neovascularization, and Cancer Coagulopathy. *Semin Thromb Hemost* (2006) 32(1):54–70. doi: 10.1055/s-2006-933341
60. Chen ZX, Jian ZW, Wu XW, Wang JC, Peng JY, Lao XM. Clinical Conditions and Treatment Requirements for Long-Term Survival Among Hepatitis B-Related Hepatocellular Carcinoma Initially Treated With Chemoembolization. *Cancer Med* (2019) 8(11):5097–107. doi: 10.1002/cam4.2380

20

Stereotactic Body Radiotherapy vs. Radiofrequency Ablation in the Treatment of Hepatocellular Carcinoma

Yang-Xun Pan [1,2,3], Yi-Zhen Fu [1,2], Dan-Dan Hu [1,2], Qian Long [1,4], Jun-Cheng Wang [1,2], Mian Xi [1,5], Shi-Liang Liu [1,4], Li Xu [1,2], Meng-Zhong Liu [1,4], Min-Shan Chen [1,2] and Yao-Jun Zhang [1,2]*

[1] Sun Yat-sen University Cancer Center, State Key Laboratory of Oncology in South China, Collaborative Innovation Center for Cancer Medicine, Guangzhou, China, [2] Department of Liver Surgery, Sun Yat-sen University Cancer Center, Guangzhou, China, [3] Department of Oncology-Pathology, Karolinska Institutet, Stockholm, Sweden, [4] Department of Experimental Research, Sun Yat-sen University Cancer Center, Guangzhou, China, [5] Department of Radiation Oncology, Sun Yat-sen University Cancer Center, Guangzhou, China

***Correspondence:**
Yao-Jun Zhang
zhangyuj@sysucc.org.cn

Background: Both stereotactic body radiotherapy (SBRT) and radiofrequency ablation (RFA) are effective local treatments for hepatocellular carcinoma (HCC), but whether RFA is superior to SBRT is still controversial. Therefore, we performed a meta-analysis to compare the treatment outcomes of SBRT with RFA as curable or bridge intention.

Methods: We searched online databases for studies that compared treatment outcomes for SBRT and RFA. Eligibility criteria included evaluation of local control, overall survival (OS), transplant rate, and post-transplant pathological necrosis.

Results: As no randomized clinical trials met the criteria, 10 retrospective studies with a total of 2,732 patients were included. Two studies were in favor of SBRT in local control, two studies preferred RFA in OS, and others reported comparable outcomes for both. SBRT demonstrated significantly higher 1- and 3-year local control than RFA [odds ratio (OR) 0.42, 95% CI 0.24–0.74, $P = 0.003$; and OR 0.54, 95% CI 0.37–0.80, $P = 0.002$, respectively]. However, SBRT reported significantly shorter 1- and 2-year OS (OR 1.52, 95% CI 1.21–1.90, $P = 0.0003$; and OR 1.66, 95% CI 1.38–2.01, $P < 0.00001$, respectively). As bridge treatment, no significant difference was shown in transplant rate and post-transplant pathological necrosis rate (OR 0.57, 95% CI 0.32–1.03, $P = 0.060$; and OR 0.49, 95% CI 0.13–1.82, $P = 0.290$, respectively).

Conclusions: This study demonstrates SBRT is able to complete a better local control for HCC than RFA, though the OS is inferior to RFA because of tumor burden or liver profiles of the enrolled studies. Well-designed, randomized, multicenter trials will be required to further investigate the conclusion.

Keywords: minimally invasive treatment, meta-analysis, hepatocellular carcinoma, stereotactic body radiotherapy, radiofrequency ablation

INTRODUCTION

Liver transplantation is the most beneficial therapy for early hepatocellular carcinoma (HCC) patients, as it removes both the tumor and the cirrhotic liver (1). However, given organ availability limitation, a number of patients who may benefit from this treatment have to stay on the waiting list for a long time. Therefore, stereotactic body radiotherapy (SBRT) and radiofrequency ablation (RFA) are offered as potential alternative local control modalities for patients in the waiting list (2, 3).

RFA induces coagulative necrosis of tumor through thermal effect and is the first-line treatment for small HCC ($\leq$3 cm), providing comparable long-term outcome with resection (4). However, RFA has several contraindications, including large tumor size and lesions adjacent to major vessels or close to the liver hilum. The above circumstances may result in incomplete ablation, which potentially leads to worse prognosis (5–9).

SBRT is an advanced technology that delivers ablative radiation doses to tumors in a few fractions while minimizing the dose to normal liver tissue. Early results with SBRT have shown considerable local control even for large tumors or HCC ineligible for surgery (10). Moreover, SBRT has been frequently used as an alternative to RFA for small HCC patients with tumors near critical anatomical structures or major vessels due to the heat sink effect that can occur with RFA (11).

Recent publications have reported either comparable outcomes between the two treatment modalities or favorable outcomes for one to the other (3, 10, 12–19). Most of the published studies retrospectively reviewed clinical data in one single center; the results of these observational studies could have been strongly affected by several biases, and hence, the efficacy of these two treatments regarding disease control, long-term survival, and treatment related complications is ununified. With the absence of randomized data, meta-analysis might be able to draw a relative objective and reliable conclusion by integrating data from different clinical centers. The aim of this meta-analysis is mainly to compare the benefits of SBRT and RFA in the local progression (LP) control and overall survival (OS) in the treatment for HCC and to further help in clinical decision making.

MATERIALS AND METHODS

Study Selection

The inclusion criteria of this meta-analysis were as follows: (1) diagnosed primary liver cancer definitively and patients diagnosed with HCC based on pathological evidence from fine-needle aspiration (FNA) or in the absence of biopsy evidence, based on imaging techniques including contrast-enhanced ultrasonography (CEUS), computed tomography (CT), and magnetic resonance imaging (MRI) companied with alpha-fetoprotein elevation; (2) no evidence of invasion into the major portal/hepatic vein branches or extrahepatic metastasis based on radiologic imaging; (3) patients without previous treatment of transcatheter arterial chemoembolization (TACE), surgery, chemotherapy, or other antitumor treatment; (4) documented indications for SBRT and RFA clearly; (5) either randomized controlled trials (RCTs) or retrospective studies were candidates; (6) patients of two groups with comparable basic clinical characters; and (7) studies with outcome information regarding LP rates, OS rates, and/or transplant rates.

Studies with following characteristics were excluded: (1) studies that did not report original data, including abstracts, case reports, expert opinions, editorials, reviews, or letters; (2) either group in the studies or combined other therapies; and (3) studies based on the same cohort.

Search Strategy

A systematic online databases search of PubMed Central, Embase, Cochrane Library, and Google Scholar was separately conducted by two reviewers to identify all relevant availability of studies until August 26, 2019.

This meta-analysis was performed consistent with the Preferred Reporting Items for Systematic Reviews and Meta-Analyses (PRISMA) statement checklist. The subject headings (MeSH) search included "radiofrequency ablation," "stereotactic radiation therapy," and "hepatocellular carcinoma"; and keywords search was used, including "radiofrequency ablation," "stereotactic body radiation therapy," and "hepatocellular carcinoma." These terms were used in different combinations. Only studies on humans and English-language studies were included. A manual research was performed by browsing all references of all identified studies. This progressed research was repeated to ensure to include the whole relevant studies. The research was completed by two reviewers before the data analysis independently (Y-XP and MX). If a study was controversial, the corresponding author was asked to judge (Y-JZ).

Data Collection

Data were extracted from the included studies, including number of patients in the SBRT and RFA groups; age; gender; primary tumor size; number of tumors; median dose of SBRT; Child–Pugh class; median follow-up time; 1-, 2-, and 3-year LP rates; 1-, 2-, 3-, and 5-year OS rates; post-transplant necrosis rates; and time to liver transplant.

Definitions

LP was defined as the recurrence of lesion in the treatment area by imaging studies. And LP time was the period from the initial treatment to the discovery of LP or last follow-up. The OS was defined the period from the date of initial treatment of the HCC to the date of death related to any cause or last follow-up. Transplant rate was the proportion of patients who received liver transplantation after SBRT or RFA therapies. Post-transplant pathological necrosis was evaluated by post-transplant pathology.

Statistical Analysis and Synthesis

All analyses were performed with the help of statistical software, named Review Manager, version 5.3 (Nordic Cochrane Center; Oxford, England). For data evaluation, patients were assigned into two groups: the SBRT-treated group and the RFA-treated group. The odds ratio (OR) and/or hazard ratios (HRs) accompanying 95% confidence interval (95% CI) were calculated for dichotomous and univariable analysis outcomes in terms

TABLE 1 | Characteristics of include studies.

References	Design	Group	Number of patients	Number of tumor (1/≥2)	Age (years)	Sex (M/F)	Tumor size (cm)	Median dose (Gy)	Child-Pugh class (A/B/C)	Median follow up (months)
Mohamed et al. (16) (American)	Non-RCT	SBRT	23	14/9	57.5 (44–70.2)	20/3	NR	50 (45–60)	17/0/5	41 (7.3–77.9)
		RFA	9	8/1	57.5 (44–70.2)	8/1	NR		9/0/0	41 (7.3–77.9)
Wahl et al. (10) (American)	Non-RCT	SBRT	63	49/14*	62 (35–85)	54/9*	2.2 (0–10)	50 (27–60)	43/18/2*	27 (0.5–86.5)*
		RFA	161	109/52*	60 (31–81)	117/44*	1.8 (0.6–7.0)		80/68/13*	50.9 (3.5–112.8)*
Sapisochin et al. (3) (Canada)	Non-RCT	SBRT	36	17/19*	60.4 (56.4–64.8)	30/5	4.5 (2.9–5.8)*	36 (30–40)	22/14/0*	28.1 (14.9–64.7)*
		RFA	244	156/88*	57.8 (53.5–62)	208/36	2.5 (1.9–3)*		158/68/8*	52.2 (21–90.7)*
Hara et al. (21) (Japan)	Non-RCT	SBRT	106	94/12	74 (48–93)	71/35	1.8 (1.0–3.0)	37.5 (35–40)	104/2/0	33.7 (0.5–75.0)
		RFA	106	93/13	75 (47–88)	76/30	1.7 (0.7–2.8)		105/1/0	29.9 (6.0–72.8)
Berger et al. (19) (American)	Non-RCT	SBRT	157	NR	68.61 (11.74)	113/44	4.8 (4.8)	NR	NR	NR
		RFA	627	NR	68.21 (10.00)	454/173	4.2 (4.6)		NR	NR
Duan et al. (22) (China)	Non-RCT	SBRT	37	NR	NR	NR	1–5	NR	NR	NR
		RFA	40	NR	NR	NR	1–5		NR	NR
Kim et al. (17) (Korea)	Non-RCT	SBRT	95	95/0	63.0 (35.0–85.0)	80/15	2.4 (0.7–5.5)	60 (52–60)	90/5/0	21.9 (11.8–31.2)
		RFA	95	95/0	67.0 (40.0–86.0)	83/12	2.1 (0.8–4.6)		90/5/0	21.6 (11.1–37.3)
Rajyaguru et al. (15) (American)	Non-RCT	SBRT	275	190/85	65 (55–75)	194/81	2.5 (2.5–3.5)	45 (45–55)	NR	25.3 (14.1–41.0)
		RFA	521	349/172	65 (55–75)	381/140	2.5 (2.5–3.5)		NR	25.3 (14.1–41.0)
Shiozawa et al. (16) (Japan)	Non-RCT	SBRT	35	35/0	75.1 (67–83)*	24/11	2.86 (1.2–5)*	50.6 (7.8)	28/7/0	12.6 (6.8–35.5)*
		RFA	38	38/0	68.7 (42–86)*	27/11	1.75 (0.7–2.9)*		31/7/0	18.7 (7.4–40.8)*
Parikh et al. (13) (American)	Non-RCT	SBRT	32	NR	77 (72–81.25)	20/12	NR	NR	NR	NR
		RFA	32	NR	79 (76–82)	22/10	NR		NR	NR
Total		SBRT	859							
		RFA	1,873							

*SBRT, stereotactic body radiotherapy; RFA, radiofrequency ablation; NR, not reported; RCT, randomized controlled trial. *Statistically significant ($P < 0.05$).*

of LP, OS, and prognostic factor on treatment allocation. Meanwhile, we assessed the heterogeneity among trials according to the chi-squared (χ^2) test including the inconsistency factor (I^2). The heterogeneity was defined as a $P < 0.05$ or an $I^2 > 40\%$ (20). Given the small number of included studies, though the heterogeneity was not high, the random effects model was applied throughout to enhance the reliability of results. A potential publication bias was assessed by visually inspecting the Begg funnel plots in which the standard error (SE) of log OR or log HR was plotted against the OR or HR, respectively.

RESULTS

Search Results and Quality Assessment

A total of 440 studies were identified for the first time from PubMed by the search strategy previously established, and 269 studies were identified *via* other sources or review. Subsequently, 11 studies were deleted for duplication with the help of Mendeley (Elsevier Inc., Atlanta, GA, USA). The titles and abstracts of 270 studies were then screened for inclusion. The full texts of 36 studies were read; and, finally, we included 10 non-RCT studies that met the present meta-analysis criteria (3, 10, 13–16, 18, 19, 21, 22). The details of the PRISMA flow diagram of the literature for meta-analysis is shown in **Supplementary Figure 1** (23).

In the present analysis, three studies were based on already existing database (13, 15, 19), and the remaining seven studies were based on retrospective studies (3, 10, 16–18, 21, 22). Two studies conducted SBRT or RFA for transplant intent. Five studies were performed in the USA (10, 13, 15, 18, 19), two in Japan (12, 16), one in Canada (3), one in South Korea (17), and one in China (22). Out of 2,732 patients from the 10 included studies, 859 patients were classified into the SBRT group, and the rest of the 1,873 patients were classified into the RFA group. The Newcastle Ottawa Scale (NOS) (24) were used to assess the quality of non-randomized studies. Although the qualities of selections and outcomes were relatively appropriate in terms of each study, over 50% of included studies were medium-score studies because of inconsistent comparability. Therefore, we believed that the present meta-analysis possesses a medium class of quality (**Supplementary Table 1**).

Among included studies, two studies were in favor of SBRT on local control (10, 21), two studies preferred RFA on OS (15, 19), and others reported comparable outcomes between groups (3, 13, 16–18, 22). Notably, according to baseline characteristics, several studies enrolled patients in SBRT group were prone to suffer from larger tumor diameter (3, 10, 16, 19) and higher proportion of Child–Pugh C patients [(18); **Table 1**]. These groups were evaluated for therapeutic efficacy in treating HCC patients. The details of the studies included in the present meta-analysis are listed in **Table 1**.

Local Progression Rates

Six out of the 10 studies illustrated 1-, 2-, and 3-year LP rates (10, 16–18, 21, 22). Our pooled results showed that the SBRT

Study or Subgroup	SBRT Events	SBRT Total	RFA Events	RFA Total	Weight	Odds Ratio M-H, Random, 95% CI
Duan 2016	2	37	4	40	10.6%	0.51 [0.09, 2.99]
Kim 2019	15	95	23	95	62.7%	0.59 [0.28, 1.21]
Mohamed 2016	2	23	2	9	7.2%	0.33 [0.04, 2.83]
Shiozawa 2015	1	35	1	38	4.2%	1.09 [0.07, 18.09]
Wahl 2016	2	63	27	161	15.3%	0.16 [0.04, 0.71]
Total (95% CI)		**253**		**343**	**100.0%**	**0.47 [0.26, 0.83]**
Total events	22		57			

Heterogeneity: Tau² = 0.00; Chi² = 2.93, df = 4 (P = 0.57); I² = 0%
Test for overall effect: Z = 2.59 (P = 0.010)

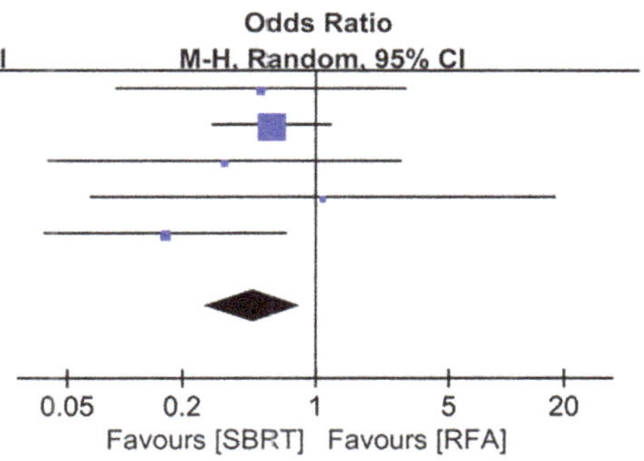

Study or Subgroup	SBRT Events	SBRT Total	RFA Events	RFA Total	Weight	Odds Ratio M-H, Random, 95% CI
Duan 2016	3	37	6	40	9.2%	0.50 [0.12, 2.16]
Kim 2019	24	95	33	95	50.3%	0.64 [0.34, 1.19]
Shiozawa 2015	3	35	4	38	8.0%	0.80 [0.17, 3.84]
Wahl 2016	10	63	32	161	32.5%	0.76 [0.35, 1.66]
Total (95% CI)		**230**		**334**	**100.0%**	**0.67 [0.43, 1.05]**
Total events	40		75			

Heterogeneity: Tau² = 0.00; Chi² = 0.33, df = 3 (P = 0.95); I² = 0%
Test for overall effect: Z = 1.76 (P = 0.08)

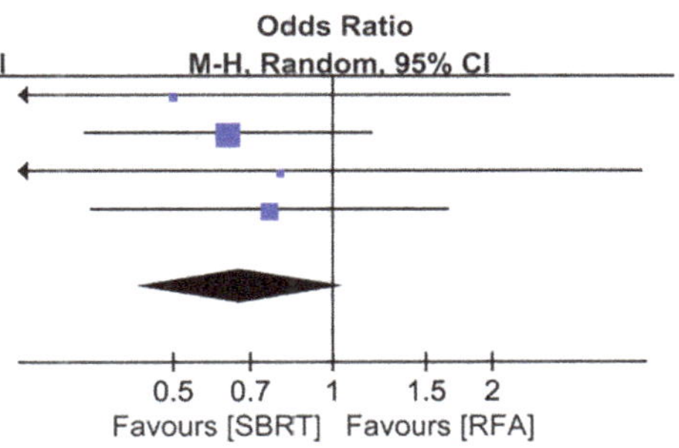

Study or Subgroup	SBRT Events	SBRT Total	RFA Events	RFA Total	Weight	Odds Ratio M-H, Random, 95% CI
Duan 2016	4	37	7	40	9.0%	0.57 [0.15, 2.14]
Hara 2019	7	106	21	106	19.2%	0.29 [0.12, 0.71]
Kim 2019	32	95	40	95	45.1%	0.70 [0.39, 1.26]
Wahl 2016	10	63	40	161	26.8%	0.57 [0.27, 1.23]
Total (95% CI)		**301**		**402**	**100.0%**	**0.55 [0.37, 0.81]**
Total events	53		108			

Heterogeneity: Tau² = 0.00; Chi² = 2.66, df = 3 (P = 0.45); I² = 0%
Test for overall effect: Z = 2.98 (P = 0.003)

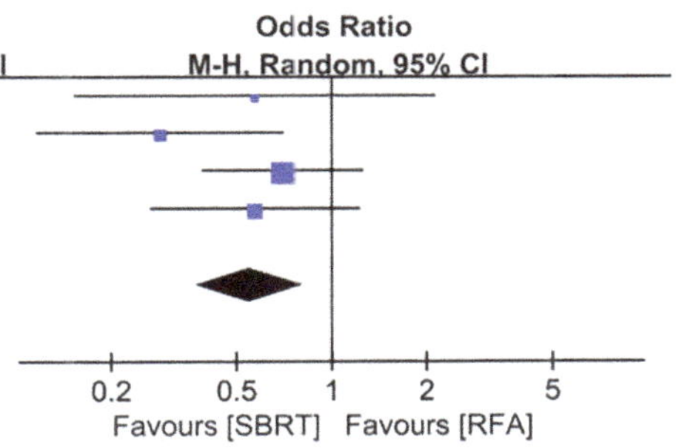

FIGURE 1 | Forest plots demonstrating 1-, 2-, and 3-year LP in SBRT and RFA for HCC. LP, local progression; SBRT, stereotactic body radiotherapy; RFA, radiofrequency ablation; HCC, hepatocellular carcinoma.

group had significantly better 1- and 3-year local control rates than the RFA group (OR 0.47, 95% CI 0.26–0.83, $P = 0.010$; and OR 0.55, 95% CI 0.37–0.81, $P = 0.003$, respectively). However, the 2-year LP rate showed marginal benefit of SBRT group than the RFA group (OR 0.67, 95% CI 0.43–1.05, $P = 0.080$). No heterogeneity was shown among the studies of 1-, 2-, and 3-year LP rates ($\chi^2 = 2.93$, $I^2 = 0\%$; $\chi^2 = 0.33$, $I^2 = 0\%$; and $\chi^2 = 2.66$, $I^2 = 0\%$, respectively) (**Figure 1**).

Overall Survival

Nine studies with 2,700 patients compared OS rates of SBRT group with RFA group (3, 10, 13, 15–17, 19, 21, 22), one study with 280 patients were excluded as both SBRT and RFA were applied as bridge therapies before transplantation, and the actual OS rates of SBRT or RFA might be affected by subsequent transplantation (3). The pool results showed that 2-year OS rates of RFA group were better than those of the SBRT group (OR 1.57, 95% CI 1.23–2.00, $P < 0.0003$), whereas there were no differences for 1-, 3-, and 5-year OS rates in both groups (OR 1.38, 95% CI 1.00–1.93, $P = 0.050$; OR 1.44, 95% CI 0.90–2.33, $P = 0.130$; and OR 1.35, 95% CI 0.81–2.26, $P = 0.250$, respectively; **Figure 2**).

Additionally, a secondary analysis was performed to control the potential report bias, and we enrolled the studies that reported outcomes of both LP and OS. As a result, the 1-, 2-, 3-, and 5-year OS rates indicated no significant difference between both groups (OR 0.96, 95% CI 0.59–1.57, $P = 0.870$; OR 1.35, 95% CI 0.89–2.03, $P = 0.160$; OR 0.97, 95% CI 0.28–3.36, $P = 0.960$; and OR 0.65, 95% CI 0.37–1.16, $P = 0.150$, respectively; **Supplementary Figure 2**).

Prognosis for Treatment Allocation

Three and five studies evaluated the results of treatment allocation as a prognostic factor for LP (10, 16, 17) and OS (13, 15, 17, 19, 21), respectively. The treatment allocation was

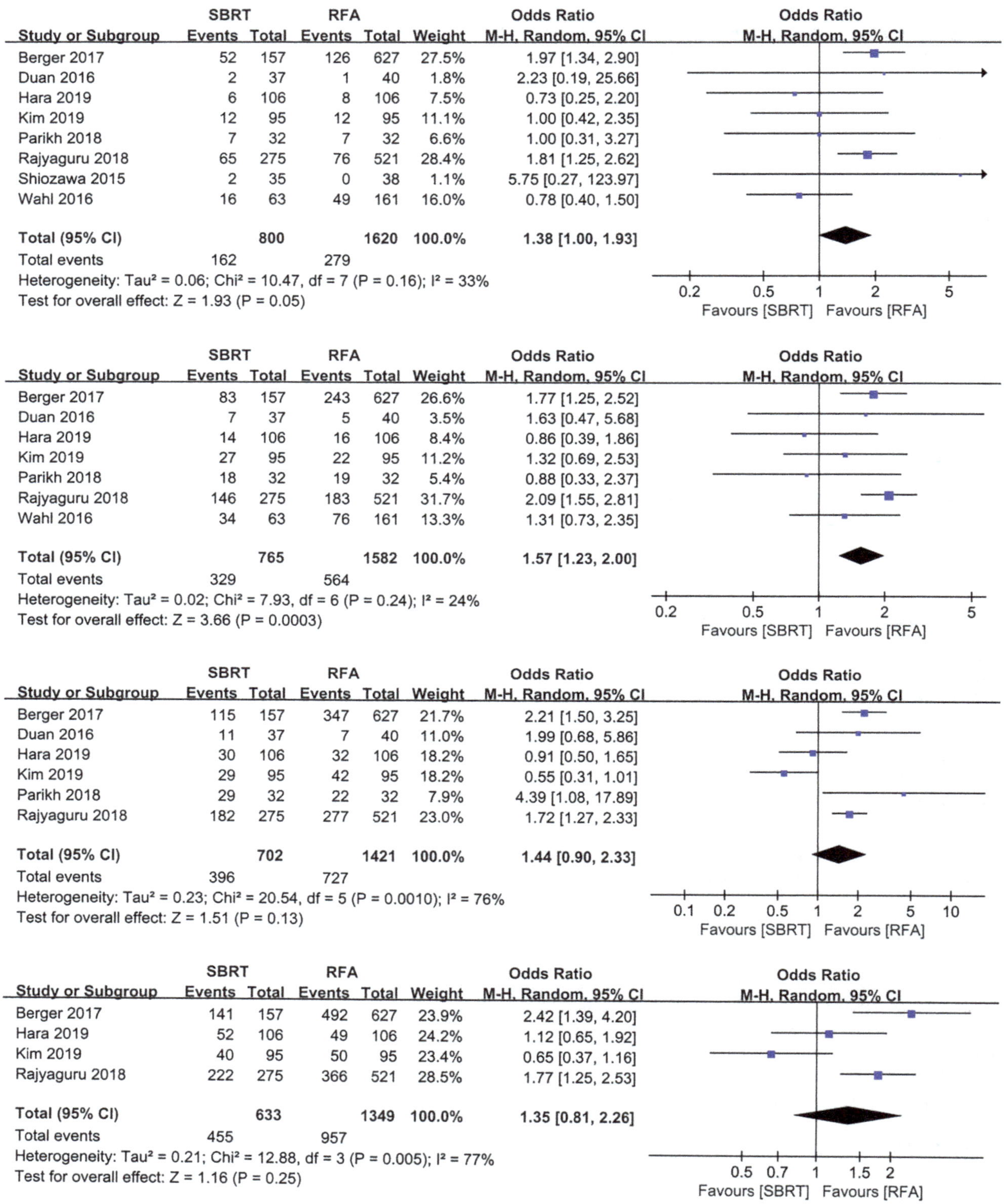

FIGURE 2 | Forest plots demonstrating 1-, 2-, 3-, and 5-year LP in SBRT and RFA for HCC. LP, local progression; SBRT, stereotactic body radiotherapy; RFA, radiofrequency ablation; HCC, hepatocellular carcinoma.

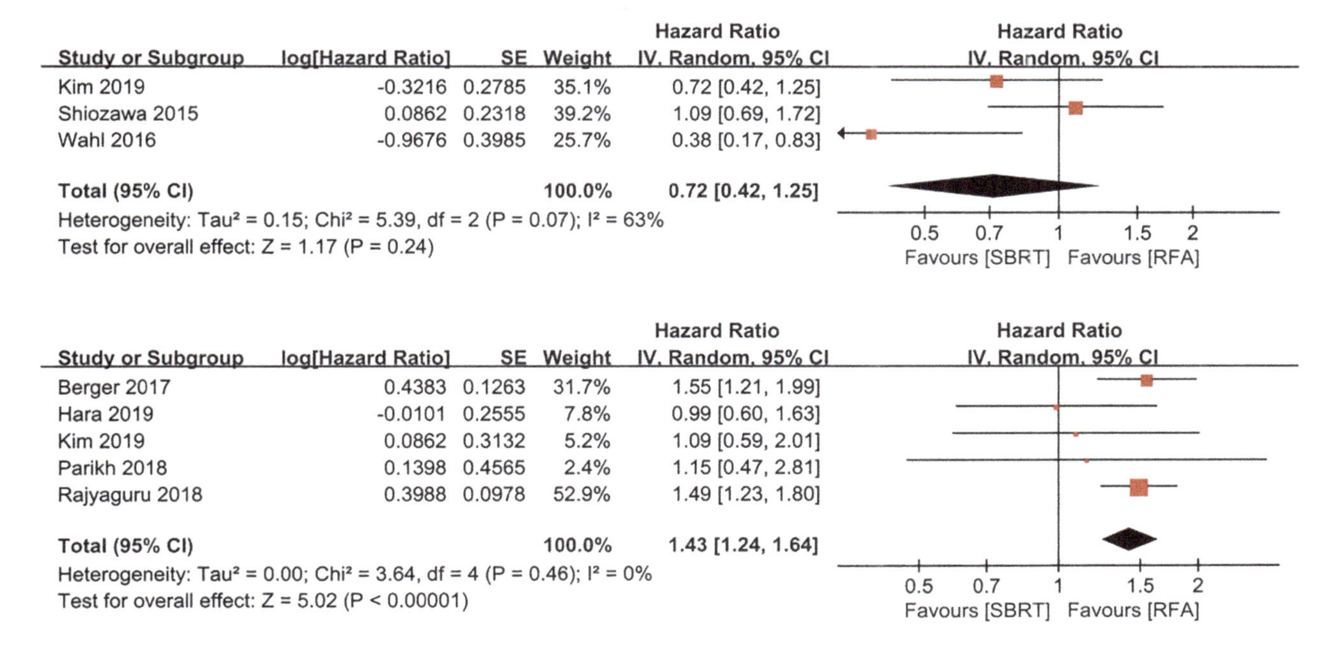

FIGURE 3 | Forest plots demonstrating prognostic factor for LP and OS regarding to treatment allocation. LP, local progression; OS, overall survival.

not a prognostic factor for LP (HR 0.72, 95% IC 0.42–1.25, $P = 0.240$). However, RFA group was more favorable than SBRT group for OS benefits (HR 1.43, 95% IC 1.24–1.64, $P < 0.00001$; **Figure 3**).

Transplant and Post-transplant Pathological Necrosis Rate

Three and two studies reported the transplant rate and post-transplant pathological necrosis rate, respectively (3, 10, 18). There were no significant differences in transplant rate and post-transplant pathological necrosis rate for both SBRT and RFA (OR 0.65, 95% CI 0.24–1.79, $P = 0.040$; and OR 0.46, 95% CI 0.13–1.63, $P = 0.230$, respectively; **Figure 4**).

Publication Bias

The Begg funnel plot was used to evaluate the reliability of publication bias in our meta-analysis (25). The shape of 11 funnel plots was basically inverted and bilateral symmetry. Therefore, these results indicated that there was little publication bias among all comparisons in this meta-analysis (**Supplementary Figure 3**).

DISCUSSION

The main finding of this meta-analysis is that SBRT showed a better local control than RFA for patients with HCC, though the 2-year OS rates of SBRT were inferior because of the tumor burden and liver profiles. Recently, RFA, as a traditional curable treatment, was challenged by SBRT (15, 21, 22). With the development of imaging technique, such as four-dimensional CT (4DCT), SBRT is able to provide a more precise picture of HCC for treatment design (26). This improvement of SBRT effectively fixed the deficiencies of the high incomplete ablation rate of RFA under several specific conditions (7).

In 2006, Romero et al. (27) firstly applied the radiational technique of SBRT as a salvage treatment to control the primary and metastatic liver tumors. Although only 25 patients with 45 lesions that were unfit for other local control treatment were included in this study, the results preliminarily indicated that SBRT was feasible with acceptable toxicity and local control efficacy. They additionally pointed out that patients with Child B level were accompanied by high toxicity risks, and the optimal dose-fractionation schemes had to be found. Inspired by Romero et al., other investigators mainly focused on the application of SBRT on unresectable HCC and its effect in combination with other therapies (28–30). All these studies proved that SBRT was safe and provided satisfying local control for HCC, and this encouraged the temptation of expanding the indications of SBRT from a salvage or bridge treatment to curable intention.

RFA has long been applied as the first-line treatment for small HCC according to several clinical practice guidelines, including the European Society for Medical Oncology (ESMO) and American Association for the Study of Liver Disease (AASLD) (31, 32). However, RFA still suffers from high incidence of local incomplete ablation because of technical limitations [varies from 2 to 60% (5–9)], and it required additional or combinational therapies (33). As an advanced technique that shows reliable local control and safety on HCC, SBRT has been considered as a potential alternative therapy to RFA.

Many observational or retrospective studies in recent years have indicated that SBRT showed a non-inferior local control rate as compared with RFA (10, 16–18, 22). Shiozawa et al. (16) first compared the clinical outcomes between SBRT and

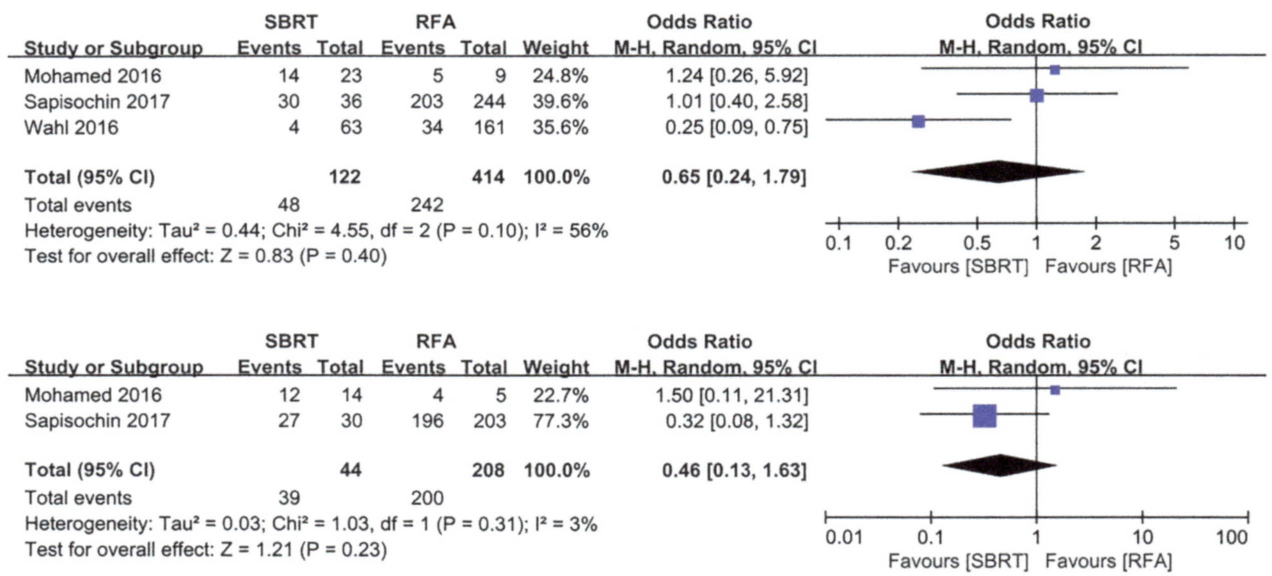

FIGURE 4 | Forest plot demonstrating transplant rate and post-transplant pathologic necrosis in SBRT and RFA for HCC. SBRT, stereotactic body radiotherapy; RFA, radiofrequency ablation; HCC, hepatocellular carcinoma.

RFA for HCC patients in a pilot study in 2015 and reported that SBRT was likely to become an important option for local treatment of early HCC. The subsequent studies indicated that SBRT appeared to be a reasonable alternative treatment of inoperable HCC in 2016 (10, 22). Subsequently, several large-volume validation studies based on online database had also proved comparable outcomes between SBRT and RFA regarding local control (13, 19). Moreover, in 2019, Kim et al. (17) retrospectively reviewed the institutional database for RFA and SBRT with curative intent, and they revealed that SBRT appears to be an effective alternative treatment for HCC when RFA is not feasible due to tumor location or size. However, another database validation from the American National Cancer Database revealed better OS of RFA than SBRT (15). A meta-analysis is needed to attain definitive proof to solve these debates. Thus, we performed this meta-analysis to help identify the advantages and disadvantages of SBRT and RFA in HCC.

In the present meta-analysis, with respect to local control, SBRT showed significantly lower 1- and 3-year LP rates, which indicated that SBRT achieved superior local control to RFA in treating HCC. In detail, there were five and four studies that enrolled the 1- and 3-year LP rate analyses, respectively. Among these studies, studies from Wahl et al. (10) and Duan et al. (22) were based on patients with inoperable HCC, studies of Shiozawa et al. (16) and Hara et al. (21) were based on patients with early-stage HCC, and studies from Kim et al. (17) and Mohamed et al. (18) did not specify patients characteristics. Most of the enrolled studies tended to draw the conclusions with respect to local control that supported SBRT. Moreover, Wahl et al. (10) and Hara et al. (21) reached significantly favorable results for SBRT in treating inoperable and early-stage HCC, respectively. However, only Kim et al. (17) clarified the information of HCC location; others did not refer to this critical factor, which might influence the local control of RFA in our previous study (34). Additionally, treatment allocation was not a significance prognostic factor on the basis of prognostic analysis. Therefore, further studies are needed to guarantee the appropriate individual treatment allocation.

Although SBRT enjoyed higher local control rates than RFA in the present study, the 2-year OS rates of SBRT were significantly lower than RFA. Notably, Berger et al. (19) and Rajyaguru et al. (15), who reported favorable OS rates of RFA with large sample volume, did not illustrate the LP rates correspondingly. There were two main reasons to the contradictory results between OS rates and LP rates. Firstly, there might be report bias when analyzing LP rates for both groups, which might result in inconsistent outcomes between LP rates and OS rates because of unreported LP. Therefore, we conducted the secondary analysis on OS rates that included the studies that reported both LP rates and OS rates, and we found that the 1-, 2-, 3-, and 5-year OS rates were comparable between SBRT and RFA (**Supplementary Figure 2**). Secondly, as the first-line treatment, RFA is more likely to be assigned to patients with better conditions. Patients who underwent SBRT were prone to suffer from larger tumor size and worse liver function, which indicated worse prognosis and decreased OS. Interestingly, the 3- and 5-year OS rates showed no significance in both groups, indicating that patients who did not die of tumor burden or liver functions in a short time might finally benefit from both treatments similarly. Meanwhile, RFA showed significant survival benefit for prognostic analysis on treatment allocation, which also could be explained by the reasons above. Therefore, we believed that the real effects of SBRT and RFA on long-term survival need to be further validated by high-level evidence, including RCTs.

As for bridge therapies to transplant, both SBRT and RFA provided a similar effect on patients waiting for transplantation. And the post-transplant pathological necrosis rate was comparable between both groups. These outcomes indicated that SBRT can be safely utilized as a bridge treatment to patients in the waiting list for transplantation with HCC, as an alternative to conventional bridging therapies. However, only three studies and 536 patients in total compared these parameters, and more solid studies were needed to be enrolled in the future.

This meta-analysis suffered from several limitations. First of all, only retrospective studies were available, resulting in relatively low quality of the evidence for the whole pooled results. Secondly, the results from this study should be interpreted carefully, because the sample sizes of four studies were relatively small, which is supposed to affect the reliability. And a further sensitivity analysis on the factors affecting outcomes could not be applied. Additionally, some studies were shorter follow-up in the SBRT group, which could result in obscuring late effects. Therefore, some well-designed, large, prospective, and multicenter studies are desperately needed to obtain more solid evidence.

CONCLUSIONS

In sum, our meta-analysis shows that SBRT provided better local control than RFA, and it could be used as a potential alternative local control treatment for HCC.

AUTHOR CONTRIBUTIONS

Y-XP and D-DH designed the experiments and drafted the manuscript. Y-ZF, QL, J-CW, and MX were responsible for data collection and statistical analysis. S-LL, LX, and M-ZL helped revise the manuscript. M-SC and Y-JZ approved the final version. All authors contributed to the article and approved the submitted version.

ACKNOWLEDGMENTS

The authors acknowledge and express their deepest gratitude to the participants of this study. This manuscript has been revised by a native English speaker for effective communication to a professional medical audience.

REFERENCES

1. Sapisochin G, Bruix J. Liver transplantation for hepatocellular carcinoma: outcomes and novel surgical approaches. *Nat Rev Gastroenterol Hepatol.* (2017) 14:203–17. doi: 10.1038/nrgastro.2016.193
2. Panel NHC. Hepatobiliary cancers, V.1.2010. *Nccn Guidelines.* (2019) 1:1–142. doi: 10.6004/jnccn.2019.0019
3. Sapisochin G, Barry A, Doherty M, Fischer S, Goldaracena N, Rosales R, et al. Stereotactic body radiotherapy vs. TACE or RFA as a bridge to transplant in patients with hepatocellular carcinoma. An intention-to-treat analysis. *J Hepatol.* (2017) 67:92–99. doi: 10.1016/j.jhep.2017.02.022
4. Chen M-S, Li J-Q, Zheng Y, Guo R-P, Liang H-H, Zhang Y-Q, et al. A prospective randomized trial comparing percutaneous local ablative therapy and partial hepatectomy for small hepatocellular carcinoma. *Ann Surg.* (2006) 243:321–8. doi: 10.1097/01.sla.0000201480.65519.b8
5. N'Kontchou G, Mahamoudi A, Aout M, Ganne-Carrie N, Grando V, Coderc E, et al. Radiofrequency ablation of hepatocellular carcinoma: long-term results and prognostic factors in 235 Western patients with cirrhosis. *Hepatology.* (2009) 50:1475–83. doi: 10.1002/hep.23181
6. Tateishi R, Shiina S, Teratani T, Obi S, Sato S, Koike Y, et al. Percutaneous radiofrequency ablation for hepatocellular carcinoma. An analysis of 1000 cases. *Cancer.* (2005) 103:1201–9. doi: 10.1002/cncr.20892
7. Waki K, Aikata H, Katamura Y, Kawaoka T, Takaki S, Hiramatsu A, et al. Percutaneous radiofrequency ablation as first-line treatment for small hepatocellular carcinoma: results and prognostic factors on long-term follow up. *J Gastroenterol Hepatol.* (2010) 25:597–604. doi: 10.1111/j.1440-1746.2009.06125.x
8. Granata V, Petrillo M, Fusco R, Setola SV, de Lutio di Castelguidone E, Catalano O, et al. Surveillance of HCC patients after liver RFA: role of MRI with hepatospecific contrast versus three-phase CT scan-experience of high volume oncologic institute. *Gastroenterol Res Pract.* (2013) 2013:469097. doi: 10.1155/2013/469097
9. Doyle A, Gorgen A, Muaddi H, Aravinthan AD, Issachar A, Mironov O, et al. Outcomes of radiofrequency ablation as first-line therapy for hepatocellular carcinoma less than 3 cm in potentially transplantable patients. *J Hepatol.* (2019) 70:866–73. doi: 10.1016/j.jhep.2018.12.027
10. Wahl DR, Stenmark MH, Tao Y, Pollom EL, Caoili EM, Lawrence TS, et al. Outcomes after stereotactic body radiotherapy or radiofrequency ablation for hepatocellular carcinoma. *J Clin Oncol.* (2016) 34:452–9. doi: 10.1200/JCO.2015.61.4925
11. Feng M, Suresh K, Schipper MJ, Bazzi L, Ben-Josef E, Matuszak MM, et al. Individualized adaptive stereotactic body radiotherapy for liver tumors in patients at high risk for liver damage: a phase 2 clinical trial. *JAMA Oncol.* (2018) 4:40–47. doi: 10.1001/jamaoncol.2017.2303
12. Hara K, Takeda A, Tsurugai Y, Sanuki N, Saigusa Y, Maeda S, et al. Clinical outcomes after treatment for hepatocellular carcinoma, stereotactic body radiotherapy vs radiofrequency ablation: a propensity score-matched analysis. *Hepatology.* (2018) 68:848A. doi: 10.1002/hep.30257
13. Parikh ND, Marshall VD, Green M, Lawrence TS, Razumilava N, Owen D, et al. Effectiveness and cost of radiofrequency ablation and stereotactic body radiotherapy for treatment of early-stage hepatocellular carcinoma: an analysis of SEER-medicare. *J Med Imaging Radiat Oncol.* (2018) 62:673–81. doi: 10.1111/1754-9485.12754
14. Wahl D, Stenmark M, Pollom E, Tao Y, Lee O, Schipper M, et al. SBRT provides equivalent local control compared to RFA for the treatment of hepatocellular carcinoma with minimal toxicity. *Int J Radiat Oncol Biol Phys.* (2014) 90:S378–9. doi: 10.1016/j.ijrobp.2014.05.1218
15. Rajyaguru DJ, Borgert AJ, Smith AL, Thomes RM, Conway PD, Halfdanarson TR, et al. Radiofrequency ablation versus stereotactic body radiotherapy for localized hepatocellular carcinoma in nonsurgically managed patients: analysis of the national cancer database. *J Clin Oncol.* (2018) 36:600–8. doi: 10.1200/JCO.2017.75.3228
16. Shiozawa K, Watanabe M, Ikehara T, Matsukiyo Y, Kogame M, Kishimoto Y, et al. Comparison of percutaneous radiofrequency ablation and CyberKnife® for initial solitary hepatocellular carcinoma: a pilot study. *World J Gastroenterol.* (2015) 21:13490–9. doi: 10.3748/wjg.v21.i48.13490
17. Kim N, Kim HJ, Won JY, Kim DY, Han K-H, Jung I, et al. Retrospective analysis of stereotactic body radiation therapy efficacy over radiofrequency ablation for hepatocellular carcinoma. *Radiother Oncol.* (2019) 131:81–87. doi: 10.1016/j.radonc.2018.12.013
18. Mohamed M, Katz AW, Tejani MA, Sharma AK, Kashyap R, Noel MS, et al. Comparison of outcomes between SBRT, yttrium-90 radioembolization, transarterial chemoembolization, and radiofrequency ablation as bridge to transplant for hepatocellular carcinoma. *Adv Radiat Oncol.* (2016) 1:35–42. doi: 10.1016/j.adro.2015.12.003
19. Berger NG, Tanious MN, Hammad AY, Miura JT, Mogal H, Clarke CN, et al. External radiation or ablation for solitary hepatocellular carcinoma: a survival analysis of the SEER database. *J Surg Oncol.* (2017) 116:307–12. doi: 10.1002/jso.24661

20. Melsen WG, Bootsma MCJ, Rovers MM, Bonten MJM. The effects of clinical and statistical heterogeneity on the predictive values of results from meta-analyses. *Clin Microbiol Infect.* (2014) 20:123–9. doi: 10.1111/1469-0691.12494
21. Hara K, Takeda A, Tsurugai Y, Saigusa Y, Sanuki N, Eriguchi T, et al. Radiotherapy for hepatocellular carcinoma results in comparable survival to radiofrequency ablation: a propensity score analysis. *Hepatology.* (2019) 69:2533–45. doi: 10.1002/hep.30591
22. Duon X, Zhang T, Xie H, Sun J, He W, Xu H. Stereotactic body radiotherapy vs. radiofrequency ablation in the Treatment of small hepatocellular Carcinoma. *Hepatology.* (2016) 64:653–4A. doi: 10.1002/hep.28799
23. Tian J, Zhang J, Ge L, Yang K, Song F. The methodological and reporting quality of systematic reviews from China and the USA are similar. *J Clin Epidemiol.* (2017) 85:50–58. doi: 10.1016/j.jclinepi.2016.12.004
24. Stang A. Critical evaluation of the Newcastle-Ottawa scale for the assessment of the quality of nonrandomized studies in meta-analyses. *Eur J Epidemiol.* (2010) 25:603–5. doi: 10.1007/s10654-010-9491-z
25. Higgins JPT, Altman DG, Gotzsche PC, Juni P, Moher D, Oxman AD, et al. The cochrane collaboration's tool for assessing risk of bias in randomised trials. *BMJ.* (2011) 343:d5928. doi: 10.1136/bmj.d5928
26. Couri T, Pillai A. Goals and targets for personalized therapy for HCC. *Hepatol Int.* (2019) 13:125–37. doi: 10.1007/s12072-018-9919-1
27. Romero AM, Wunderink W, Hussain SM, De Pooter JA, Heijmen BJ, Nowak PC, et al. Stereotactic body radiation therapy for primary and metastatic liver tumors: a single institution phase i-ii study. *Acta Oncol.* (2006) 45:831–7. doi: 10.1080/02841860600897934
28. Goyal K, Einstein D, Yao M, Kunos C, Barton F, Singh D, et al. Cyberknife stereotactic body radiation therapy for nonresectable tumors of the liver: preliminary results. *HPB Surgery.* (2010) 2010:309780. doi: 10.1155/2010/309780
29. Bae SH, Kwon JH, Jang JW, Song MJ, Choi JY, Yoon SK. Stereotactic body radiation therapy using Cyberknife for primary hepatocellular carcinoma ineligible for local ablation therapy or surgical resection. *Hepatology.* (2009) 50:1100A. doi: 10.1002/hep.23307
30. Choi BO, Choi IB, Jang HS, Kang YN, Jang JS, Bae SH, et al. Stereotactic body radiation therapy with or without transarterial chemoembolization for patients with primary hepatocellular carcinoma: Preliminary analysis. *BMC Cancer.* (2008) 8:351. doi: 10.1186/1471-2407-8-351
31. Heimbach JK, Kulik LM, Finn RS, Sirlin CB, Abecassis MM, Roberts LR, et al. AASLD guidelines for the treatment of hepatocellular carcinoma. *Hepatology.* (2018) 67:358–80. doi: 10.1002/hep.29086
32. Vogel A, Cervantes A, Chau I, Daniele B, Llovet J, Meyer T, et al. Hepatocellular carcinoma: ESMO clinical practice guidelines for diagnosis, treatment and follow-up†. *Ann Oncol.* (2018) 29:iv238–55. doi: 10.1093/annonc/mdy308
33. Peng Z-W, Zhang Y-J, Chen M-S, Xu L, Liang H-H, Lin X-J, et al. Radiofrequency ablation with or without transcatheter arterial chemoembolization in the treatment of hepatocellular carcinoma: a prospective randomized trial. *J Clin Oncol.* (2013) 31:426–32. doi: 10.1200/JCO.2012.42.9936
34. Chen J, Peng K, Hu D, Shen J, Zhou Z, Xu L, et al. Tumor location influences oncologic outcomes of hepatocellular carcinoma patients undergoing radiofrequency ablation. *Cancers.* (2018) 10:1–14. doi: 10.3390/cancers10100378

21

Magnetic Resonance-Guided Stereotactic Body Radiotherapy of Liver Tumors: Initial Clinical Experience and Patient-Reported Outcomes

Fabian Weykamp[1,2,3], Philipp Hoegen[1,2,3], Sebastian Klüter[1,2,3], C. Katharina Spindeldreier[1,2,3], Laila König[1,2,3], Katharina Seidensaal[1,2,3], Sebastian Regnery[1,2,3], Jakob Liermann[1,2,3], Carolin Rippke[1,2,3], Stefan A. Koerber[1,2,3], Carolin Buchele[1,2,3], Jürgen Debus[1,2,3,4,5,6] and Juliane Hörner-Rieber[1,2,3,5]*

[1] Department of Radiation Oncology, Heidelberg University Hospital, Heidelberg, Germany, [2] Heidelberg Institute of Radiation Oncology (HIRO), Heidelberg, Germany, [3] National Center for Tumor Diseases (NCT), Heidelberg, Germany, [4] Heidelberg Ion-Beam Therapy Center (HIT), Department of Radiation Oncology, Heidelberg University Hospital, Heidelberg, Germany, [5] Clinical Cooperation Unit Radiation Oncology, German Cancer Research Center (DKFZ), Heidelberg, Germany, [6] German Cancer Consortium (DKTK), Heidelberg, Germany

Correspondence:
Juliane Hörner-Rieber
juliane.hoerner-rieber@med.uni-heidelberg.de

Purpose/Objective: Stereotactic body radiation therapy (SBRT) has emerged as a valid treatment alternative for non-resectable liver metastases or hepatocellular carcinomas (HCC). Magnetic resonance (MR) guided SBRT has a high potential of further improving treatment quality, allowing for higher, tumoricidal irradiation doses whilst simultaneously sparing organs at risk. However, data on treatment outcome and patient acceptance is still limited.

Material/Methods: We performed a subgroup analysis of an ongoing prospective observational study comprising patients with liver metastases or HCC. Patients were treated with ablative MR-guided SBRT at the MRIdian Linac in the Department of Radiation Oncology at Heidelberg University Hospital between January 2019 and February 2020. Local control (LC) and overall survival (OS) analysis was performed using the Kaplan–Meier method. An in-house designed patient-reported outcome questionnaire was used to measure patients' experience with the MR-Linac treatment. Toxicity was evaluated using the Common Terminology Criteria for Adverse Events (CTCAE v. 5.0).

Results: Twenty patients (with n = 18 metastases; n = 2 HCC) received MR-guided SBRT for in total 26 malignant liver lesions. Median biologically effective dose (BED at $\alpha/\beta = 10$) was 105.0 Gy (range: 67.2–112.5 Gy) and median planning target volume was 57.20 ml (range: 17.4–445.0 ml). Median treatment time was 39.0 min (range: 26.0–67.0 min). At 1-year, LC was 88.1% and OS was 84.0%. Grade I° gastrointestinal toxicity °occurred in 30.0% and grade II° in 5.0% of the patients with no grade III° or higher toxicity. Overall treatment experience was rated positively, with items scoring MR-Linac staff's performance and items concerning the breath hold process being among the top positively rated elements. Worst scored items were treatment duration, positioning and low temperature.

Conclusion: MR-guided SBRT of liver tumors is a well-tolerated and well-accepted treatment modality. Initial results are promising with excellent local control and only mildest toxicity. However, prospective studies are warranted to truly assess the potential of MR-guided liver SBRT and to identify which patients profit most from this new versatile technology.

Keywords: stereotactic body radiotherapy, liver metastases, MR-guided, hepatocellular carcinoma, patient reported outcomes

BACKGROUND AND PURPOSE

Surgical resection was one of the first local ablative treatment options for selected patients with hepatic oligometastases (1). In a retrospective cohort of 612 patients, resection of colorectal liver metastases led to a remarkable long-term survival of 17% after 10 years (2). However, only up to 20% of patients with hepatic oligometastases are initially amenable for surgery (3, 4). In case of reduced general condition, insufficient liver function or critical localization of the liver tumor, cryoablation, radiofrequency- and microwave ablation as well as transarterial chemoembolization are treatment alternatives for local therapy of both hepatic metastases and also primary liver tumors (5, 6). Lately, stereotactic body radiotherapy (SBRT) has been proven as a further safe and effective non-invasive treatment option (7–10).

In case of limited tumor burden, modern radiotherapy evolved from treatment of a whole organ to targeting specific lesions within the organ. In the last century, irradiation of the liver was therefore predominantly used to for palliation, due to dose limiting toxicity together with the fear of radiation-induced liver disease (RILD) (11–14). Nowadays, SBRT offers application of highly conformal tumoricidal irradiation doses whilst sparing surrounding organs at risk (OAR) due to a steep dose gradient. However, adjacent stomach, duodenum and small bowel still represent dose limiting OAR, which impede the goal of achieving ablative irradiation doses (15–18). Standard image guidance with cone beam CT scans only offers a limited soft tissue contrast impairing differentiation between tumor lesions and surrounding radiosensitive OAR (19). Additionally, respiratory motion of the liver causes anatomic changes of up to several centimeters, which can lead to inferior local control, if not adequately accounted for (20–23). Traditionally, motion management includes the usage of an internal target volume (ITV) concept resulting in larger, unnecessary target volumes which might further harm OAR (24). Advanced motion management strategies comprise gating and tracking of the target lesion: surface-guided (SG) SBRT uses the body surface as a surrogate structure for image guidance including patient positioning, intra-fraction motion monitoring and respiratory gating (25–28), while the Cyberknife system can track invasively implanted fiducials using frequent noncoplanar X-ray scans (29). MR-guided radiotherapy has recently become clinically available offering additional superior soft-tissue contrast for precise identification of liver lesions and adjacent OAR. Furthermore, some MR-Linac systems also enable gated dose delivery which offers the possibility to further reduce safety margins (30). Available literature on MR-guided SBRT for malignant liver lesions is growing, but still limited. Especially, patient acceptance needs to be evaluated, considering the long treatment time of MR-guided irradiation of the liver, which is further prolonged through online treatment adaptation (31, 32).

METHODS

The presented study is a subgroup analysis from a prospective observational trial comprising cancer patients with liver metastases or primary hepatocellular carcinoma (HCC), who were referred to our institution because they were deemed medically or functional inoperable or refused resection. Patients were treated with ablative MR-guided SBRT at the MRIdian Linac (ViewRay Inc., Mountain View, CA) in the Department of Radiation Oncology at Heidelberg University Hospital between January 2019 and February 2020. According to the guideline of the working group "Stereotactic Radiotherapy" of the German Society of Radiation Oncology (DEGRO), SBRT was defined as single fraction doses ≥ 4 Gy and number of fractions ≤12 (33).

Treatment Characteristics

A detailed description of our treatment simulation and planning has been published previously (31). Four of our analyzed patients had already been previously included and published in this referenced study. In short, treatment simulation at the MR-Linac was performed to both acquire MR image data and to check for patients' compliance. Three-dimensional (3D) simulation MR images, using the TrueFISP sequence (a steady-state coherent MRI sequence) with an acquisition time of 17 to 25 s were obtained in deep inspiration breath-hold, followed by planar cine-MRI in a sagittal plane to evaluate target motion characteristics (34). For the 3D simulation MRI, in-plane resolutions of either $1.5 \times 1.5\ mm^2$ or $1.6 \times 1.6\ mm^2$ and slice thicknesses of 3 mm with varying fields-of-view were used. No MR contrast fluid was administered. The acquired MR image data was used as the primary image set for treatment planning.

All patients received additional diagnostic, contrast-enhanced MRIs for treatment planning. Furthermore, a planning CT scan with and without contrast enhancement was performed to also obtain data on electron density information for dose calculation. The gross tumor volume (GTV) was delineated as the macroscopic tumor volume on all available co-registered planning imaging modalities, with a clinical target volume (CTV) expansion of 5 mm and additional 3 mm for creating the planning target volume (PTV) due to technical uncertainties.

Daily image guidance was performed for each fraction by onboard 3D MRI using identical settings (field of view, duration, pulse sequence, breathing instructions) as during MR simulation. Soft-tissue based registration with the reference MR scan was applied, always registered directly on the GTV.

Gated dose delivery in breath hold was performed. The TrueFISP sequence was applied for real time MR-gating (cine-MRI scan) within one sagittal slice and four frames per second. If the liver lesion was visible on the TrueFISP sequence, the lesion was used as the gating structure (region of interest; ROI). This was the case in 14 of the 20 analyzed patients. Otherwise, an anatomical surrogate structure in proximity of the target lesion was defined as the gating target. In five patients, the nearest surface of the respective liver segment was used for this purpose. In one patient, a prominent adjacent liver vessel was defined as the surrogate structure. The predefined ROI (either the GTV or the surrogate structure) was expanded by 3 mm in every direction, which formed the gating boundary. The irradiation beam was automatically shut off, if the target structure (usually the GTV) left the gating boundary, including a tolerance threshold of mostly 3%, with a maximum of 7% in very rare cases. During gated dose delivery, patients were offered visual guidance *via* an in-room monitor displaying the live sagittal cine-MR image with an overlay of the gating target and the boundary. A video of this process can be found in the supplementary material section. If an intrafractional GTV deviation occurred and the patient could therefore no longer keep the ROI within the boundary, a table correction including a subsequent new MRI scan had to be performed. This procedure was mandatory to allow for a 3D table correction, since the cine-MRI only provides a 2D image control (in the sagittal plane). No online treatment adaptation was performed, as this technique had not yet been implemented, when the patients were treated.

Doses and fractionation schemes depended on the size and localization of the hepatic lesion as well as patients' breath holding capability. In general, small and centrally located lesions were treated with three fractions of 15 Gy, prescribed to the conformally enclosing 65% isodose, while larger lesions (>5 cm) were irradiated with eight fractions of 7.5 Gy or five fractions of 10Gy prescribed to the conformally enclosing 80% isodose. Hepatic lesions in close proximity to radiosensitive OAR were usually treated with ten fractions of 5 Gy prescribed to the conformally enclosing 80%-isodose. One hepatic metastasis was treated with twelve fractions of 4 Gy prescribed to the conformally enclosing 95% isodose as the patient had been treated with prior hemihepatectomy and the lesion was diagnosed at the liver margin which had been sutured to the small bowel.

Target coverage was comprised if required OAR dose constraints could not be met. Applied dose constraints were the following (for five fractions):

–esophagus: 0.5 cc <34 Gy
–stomach/intestine: 0.5 cc <35 Gy
–liver minus CTV: ≥700 cc <24 Gy
–kidney: mean dose <10 Gy
–spinal cord 0.1 cc <27 Gy
–heart: 0.5 cc <29 Gy.

An in-house designed patient-reported outcome questionnaire (PRO-Q) was used to measure patients' experience with the MR-Linac treatment (grades from 1–5, where 1 represents a completely positive and 5 a completely negative experience) (31). Patients were additionally asked, how many minutes it took to fully mentally and physically recover after their effort during the respective treatment session. Furthermore, our staff was surveyed about their opinion on each patient's treatment performance (grades from 1–10, where 1 represents a completely easy and 10 an almost inacceptable expenditure).

Endpoints and Statistical Methods

LC and OS were estimated starting from the first day of the SBRT. LC was calculated based on each lesion, whereas OS was calculated per patient. The Response Evaluation Criteria in Solid Tumors (RECIST 1.1) was used to asses tumor response. Toxicity was described using the Common Terminology Criteria for Adverse Events (CTCAE v. 5.0).

In accordance with the study protocol, each patient was specifically assessed for presence of fatigue, nausea, vomiting, diarrhea, constipation, dyspnea, cough, skin disorder and pain. This evaluation was performed before irradiation, at the last treatment day and at first follow-up. Follow-up consisted of a contrast fluid enhanced MRI or CT scan of the liver, performed six to eight weeks after completion of the SBRT together with a clinical examination. Further imaging follow-up was performed every three months afterwards and consisted of a contrast fluid enhanced CT of the thorax and the abdomen or a contrast-enhanced MRI, but was not part of the prospective study. The Child–Pugh score was assessed within four weeks prior to the SBRT and at the first follow-up examination.

LC and OS were estimated using the Kaplan–Meier method. The biologically effective dose (BED) was calculated applying the linear-quadratic model (35). An α/β ratio of 10 was assumed for liver metastases and HCC.

$$BED(Gy) = \text{single } dose \times number\ of\ fractions\left(1 + \frac{\text{single } dose}{\alpha/\beta}\right)$$

All statistical analyses were performed with SPSS software (IBM SPSS Version 24.0). A p-value of <0.05 was defined significant. The MR-Linac observational study was approved by the Ethics committee of the University Hospital Heidelberg (S-543/2018). Written informed consent was obtained from all patients included into the study.

Two Selected Cases From Daily Routine

For providing detailed clinical inside into treatment reality at the MR-Linac, two characteristic patients were selected for in-detail description. Since gated dose delivery in breath hold is challenging, as it demands a certain amount of treatment compliance and the bore of the MR-Linac is relatively narrow (70 cm), the oldest patient and the patient with the highest body mass index were selected for further description.

RESULTS

Patient characteristics are described in **Table 1**. Median age of the 20 patients was 61 years. Most patients had a very good performance status and a non-obese body mass index. Most irradiated liver lesions were metastases from colorectal carcinoma. Two patients suffered from HCC. Systemic therapy was administered in most patients before (75%) and after (55%) radiotherapy. One patient underwent hemihepatectomy prior to radiotherapy. Twelve patients had already complained of grades I–II° adverse events before starting hepatic SBRT, mostly grade I° fatigue.

Most patients were treated with hepatic SBRT for one single liver lesion (n = 18), while two patients had four lesions irradiated. Median PTV size was 57.2 ml (17.4–445.0 ml). Median dose was 50 Gy (45–60 Gy) with a calculated BED of 105.0 Gy (67.2–112.5 Gy).

Further treatment characteristics are listed in **Table 2**. **Figure 1** shows a characteristic treatment plan, where maximum sparing of the neighboring small bowl and stomach could be achieved.

TABLE 1 | Patient characteristics (n = 20).

median age	61 years	range 37–78 years
median Karnofsky Score	90%	range 70–100%
median Body Mass Index	23.8 kg/m²	range 18.0–42.3 kg/m²
female/male	10/10	50.0%/50.0%
Hepatocellular Carcinoma	2	10.0%
Metastases	18	90.0%
n = 5 colorectal carcinoma; n = 4 breast cancer; n = 3 malignant melanoma; n = 1 adenoid cystic carcinoma; n = 1 cholangiocellular carcinoma; n = 1 urinary bladder carcinoma; n = 1 papillary carcinoma; n = 1 pancreatic cancer; n = 1 prostate cancer.		
distant metastases present (apart from the irradiated liver metastases)		
n = 0	9	45.0%
n = 1–5	5	25.0%
n > 5	6	30.0%
prior hemihepatectomy	1	4.7%
median Child–Pugh-Score[1]	5	range 5–7
extrahepatic disease progression within four weeks before irradiation	2	10.0%
systemic therapy within 4 weeks before irradiation	15	75.0%
n = 10 chemotherapy; n = 3 checkpoint inhibition; n = 2 hormonal therapy		
systemic therapy within 4 weeks after irradiation	11	55.0%
n = 5 chemotherapy; n = 3 checkpoint inhibition; n = 2 hormonal therapy; n = 1 targeted therapy		
Adverse events before radiotherapy		
I°	10	50.0%
n = 6 fatigue; n = 2 fatigue + diarrhea; n = 2 pain + cough		
II°	2	10.0%
n = 1 nausea; n = 1 fatigue		
≥III°	0	0
Adverse events at last treatment day		
I°	12	60.0%
n = 5 fatigue; n = 1 nausea; n = 1 diarrhea + nausea + fatigue; n = 1 fatigue + dysphagia +erythema; n = 1 flatulence + fatigue; n = 1 fatigue + dyspepsia; n = 1 fatigue + nausea; n = 1 fatigue + dizziness		
II°	1	5.0%
n = 1 fatigue + diarrhea		
≥III°	0	0
Adverse events at first follow-up		
I°	8	40.0%
n = 3 fatigue; n = 1 pain; n = 1 fatigue + nausea; n = 1 nausea + diarrhea; n = 1 nausea + dyspepsia; n = 1 fatigue + pain		
II°	0	0
≥III°	0	0

[1]available data for n = 15 patients.

Outcome

Median follow-up was 9.4 months. Estimated local control was 88.1% at 12 months (**Figure 2A**). All irradiated liver lesions were stable or had a decrease in size at first follow-up (**Table 2**). Two patients (10%) died during follow-up time. Estimated OS at 12 months was 84.0% (**Figure 2B**). Child–Pugh score (available for n = 15 patients) did not decrease after irradiation. **Figure 3** illustrates a representative patient case, where additional pre-

TABLE 2 | Irradiation treatment characteristics.

total number of irradiated liver targets per patient		
n = 1	18	90.0%
n = 4	2	10.0%
localization of liver targets	Segment I (7.7%) II (23.1%) III (0%) IV (15.3%) V (7.7%) VI (7.7%) VII (23.1%) VIII (15.4%)	
response to irradiation in first follow-up examination		
partial remission	15	57.6%
stable disease	11	42.4%
	median	range
largest axial diameter	21 mm	8–77 mm
GTV	15.5 mL	1.4–255.0 mL
CTV	36.4 mL	6.4–349.3 mL
PTV	57.2 mL	17.4–445.0 mL
prescribed total dose	50 Gy	45–60 Gy
fractions	8	3–12
dose inhomogeneity	80%	65–80%
EQD2(α/β = 10)	87.5 Gy	56.0–93.8 Gy
BED (α/β = 10)	105.0 Gy	67.2–112.5 Gy
monitor units per fraction	2,403.9	1,155.4–6,309.7
number of beams that are on	11	7–15
duration of the session ("on table")	39.0 min	26.0–67.0 min
-radiation time	15.8 min	10.3–38.2 min
-pure beam on time	3.8 min	1.83–10.0 min

BED, biologically effective dose; CTV, clinical target volume; EQD2, equivalent dose at 2 Gy; GTV, gross tumor volume; PTV, planning target volume.

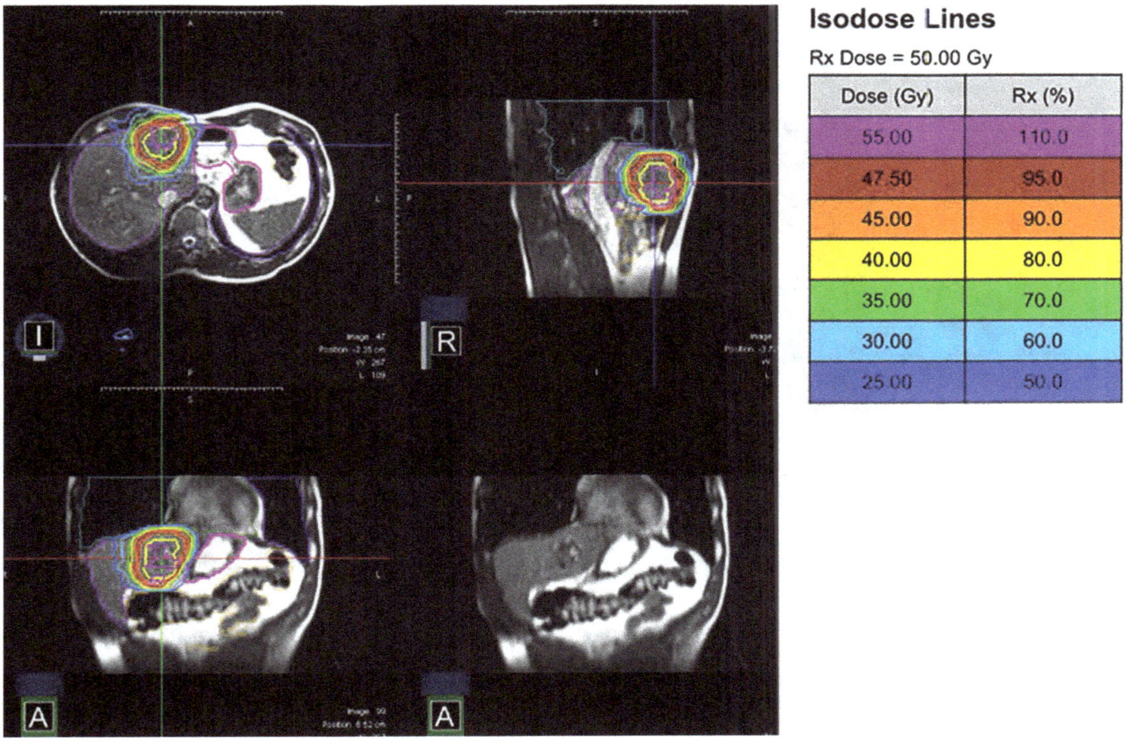

FIGURE 1 | MR-Linac treatment plan (10 fractions of 5 Gy prescribed to the conformally enclosing 80%-isodose) from different perspectives (I, inferior; A, anterior; R, right) with and without isodose lines.

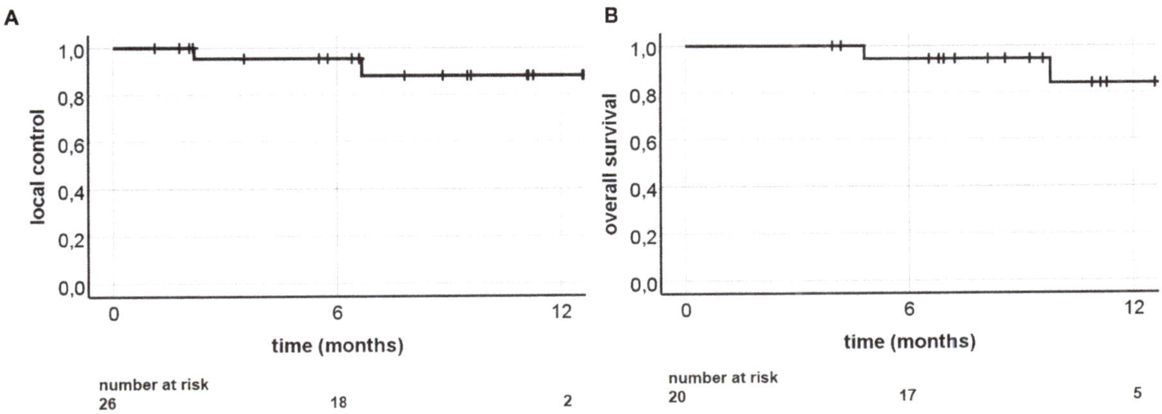

FIGURE 2 | **(A)** Local control and **(B)** overall survival following MR-guided liver SBRT.

and post-radiotherapy FDG PET-CT scans were performed, which revealed only residual activity of the liver metastasis after MR-guided hepatic SBRT. Later hemihepatectomy due to disease progression in the right liver lobe outside the irradiated area revealed complete pathological remission of the irradiated lesion.

Toxicity

Acute toxicity was mild with thirteen patients describing grades I–II° adverse events on the last day of radiotherapy, including mostly grade I° fatigue. Six patients suffered from grade I° gastrointestinal side effects and one patient was diagnosed with grade II° gastrointestinal side effects (diarrhea). Eight patients

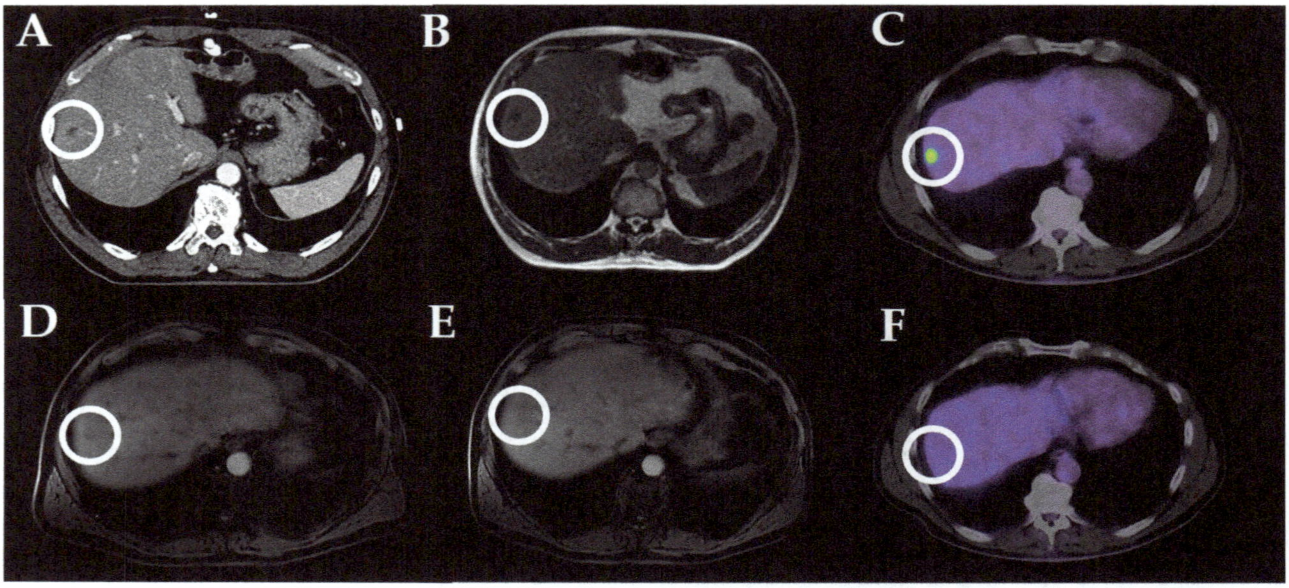

FIGURE 3 | Stereotactic MR guided radiotherapy of a hepatic metastasis in a patient with pancreatic cancer (10 × 5 Gy): **(A)** planning CT scan (portal venous phase); **(B)** online liver simulation at the MR-Linac; **(C)** pre-radiotherapy FDG-PET CT scan; **(D)** first (3 months after radiotherapy) post-radiotherapy MRI scan (liver imaging with volume acceleration-flexible MRI); **(E)** second (4 months) post-radiotherapy MRI (liver imaging with volume acceleration-flexible MRI); **(F)** post-radiotherapy (4 months) FDG-PET CT scan. Comment: later hemihepatectomy revealed complete remission of the radiated liver metastasis.

complained of grade I° adverse events at first follow-up examination, mainly fatigue. No grade III° adverse event ore higher was reported at any time.

Patient and Staff Reported Outcome

Table 3 displays the personal subjective experience of the treated patients. Overall treatment experience was rated positively, with items scoring MR-Linac staff's performance and items concerning the breath hold process being among the top positively rated items (each median 1 point). Worst scored elements were treatment duration, positioning and temperature of body parts (each median 3 points). The whole treatment processes, including breathing instructions, were challenging for some patients, both mentally and physically. Median time to full mental and physical recovery after the first treatment session was 20 min (range 0–360 min). Median complexity of radiotherapy at the MR-Linac was rated as average by the staff (**Table 3**).

Two Selected Cases From Daily Routine

The most obese patient (187 cm, 148 kg, body mass index = 42 kg/m^2; ventrodorsal abdominal diameter = 35 cm; 52 years, Karnofsky Performance Score 70%) was treated for a single liver metastasis of a rectum carcinoma (three fractions of 15 Gy). The duration of the treatment session (40 min; "on table", including patient positioning), was comparable to the study median (39 min). Mere radiation time (16 min) was below the median of the study cohort (22 min). Recovery time after radiotherapy (10 min) was below the study median of 20 min. No patient reported outcome item was rated worse than average. MR-Linac staff documented average complexity of the irradiation process.

The oldest patient (78 years; Karnofsky Performance Score 80%; body mass index = 30 kg/m^2, no reported lung disease) was treated for a single liver metastasis of a cholangiocellular carcinoma (three fractions of 15 Gy). Duration of the treatment session (38 min) and pure radiation time (21 min) were comparable to the median of the study cohort (39 and 22 min). Recovery time after radiotherapy (90 min) was more than four times the study median of 20 min. Patient reported outcome items were among the worst of the study population (treatment duration rated with 5; breath holding rated with 4). MR-Linac staff documented maximum complexity of the irradiation process.

DISCUSSION

In this subgroup analysis of a prospective observational study, 20 patients received MR-guided SBRT for in total 26 malignant liver lesions at Heidelberg University Hospital from January 2019 to February 2020. MR-guided SBRT for tumors in the abdomen was described to be safe in a phase-I study as well as in a study by Hal et al. with no higher-grade toxicities (36, 37). However, these studies included patients with different abdominal malignancies. Experience with MR-guided radiotherapy of malignant lesions of the liver is growing, yet still scarce (**Table 4**). Gani et al. published one of the first prospective studies investigating the MR-guided liver SBRT using a high-field MR-Linac (32). Patient acceptance was high with very low toxicity burden. As far as

TABLE 3 | Patient (positions 1–18) and staff (position 19) reported outcome (available for n = 18 patients).

	categorical point scale form 1–5, where 1 equals very positive and 5 equals very negative median	range
1. Overall treatment experience	2	1–5
2. Information provided by the staff	1	1–5
3. Friendliness of the staff	1	1–5
4. Duration of the treatment	3	1–5
5. Size of the MRI bore	2	1–5
6. Positioning during radiotherapy	3	1–5
7. Having to lie still	3	1–5
8. Noise in the MR-Linac	2	1–4
9. Temperature in the MR-Linac	3	1–5
10. Local temperature of body parts	3	1–5
11. Tingling sensations in fingers and toes	2	1–5
12. Breathing instructions	1	1–5
13. Breath holding	2	1–5
14. Anxiousness during treatment session	1	1–5
15. Reported time until full mental and physical recovery after the radiotherapy session	20 min	0–360 min
16. Difficulty to hold the target with one´s own breath	1	1–4
17. Ability to watch one´s own treatment *via* monitor	1	1–2
18. Feeling of having active control over the treatment duration	1	1–3
19. Treatment complexity from the perspective of the staff	categorical point scale form 1–10, where 1 equals very positive and 10 equals very negative	
	5	2–10

described, treatment toxicity was rather low in all larger studies in the field. Only two grade III° toxicities were described by Rosenberg and colleagues (40). No grade III° toxicity was reported in our study cohort, even though patients were prospectively evaluated for side effects.

The higher proportion of patients with HCC in the two US-American studies can be explained by epidemiology as well as the higher prevalence of viral hepatitis and obesity compared to Germany (38, 40, 42). Furthermore, in our study, estimated LC was excellent, with 88% at 1 year. However, with a median of 9.4 months, follow-up of our cohort is still rather short. One of the previously mentioned US-American studies provided data on treatment outcome: Rosenberg et al. reported a LC of 80% at the median follow-up of 21.2 months (40). Furthermore, Rogowski et al. described a local control rate of 100%, however with a median follow-up of 5 months (41). Preliminary LC results are therefore so far comparable to non-MRI-guided liver SBRT, as recently described in a systematic review by Ohri et al. with a LC after 1- and 2-years of 90 and 79% (43). Our estimated 1-year OS was higher than described by Rosenberg et al. (84% *vs.* 69%) and might be explained by the younger median age in our cohort (61 years *vs.* 70 years). The proportion of different primary tumors (mainly colorectal) was comparable as well as the median prescribed irradiation dose (**Table 4**). Nonetheless, Rosenberg et al. used cobalt sources instead of a linear accelerator. Furthermore, median PTV was nearly half the size as in our study cohort (38). Future follow-up will show, whether these circumstances will lead to a differing LC or OS.

An essential part of improving treatment quality at the MR-Linac is to assess patients' perspectives. Wearing headphones in an MRI scanner is a common and easy procedure to cope for the operating noise. This procedure seems to be sufficient in our study cohort as reflected by the positive patient reported outcome, in contrast to the room temperature. For optimal functionality of both MRI scanner and linear accelerator, the room temperature is leveled down. Moreover, to reduce the risk of metal items being accidentally taken into the vicinity of the magnetic field, patients wear hospital provided medical scrubs during the irradiation sessions, which are rather thin. Both circumstances explain the negative patient reported results concerning the temperature. As a reaction to our study results, we began to ask patients immediately before the irradiation session, whether they tend to feel cold easily. If so, patients are provided with additional blankets.

Surprisingly, patients were not disturbed by their own tumor being displayed on a monitor. Correspondingly, our data reveal that the breath hold procedure as a whole is perceived very positively by the patients. A more difficult terrain for improvement is patient positioning, treatment duration and the fact that patients have to lie still on the treatment couch for a relatively long time. Devices for patient immobilization are more challenging to be developed for the MR-Linac because they have to be both non-magnetic and adequate for the rather small bore (44). Treatment duration and not being allowed to move were perceived rather negative. Our practice to play radio music to the patients *via* headphones seems not to be sufficient to guarantee full patient comfort. One must keep in mind, that our presented patient cohort had been treated before daily online plan adaption was implemented at our MR-Linac, which surely further prolongs treatment duration. Patient positioning and MR-imaging procedure consume a large amount of time. Less than half of the treatment session is used for the irradiation process itself (including the gating procedure). Beam-on time even accounts for less than a tenth of the treatment duration (**Table 2**).

Based on the benefits mentioned above, The Lancet Oncology recently dedicated a whole review to the high capability of MR-guided liver SBRT. Witt and colleagues emphasized the potential of MR-guided adaptive SBRT to become a practice changing technology for irradiation of the liver (44). However, radiotherapy with the MR-Linac is resource intensive in terms of personnel, time, money and required patient compliance. Hence, it is of the utmost importance to identify the ideal patients for receiving MR-guided SBRT. To date, three prospective trials are going to investigate the potential of online adaptation in SBRT for liver malignancies. An US-American phase-I study aims to reveal the safe maximum tolerated dose for MR-guided SBRT treatment liver metastases through real time adaptation (45). The French phase-II RASTAF study will investigate Adaptative MR-Guided Stereotactic Body Radiotherapy of Liver Tumors (46). Our planned phase-II MAESTRO trial (magnetic resonance-guided stereotactic radiotherapy for hepatic metastases) is going to evaluate, if a higher proportion of liver lesions can be treated with locally

TABLE 4 | Studies on radiotherapy of liver lesions with a magnetic resonance imaging linear accelerator.

	patients, characteristics, design	radiation technique	Toxicity	LC	OS
Feldman et al. (38)	patients: n = 29 (n = 26 HCC, n = 2 cholangiocarcinoma, n = 1 metastatic colon cancer) irradiated lesions n = 34 median age: NA gender: NA Child–Pugh-Class: NA retrospective design	MRIdian Linac (ViewRay, Oakwood Village, OH) 0.35 T step-and-shoot IMRT; utilization of gating 27–50 Gy prescribed to at least 95% of the PTV in three or five fractions PTV margin: 5 mm mean number of beams: 10.8 (range 6–16) adaptive technique: n = 1 (3.4%) average treatment time: 34 min beam-on time: NA mean monitor units per fraction: 2,538.9 (range 1,549.1–5,737.4) median PTV volume: NA	constraints: American Association of Physicists in Medicine Task Group 101 (39) general toxicity: n = 1 nausea and vomiting n = 1 abdominal pain with bloody diarrhea (n = 4 deaths due to liver cirrhosis, unrelated to radiation effect)	–	–
Rosenberg et al. (40)	patients: n = 26 (n = 8 colorectal adenocarcinoma, n = 6 HCC, n = 3 lung, n = 2 cholangiocellular, n = 1 pancreas, n = 1 sarcoma, n = 1 head and neck, n = 4 others) liver lesions present: 1–3 per patient median age: 70 y (30–90 y) female: n = 9 (35%) Child–Pugh-Class: A (76,9%); NA (23,1%) retrospective design	MRIdian System (ViewRay Inc., Mountain View, CA) 0.35 T MRI scanner combined with 3 co-planar cobalt sources; utilization of gating median dose 50 Gy (range 30–60 Gy) in five fractions (6–12 Gy/fraction) PTV margin: 2–5 mm number of beams: 12–15 adaptive technique: no range of treatment time: 40–60 min range of beam-on time: 20–30 min occasional use of gadoxetic acid 20 min before treatment as contrast fluid median PTV volume: 98.2 cm^3 (13–2,034 cm^3)	constraints: –mean liver dose: <13 to 15 Gy, >700 cm^3 of liver receiving less than 15 Gy (liver-GTV), –stomach and bowel: V32–33 <0.5 cm^3 gastrointestinal toxicity: I–II°: NA III°: 7.7% ≥IV°: 0% n = 2 decrease in Child–Pugh-Class n = 1 significant hilar stricture n = 1 portal hypertension	80,4%@21m (100% in case of HCC)	69.0% @ 1 y
Gani et al. (32)	Patients: n = 10 (metastases of n = 5 colorectal adenocarcinoma, n = 1 esophageal, n = 1 melanoma, n = 1 cystic duct, n = 1 GIST, n = 1 ACC) no patients with Child B or Child C cirrhotic liver disease median age: 68 y (48–86 y) female: n = 5 (50%) sub-study of a basket phase 2 feasibility trial (NCT04172753)	1.5 T MR-Linac (Unity, Elekta, Crawley, UK) median dose 38.5 Gy to 98% of the GTV internal target volume concept PTV margin: 3–6 mm adaptive technique: yes range of treatment time: 26 -36min median beam-on time: 9.6min median PTV volume: 96.2 cm^3 (11.3-399.5cm^3)	constraints: based on the UKSABR guidelines (Version 6.1) no increase in transaminases >I° or gastrointestinal toxicity with the necessity of medical intervention	–	–
Rogowski et al. (41)	Patients: n = 11 Lesions: n = 15 (n = 2 Cholangiocarcinoma; metastases of n = 6 neuroendocrine tumor, n = 4 colorectal adenocarcinoma, n = 2 sarcoma, n = 1 GIST)	0.35T hybrid MR-Linac (Viewray Inc., Mountain View, CA, USA) mainly 12.5 Gy in three fractions PTV margin: 3–5 mm adaptive technique: yes	toxicity: I°: 55% ≥II°: 0%	100% @me-dian follow-up of 5 m	–

(Continued)

TABLE 4 | Continued

	patients, characteristics, design	radiation technique	Toxicity	LC	OS
	median age 66 y (47–86 y) female: n = 5 (46%) prospective observational clinical trial	median treatment time: 53 min median beam-on time: 10 min median PTV volume: 39.1 cm³ (8.3–411.3 cm³)			
Weykamp et al. (present study)	Patients: n = 20 (n = 2 HCC; metastases of: n = 5 colorectal, n = 4 breast cancer, n = 3 melanoma, n = 1 adenoid cystic carcinoma, n = 1 cholangiocellular carcinoma, n = 1 urinary bladder, n = 1 papillary carcinoma, n = 1 pancreatic cancer, n = 1 prostate cancer) median age: 61 y (37–78 y) female: n = 10 (50%) Child–Pugh-Class: A (70,0%); B (5%); NA (25,0%) subgroup analysis of a prospective observational study	MRIdian Linac (ViewRay, Oakwood Village, OH) 0.35 T step-and-shoot IMRT; utilization of gating median dose 50 Gy (range 45–60Gy) in eight fractions (3–12 Gy/fraction) CTV margin 5 mm PTV margin: 3 mm number of beams: 7–15 adaptive technique: no median duration of the session ("on table"): 39.0 min (26.0–67.0 min) median radiation time: 15.8 min (10.3–38.2 min) median monitor units per fraction: 2,403.9 (1,155.4–6,309.7) no MRI contrast fluid median PTV volume: 57.2 cm³ (17.4–445.0 cm³) median liver dose: 12.7 Gy (3.2–21.9 Gy)	constraints (for five fractions): –esophagus: 0.5 cc <34 Gy –stomach/intestine: 0.5 cc <35 Gy –liver minus CTV: ≥700 cc <24 Gy –kidney: mean dose <10 Gy –spinal cord 0.1 cc <27 Gy –heart: 0.5 cc <29 Gy gastrointestinal toxicity: I°: 30.0% II°: 5.0% ≥III°: 0% n = 0 decrease in Child–Pugh-Class	88.1% @ 1y	84.0% @ 1y

ACC, adenoid cystic carcinoma; GIST, gastrointestinal stroma tumor; HCC, hepatocellular carcinoma; m, months; min, minute; mm, millimeter; MRI, magnetic resonance imaging; NA, not available; y, years.

ablative doses of a biologic effective dose ≥100 Gy when applying MR-guided adaptive compared to standard ITV-based-SBRT.

The main limitation of the presented study is its small sample size. It was statistically not possible to detect factors which estimate patient acceptance. Instead, we provided a detailed description of the oldest patient and the patient with the highest body mass index. Obesity led to average treatment expenditure as rated by patient and staff. On the contrary, the oldest patient reported the worst negative scores, which was in accordance with the judgement by the staff. This might be explained by the exhausting breathing commands while observing the monitor carefully, leading to a demanding multitasking treatment environment. As a rule of thumb, patients at our clinic are asked if they can hold their breath for at least 25 s and whether they can picture themselves repeating this breath-holding several times whilst lying on a non-padded surface for about an hour. The evaluation of both the friendliness of our staff and the treatment expenditure appear to be highly subjective question items. However, since treatment at the MR-Linac is complex and demanding for the patient, guaranteeing an environment of thrust is highly important to ensure compliance, especially when breathing instructions are involved. Furthermore, the subjective rating of the treatment expenditure will help to identify patient characteristics, which may disqualify patients for treatment at the MR-Linac in the first place. Follow-up was rather short. Since the majority of radiation-induced liver diseases occur within the first three to four months after treatment, long-term toxicity might be underestimated to a certain degree (12).

We demonstrated that MR-guided SBRT of liver malignancies is a resource intensive treatment method both for the patient and the radio-oncology department. Further follow-up will reveal whether MR-guided SBRT will significantly improve clinical results compared to conventional techniques. Using the body surface as a surrogate parameter for image guidance, SG-SBRT might be even faster and more convenient than MR-guided SBRT. Albeit, the movement of the liver is not directly monitored (25–27) and the correlation of skin to tumor is not always constant especially for liver and pancreatic tumors (47, 48). Furthermore, Stick et al. investigated intrafractional fiducial marker position variations during visually guided, deep-inspiration breathhold (DIBH) SBRT of liver metastases and reported deviations of up to 10 mm. Based on those findings, the colleagues concluded that for ensuring accurate dose delivery real-time monitoring during treatment, e.g. MR-guided SBRT, is necessary and now apply MR-guided radiotherapy for liver metastases (49). Another option might be the additional application of ultrasound monitoring applied during SBRT with active breathhold control, which has been reported to reduce residual motion to <5 mm in most cases (50). Fiducials enable the Cyberknife system to directly track the immediate treatment area, however fiducial placement is an invasive procedure, which can cause liver trauma, bleedings or a pneumothorax (51, 52). Furthermore, treatment duration of hepatic SBRT applying tumor tracking at the Cyberknife might also easily exceed 30 min. MR-guided hepatic SBRT offers a non-invasive treatment alternative with direct intrafractional visualization of the tumor hereby ensuring optimal target coverage.

Since late February 2020, our clinic has been using online adaptation. Daily SBRT treatment can now be prescribed to the anatomy of the day, taking into account interfractional and even intrafractional changes, due to organ motion (53–56). Therefore, OAR can be superiorly spared and higher irradiation doses can be achieved (36, 40, 54). However, online adaptation further prolongs the duration of the treatment session and has already needed to be omitted in a few cases during our first clinical experience to secure compliance.

We showed that MR-guided SBRT is safe and effective, even without online adaptation. It might be especially adequate for selected patients with liver malignancies very close to OAR who refuse the invasive placement of fiducials.

CONCLUSION

We demonstrated that MR-guided SBRT of malignant liver lesions is a well-tolerated and well-accepted non-invasive treatment modality with only mild toxicity. Moreover, we provided insights into patient reported outcomes, which might support patient selection for this highly promising but nonetheless resource intensive treatment modality.

AUTHOR CONTRIBUTIONS

FW performed the data collection and the statistical analysis and drafted the manuscript. SAK, PH, LK, KS, SR, JL, and SK helped with data collection as well as figure and table preparation. SK, CS, CR, and CB performed treatment planning and contributed the medical physicist expertise. JH-R and JD participated in the study design and helped to draft the manuscript. All authors contributed to the article and approved the submitted version.

REFERENCES

1. Bartlett EK, Simmons KD, Wachtel H, Roses RE, Fraker DL, Kelz RR, et al. The Rise in Metastasectomy Across Cancer Types Over the Past Decade. *Cancer* (2015) 121(5):747–57. doi: 10.1002/cncr.29134
2. Tomlinson JS, Jarnagin WR, DeMatteo RP, Fong Y, Kornprat P, Gonen M, et al. Actual 10-Year Survival After Resection of Colorectal Liver Metastases Defines Cure. *ASCO Publication - JCO* (2007) 25(29):4575–80. doi: 10.1200/JCO.2007.11.0833
3. Smith JJ, D'Angelica MI. Surgical Management of Hepatic Metastases of Colorectal Cancer. *Hematol Oncol Clinics North Am* (2015) 29(1):61–84. doi: 10.1016/j.hoc.2014.09.003
4. Cummings LC, Payes JD, Cooper GS. Survival After Hepatic Resection in Metastatic Colorectal Cancer: A Population-Based Study. *Cancer* (2007) 109 (4):718–26. doi: 10.1002/cncr.22448
5. Izzo F, Granata V, Grassi R, Fusco R, Palaia R, Delrio P, et al. Radiofrequency Ablation and Microwave Ablation in Liver Tumors: An Update. *Oncologist* (2019) 24(10):e990–1005. doi: 10.1634/theoncologist.2018-0337
6. Sim H-W, Knox J, Dawson LA. An Update on Randomized Clinical Trials in Hepatocellular Carcinoma. *Surg Oncol Clinics North Am* (2017) 26(4):647–66. doi: 10.1016/j.soc.2017.05.006
7. Goodman BD, Mannina EM, Althouse SK, Maluccio MA, Cárdenes HR. Long-Term Safety and Efficacy of Stereotactic Body Radiation Therapy for Hepatic Oligometastases. *Pract Radiat Oncol* (2016) 6(2):86–95. doi: 10.1016/j.prro.2015.10.011
8. Andratschke N, Alheid H, Allgäuer M, Becker G, Blanck O, Boda-Heggemann J, et al. The SBRT Database Initiative of the German Society for Radiation Oncology (DEGRO): Patterns of Care and Outcome Analysis of Stereotactic Body Radiotherapy (SBRT) for Liver Oligometastases in 474 Patients With 623 Metastases. *BMC Cancer* (2018) 18(1):283. doi: 10.1186/s12885-018-4191-2
9. Joo JH, Park J-H, Kim JC, Yu CS, Lim S-B, Park IJ, et al. Local Control Outcomes Using Stereotactic Body Radiation Therapy for Liver Metastases From Colorectal Cancer. *Int J Radiat Oncol Biol Phys* (2017) 99(4):876–83. doi: 10.1016/j.ijrobp.2017.07.030
10. Zeng Z-C, Fan J, Tang Z-Y, Zhou J, Qin L-X, Wang J-H, et al. A Comparison of Treatment Combinations With and Without Radiotherapy for Hepatocellular Carcinoma With Portal Vein and/or Inferior Vena Cava Tumor Thrombus. *Int J Radiat Oncol Biol Phys* (2005) 61(2):432–43. doi: 10.1016/j.ijrobp.2004.05.025
11. Munoz-Schuffenegger P, Ng S, Dawson LA. Radiation-Induced Liver Toxicity. *Semin Radiat Oncol* (2017) 27(4):350–7. doi: 10.1016/j.semradonc.2017.04.002
12. Pan CC, Kavanagh BD, Dawson LA, Li XA, Das SK, Miften M, et al. Radiation-Associated Liver Injury. *Int J Radiat Oncol Biol Phys* (2010) 76(3 Suppl):S94–100. doi: 10.1016/j.ijrobp.2009.06.092
13. Greco C, Catalano G, Di Grazia A, Orecchia RJTJ. Radiotherapy of Liver Malignancies. From Whole Liver Irradiation to Stereotactic Hypofractionated Radiotherapy. *Tumori J* (2004) 90(1):73–9. doi: 10.1177/030089160409000116
14. Dawson LA, Normolle D, Balter JM, McGinn CJ, Lawrence TS, Ten Haken RK. Analysis of Radiation-Induced Liver Disease Using the Lyman NTCP Model. *Int J Radiat Oncol Biol Phys* (2002) 53(4):810–21. doi: 10.1016/S0360-3016(02)02846-8
15. Doi H, Shiomi H, Masai N, Tatsumi D, Igura T, Imai Y, et al. Threshold Doses and Prediction of Visually Apparent Liver Dysfunction After Stereotactic Body Radiation Therapy in Cirrhotic and Normal Livers Using Magnetic Resonance Imaging. *J Radiat Res* (2016) 57(3):294–300. doi: 10.1093/jrr/rrw008
16. Kavanagh BD, Pan CC, Dawson LA, Das SK, Li XA, Ten Haken RK, et al. Radiation Dose-Volume Effects in the Stomach and Small Bowel. *Int J Radiat Oncol Biol Phys* (2010) 76(3 Suppl):S101–7. doi: 10.1016/j.ijrobp.2009.05.071
17. Miften M, Vinogradskiy Y, Moiseenko V, Grimm J, Yorke E, Jackson A, et al. Radiation Dose-Volume Effects for Liver Sbrt. *Int J Radiat Oncol Biol Phys* (2021) 17(1):196–205. doi: 10.1016/j.ijrobp.2017.12.290
18. Bae SH, Kim M-S, Cho CK, Kang J-K, Lee SY, Lee K-N, et al. Predictor of Severe Gastroduodenal Toxicity After Stereotactic Body Radiotherapy for Abdominopelvic Malignancies. *Int J Radiat Oncol Biol Phys* (2012) 84(4): e469–74. doi: 10.1016/j.ijrobp.2012.06.005
19. Noel CE, Parikh PJ, Spencer CR, Green OL, Hu Y, Mutic S, et al. Comparison of Onboard Low-Field Magnetic Resonance Imaging Versus Onboard Computed Tomography for Anatomy Visualization in Radiotherapy. *Acta Oncol* (2015) 54(9):1474–82. doi: 10.3109/0284186X.2015.1062541
20. Van den Begin R, Engels B, Gevaert T, Duchateau M, Tournel K, Verellen D, et al. Impact of Inadequate Respiratory Motion Management in SBRT for Oligometastatic Colorectal Cancer. *Radiother Oncol* (2014) 113(2):235–9. doi: 10.1016/j.radonc.2014.11.005
21. Bertholet J, Worm ES, Fledelius W, Hoyer M, Poulsen PR. Time-Resolved Intrafraction Target Translations and Rotations During Stereotactic Liver Radiation Therapy: Implications for Marker-based Localization Accuracy. *Int J Radiat Oncol Biol Phys* (2016) 95(2):802–9. doi: 10.1016/j.ijrobp.2016.01.033
22. Poulsen PR, Worm ES, Petersen JB, Grau C, Fledelius W, Hoyer M. Kilovoltage Intrafraction Motion Monitoring and Target Dose Reconstruction for Stereotactic Volumetric Modulated Arc Therapy of Tumors in the Liver. *Radiother Oncol: J Eur Soc Ther Radiol Oncol* (2014) 111(3):424–30. doi: 10.1016/j.radonc.2014.05.007
23. Worm ES, Hoyer M, Fledelius W, Hansen AT, Poulsen PR. Variations in Magnitude and Directionality of Respiratory Target Motion Throughout Full Treatment Courses of Stereotactic Body Radiotherapy for Tumors in the Liver. *Acta Oncol* (2013) 52(7):1437–44. doi: 10.3109/0284186X.2013.813638

24. Sterzing F, Brunner TB, Ernst I, Baus WW, Greve B, Herfarth K, et al. Stereotactic Body Radiotherapy for Liver Tumors. *Strahlenther und Onkol* (2014) 190(10):872–81. doi: 10.1007/s00066-014-0714-1
25. Boda-Heggemann J, Knopf AC, Simeonova-Chergou A, Wertz H, Stieler F, Jahnke A, et al. Deep Inspiration Breath Hold-Based Radiation Therapy: A Clinical Review. *Int J Radiat Oncol Biol Phys* (2016) 94(3):478–92. doi: 10.1016/j.ijrobp.2015.11.049
26. Alderliesten T, Sonke JJ, Betgen A, van Vliet-Vroegindeweij C, Remeijer P. 3D Surface Imaging for Monitoring Intrafraction Motion in Frameless Stereotactic Body Radiotherapy of Lung Cancer. *Radiother Oncol: J Eur Soc Ther Radiol Oncol* (2012) 105(2):155–60. doi: 10.1016/j.radonc.2012.08.016
27. Hughes S, McClelland J, Tarte S, Lawrence D, Ahmad S, Hawkes D, et al. Assessment of Two Novel Ventilatory Surrogates for Use in the Delivery of Gated/Tracked Radiotherapy for non-Small Cell Lung Cancer. *Radiother Oncol: J Eur Soc Ther Radiol Oncol* (2009) 91(3):336–41. doi: 10.1016/j.radonc.2009.03.016
28. Freislederer P, Kügele M, Öllers M, Swinnen A, Sauer TO, Bert C, et al. Recent Advances in Surface Guided Radiation Therapy. *Radiat Oncol* (2020) 15 (1):187. doi: 10.1186/s13014-020-01629-w
29. Brock KK, Dawson LA. Adaptive Management of Liver Cancer Radiotherapy. *Semin Radiat Oncol* (2010) 20(2):107–15. doi: 10.1016/j.semradonc.2009.11.004
30. van Sörnsen de Koste JR, Palacios MA, Bruynzeel AME, Slotman BJ, Senan S, Lagerwaard FJ. MR-Guided Gated Stereotactic Radiation Therapy Delivery for Lung, Adrenal, and Pancreatic Tumors: A Geometric Analysis. *Int J Radiat Oncol Biol Phys* (2018) 102(4):858–66. doi: 10.1016/j.ijrobp.2018.05.048
31. Klüter S, Katayama S, Spindeldreier CK, Koerber SA, Major G, Alber M, et al. First Prospective Clinical Evaluation of Feasibility and Patient Acceptance of Magnetic Resonance-Guided Radiotherapy in Germany. *Strahlenther und Onkol* (2020) 196:691–8.
32. Gani C, Boeke S, McNair H, Ehlers J, Nachbar M, Mönnich D, et al. Marker-Less Online MR-Guided Stereotactic Body Radiotherapy of Liver Metastases at a 1.5 T MR-Linac – Feasibility, Workflow Data and Patient Acceptance. *Clin Trans Radiat Oncol* (2021) 26:55–61. doi: 10.1016/j.ctro.2020.11.014
33. Guckenberger M, Baus WW, Blanck O, Combs SE, Debus J, Engenhart-Cabillic R, et al. Definition and Quality Requirements for Stereotactic Radiotherapy: Consensus Statement From the DEGRO/DGMP Working Group Stereotactic Radiotherapy and Radiosurgery. *Strahlenther und Onkol* (2020) 196(5):417–20. doi: 10.1007/s00066-020-01603-1
34. Klüter S. Technical Design and Concept of a 0.35 T Mr-Linac. *Clin Trans Radiat Oncol* (2019) 18:98–101. doi: 10.1016/j.ctro.2019.04.007
35. Park C, Papiez L, Zhang S, Story M, Timmerman RD. Universal Survival Curve and Single Fraction Equivalent Dose: Useful Tools in Understanding Potency of Ablative Radiotherapy. *Int J Radiat Oncol Biol Phys* (2008) 70 (3):847–52. doi: 10.1016/j.ijrobp.2007.10.059
36. Henke L, Kashani R, Robinson C, Curcuru A, DeWees T, Bradley J, et al. Phase I Trial of Stereotactic MR-guided Online Adaptive Radiation Therapy (SMART) for the Treatment of Oligometastatic or Unresectable Primary Malignancies of the Abdomen. *Radiother Oncol* (2018) 126(3):519–26. doi: 10.1016/j.radonc.2017.11.032
37. Hal WA, Straza MW, Chen X, Mickevicius N, Erickson B, Schultz C, et al. Initial Clinical Experience of Stereotactic Body Radiation Therapy (SBRT) for Liver Metastases, Primary Liver Malignancy, and Pancreatic Cancer With 4D-MRI Based Online Adaptation and Real-Time MRI Monitoring Using a 1.5 Tesla Mr-Linac. *PLOS ONE* (2020) 15(8):e0236570. doi: 10.1371/journal.pone.0236570
38. Feldman AM, Modh A, Glide-Hurst C, Chetty IJ, Movsas B. Real-Time Magnetic Resonance-Guided Liver Stereotactic Body Radiation Therapy: An Institutional Report Using a Magnetic Resonance-Linac System. *Cureus* (2019) 11(9):e5774. doi: 10.7759/cureus.5774
39. Benedict SH, Yenice KM, Followill D, Galvin JM, Hinson W, Kavanagh B, et al. Stereotactic Body Radiation Therapy: The Report of AAPM Task Group 101. *Med Phys* (2010) 37(8):4078–101. doi: 10.1118/1.3438081
40. Rosenberg SA, Henke LE, Shaverdian N, Mittauer K, Wojcieszynski AP, Hullett CR, et al. A Multi-Institutional Experience of MR-Guided Liver Stereotactic Body Radiation Therapy. *Adv Radiat Oncol* (2019) 4(1):142–9. doi: 10.1016/j.adro.2018.08.005
41. Rogowski P, von Bestenbostel R, Walter F, Straub K, Nierer L, Kurz C, et al. Feasibility and Early Clinical Experience of Online Adaptive MR-Guided Radiotherapy of Liver Tumors. *Cancers* (2021) 13(7):1523. doi: 10.3390/cancers13071523
42. Mittal S. El-Serag Hbjjocg. *Epidemiol HCC: Consider Popul* (2013) 47:S2. doi: 10.1097/MCG.0b013e3182872f29
43. Ohri N, Tome WA, Mendez Romero A, Miften M, Ten Haken RK, Dawson LA, et al. Local Control After Stereotactic Body Radiation Therapy for Liver Tumors. *Int J Radiat Oncol Biol Phys* (2018) 21(2):e74–82. doi: 10.1016/S1470-2045(20)30034-6
44. Witt JS, Rosenberg SA, Bassetti MF. MRI-Guided Adaptive Radiotherapy for Liver Tumours: Visualising the Future. *Lancet Oncol* (2020) 21(2):e74–82. doi: 10.1016/S1470-2045(20)30034-6
45. University of Wisconsin M. *OAR-Based, Dose Escalated SBRT With Real Time Adaptive MRI Guidance for Liver Metastases ClinicalTrials.gov* (2020). Available at: https://clinicaltrials.gov/ct2/show/NCT04020276.
46. Leclerc CGF. *Adaptative MR-Guided Stereotactic Body Radiotherapy of Liver Tumors (RASTAF) ClinicalTrials.gov* (2020). Available at: https://clinicaltrials.gov/ct2/show/NCT04242342.
47. Velec M, Moseley JL, Craig T, Dawson LA, Brock K. Accumulated Dose in Liver Stereotactic Body Radiotherapy: Positioning, Breathing, and Deformation Effects. *Int J Radiat Oncol Biol Phys* (2012) 83(4):1132–40. doi: 10.1016/j.ijrobp.2011.09.045
48. Minn AY, Schellenberg D, Maxim P, Suh Y, McKenna S, Cox B, et al. Pancreatic Tumor Motion on a Single Planning 4D-CT Does Not Correlate With Intrafraction Tumor Motion During Treatment. *Am J Clin Oncol* (2009) 32(4):364–8. doi: 10.1097/COC.0b013e31818da9e0
49. Stick LB, Vogelius IR, Risum S, Josipovic M. Intrafractional Fiducial Marker Position Variations in Stereotactic Liver Radiotherapy During Voluntary Deep Inspiration Breath-Hold. *Br J Radiol* (2020) 93(1116):20200859. doi: 10.1259/bjr.20200859
50. Vogel L, Sihono DSK, Weiss C, Lohr F, Stieler F, Wertz H, et al. Intra-Breath-Hold Residual Motion of Image-Guided DIBH Liver-SBRT: An Estimation by Ultrasound-Based Monitoring Correlated With Diaphragm Position in CBCT. *Radiother Oncol* (2018) 129(3):441–8. doi 10.1016/j.radonc.2018.07.007
51. Wurm RE, Gum F, Erbel S, Schlenger L, Scheffler D, Agaoglu D, et al. Image Guided Respiratory Gated Hypofractionated Stereotactic Body Radiation Therapy (H-SBRT) for Liver and Lung Tumors: Initial Experience. *Acta Oncol (Stockholm Sweden)* (2006) 45(7):881–9. doi: 10.1080/02841860600919233
52. Bahig H, Campeau M-P, Vu T, Doucet R, Nadeau DB, Fortin B, et al. Predictive Parameters of CyberKnife Fiducial-Less (Xsight Lung) Applicability for Treatment of Early Non-Small Cell Lung Cancer: A Single-Center Experience. *Int J Radiat Oncol Biol Phys* (2013) 87(3):583–9. doi: 10.1016/j.ijrobp.2013.06.2048
53. Henke LE, Olsen JR, Contreras JA, Curcuru A, DeWees TA, Green OL, et al. Stereotactic MR-Guided Online Adaptive Radiation Therapy (SMART) for Ultracentral Thorax Malignancies: Results of a Phase 1 Trial. *Adv Radiat Oncol* (2019) 4(1):201–9. doi: 10.1016/j.adro.2018.10.003
54. Bohoudi O, Bruynzeel AME, Senan S, Cuijpers JP, Slotman BJ, Lagerwaard FJ, et al. Fast and Robust Online Adaptive Planning in Stereotactic MR-guided Adaptive Radiation Therapy (SMART) for Pancreatic Cancer. *Radiother Oncol* (2017) 125(3):439–44. doi: 10.1016/j.radonc.2017.07.028
55. Acharya S, Fischer-Valuck BW, Kashani R, Parikh P, Yang D, Zhao T, et al. Online Magnetic Resonance Image Guided Adaptive Radiation Therapy: First Clinical Applications. *Int J Radiat Oncol Biol Phys* (2016) 94(2):394–403. doi: 10.1016/j.ijrobp.2015.10.015
56. Henke LE, Contreras JA, Green OL, Cai B, Kim H, Roach MC, et al. Magnetic Resonance Image-Guided Radiotherapy (Mrigrt): A 4.5-Year Clinical Experience. *Clin Oncol* (2018) 30(11):720–7. doi: 10.1016/j.clon.2018.08.010

Permissions

All chapters in this book were first published Frontiers; hereby published with permission under the Creative Commons Attribution License or equivalent. Every chapter published in this book has been scrutinized by our experts. Their significance has been extensively debated. The topics covered herein carry significant findings which will fuel the growth of the discipline. They may even be implemented as practical applications or may be referred to as a beginning point for another development.

The contributors of this book come from diverse backgrounds, making this book a truly international effort. This book will bring forth new frontiers with its revolutionizing research information and detailed analysis of the nascent developments around the world.

We would like to thank all the contributing authors for lending their expertise to make the book truly unique. They have played a crucial role in the development of this book. Without their invaluable contributions this book wouldn't have been possible. They have made vital efforts to compile up to date information on the varied aspects of this subject to make this book a valuable addition to the collection of many professionals and students.

This book was conceptualized with the vision of imparting up-to-date information and advanced data in this field. To ensure the same, a matchless editorial board was set up. Every individual on the board went through rigorous rounds of assessment to prove their worth. After which they invested a large part of their time researching and compiling the most relevant data for our readers.

The editorial board has been involved in producing this book since its inception. They have spent rigorous hours researching and exploring the diverse topics which have resulted in the successful publishing of this book. They have passed on their knowledge of decades through this book. To expedite this challenging task, the publisher supported the team at every step. A small team of assistant editors was also appointed to further simplify the editing procedure and attain best results for the readers.

Apart from the editorial board, the designing team has also invested a significant amount of their time in understanding the subject and creating the most relevant covers. They scrutinized every image to scout for the most suitable representation of the subject and create an appropriate cover for the book.

The publishing team has been an ardent support to the editorial, designing and production team. Their endless efforts to recruit the best for this project, has resulted in the accomplishment of this book. They are a veteran in the field of academics and their pool of knowledge is as vast as their experience in printing. Their expertise and guidance has proved useful at every step. Their uncompromising quality standards have made this book an exceptional effort. Their encouragement from time to time has been an inspiration for everyone.

The publisher and the editorial board hope that this book will prove to be a valuable piece of knowledge for researchers, students, practitioners and scholars across the globe.

List of Contributors

Kongying Lin, Jianxing Zeng, Zongren Ding, Hongzhi Liu, Jun Fu and Yongyi Zeng
Department of Hepatopancreatobiliary Surgery, Mengchao Hepatobiliary Hospital of Fujian Medical University, Fuzhou, China

Qizhen Huang
Department of Radiation Oncology, Mengchao Hepatobiliary Hospital of Fujian Medical University, Fuzhou, China

Lei Wang
Department of Radiation Oncology, Fujian Medical University Cancer Hospital, Fujian Cancer Hospital, Fuzhou, China

Jingfeng Liu
Department of Hepatopancreatobiliary Surgery, Mengchao Hepatobiliary Hospital of Fujian Medical University, Fuzhou, China
Department of Radiation Oncology, Fujian Medical University Cancer Hospital, Fujian Cancer Hospital, Fuzhou, China

Pengfei Guo and Zhenwei Chen
The Big Data Institute of Southeast Hepatobiliary Health Information, Mengchao Hepatobiliary Hospital of Fujian Medical University, Fuzhou, China

Weiping Zhou
The Third Department of Hepatic Surgery, Eastern Hepatobiliary Surgery Hospital, Second Military Medical University, Shanghai, China

Cheng Guo, Jie Zhou, Boyu Ma, Rui Wang, Yanli Ge, Zhe Wang, Bing Ji, Wei Wang, Junjie Zhang and Zhirong Wang
Department of Gastroenterology, Tongji Hospital, Tongji University School of Medicine, Shanghai, China

Junsheng Yang, Yongjin Bao, Weibo Chen, Yunfei Duan and Donglin Sun
Department of Hepatopancreatobiliary Surgery, The Third Affiliated Hospital of Soochow University, Changzhou, China

Qiongxuan Fang, Ruifeng Yang, Dongbo Chen, Ran Fei and Hongsong Chen
Beijing Key Laboratory of Hepatitis C and Immunotherapy for Liver Diseases, Peking University Hepatology Institute, Peking University People's Hospital, Beijing, China

Pu Chen and Kangjian Deng
Laboratory of Hepatobiliary and Pancreatic Surgery, Affiliated Hospital of Guilin Medical University, Guilin, China

Jie Gao
Department of Hepatobiliary Surgery, Peking University People's Hospital, Beijing, China

Dengliang Lei, Yang Zhou, Gangli Hu and Fang Luo
Department of Hepatobiliary Surgery, The First Affiliated Hospital of Chongqing Medical University, Chongqing, China

Yue Chen
Central Laboratory, The First Affiliated Hospital of Chongqing Medical University, Chongqing, China

Minjun Liao, Jiarun Sun, Cuirong Tang, Chengguang Hu, Yangda Song, Meng Li and Yuanping Zhou
Guangdong Provincial Key Laboratory of Gastroenterology, Department of Gastroenterology and Hepatology Unit, Nanfang Hospital, Southern Medical University, Guangzhou, China

Qifan Zhang
Department of Hepatobiliary Surgery, Nanfang Hospital, Southern Medical University, Guangzhou, China

Yuchen Zhou
Department of Hepatobiliary Surgery, Nanfang Hospital, Southern Medical University, Guangzhou, China
Department of General Surgery, Integrated Hospital of Traditional Chinese Medicine, Southern Medical University, Guangzhou, China

Mingrong Cao
Department of Hepatobiliary Surgery, the First Affiliated Hospital of Jinan University, Guangzhou, China

Tao Chen
Department of Hepatobiliary Surgery, Sun Yat-Sen Memorial Hospital, Sun Yat-Sen University, Guangzhou, China

Junxiong Yu and Weijia Liao
Laboratory of Hepatobiliary and Pancreatic Surgery, Affiliated Hospital of Guilin Medical University, Guilin, China

Han Xiao and Shu-Ling Chen
Division of Interventional Ultrasound, The First Affiliated Hospital of Sun Yat-sen University, Guangzhou, China

Jia-Li Li
Department of Liver Surgery, Dongguan People's Hospital, Dongguan, China

Mi-Mi Tang and Shi-Ting Feng
Department of Medical Imaging, The First Affiliated Hospital of Sun Yat-sen University, Guangzhou, China

Qian Zhou
Clinical Trials Unit, The First Affiliated Hospital of Sun Yat-sen University, Guangzhou, China

Ting-Fan Wu
Clinical Education Team, GE Healthcare, Beijing, China

Xin Li
Global Research, GE Healthcare, Beijing, China

Zhen-Wei Peng
Clinical Trials Unit, The First Affiliated Hospital of Sun Yat-sen University, Guangzhou, China
Department of Radiotherapy, The First Affiliated Hospital of Sun Yat-sen University, Guangzhou, China

Sui Peng
Clinical Trials Unit, The First Affiliated Hospital of Sun Yat-sen University, Guangzhou, China
Department of Gastroenterology, The First Affiliated Hospital of Sun Yat-sen University, Guangzhou, China

Ming Kuang
Division of Interventional Ultrasound, The First Affiliated Hospital of Sun Yat-sen University, Guangzhou, China
Department of Liver Surgery, The First Affiliated Hospital of Sun Yat-sen University, Guangzhou, China

Wang Yao, Miao Xue, Yu Wang, Yue Zhao, Yanqin Wu, Wenzhe Fan and Jiaping Li
Department of Interventional Oncology, the First Affiliated Hospital of Sun Yat-Sen University, Guangzhou, China

Mingjian Lu
Department of Radiology, Affiliated Cancer Hospital & Institute of Guangzhou Medical University, Guangzhou, China

Yu Pan, Shunjie Xia, Ke Chen and Xiujun Cai
Department of General Surgery, Sir Run Run Shaw Hospital, School of Medicine, Zhejiang University, Zhejiang, China
Key Laboratory of Endoscopic Technique Research of Zhejiang Province, Hangzhou, China

Jiaqin Cai
Department of Plastic Surgery, Sir Run Run Shaw Hospital, School of Medicine, Zhejiang University, Zhejiang, China

Jialiang Wei
Department of Interventional Oncology, The First Affiliated Hospital, Sun Yat-sen University, Guangzhou, China

Wei Cui
Department of Interventional Therapy, Cancer Center, Guangdong Provincial People's Hospital, Guangdong Academy of Medical Sciences, School of Medicine, South China University of Technology, Guangzhou, China

Haoyu Hu, Shuo Qi, Silue Zeng, Peng Zhang, Linyun He, Sai Wen and Weiqi Zhang
Department of Hepatobiliary Surgery, Zhujiang Hospital, Southern Medical University, Guangzhou, China

Ning Zeng, Jian Yang, Wen Zhu, Nan Xiang and Chihua Fang
Department of Hepatobiliary Surgery, Zhujiang Hospital, Southern Medical University, Guangzhou, China
Guangdong Provincial Clinical and Engineering Center of Digital Medicine, Guangzhou, China

Guozhi Wu, Yuan Yang, Yemao Li, Zipeng Zhai and Lina An
The First Clinical Medical College, Lanzhou University, Lanzhou, China
Department of Gastroenterology, The First Hospital of Lanzhou University, Lanzhou, China
Gansu Key Laboratory of Gastroenterology, Lanzhou University, Lanzhou, China

Min Liu, Ya Zheng, Yuping Wang, Yongning Zhou and Qinghong Guo
Department of Gastroenterology, The First Hospital of Lanzhou University, Lanzhou, China
Gansu Key Laboratory of Gastroenterology, Lanzhou University, Lanzhou, China

Yu Zhu
The First Clinical Medical College, Lanzhou University, Lanzhou, China
Department of Hematology, the First Hospital of Lanzhou University, Lanzhou, China

Lawrence Lawer Atteh, Xianzhuo Zhang, Chongfei Huang, Mingzhen Bai, Haidong Ma, Chao Zhang, Wenkang Fu and Long Gao
The First Clinical Medical College, Lanzhou University, Lanzhou, China

Teng Cai
The First Clinical Medical College, Lanzhou University, Lanzhou, China
Gansu Province Key Laboratory Biotherapy and Regenerative Medicine, Lanzhou, China

Yanyan Lin
The Department of General Surgery, The First Hospital of Lanzhou University, Lanzhou, China
Gansu Province Institute of Hepatopancreatobiliary Surgery, Lanzhou, China

Wenbo Meng
The First Clinical Medical College, Lanzhou University, Lanzhou, China
The Department of General Surgery, The First Hospital of Lanzhou University, Lanzhou, China
Gansu Province Institute of Hepatopancreatobiliary Surgery, Lanzhou, China

Xiao-Lu Ma, Su-Hong Xie, Guo Lin and Ren-Quan Lu
Department of Clinical Laboratory, Shanghai Cancer Center, Fudan University, Shanghai, China
Department of Oncology, Shanghai Medical School, Fudan University, Shanghai, China

Wei-Guo Tang
Department of Liver Surgery, Liver Cancer Institute, Zhongshan Hospital, Fudan University, Shanghai, China
Department of Hepatobiliary and Pancreatic Surgery, Minhang Hospital, Fudan University, Shanghai, China

Min-Jie Yang
Department of Interventional Radiology, Zhongshan Hospital, Fudan University and Shanghai Institute of Medical Imaging, Shanghai, China

Min-Le Wu
Department of Clinical Laboratory, Shanghai Public Health Clinical Center, Fudan University, Shanghai, China

Wei Li, Haitao Xiao, Xuewen Xu and Yange Zhang
Department of Plastic and Burns Surgery, West China Hospital, Sichuan University, Chengdu, China

Hong Wu
Department of Liver Surgery & Liver Transplantation Center, West China Hospital, Sichuan University, Chengdu, China

Yannan Bai, Jiayi Wu, Jianlin Lai, Funan Qiu, Songqiang Zhou, Yifeng Tian, Yaodong Wang and Maolin Yan
Department of Hepatobiliopancreatic Surgery, Fujian Provincial Hospital, Shengli Clinical Medical College of Fujian Medical University, Fuzhou, China

Yuane Lian and Yinghong Yang
Department of Pathology, Fujian Medical University Union Hospital, Fuzhou, China

Xiaoping Chen and Zijing Zhu
Department of Statistics, College of Mathematics and Informatics & FJKLMAA, Fujian Normal University, Fuzhou, China

Qunfang Zhou, Ruixia Li, Zhimei Huang and Jinhua Huang
Department of Minimally Invasive Interventional Therapy, Sun Yat-sen University Cancer Center, Guangzhou, China

Fei Tuo
Department of Ultrasound Diagnose, The First Hospital of Hunan University of Chinese Medicine, Changsha, China

Xiaohui Wang, Juncheng Wang and Minshan Chen
Department of Hepatobiliary Oncology, Sun Yat-sen University Cancer Center, Sun Yat-sen University, Guangzhou, China

Shilun Wu, Ruize Gao, Ruhang Zhu, Jun Gao and Wenbing Sun
Department of Hepatobiliary Surgery, Beijing Chaoyang Hospital Affiliated to Capital Medical University, Beijing, China

Tao Yin
Department of General Surgery, Affiliated Hospital of Chifeng University, Chifeng, China

Shigang Guo
Department of General Surgery, Chaoyang Central Hospital, Chaoyang, China

Zonghai Xin
Department of General Surgery, Binzhou Second People's Hospital, Binzhou, China

Aolei Li
Department of General Surgery, Chaoyang Second Hospital, Chaoyang, China

Xinliang Kong
Department of Hepatobiliary Surgery, Rizhao Central Hospital, Rizhao, China

Mingyang Bao
State Key Laboratory of Genetic Engineering, Institute of Biostatistics, School of Life Sciences, Fudan University, Shanghai, China

Xiaoyi Hu
Division of Hepatobiliary and Pancreatic Surgery, Department of Surgery, The First Affiliated Hospital, Zhejiang University School of Medicine, Hangzhou, China

Qiuyu Zhu
Division of Hepatobiliary and Pancreatic Surgery, Department of Surgery, The First Affiliated Hospital, Zhejiang University School of Medicine, Hangzhou, China
Department of Surgery, Shanghai Jiaotong University School of Medicine, Shanghai, China

Tuerganaili Aji, Talaiti Tuergan and Alimu Tulahong
Department of Hepatobiliary and Hydatid Surgery, The First Affiliated Hospital of Xinjiang Medical University, Urumqi, China

Shuyao Wei
Clinical Laboratory Diagnostics, School of Public Health, Gansu University of Chinese Medicine, Lanzhou, China

Xiaoqin Ha
Department of Clinical Laboratory, The 940th Hospital of Joint Logistics Support Force of Chinese People's Liberation Army, Lanzhou, China

Yueqing Hu
State Key Laboratory of Genetic Engineering, Institute of Biostatistics, School of Life Sciences, Fudan University, Shanghai, China
Shanghai Center for Mathematical Sciences, Fudan University, Shanghai, China

Yi-Zhen Fu, Dan-Dan Hu, Jun-Cheng Wang, Li Xu, Min-Shan Chen and Yao-Jun Zhang
Sun Yat-sen University Cancer Center, State Key Laboratory of Oncology in South China, Collaborative Innovation Center for Cancer Medicine, Guangzhou, China
Department of Liver Surgery, Sun Yat-sen University Cancer Center, Guangzhou, China

Yang-Xun Pan
Sun Yat-sen University Cancer Center, State Key Laboratory of Oncology in South China, Collaborative Innovation Center for Cancer Medicine, Guangzhou, China
Department of Liver Surgery, Sun Yat-sen University Cancer Center, Guangzhou, China
Department of Oncology-Pathology, Karolinska Institutet, Stockholm, Sweden

Qian Long, Shi-Liang Liu and Meng-Zhong Liu
Sun Yat-sen University Cancer Center, State Key Laboratory of Oncology in South China, Collaborative Innovation Center for Cancer Medicine, Guangzhou, China
Department of Experimental Research, Sun Yat-sen University Cancer Center, Guangzhou, China

Mian Xi
Sun Yat-sen University Cancer Center, State Key Laboratory of Oncology in South China, Collaborative Innovation Center for Cancer Medicine, Guangzhou, China
Department of Radiation Oncology, Sun Yat-sen University Cancer Center, Guangzhou, China

Fabian Weykamp, Philipp Hoegen, Sebastian Klüter, C. Katharina Spindeldreier, Laila König, Katharina Seidensaal, Sebastian Regnery, Jakob Liermann, Carolin Rippke, Stefan A. Koerber and Carolin Buchele
Department of Radiation Oncology, Heidelberg University Hospital, Heidelberg, Germany
Heidelberg Institute of Radiation Oncology (HIRO), Heidelberg, Germany
National Center for Tumor Diseases (NCT), Heidelberg, Germany

Juliane Hörner-Rieber
Department of Radiation Oncology, Heidelberg University Hospital, Heidelberg, Germany
Heidelberg Institute of Radiation Oncology (HIRO), Heidelberg, Germany
National Center for Tumor Diseases (NCT), Heidelberg, Germany
Clinical Cooperation Unit Radiation Oncology, German Cancer Research Center (DKFZ), Heidelberg, Germany

Jürgen Debus
Department of Radiation Oncology, Heidelberg University Hospital, Heidelberg, Germany
Heidelberg Institute of Radiation Oncology (HIRO), Heidelberg, Germany
National Center for Tumor Diseases (NCT), Heidelberg, Germany
Heidelberg Ion- Beam Therapy Center (HIT), Department of Radiation Oncology, Heidelberg University Hospital, Heidelberg, Germany
Clinical Cooperation Unit Radiation Oncology, German Cancer Research Center (DKFZ), Heidelberg, Germany
German Cancer Consortium (DKTK), Heidelberg, Germany

Index

O

P

R

S

T

U

V